Handbook of Experimental Pharmacology

Volume 96

Chemotherapy of Fungal Diseases

Contributors

Donald Armstrong, F. Thomas Boyle, Manuel Debono
Bertrand Dupont, Sarah C. Eardley, Oliver P. Flint
Robert S. Gordee, John R. Graybill, Heinz Hänel
Thomas C. Jones, David Kerridge, Ann Lambert
David Loebenberg, Philip A. Pizzo, Annemarie Polak
Wolfgang Ritter, Marguerite M. Roberts
William R. Robertson, John F. Ryley, Heinz J. Schmitt
Jack D. Sobel, John J. Stern, Alan M. Sugar, Michael H. Tarbit
Hugo Vanden Bossche, Violette V. Villars, Thomas J. Walsh
Robert G. Wilson, Michel Zaug

Editor
John F. Ryley

Springer-Verlag
Berlin Heidelberg New York
London Paris Tokyo
Hong Kong Barcelona

JOHN F. RYLEY

ICI Pharmaceuticals
Mereside, Alderley Park,
Macclesfield, Cheshire SK10 4TG
England

With 72 Figures

ISBN 3-540-52232-8 Springer-Verlag Berlin Heidelberg New York
ISBN 0-387-52232-8 Springer-Verlag New York Berlin Heidelberg

Library of Congress Cataloging-in-Publication Data. Chemotherapy of fungal diseases/contributors, Donald Armstrong . . . [et al.]; editor, John F. Ryley. p. cm. – (Handbook of experimental pharmacology: v. 96) Includes bibliographical references. ISBN 0-387-52232-8 (U.S.: alk. paper): 1. Antifungal agents. 2. Mycoses – Chemotherapy. I. Armstrong, Donald, 1931– . II. Ryley, J. F. (John Frederick), 1928– . III. Series. [DNLM: 1. Antifungal Agents – therapeutic use. 2. Mycoses – drug therapy. W1 HA51L v. 96/WC 450 C517] QP905.H3 vol. 96 [RM410] 615'. 1 s-dc20 [616.9'69061] DNLM/DLC for Library of Congress 90-9471 CIP

Typesetting: Best-set Typesetter Ltd., Hong Kong
Printing and bookbinding: Brühlsche Universitätsdruckerei, Giessen
2127/3130-543210 – Printed on acid-free paper

List of Contributors

DONALD ARMSTRONG, Infectious Disease Section, Memorial Sloan–Kettering Cancer Center, 1275 York Avenue, New York, NY 10021, USA

F. THOMAS BOYLE, ICI Pharmaceuticals, Mereside, Alderley Park, Macclesfield, Cheshire SK10 4TG, England

MANUEL DEBONO, Lilly Research Laboratories, Lilly Corporate Center, Indianapolis, IN 46285, USA

BERTRAND DUPONT, Pasteur Institute, Infectious Disease Unit and Mycology Unit, 25 Rue du Dr. Roux, F-75015 Paris, France

SARAH C. EARDLEY, ICI Pharmaceuticals, Mereside, Alderley Park, Macclesfield, Cheshire SK10 4TG, England.

OLIVER P. FLINT, ICI Pharmaceuticals, Mereside, Alderley Park, Macclesfield, Cheshire SK10 4TG, England. *Present address:* Bristol–Myers Squibb PRDD, P.O. Box 4755, Syracuse, NY 13221–4755, USA

ROBERT S. GORDEE, Lilly Research Laboratories, Lilly Corporate Center, Indianapolis, IN 46285, USA

JOHN R. GRAYBILL, Audie L. Murphy Memorial Veterans Hospital, 7400 Merton Minter Boulevard, San Antonio, TX 78284, USA

HEINZ HÄNEL, Hoechst Aktiengesellschaft, Postfach 80 03 20, 6230 Frankfurt am Main 80, FRG

THOMAS C. JONES, Allergy and Infectious Diseases, Clinical Research, Sandoz Ltd., Basle 4002, Switzerland

DAVID KERRIDGE, Department of Biochemistry, Tennis Court Road, Cambridge CB2 1QW, England

ANN LAMBERT, Department of Medicine (Clinical Biochemistry), Hope Hospital, Eccles Old Road, Salford M6 8HD, England

DAVID LOEBENBERG, Schering Research, Schering-Plough Corporation, 60 Orange Street, Bloomfield, NJ 07003, USA

PHILIP A. PIZZO, Infectious Diseases Section, Pediatric Branch, National Cancer Institute, Bethesda, MD 20892, USA

ANNEMARIE POLAK, Pharmaceutical Research Division, F. Hoffmann-La Roche Ltd., 124 Grenzacherstrasse, 4002 Basel, Switzerland

WOLFGANG RITTER, Bayer AG, Institut für Klinische Pharmakologie, Aprather Weg, Postfach 10 17 09, 5600 Wuppertal 1, FRG

MARGUERITE M. ROBERTS, The Skin Hospital, Out-Patients Department (University of Manchester School of Medicine), Chapel Street, Salford, Lancs M60 9EP, England

WILLIAM R. ROBERTSON, Department of Medicine (Clinical Biochemistry), Hope Hospital, Eccles Old Road, Salford M6 8HD, England

JOHN F. RYLEY, ICI Pharmaceuticals, Mereside, Alderley Park, Macclesfield, Cheshire SK10 4TG, England

HEINZ J. SCHMITT, Kinderklinik der Universität, Langenbeckstrasse, 6500 Mainz, FRG

JACK D. SOBEL, Division of Infectious Diseases, Suite 202 Professional Building, Harper Hospital, 4160 John R, Detroit, MI 48201, USA

JOHN J. STERN, Buckley Medical Associates, Pennsylvania Hospital, 822 Pine Street, Philadelphia, PA 19107, USA

ALAN M. SUGAR, Section of Infectious Diseases, Evans Memorial Department of Clinical Research, The University Hospital, 88 East Newton Street, Boston, MA 02118–2393, USA

MICHAEL H. TARBIT, Department of Bichemical Pharmacology, Glaxo Group Research, Ware, Hertfordshire SG12 ODP, England

HUGO VANDEN BOSSCHE, Department of Comparative Biochemistry, Janssen Research Foundation, Turnhoutseweg 30, B-2340 Beerse, Belgium

VIOLETTE V. VILLARS, Allergy and Infectious Diseases, Clinical Research, Sandoz Ltd., Basle 4002, Switzerland

THOMAS J. WALSH, Infectious Diseases Section, Pediatrics Branch, National Cancer Institute, Bethesda, MD 20892, USA

ROBERT G. WILSON, ICI Pharmaceuticals, Mereside, Alderley Park, Macclesfield, Cheshire SK10 4TG, England

MICHEL ZAUG, Pharmaceutical Research Division, F. Hoffmann-La Roche Ltd., 124 Grenzacherstrasse, 4002 Basel, Switzerland

Preface

Fungal diseases have been with us from antiquity; interest in the chemotherapy of fungal disease has exploded in the past decade. To plan and produce a book on the topic of antifungal chemotherapy has come as a personal challenge – and something of an eye-opener – towards the end of my research career. A landmark publication which still merits reading is *Antifungal Chemotherapy* (John Wiley & Sons, Chichester, UK), edited by David Speller, which appeared in 1980. However, the fact that ketoconazole, the first of the modern, orally active, wide-spectrum antifungals, attracted no more than two sentences in it indicates just how far we have come in the 1980s. A steady stream of original papers and a number of conference proceedings have chronicled this progress in drug research; outstanding among the latter are the proceedings of an international telesymposium, entitled *Recent Trends in the Discovery, Development and Evaluation of Antifungal Agents*, edited by Robert Fromtling (J.R. Prous, Barcelona, 1987) and volume 544 of the Annals of the New York Academy of Sciences, entitled *Antifungal Drugs*, edited by Vassil St. Georgiev, and containing papers and posters presented at a most enjoyable 3-day conference held at Garden City, New York, in the autumn of 1987.

Why then a new book? The Telesymposium Proceedings, and to a lesser extent the New York Academy of Sciences volume, are product-oriented works dealing with recently marketed compounds and some still in development. Although tremendous strides in antifungal chemotherapy have been made during the last decade, and although many conditions can now be successfully treated, the problems of fungal disease remain and are, in fact, increasing. This is because potential sources of infection are widespread, and fungal infection is often the consequence of another illness or predisposing cause in the patient. Advances in high-technology medicine, a greater use of antibiotics, increasingly aggressive chemotherapy of malignant conditions, organ transplantation with its associated immunosuppression and the ever-growing incidence of AIDS have all contributed to the burgeoning prevalence of opportunistic mycoses. Against this background of continuing need, I have tried to produce a volume which will chart the processes involved in the discovery, development and final clinical utilisation of a new drug. My aim has not been to produce a series of specialist chapters for specialists but rather a volume which will help the specialist involved at just one stage of the complex process of drug discovery and development to appreciate the need for and contributions to be made by the many others involved in the overall process before a new drug is successfully established.

In planning this volume I have particularly had in mind five groups of people: the experimentalist, the "middleman", the clinician, the manager and the academic. In the first group I hope to stimulate a reappraisal of screening methodology based on recent experience, suggest new approaches to drug discovery, make them more aware of the complex processes involved before a product of their research can become an acceptable drug and present the challenges of the ever-changing clinical needs. I trust the experts involved in the various stages of drug development, who are not necessarily experts in matters mycological, might find useful background information on both research and clinical matters which would stimulate them as they make their vital contribution to the complete scheme. It is easy for a clinician to prescribe a drug in areas of medicine for which plenty of alternative therapies are available. I hope the clinician faced with fungal diseases, perhaps frustrated by the limited choices available, will find in this volume some reminder of the cost both in terms of money, time and scientific effort required before a new drug can be added to his armamentarium. It must be an awesome decision for any management to take to enter a new area of medicinal research; to discover, develop and launch a new drug might cost at today's prices something in the region of £100 million, money which will have to be recouped from sales before any hope of profit is possible. My wish is that this book will remind managers of the urgent needs and opportunities in the field of antifungal chemotherapy as well as of the ideas and processes by which these needs might be met. Often with little experience or understanding of the pressures and issues in industry, academics will hopefully come to appreciate better the complexity and cost of the processes of drug discovery, and particularly of drug development, and to see where in the general scheme of things they can make their most valuable contribution.

I am most grateful to the many friends from academic and clinical situations who have so readily come to my rescue and written chapters on their own particular specialities. Two pharmaceutical companies in particular have had a great deal of recent experience taking new compounds from the laboratory to the clinic. I had planned for the drug development section of this book to have a series of chapters written jointly by experts from these two establishments based on their recent experiences. In the event collaboration was not forthcoming, and my grand design was frustrated. I am particularly grateful, therefore, to the friends and colleagues from other parts of industry – and to their helpful and co-operative managements – who have not only rescued me from my predicament but have also contributed so generously to the other two sections of the book.

As so as we begin the last decade of the twentieth century, it is my hope that this volume will in some way stimulate research into new ways of meeting the continuing challenge of fungal diseases and promote better understanding between those involved at the practical level in discovering and progressing a new treatment.

Alderley Park

JOHN F. RYLEY

Contents

SECTION I. Drug Discovery

CHAPTER 12

Clinical Trials

SECTION III. Clinical Usage

CHAPTER 15

An Infectious Disease Specialist's Viewpoint

CHAPTER 16

Management of Fungal Infections in Patients with Neoplastic Diseases

CHAPTER 19

Systemic Azole Antifungal Drugs — Into the 1990s

CHAPTER 20

Terbinafine

CHAPTER 21

Amorolfine

Section I. Drug Discovery

Introduction

JOHN F. RYLEY

Once management has made that brave decision to embark on a programme aimed at discovering a new antifungal agent, how does the research scientist *actually* set about the process of drug discovery? Past experience suggests that the empirical approach has much to recommend it; lurking in some vast chemical collection somewhere or being constantly produced by some strange microorganism in some far corner of the world are surely new antifungal agents just waiting to be recognised. But how can we identify them? It is a continuing source of irritation and challenge to the modern scientist that the rational approach to chemotherapy has not been more successful. Perhaps next year? Tom BOYLE has collaborated with me for a number of years in our search at ICI for a new antifungal agent. He opens the volume with a chapter which tries to explain to the non-chemists among us how the chemical mind operates as he hovers over his retort planning what to brew up next. His thinking may be directed by analogy with known active structures or by fashionable biochemical pathways, but beyond this the medicinal chemist needs a vision and a feel for the target.

It is often possible in retrospect to explain in biochemical terms how a particular drug works. What is needed is to make this process work in reverse – to define the target and then design the drug. My good friends David KERRIDGE and Hugo VANDEN BOSSCHE have put together their considerable experience in academia and industry to illustrate ways in which the biochemist can feed the chemist with rational ideas aimed at drug discovery. For those who have more faith in Nature, Bob GORDEE and his colleague Manuel DEBONO discuss some of the ways in which one can look for natural product activity. In terms of active molecules turned up over the years, the natural product approach is attractive. In so many cases, however, activity in vivo and/or freedom from toxicity have been elusive, but their efforts have at last been rewarded by the discovery of cilofungin, recorded later in this book.

With productive chemists spurred on by idea-rich biochemists and natural product samples in abundance, problems can arise with detecting and evaluating antifungal activity. Geoff WILSON and I have gained a fair amount of experience during the past decade attacking a collection of around 200 000 chemicals as well as dealing with the output of a number of dedicated synthetic and natural product chemists. In the last two chapters of this section we discuss some of the methods, problems and pitfalls associated with screening for antifungal activity both in vitro and in vivo.

CHAPTER 1

Drug Discovery: A Chemist's Approach

F. THOMAS BOYLE

A. Introduction

The medicinal chemist's role in the multidisciplinary team involved in the modern day drug discovery process is to furnish agents for biochemical and biological experimentation and ultimately for therapeutic or prophylactic use in disease. In the antifungal area, the complexity of drug-fungal interactions and the intensity of the drug effect depend to a large extent on the concentration of drug in the active biophase (e.g. cell membrane), whereas the duration of the effect is determined by its persistence in a sufficient concentration at the active site. Drug molecules, therefore, owe much of their effect to interaction with biological structures, e.g. lipoprotein receptors, biomembranes and nucleic acids. This interaction triggers a series of steps, ultimately resulting in a macroscopic physiological change that constitutes the pharmacological effect. Ideally, only by first unravelling the relatively simple primary interaction between the drug molecule and a macromolecular structure can drug activity at the molecular level be understood. The increasing complexity of the whole organism, and then the animal model, requires an understanding of many more parameters – including some not always available to the chemist in the early phase of the programme.

Not surprisingly, therefore, much of the early literature and history of drug discovery stems from a process of trial and error, or even serendipity. These methods, though somewhat wasteful, have stood us in good stead, particularly when augmented by intuition and experience within the specialised confines of a particular chemical series.

The most difficult problem for the medicinal chemist is the discovery of a 'lead' compound. Only in a few cases have lead compounds been found by deliberate design. In most cases random screening has been the major source, particularly when related to some idea of the biological locus of intervention. It follows that a valid biochemical working hypothesis is essential to the establishment of a more rational screening approach. In this way lead compounds from screening programmes will continue to identify classes of compounds which allow the medicinal chemist the opportunity to expore many of the limitations and biochemical requirements for activity. In the antifungal area there is much precedent for this approach; I will illustrate it from the azole series of inhibitors for which much biochemical/mode of action information is available. The example of the identification and development of ICI 195,739 is useful for this purpose. In the second part of this chapter I will attempt to consider the more complex issues involved in the identification of a lead compound, and in particular detail the process requirements placed on the medicinal chemist to identify an alternative locus in the sterol metabolic pathway. At the outset the locus had to be unique to fungi, free from the potential toxicological complications of cytochrome P-450 interaction and suitable for chemical exploitation. We chose to consider the inhibition of the C_{24}-transmethylation process. There are clearly many other targets, all with their unique problems, but in constructing the chapter in this way I hope to illustrate many of the underlying problems facing the medicinal chemist.

B. Development of a Lead

Examples of compound development now exist based on the impairment of steroidal biosynthesis in the fungal cell membrane. Recent examples from Pfizer (fluconazole, MARRIOTT and RICHARDSON 1987), Janssen (intraconazole, VAN CUTSEM et al. 1987), Bayer (bifonazole, PLEMPEL et al. 1987) and Sandoz (terbinafine, RYDER 1988) have illustrated developments and improvements in the properties of antifungal agents. These improvements, highlighted after several years' clinical experience with ketoconazole, include:

1. A broad antimycotic spectrum against dermatophytes, yeasts, and filamentatous and dimorphic fungi
2. Orally effective with a pharmacokinetic profile suitable to once daily dosing
3. A reduced risk of side effects involving the liver
4. A reduced interference with gonadal and adrenal hormone biosynthesis
5. Non-teratogenic

The first experience of an azole antifungal within ICI was with ICI 153,066 (I), which was reported by RYLEY and WILSON (1982) to have therapeutic activity against vaginal candidosis in mice and rats and against dermatophyte lesions in mice and guinea pigs following oral administration. Although the compound was shown to have 10–100 times the potency of ketoconazole in these models, subsequent toxicological investigations precluded further development. The main concerns centred on effects in reproductive toxicology in the rat and rabbit and unacceptable toxicity in the dog. The latter problem stemmed from an extended elimination half-life, a feature not seen in the rat.

For the synthetic chemist developing an alternative compound using ICI 153,066 as an existing lead – a compound generated in part as a result of a joint programme targeted at human and plant pathogens – the prime need is the development of worthwhile correlations which allow the processing of in vitro potency into in vivo activity. In this two major problems have to be

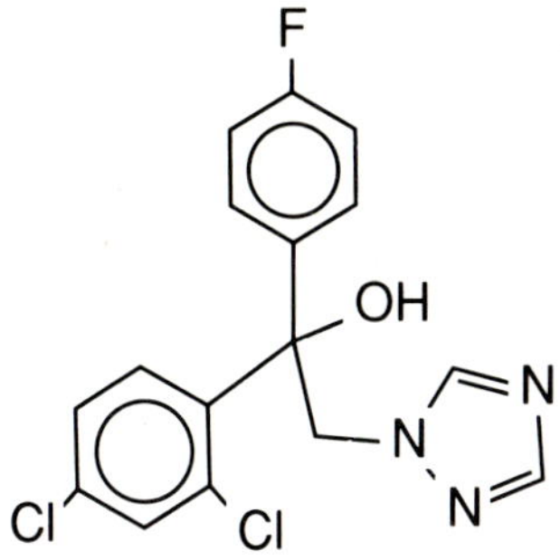

ICI 153,066 (I)

addressed: the first stems from the observation that the susceptibility of fungi to azoles in vitro is notoriously dependent on media composition, inoculum effects, growth conditions, etc. (ODDS 1985); the second arises from attempting to extend this to predicting and correlating with the activity in vivo.

In extending the initial in vitro activity against a target organism to worthwhile in vivo activity, the synthetic chemist is faced with overcoming several extra barriers to the expression of the drug-active site interaction. Information on such factors as absorption rates from the site of administration, the manner in which the drug is distributed within the body, the results of lipid binding, and hence the rate and route of elimination from the body is invariably unavailable. Studies aimed at determining these factors are rare, and in an integrated research programme are often too cumbersome, time-consuming and resource-demanding to be available for other than the final drug candidate. A further complicating factor is the host's metabolic capacity to modify the structural integrity of the dosed compound. This can – and often does – markedly affect the levels of bioavailable material, and as a consequence the medicinal chemist is required to make step-jumps in synthetic judgement in attempting to define those factors controlling the eventual disposition of sufficient levels of drug to the target site. With these problems in mind a reassessment of the monotriazole tertiary alcohols was undertaken using standardised testing procedures – determination of IC_{50} in yeast nitrogen base (YNB) broth and activity against a *Candida albicans* infection of the mouse vagina (BOYLE et al. 1987). A conventional plot of log oral activity against log in vitro activity (Fig. 1) suggested that no worthwhile correlation existed. However, three sub-series of compounds were identified which illustrate many of the biopharmaceutical problems encountered by the medicinal chemist in such correlations.

Irrespective of in vitro potency, compounds with unsubstituted aromatic nuclei were inactive in vivo – reflecting the metabolic vulnerability of such systems to the P-450-mediated epoxidase/hydroxylase systems of the host.

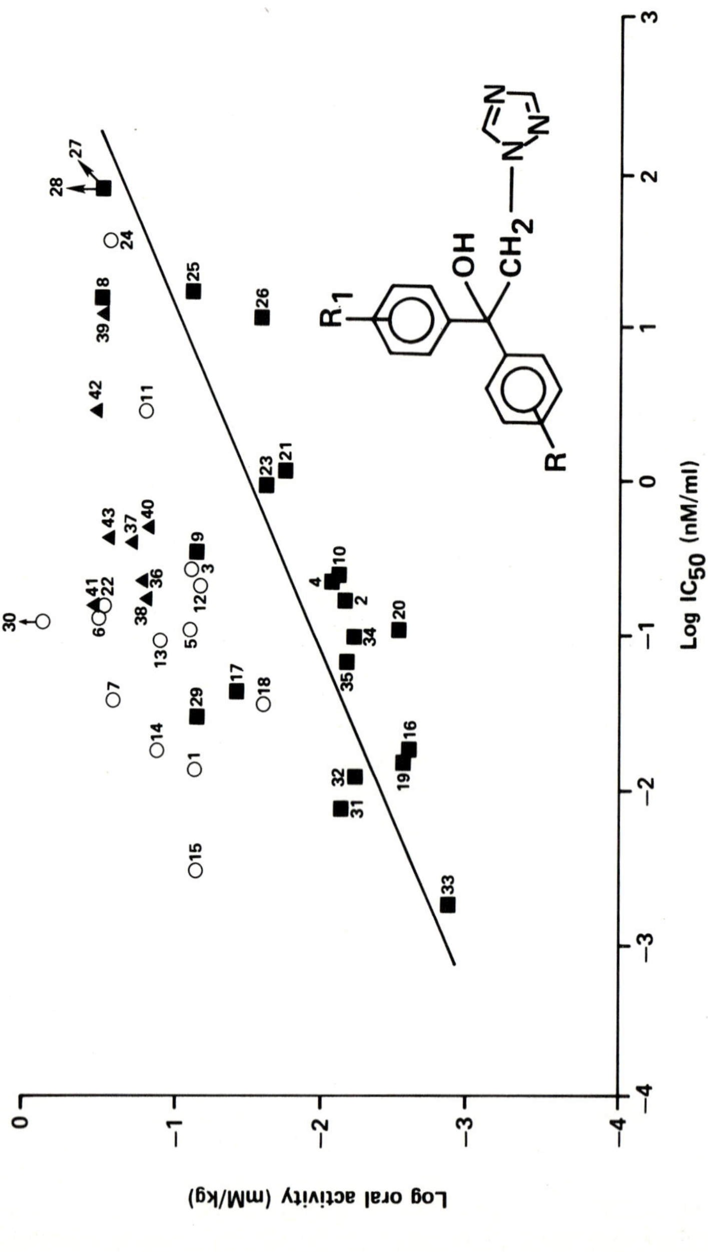

Fig. 1. Correlations of in vitro with in vivo activity for monotriazole tertiary alcohols

Compounds with an exposed *para* position in at least one ring gave no correlation between in vitro and in vivo activity, although marginal levels of activity (50–100 mg/kg) were observed. A final series of some 20 compounds could be subdivided into compounds bearing metabolically vulnerable substituents (OH or NH_2) in which no in vivo activity was observed and a further set which contained substituents with metabolic stability and which showed similar biopharmaceutical properties. In this latter subset a highly significant correlation of in vitro potency with in vivo activity was observed. This analysis supported (from an activity viewpoint only) the decision to proceed with ICI 153,066 to extended evaluation. However, the toxicological problems led to a need for an alternative agent.

The regulatory demands for the reporting of all observable effects of a potential drug candidate have alerted experimental biologists to look out for properties which might modify or detract from its primary utility. Azole antifungals interfere primarily at low concentrations with the microsomal P-450-dependent $C_{14}\alpha$-demethylation of lanosterol (SISLER and RAGSDALE 1984) although other biochemical targets are affected at higher drug concentrations (e.g. fatty acid disturbance, BORGERS and WALDRON 1981). Cytochromes P-450 are ubiquitous haemoproteins and are recognised as having a key role in the metabolism of lipids, in xenobiotic degradation in the liver and in many other processes (CONNEY 1986). Azoles like ketoconazole are known to have the potential for inhibition of host P-450 systems, particularly those enzymes involved in steroidogenesis (KOWAL 1983). In a similar way part of the toxicology associated with ICI 153,066 could be accounted for by interference with the ovarian aromatase enzyme complex. Resolution of the compound and assaying the individual enantiomers in vitro and in vivo displayed a clear separation of the antifungal and aromatase activities, the antifungal R isomer (ICI 171,692) being the less potent aromatase inhibitor (BOYLE et al. 1988).

Development of a synthetic programme aimed at an alternative to ICI 153,066 was aided in the first instance by a self-consistent concept of azole-haem protein interaction at the $C_{14}\alpha$-demethylase complex for a range of inhibitors. A computer graphics model was established, and mutually exclusive fits of the R and S isomers of ICI 153,066 within the Van der Waal surface of the lanosterol or testosterone substrates increased confidence in the utility of this approach (Fig. 2). At the same time, the establishment of an expanded test cascade to monitor compound effects against fungal sterol demethylation and aromatase (BARRETT-BEE et al. 1988) allowed assessment of a structural series for maximal separation of these two activities. Attention was focussed on the bistriazole tertiary alcohol series, the initial samples of which were supplied by colleagues at ICI Agriculturals (WORTHINGTON 1982). As well as showing good separation in the biochemical marker screens, these compounds were attractive for two reasons: they were orally effective in the screening cascade, and they had low partition coefficients. This latter property was considered to be important since the relatively high log P (3.11) of ICI 153,066 together with the metabolically stable nature of the substitu-

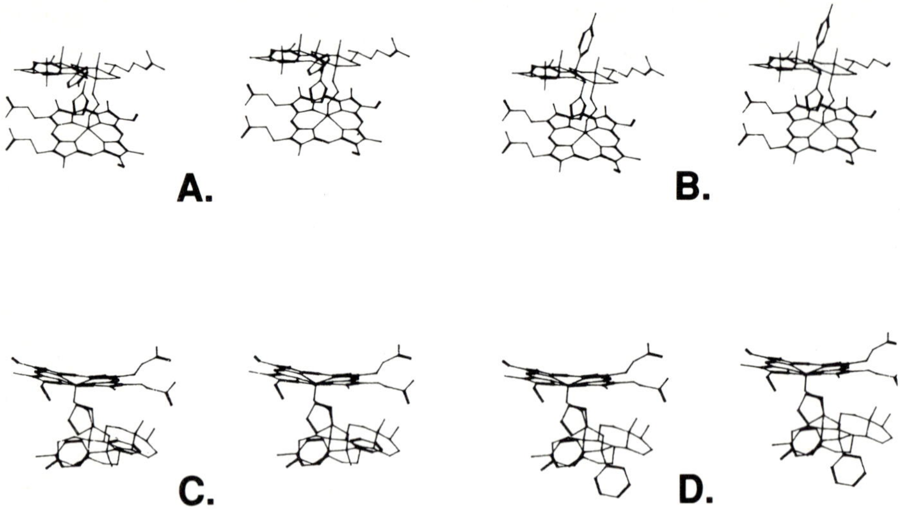

Fig. 2A–D. Stereo-pair computer graphics overlays of the enantiomers of ICI 153,066 on the (**A**, **B**) $C_{14}\alpha$-demethylase model of the lanosterol-dioxyporphyrin complex and on the (**C**, **D**) $C_{19}\beta$-demethylase model of the testosterone-dioxyporphyrin complex

tion pattern in the molecule were responsible for its unacceptable pharmacokinetic profile.

From a structure-activity point of view, this more hydrophilic series of compounds proved simpler to analyse. Interestingly, whilst the lower in vitro potency of this series required modification of the test system, an extremely good in vitro-in vivo activity correlation was developed (Fig. 3); fluconazole (compound II) was identified from this series of compounds (Marriott and Richardson 1987). In extending this process, a further structural feature of the bistriazole nucleus – namely the two azole rings – was intriguing. If only

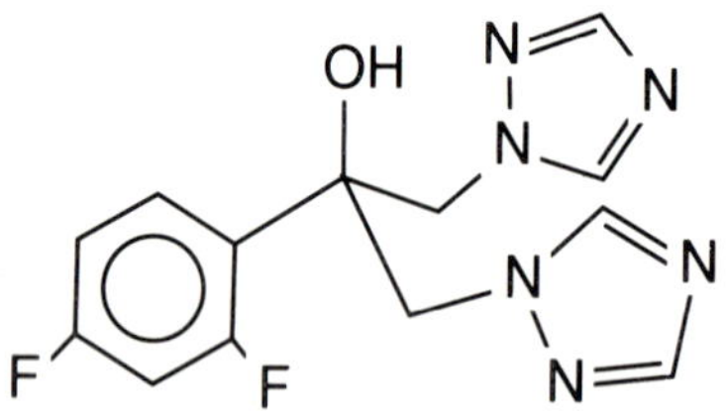

Fluconazole (II)

one azole was required for P-450 binding, what function did the second azole nucleus fulfil? Various theoretical options were: was it providing a specific intermolecular hydrogen bonding locus within the enzyme site, or was it just a

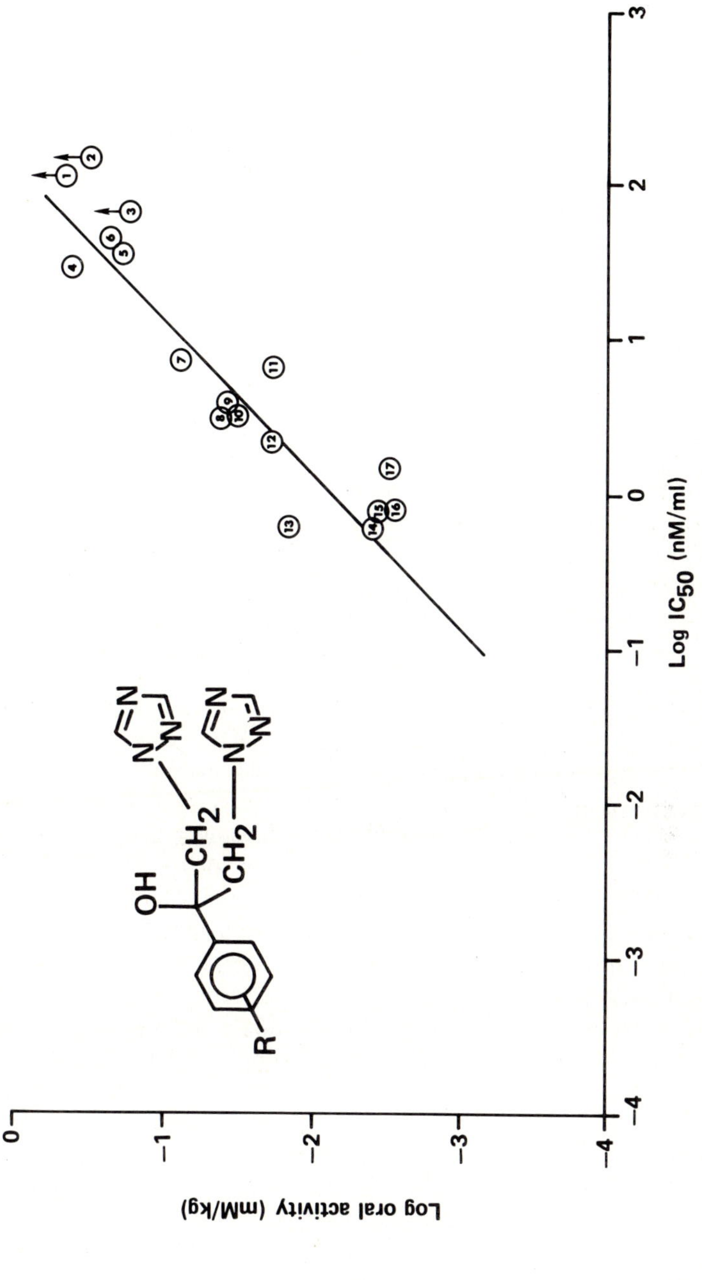

Fig. 3. Correlations of in vitro with in vivo activity for bistriazole tertiary alcohols

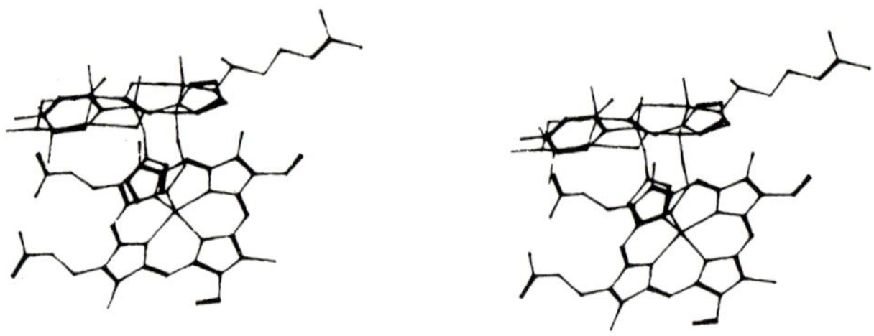

Fig. 4. Stereo-pair computer graphics overlay of a bistriazole tertiary alcohol on the $C_{14}\alpha$-demethylase model

more general polar function for membrane interactions? A third alternative existed: the ring may be interacting with the tertiary protein complex by mimicking the D-ring of the steroid (Fig. 4). If this were the case, then in attempting to increase the antifungal specificity of the inhibitor by the identification of extra receptor binding sites within the type 1 binding region of the enzyme complex, potential lanosterol mimics (rather than, for example, testosterone) should be synthesised.

Early results from compounds aimed at addressing the fundamental question of how much substitution (if any) in the azole nucleus the $C_{14}\alpha$-demethylase enzyme complex would tolerate were not encouraging. However, the observation that a 3′-phenethyl derivative (VII) increased in vitro activity, which was subsequently substantiated by the heteroalkyl (V and VI) isosteres (Table 1), encouraged continued synthesis.

With the aid of the computer graphics model, more rational side chain mimics were assembled. Synthetic difficulties prevented the lanosterol side chain bistriazole derivative being assembled; however, a subsequent aim to locate a π-bonding system in the Δ_{24} region predicted the 3′-styryl functionality to be a key structural element from this analysis. Graphics also suggested a strong preference for Z-stereochemistry (Fig. 5).

Examples of the main structure-activity patterns are presented in Table 2. In vitro potencies against *C. albicans* show a 2–3 order of magnitude increase over the parent fluconazole except when strongly hydrophilic or hydrogen bond acceptor substituents are present (compound XVI). In general there was good in vitro-in vivo correlation except when metabolic vulnerability existed in the molecule (VIII and XIII), confirming that the host metabolic P-450-mediated hydroxylase/demethylase and secondary conjugative mechanisms play a key role in the expression of the in vitro potential. Later we were forced to use this phenomenon to our advantage.

In the 4-CF_3 (XI) and 4-OCF_3 (XII) derivatives, antifungal agents of significant interest were realised, but although both compounds satisfied teratological and toxicological requirements, long elimination half-lives in both the rat and the dog prevented their further advancement to the clinic. The lesson was clear: as the direction of chemistry had moved from the parent bis-triazole structure to the 3′-styryl substituted series in optimising oral

Table 1. Biological consequences of 3′-substitution in bistriazole tertiary alcohols

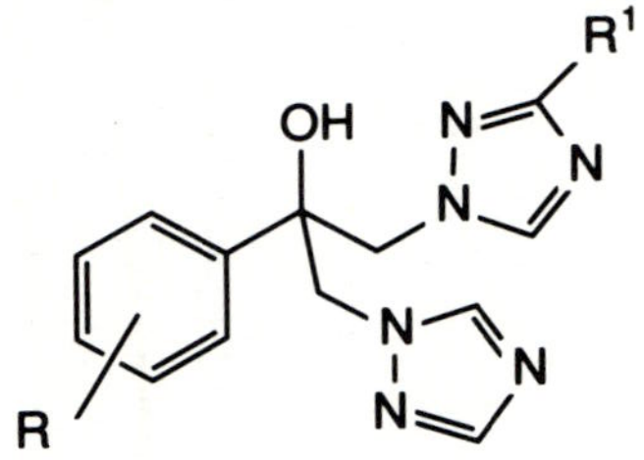

Compound No.	R	R′	*Candida albicans* (broth-dilution) IC_{50} (μg/ml)	Antifungal spectrum (agar-dilution) (MIC in μg/ml) *Candida albicans* Yeast	*Candida albicans* Mycelium	Dermat-ophytes	*Candida albicans* in vivo (mg/kg)
II	2,4F	H	0.62	100	0.1	(100)	5.0
III	2,4F	$C_6H_4CF_3$	0.94	(100)	<0.01	(100)	10
IV	2,4Cl	$CH_2CH(Me)_2$	0.95	100-6.2	<0.01	100	25
V	2,4Cl	$CH_2OC_6H_4Cl$	–	100-1.6	<0.01	6.2-1.6	>50
VI	2,4F	$SCH_2C_6H_4CF_3$	–	100-6.2	0.01	25-6.2	>50
VII	2,4Cl	$CH_2CH_2C_6H_5$	0.02	100-1.6	<0.01	25-1.6	>25

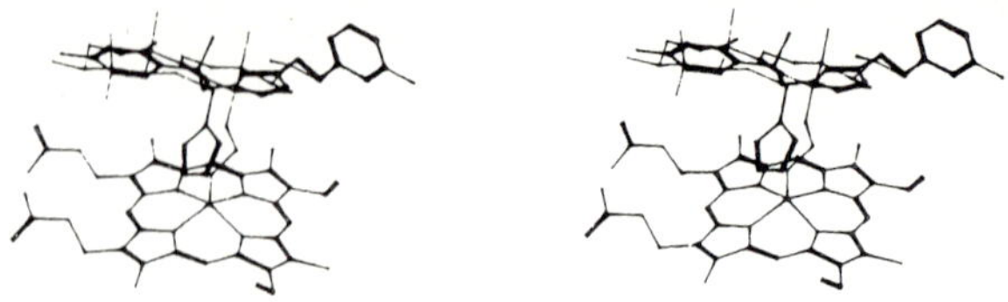

Fig. 5. Stereo-pair computer graphics overlay of a 3′-styryl bistriazole tertiary alcohol on the $C_{14}\alpha$-demethylase model

activity, by utilising metabolically stable substrates, compounds of profound metabolic stability had been produced. The challenge to the medicinal chemist was equally clear: identification of a compound possessing the pharmacological and toxicological properties of compounds (XI) and (XII) but with a much reduced elimination half-life.

In this particular example, clues existed: the biological data presented in Table 2 suggest that in pairs of structural isosteres with metabolic *non*-equivalence ($CN/CONH_2$:OCH_3/OCF_3) resistance to metabolism correlated with in vivo activity. An initial approach based on the $CN/CONH_2$ isosteres attempted to modulate the rate of amide metabolism by the host deaminase-amidase cleavage enzymes. This failed even with highly blocked amide derivatives; rapid metabolic clearance still prevented complete expression of the in vitro potential because no elimination half-life could be measured. An alternative approach based on metabolic modulation of the simple OCH_3/OCF_3 isosteres proved more successful. In analysing the problem, two potential centres for metabolism were postulated – ring and substituent. At this level of the testing cascade, evidence for these centres being metabolically vulnerable was not available to the medicinal chemist since detailed metabolic studies could not be justified. From a chemical standpoint this analysis was further complicated by the changed electronic character of the substituent on metabolic stabilisation, the subsequent effect on the ring's electronic character and hence its susceptibility to an epoxidase-hydroxylase enzyme system. However, on going from OCF_3 to OCH_2CF_3, exposure of both the

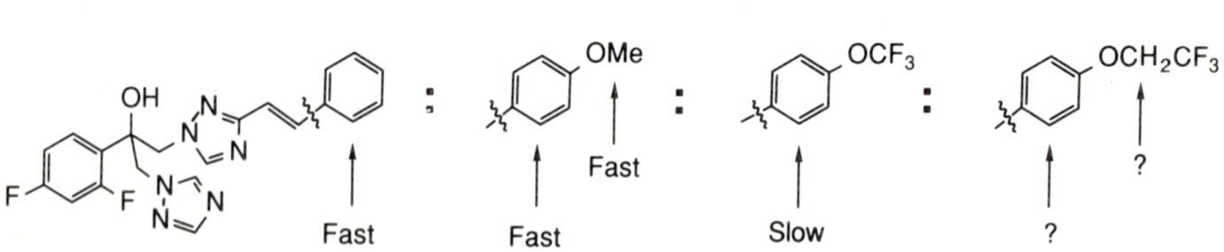

Fig. 6. Different substituents at metabolic sites and their effects on rates of metabolism

ring and the side chain to metabolic attack was anticipated, leading to a modification of the elimination half-life (Fig. 6). The biological/pharmacokinetic consequences of this approach are summarised in Table 3. In vitro

Table 2. Biological consequences of 4-substitution in 3′-styryl triazole tertiary alcohols

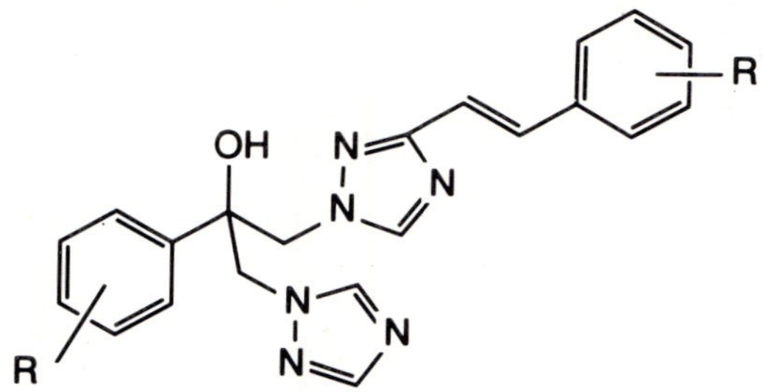

Compound No.	R	R′	*Candida albicans* (broth-dilution) IC_{50} (μg/ml)	Antifungal spectrum (agar-dilution) (MIC in μg/ml) *Candida albicans* Yeast	*Candida albicans* Mycelium	Dermatophytes	*Candida albicans* in vivo (mg/kg)
VIII	2,4Cl	H	0.06	100-6.2	<0.1	25-6.2	>50
IX	2,4F	4F	0.05	25	<0.1	25	10
X	2,4F	4Br	0.001	25-1.6	<0.1	6.2	0.25
XI	2,4F	$4CF_3$	0.09	6.2-1.6	<0.1	6.2	1-0.5
XII	2,4F	$4OCF_3$	0.05	6.2-1.6	<0.001	1.6	0.25
XIII	2,4F	$4OCH_3$	0.001	100-1.6	<0.01	25-1.6	>25
XIV	2,4F	$4NO_2$	0.14	100-1.6	0.01	>100	5
XV	2,4F	4CN	0.12	100-1.6	0.01	100-1.6	1
XVI	2,4F	$4CONH_2$	0.53	>100	0.01	(100)	>25

potency covered a wide range of substituents and did not limit the chemical exploitation of this area.

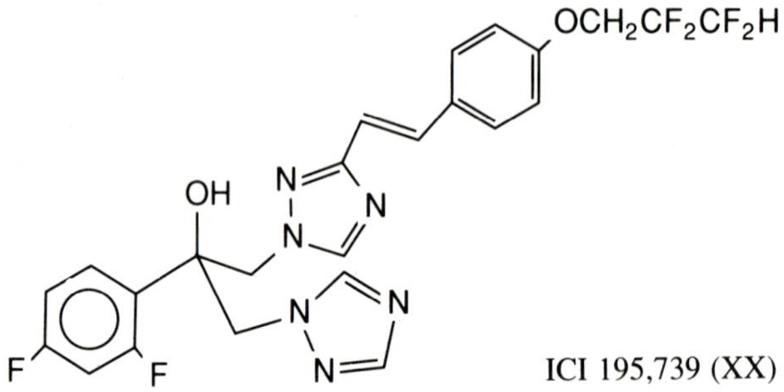

ICI 195,739 (XX)

Success was achieved with fluorinated side chain derivatives of which the methylene homologue (XIX) showed good oral activity with the desired reduction in elimination half-life. The tetrafluoroethoxy derivative (XVIII) showed increased in vitro potency and oral activity but retained a long elimination half-life; homologation of this to ICI 195,739 (XX) gave a compound with a near optimal profile of increased in vitro potency, broad spectrum of activity, oral activity and an elimination half-life of approximately 24 h. Subsequent studies confirming the value of this compound have been presented by RYLEY et al. (1988).

C. Identification of a Lead

I. Fungal Sterol Metabolism – A Target for Lead Identification

Lead compound identification is the most difficult problem facing the medicinal chemist. We have not yet reached the level of sophistication at which an intimate knowledge of receptor mechanisms allows us to design novel compounds without a previous model. There are obviously several well-tested methods for uncovering such leads other than de novo design – the previous section provides one particular illustration of such a process. Extending these processes to allow the medicinal chemist to consider alternative sites of intervention in, for example, the fungal sterol metabolic pathway forces a heavy reliance on the biochemical knowledge available. The mechanisms by which perturbation of the sterol balance in fungi (e.g. *C. albicans*) leads to fungiotoxicity have not so far been satisfactorily elucidated. In the squalene epoxidase and $C_{14}\alpha$-demethylation inhibition areas, for example, significant advances have been made in our understanding (RYDER 1988; VANDEN BOSSCHE et al. 1984; VANDEN BOSSCHE 1987). From studies with azoles, the $C_{14}\alpha$-demethylase area is probably the best defined. There exists a close interrelationship between sterol composition and content, fatty acid composition, the activation of normal surface-bound cellular enzymes, e.g. chitin synthase, and the fungiotoxicity observed with these agents.

Table 3. Elimination half-life and biological activity of 3′-styryl triazoles

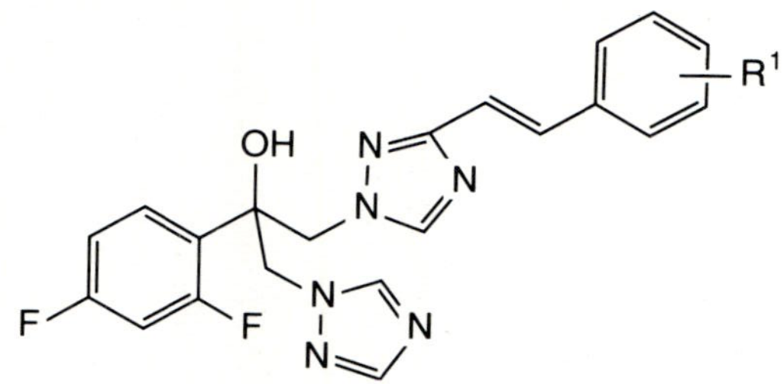

Compound No.	R′	*Candida albicans* (broth-dilution) IC_{50} (μg/ml)	Antifungal spectrum (agar-dilution) (MIC in μg/ml): *Candida albicans* Yeast	Antifungal spectrum (agar-dilution) (MIC in μg/ml): *Candida albicans* Mycelium	Antifungal spectrum (agar-dilution) (MIC in μg/ml): Dermat-ophytes	*Candida albicans* in vivo (mg/kg)	Rat $t_{1/2}$ (days)
XV	4CN	0.12	100-1.6	0.01	100-1.6	1	2
XVI	$4CONH_2$	0.53	>100	0.01	(100)	>25	ND
XVII	$4CON(CH_3)CH_2C_3F_7$	0.006	25-6.2	<0.01	≤1.6	10	ND
XII	$4OCF_3$	0.05	6.2-1.6	<0.001	1.6	0.25	6.5
XVIII	$4OCF_2CF_2H$	0.004	100-1.6	<0.01	6.2-1.6	0.25	9
XIX	$4OCH_2CF_3$	0.03	1.6	<0.01	1.6	0.5	1.5
XX	$4OCH_2CF_2CF_2H$	0.003	6.2-1.6	<0.01	≤1.6	0.25	1
XXI	$4OCH_2CH_2F$	0.003	25-1.6	<0.001	1.6	25	–
XIII	$4OCH_3$	0.001	100-1.6	<0.01	25-1.6	>25	–

ND, not done.

The inhibition of sterol biosynthesis is a proven therapeutic target, and to the medicinal chemist looking for new approaches to sterol inhibitors it is logical to consider sites of interventioin which are unique to this aspect of fungal metabolism. There are volumes of literature on ergosterol biosynthesis inhibitors applied to non-medical pathogens. However, the amount of data available concerning human pathogens, and more particularly compound intervention studies, is sparse. Ergosterol, the most dominant and biologically important product of sterol biosynthesis in fungi, corresponds to cholesterol in animals. The biosynthetic pathway from mevalonic acid to lanosterol is well established and is essentially similar in fungi and mammals (Mercer 1984), whilst the biosynthetic pathways post lanosterol diverge. In most fungi the following key transformations from lanosterol take place:

In *most fungi*, the steps are:

1. Methylation at C-24
2. Demethylation at C-4 and C-14:
   (i) at C-14;
   (ii) at C-4.

   (Yeast: order of steps 1 and 2 reversed, as indicated by dashed arrow)

3. Double bond transformations
   in nucleus ($\Delta_8 \rightarrow \Delta_7 \rightarrow \Delta_{5,7}$;
   in side chain:
   (i) saturation of 24 (28) double bond;
   (ii) formation of 22 (23) double bond.

The sequence of these events, however, seems to vary between fungi, and these route differences may account for the claimed different modes of action reported with some antifungal agents. The generalised transition matrix for lanosterol to ergosterol developed by Pierce et al. (1979) provides a good overview of the potential biosynthetic interconversions. Variations in the pathway, while academically interesting, are not too surprising when one considers the diverse environments of plant and mammalian fungal parasites.

The enzymic systems responsible for sterol modification are able to accept a variety of closely related substrates; what determines the major synthetic sequence is the relative efficiencies with which these systems operate on them. From a compound intervention standpoint, optimum activity would be expected when substrates are produced on which the enzymes are *incapable* of operating. Thus, for example, in *C. albicans* the primary substrate for Δ_{24}-methyl transfer is zymosterol (XXII; Parks et al. 1979); in *Ustilago* it is lanosterol (XXIII; Sisler and Ragsdale 1984). However, when $C_{14}\alpha$-demethylation is blocked by azole inhibitors, *C. albicans* will, in an attempt to bypass the consequences of compound intervention, operate with a much reduced efficiency on lanosterol to produce 24-methylene lanosterol (Barrett-Bee, personal communication).

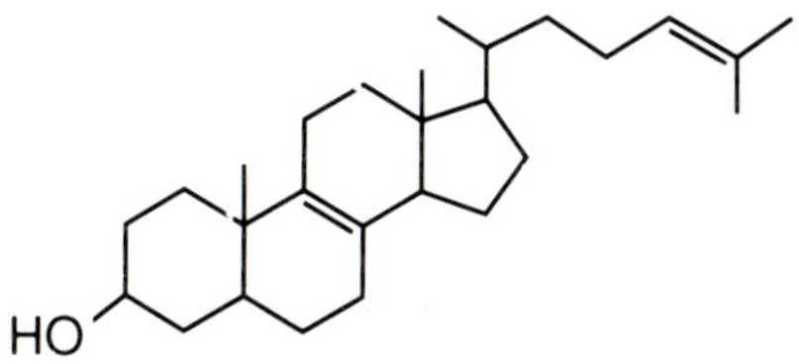

Zymosterol (XXII)

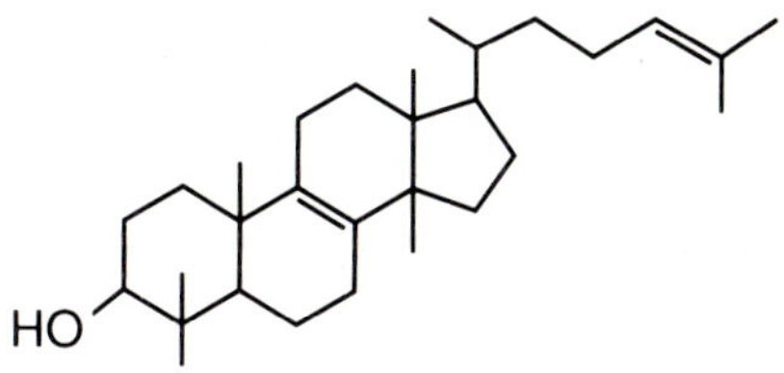

Lanosterol (XXIII)

With human fungal pathogens, investigations aimed specifically at sterol structure and the support of fungal growth do not exist. However, in *Saccharomyces cerevisiae*, from studies using either induced antibiotic resistance (THOMPSON and PARKS 1974) or its ability to grow anaerobically under certain conditions (and thus preclude the oxidative conversion of squalene to lanosterol), the requirement for different sterols to support fungal growth have been investigated (NES et al. 1978). Accepting the limitation that in such studies it is difficult to ascribe no fungal growth to direct sterol toxicity or poor substrate specificity, the results allow the marked dependence of precise structural features within the lanosterol to ergosterol biosynthetic sequence to be identified. From the medicinal chemist's viewpoint the structural features can be divided into ring and side chain requirements. For the ring the 3β-OH is obligatory for growth, whereas the presence of C_{14} and C_4 methyl groups in the nucleus did not allow growth. There appeared to be little advantage in the $\Delta_5\Delta_7$-conjugated diene over the Δ_5 olefin or even the fully saturated B ring sterols. In the side-chain the 24β-methyl was obligatory for growth, but better growth still was observed with the 24β-methyl Δ_{22} double-bonded side chain. A *trans* Δ_{22} double bond was essential since *cis* stereochemistry at this position did not support growth. From fixed E and Z Δ_{20} olefins the natural sterol probably acts in the form of a preferred linear conformer (Z) since only this form supported growth. Finally, stereoselective reduction of the C_{24}-methenylated side chain to produce the β-methyl epimer gave optimal support of growth, the α-epimer being extremely poor.

These data underpin many of the published inhibitor studies and confirm that the normal biosynthetic process of removal of methyl groups from the nucleus and the introduction of one in the side chain are of profound functional significance to the integrity of normal membrane function. Also, the precise structural character of the side chain appears to be quantitatively more important than the degree of unsaturation of the nucleus. The implication of this, *if it holds true for a range of human pathogenic fungi*, is clear: an inhibitor of the biosynthetic elaboration of the sidechain of ergosterol should be a prime target. Of more questionable relevance as a target would be an specific inhibitor of the Δ_8-Δ_7 rearrangement. The value of inhibiting the Δ_{24}-transmethylation process over conventional C_{14}- and C_4-demethylation is that it offers the opportunity of a non P-450 mediated intervention mechanism. Having identified the biochemical target, what is known?

II. Δ_{24}-Transmethylation in Yeast and Fungal Sterol Synthesis

The cellular localisation and kinetic properties of the sterol Δ_{24}-methyl transferase have been thoroughly studied (PARKS et al. 1979). It is not within the scope of this chapter to review this, except in connection with the help it gives the medicinal chemist in lead generation. Mechanistically, Δ_{24}-transmethylation is accomplished by *S*-adenosyl methionine (SAM) (PARKS 1958). Subsequently LEDERER (1965), from deuterium transfer studies, showed that only two of the C_{28} methyl group hydrogens are incorporated, the third proton being introduced by a NADPH-dependent reductase.

Further data on the chirality of enzymic transmethylation, the absolute configuration of the sulphonium centre of SAM and its relation to enzymic reactivity in these processes can be derived from the work of FLOSS et al. (1979), CORNFORTH et al. (1979) and DE LA HABA (1959).

Mechanistically, the key to the methylation reaction is the positively charged sulphonium centre in SAM (XXIV) which renders the methyl group

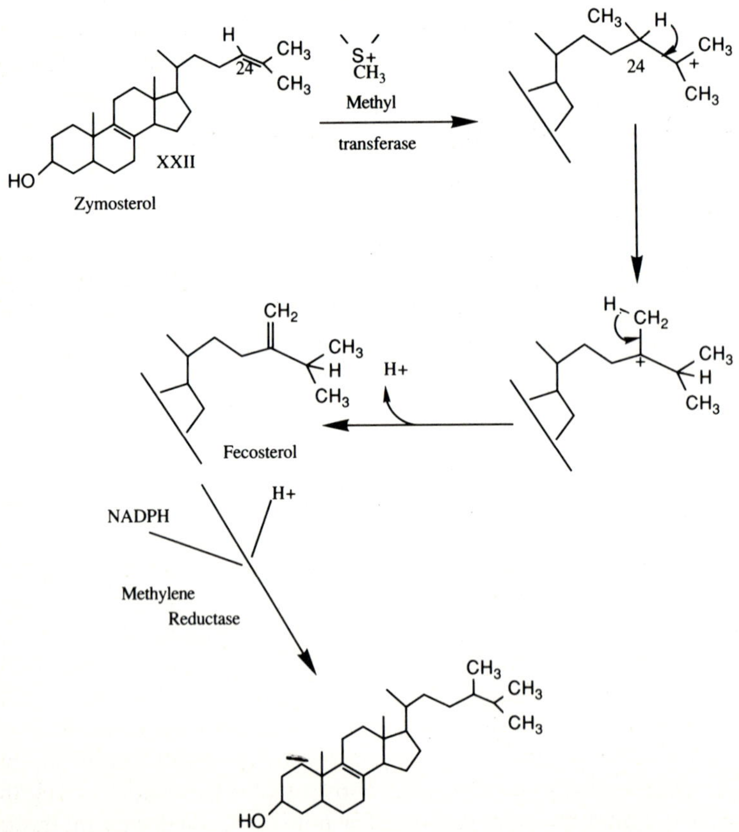

Fig. 7. Mechanism of Δ_{24}-methyltransferase in yeast sterol synthesis

electrophilic and susceptible to the relatively nucleophilic Δ_{24}-double bond (Fig. 7). The ensuing reaction results in S-CH_3 bond cleavage, formation of a C_{24}-CH_3 bond and generation of a transient carbonium ion at C_{25}. 1,2-Hydride shift gives the thermodynamically more stable C_{24} carbonium ion, which is then stabilised by proton loss from the newly introduced methyl group, resulting in the production of fecosterol. It is worthy of note that unlike in algae (WOJCIECHOWSKI et al. 1973), chirality of C_{24} is not specified until the 24(28)-double bond is saturated: in this case it is the $\Delta_{24(28)}$-sterol reductase which determines that chirality. From an intervention standpoint the medicinal chemist now needs to identify those factors which are important in the regulation of the enzyme.

III. Regulation of Δ_{24}-Transmethylation

Cellular sterol composition as a measure of Δ_{24}-transmethylation activity is affected by levels of growth nutrients in the medium, temperature of incubation and the particular yeast strain employed; oxygen availability is also important. Although sterols cannot be synthesised under anaerobic conditions, the transmethylation system is present in the non-respiratory promitochondrial structures. Non-methylated sterols accumulate under anaerobic conditions, and when the cells are returned to aerobic conditions, the methylated sterols subsequently produced are used to the exclusion of other sterols, reflecting the importance of the process.

The transmethylation systems of yeast are inhibited by monovalent cations, mitochondrial localisation presumably protecting the reaction from the high cation concentrations in the cytosol. Since inhibitions by different monovalent cations are additive, sodium and potassium ion transport through organelle membranes and subsequent accumulation at the site of methyl transferase activity have been shown to inhibit SAM activity (BAILEY et al. 1974). Competitive inhibitors of SAM have been identified.

At concentrations of 10 mM, *S*-adenosyl homocysteine (SAH; XXV) inhibits sterol Δ_{24}-transmethylation (MCCAMMON et al. 1984). In an attempt to extend this to selective inhibitors of fungal Δ_{24}-transmethylation, derivatives of SAH were produced which allowed the key structural features for inhibitory activity to be identified. Using this approach, sinefungin (XXVI) was identified as the most potent inhibitor. This had been previously shown to have growth-inhibitory activity against *C. albicans*, with minimum inhibitory concentrations (MICs) in the 3–6 μM range (GORDEE and BUTLER 1973).

From a mechanistic viewpoint, sinefungin confirms the concept that at levels at which intracellular inhibition of sterol Δ_{24}-transmethylation leads to the accumulation of zymosterol, antifungal activity can be achieved. However, the compound went no further; while it was a good enzyme inhibitor, an observed lack of specificity against other SAM-dependent transmethylation led to unacceptable toxicity (MCCAMMON et al. 1984).

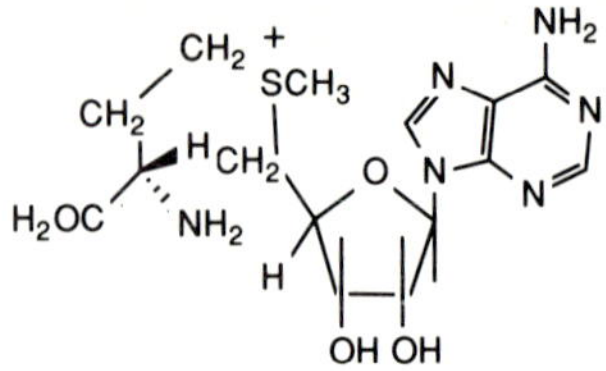

S-Adenosyl Methionine (XXIV)

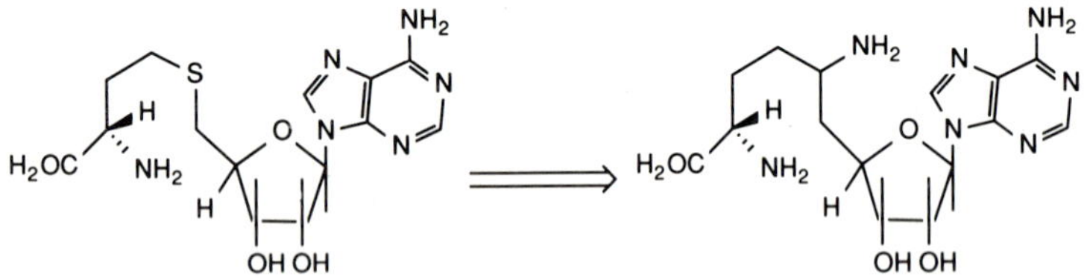

S-Adenosyl homocysteine (XXV) Sinefungin (XXVI)

An alternative approach – well developed in the $C_{14}\alpha$-demethylation area – is based on substrate-derived competitive inhibitors. Precedents in the literature from attempts to produce inhibitors of cholesterol biosynthesis by interventions in side chain biosynthesis with azasterols have been known for some 25 years (COUNSELL et al. 1962). From a series of azacholesterol derivatives the 25-aza (XXVII) was identified as the most potent. This in humans lowered cholesterol levels, with a concomitant rise in those of desmosterol, a product consistent with inhibition of the $\Delta_{24(28)}$-reductase enzyme. The triarylethane inhibitor triparinol (XXIX) similarly inhibits the $\Delta_{24(28)}$-reductase enzyme and offers the prospect of non-steroidal carrier systems being developed.

AKHTAR et al. (1969) showed that the mechanisms of $\Delta_{24(28)}$-reduction and Δ_{24}-transmethylation are essentially similar, involving attack of an electrophile (H^+ in reduction and CH_3^+ in transmethylation) on the π electron-rich centre at C_{24} of the Δ_{24}-substrate. MALHOTRA and NES (1971) substantiated this in plant cell culture, proposing that inhibition by triparinol (XXIX) was due to nitrogen lone-pair binding to the electrophilic centres in both enzymes. More recently, this work has been reviewed and extended by RAHIER et al. (1984) to the design of specific steroidal and non-steroidal Δ_{24}-transmethylation inhibitors of cycloartenol biosynthesis.

In the fungal areas precedent for the utility of azasteroid inhibitors also exists. In *S. cerevisiae* 23-aza cholesterol (XXVIII) at 0.2, 0.5 or 1 μM caused the slow accumulation of zymosterol with a concomitant decline in ergosterol synthesis (PIERCE et al. 1978); inhibition of growth occurred at approximately 5 μM. KABARA et al. (1976) in an earlier study investigated a range of 39 azasteroids. They postulated that the side-chain effects of these agents on sterol metabolism was a secondary event, and that the primary effect was due to impaired oxidative phosphorylation and/or microsomal activity. Interestingly, against both *Candida* and *Saccharomyces*, the 23-aza was significantly more active than the 25-azasterol (MICs 2.5 vs 50 μM).

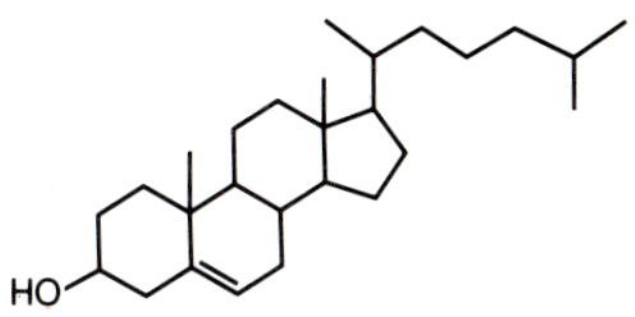

Cholesterol

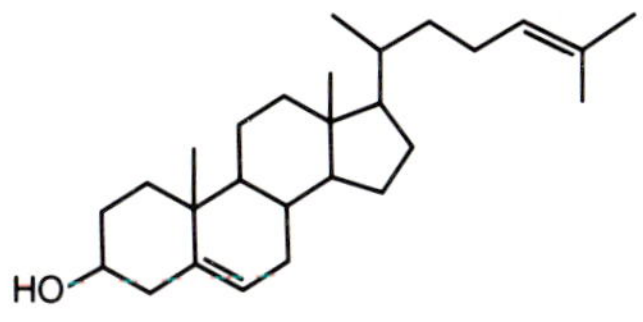

Desmosterol

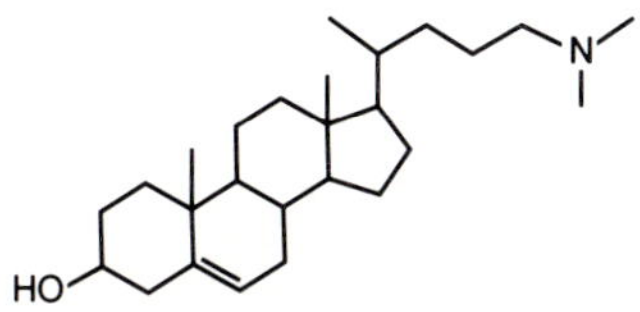

25-Azacholesterol (XXVII)

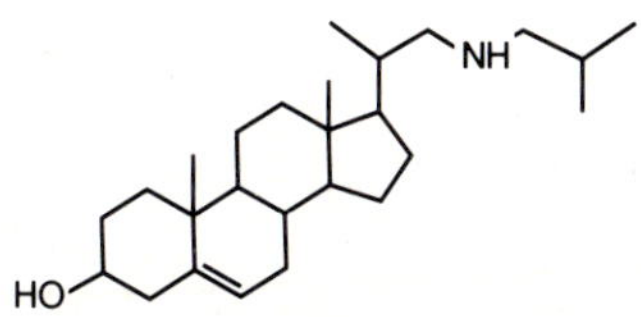

23-Azacholesterol (XXVIII)

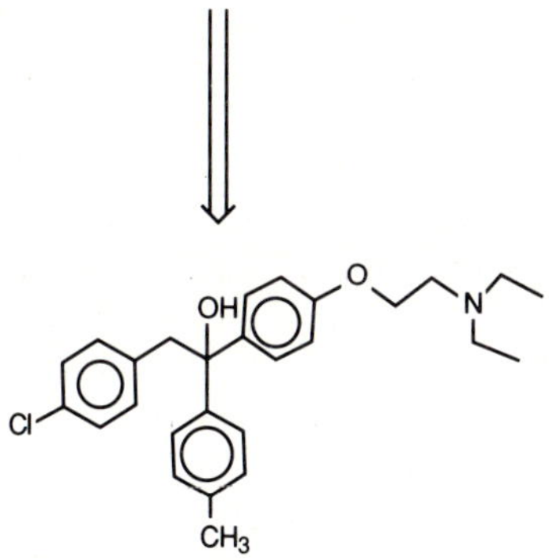

Triparinol (XXIX)

IV. In House Lead Structure Selection and Biological Investigations

From the preceding discussion, significant precedent exists to substantiate the following observations:

1. Δ_{24}-transmethylation is unique to fungi and is a key enzymic process in the biosynthetic elaboration of ergosterol
2. Δ_{24}-transmethylation is a non-cytochrome P-450-dependent process, requiring SAM as the carbon donor
3. Inhibitors of the Δ_{24}-transmethylation process have been identified – either SAM antagonists (SAH, sinefungin) or 23/25-azasterols – which cause fungiotoxicity, probably due to accumulation of atypical sterols (e.g. zymosterol) or depletion of ergosterol in the cellular membrane
4. Evidence exists suggesting that non-steroidal inhibitors of the process could be developed (e.g. triparinol)

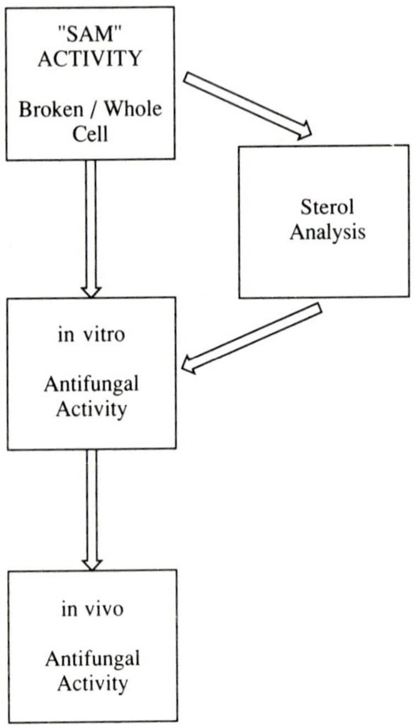

Fig. 8. Test cascade for the identification of Δ_{24}-methyltransferase inhibitors

To move the lead generation process to the next level requires the establishment of a testing cascade capable of identifying in-house chemical structures and supporting chemical synthesis. Such a cascade (Fig. 8) must contain 1. a screen capable of handling large numbers of compounds with activity against Δ_{24}-transmethylation; 2. a conventional antifungal assay; and 3. a test capable of detecting the effects of selected compounds on sterol patterns in target organisms (e.g. *C. albicans*/*Trichophyton quinckeanum*). In vivo assessment of activity would be the logical extension of this process.

Table 4. Inhibition of Δ_{24}-transmethylation by selected sterol derivatives

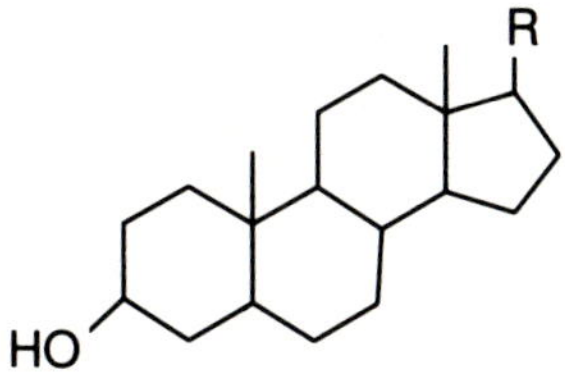

Compound No.	R	IC_{50}
XXX	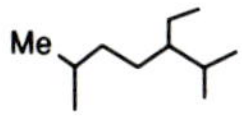	11% at 2.5 μM
XXXI	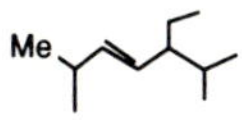	21% at 2.5 μM
XXXII	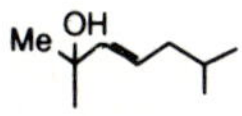	2.5 μM
XXXIII	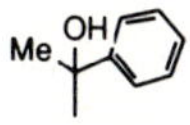	16% at 2.5 μM
XXXIV	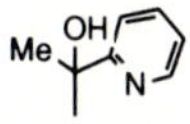	20 μM
XXXV	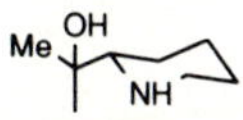	20 nM
XXXVI	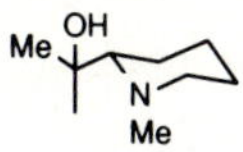	10 nM
XXXVII	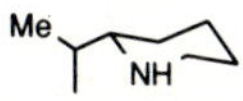	65 nM
XXXVIII	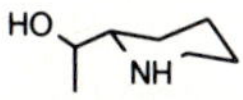	7 μM
XXXIX	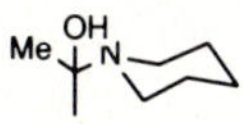	250 nM
XL	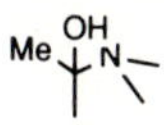	65 nM
XLI	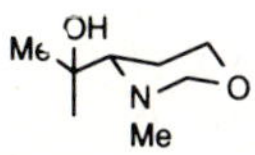	0.8 μM
XLII	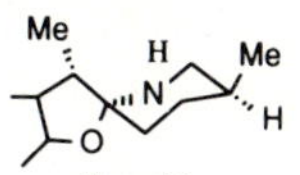 Tomatidine	40 nM
XXIII	Lanosterol	10 % at 2.5 μM
–	Cholesterol	

Table 5. Growth inhibition of *C. albicans* and sterol perturbation caused by ICI 62,965

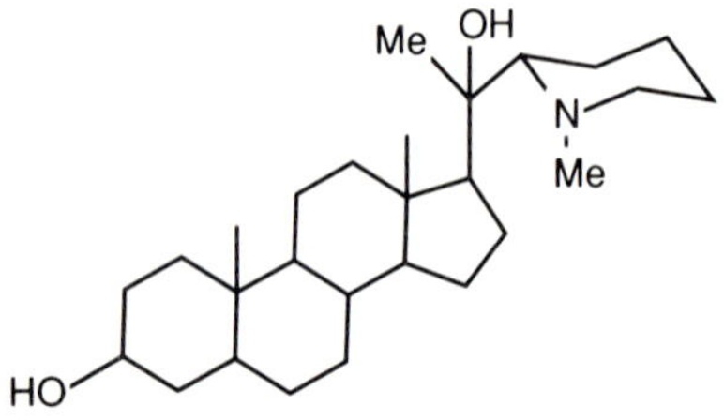

ICI 62,965 (XXXVI)

Concentration	Inhibition[a] (%)	Ergosterol[b]	Zymosterol[b]
0	0	100	0
10 nM	12	94	7
100 nM	12	83	17
1 μM	12	83	17
10 μM	50	5	95
100 μM	>70	1	99

[a] 16-h growth inhibition determined by OD at 650 nm.
[b] Percentage of total sterols by GC-MS.

Extending literature observations to the selection of compounds for screening, an approach was chosen to inhibit the enzyme competitively, based on the 23-aza steroids of Kabara et al. (1976), involving a fixed locus nitrogen lone pair to mimic the developing olefin nucleophile of zymosterol.

Azasterols were identified in the ICI company collection and were screened for their ability to inhibit the transfer of radiolabel from *S*-adenosyl-*L*-[methyl-^{3}H] methionine (SAM) to sterols in both broken and whole cell preparations of *C. albicans* and *T. quinckeanum* (Barrett-Bee, personal communication). Data generated with *C. albicans* illustrating the major structure activity relationships are presented in Table 4.

The assay showed good endogenous substrate specificity; the addition of a range of exogenous sterols (in this case illustrated by the addition of 2.5 μM lanosterol or cholesterol) had little or no effect. Sub-optimal potential suicide substrates, aromatic (XXXIII), olefinic (XXXI) or acetylenic (XXXII) C_{22-23} side-chain analogues, all gave poor inhibition (10%–50% at 2.5 μM). Secondary and tertiary C_{23}-amino derivatives in general produce the best inhibition of the enzyme, and the following structure activity patterns are worth comment:

- Linkage of the 2° or 3° amine α to nitrogen (compounds XXXV and XXXVI) generally gave better inhibitors than direct N-substitution (XXXIX; 10–20 nM vs 250 nM)

- Acyclic N-linked systems (XL) are better than cyclic piperidine (XXXIX) or morpholine (XLI)
- The C_{20} hydroxyl is not essential for activity (65 vs 20 nM); it may, however, play a secondary conformational role, an observation based mainly on the interesting results with the natural product tomatidine (XLII)
- The C_{21} methyl (XXXVIII) is essential for good activity (20 nM vs 7 μM), again confirming its strong structural requirement in the steroid side chain.

To explore further the biological utility of this series of inhibitors, ICI 62,965 (XXXVI) was selected for investigation. Results of a study to quantify the degree of inhibition of ergosterol biosynthesis/zymosterol accumulation required before inhibition of the growth of *C. albicans* was observed are presented in Table 5. The results clearly show that for inhibition over the 16 h duration of the experiment there needs to be in the order of 90% inhibition of ergosterol with a subsequent accumulation of zymosterol. Interestingly, similar levels of perturbation were observed by inhibition of the growth of *C. albicans* by the $C_{14}\alpha$-demethylase inhibitor ICI 195,739. In this case 90%–95% accumulation of lanosterol and 24-methylene lanosterol were observed before inhibition of growth occurred (Barrett-Bee et al. 1988).

The ability of the sterol metabolising enzyme complex to utilise structurally similar substrates with varying efficiencies in the support of growth has already been documented. This is particularly so in compound intervention studies and probably accounts for the fungiostasis observed with many classes of ergosterol biosynthesis inhibitors. To obtain a truly fungicidal response, a second point of intervention may be required. We therefore chose to consider the Δ_{24}-transmethylation inhibitor ICI 62,965 (XXXVI) in combination with inhibitors of the following key steps:

Biosynthetic reaction – Inhibitor
Squalene epoxidase – Terbinafine (SF-86327)
$C_{14}\alpha$-demethylase – ICI 153,066
Δ_{14}-reductase – A25882B
Δ_{8-7}-isomerase – Trifluperidol

The following test procedure was adopted. All compounds were dissolved in dimethyl sulphoxide (DMSO) at 10 mg/ml and further serially diluted in test medium to 4 times the required final concentration. The media used were YNB or Sabouraud dextrose broth (SDB). Microtitre plates (96 well) were inoculated in a 'checkerboard' fashion using 50 μl of inhibitor A plus 50 μl of inhibitor B together with 100 μl of *C. albicans* B2630 (4×10^3 organism/ml) inoculum. The plates were incubated at 37°C and examined for growth at 24 and 48 h (Multiscan MC). From the absorbance data it was possible to calculate the degree of inhibition of growth and thereby determine whether the effects observed were simply additive or synergistic.

Table 6. Combination toxicity studies of sterol inhibitors vs *C. albicans*[a]

Combination	Locus	MIC (μg/ml)	Mixed MIC		Minimum fungicidal combination		Major sterol product[b]
ICI 62,965 + ICI 153,066	A B	25 6.2-25	25 + 6.2		none	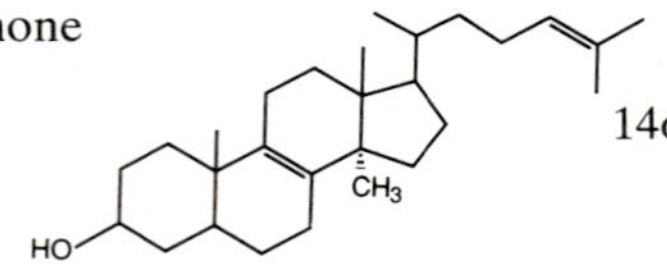	14α-methylzymosterol
ICI 62,965 + A25882B	A C	25 6.2	0.4 + 0.4	6.2 + 0.006	10 + 1	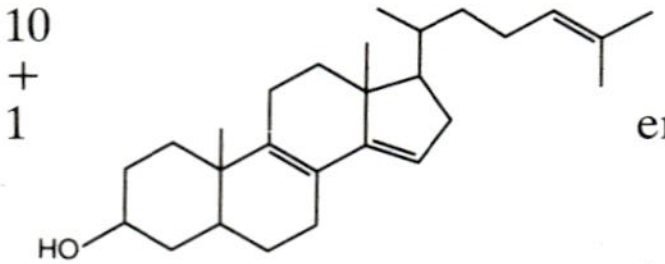	ergosta-8:14:24-triene
ICI 62,965 + Trifluperidol	A D	2.5 400	0.4 + 400	1.6 + 100	25 + 400	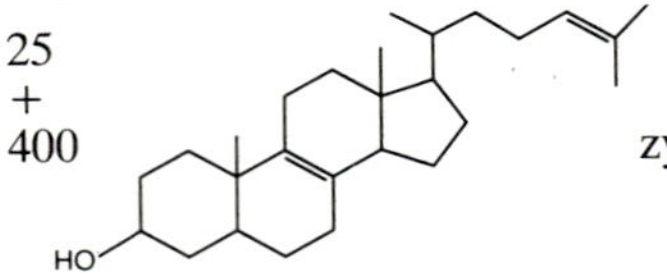	zymosterol
ICI 62,965 + Terbinafine	A E	25 100	0.4 + 6.2	6.2 + 1.6	2.5-5 + 5-10		squalene + zymosterol (trace)

A, Δ_{24}-transmethylation; B, C_{14}-demethylation; C, Δ_{14}-reductase; D, Δ_{8-7}-isomerase; E, squalene epoxidase.

[a] Minimum inhibitory concentration (MIC) determined for each inhibitor in YNB broth; the lowest concentrations which when mixed resulted in complete inhibition after 48 h and the lowest concentrations which when combined resulted in ≥90% fungicidal activity after 24 h.

[b] >90% of total sterol as determined by GC-MS.

To determine whether the inhibitory effects seen were fungistatic or fungicidal, 10 μl aliquots were removed from all wells showing no growth into 2 ml of fresh medium and further incubated for 96 h to allow any inhibited organism to grow. When no growth on subculture was observed, the activity was deemed to be fungicidal. When a fungicidal effect was seen, this was further confirmed and quantified in separate experiments. Multiple combinations of effective concentrations were prepared and added to medium containing *C. albicans* (4×10^3/ml). These mixtures were incubated at 37°C and sampled at intervals up to 48 h. The samples were plated out, and after incubation for 72 h, the number of colonies were counted and the percentage kill based on the original inoculum calculated. Table 6 presents the results of these combination studies, showing the MIC for each inhibitor after 48 h incubation in YNB broth, the lowest concentrations which when mixed resulted in complete inhibition after 48 h and the lowest concentrations which when combined resulted in ≥90% fungicidal activity after 24-h incubation.

In a parallel series of experiments the effects on sterol patterns were investigated. Based on the above results, combinations of inhibitors were chosen and incubated with *C. albicans* for 1 h. The cells were then harvested and a broken cell preparation obtained using a Braun homogeniser. Saponification with KOH followed by extraction of the free sterols into ether gave, after concentration and treatment with trimethylsilyl chloride, material suitable for GC-MS analysis; the major sterol products are shown in Table 6.

Both synergistic and fungicidal effects were obtained with all combinations except Δ_{24}-transmethylation and $C_{14}\alpha$-demethylation inhibitors. Several experiments failed to show any significant benefit of a combination of these latter inhibitors; I was unable to produce complete inhibition using any combination of concentrations below MIC levels. With this exception, it can be seen, however, that double blockade of the pathway resulted in all other cases in activity greater than that achieved by individual inhibitors. Perhaps of greatest interest from a chemotherapeutic standpoint is the potential for equimolar concentrations of a Δ_{24}-transmethylase and a Δ_{14}-reductase inhibitor, or a Δ_{24}-transmethylase and squalene epoxidase inhibitors. The chemical challenge of introducing such combinations into one molecule remains an attractive target.

D. Concluding Remarks

In this chapter I have, from personal experience, attempted to explore two approaches to the development of antifungal agents. Rather than provide an encylopaedic review of the area of antifungal chemotherapy, I initially concentrated on the extension of a conventional lead structure ICI 153,066 and highlighted the process of, and factors important to, the medicinal chemist in the development of fluconazole (ICI 178,998) and ultimately of ICI 195,739. In the second part of the chapter I presented those aspects of lead development required by the medicinal chemist in the establishment of a potential new structural series. The message is clear: conventional screening is and will continue to be very significant in the process of drug discovery. Newer targets will continue to develop; Δ_{24}-transmethylase is one such. Major challenges exist outside of the ergosterol biosynthesis area – perhaps paramount among these are approaches being developed with inhibitors of the cell wall structural elements, chitin, mannan and glucan. Particularly with chitin, progress is being made, and synthetic analogues of the polyoxin/nikkomycins class offer a major chemical fascination for the next decade.

Acknowledgements. I am grateful to Geoff Wilson, John Ryley and Keith Barrett-Bee for the biological and biochemical data given in Tables 1–6, Figs. 1 and 3, and in the text, and without whose effort the latter programme would not have been possible.

References

Akhtar M, Munday KA, Rahimtula AD, Watkinson IA, Wilton DC (1969) Mechanism of reduction of double bonds in biological systems: conversion of desmosterol into cholesterol. Chem Comms 1969:1287–1288

Bailey RB, Thompson ED, Parks LW (1974) Kinetic properties of S-adenosylmethionine: Δ^{24}-sterol methyltransferase enzyme(s) in mitochondrial structures of *Saccharomyces cerevisiae*. Biochim Biophys Acta 334:127–136

Barrett-Bee K, Lees J, Pinder P, Campbell J, Newboult L (1988) Biochemical studies with a novel antifungal agent, ICI 195,739. Ann NY Acad Sci 544:231–244

Borgers M, Waldron HA (1981) The action of ketoconazole on fungi. Clin Res Rev 1:165–171

Boyle FT, Ryley JF, Wilson RG (1987) In vitro-in vivo correlations with azole antifungals. In: Fromtling RA (ed) Recent trends in the discovery, development and evaluation of antifungal agents. J R Prous, Barcelona, pp S1:31–S1:41

Boyle FT, Gilman DJ, Gravestock MB, Wardleworth JM (1988) Synthesis and structure activity relationships of a novel antifungal agent, ICI 195,739. Ann N Y Acad Sci 544:86–100

Conney AH (1986) Induction of microsomal cytochrome P-450 enzymes. Life Sci 39:2493–2518

Cornforth JW, Carrell HL, Glusker JP, Talalay P (1979) The absolute configuration at the sulfonium center in S-adenosyl-L-methionine. In: Usdin E, Borchardt RT, Creveling CR (eds) Transmethylation. Developments in Neuroscience, vol 5. Elsevier/North Holland, New York, pp 19–25

Counsell RE, Klimstra PD, Ranney RE, Cook DL (1962) Hypocholesterolemic agents. 1. 20α-(2-dialkylaminoethyl)aminopregn-5-en-3β-ol derivatives. J Med Pharm Chem 5:720–729

De La Haba G, Jamieson GA, Mudd SH, Richards HH (1959) S-Adenosylmethionine: the relation of configuration at the sulfonium center to enzymatic reactivity. J Am Chem Soc 81:3975–3980

Floss HG, Mascaro L, Tsai M-D, Woodard RW (1979) Stereochemistry of enzymatic transmethylation. In: Usdin E, Borchardt RT, Creveling CR (eds) Transmethylation. Developments in Neuroscience, vol 5. Elsevier/North Holland, New York, pp 135–141

Gordee RS, Butler TF (1973) A9145, a new adenine-containing antifungal antibiotic. II. Biological activity.J Antibiot 26:466–470

Kabara JJ, Holzschu DL, Catsoulacos DP (1976) Structure-function activity of azasterols and nitrogen-containing steroids. Lipids 11:755–762

Kowal J (1983) The effect of ketoconazole on steroidogenesis in cultured mouse adrenal cortex tumor cells. Endocrinology 112:1541–1543
Lederer E (1965) C-methylations in biological systems. Israel J Med Sci 1:1129–1147
Malhotra HC, Nes WR (1971) The mechanism of introduction of alkyl groups at C-24 of sterols. J Biol Chem 246:4934–4937
Marriott MS, Richardson K (1987) The discovery and mode of action of fluconazole. In: Fromtling RA (ed) Recent trends in the discovry, development and evaluation of antifungal agents. J R Prous, Barcelona, pp 81–92
McCammon MT, Hartmann M-A, Bottema CDK, Parks LW (1984) Sterol methylation in *Saccharomyces cerevisiae*. J Bacteriol 157:475–483
Mercer EI (1984) The biosynthesis of ergosterol. Pestic Sci 15:133–155
Nes WR, Sekula BC, Nes WD, Adler JH (1978) The functional importance of strctural features of ergosterol in yeast. J Biol Chem 253:6218–6225
Odds FC (1985) Laboratory tests for the activity of imidazole and triazole antifungal agents in vitro. Semin Dermatol 4:260–270
Parks LW (1958) S-Adenosylmethionine and ergosterol synthesis. J Am Chem Soc 80:2023–2024
Parks LW, McLean-Bowen C, McCammon M, Hays PR (1979) S-Adenosylmethionine: Δ^{24}-sterol methyltransferase: studies on its regulation and physiological role. In: Usdin E, Borchardt RT, Creveling CR (eds) Transmethylation. Developments in neuroscience, vol 5. Elsevier/North Holland, New York, pp 319–327
Pierce AM, Unrau AM, Oehlschlager AC, Woods RA (1979) Azasterol inhibitors in yeast. Inhibition by the Δ^{24}-sterol methyltransferase and the 24-methylene sterol $\Delta^{24(28)}$-reductase in sterol mutants of *Saccharomyces cerevisiae*. Can J Biochem 57:201–208
Pierce HD, Pierce AM, Srinivasan R, Unrau AM, Oehlschlager AC (1978) Azasterol inhibitors in yeast. Inhibition of the 24-methylene sterol $\Delta^{24(28)}$-reductase and Δ^{24}-sterol methyltransferase of *Saccharomyces cerevisiae* by 23-azacholesterol. Biochim Biophys Acta 529:429–437
Plempel M, Berg D, Abbink J (1987) Antimycotic characteristics of bifonazole. In: Fromtling RA (ed) Recent trends in the discovery, development and evaluation of antifungal agents. J R Prous, Barcelona, pp 287–312
Rahier A, Genot J-C, Schuber F, Benveniste P, Narula AS (1984) Inhibition of S-adenosyl-L-methionine sterol-C-24-methyltransferase by analogues of a carbocationic ion high-energy intermediate. J Biol Chem 259:15215–15223
Ryder NS (1988) Mechanism of action and biochemical selectivity of allylamine antimycotic agents. Ann N Y Acad Sci 544:208–220
Ryley JF, Wilson RG (1982) ICI 153,066, a new orally active antifungal agent. 22nd Intersci Conf Antimicrob Agents Chemother, Miami Beach, Abstr 477
Ryley JF, McGregor S, Wilson RG (1988) Activity of ICI 195,739 – a novel, orally active bistriazole – in rodent models of fungal and protozoal infections. Ann NY Acad Sci 544:310–328
Sisler HD, Ragsdale NN (1984) Biochemical and cellular aspects of the antifungal action of ergosterol biosynthesis inhibitors. In: Trinci APJ, Ryley JF (eds) Mode of action of antifungal agents. British Mycological Society Symposium 9. Cambridge University Press, Cambridge, pp 257–282
Thompson ED, Parks LW (1974) Effect of altered sterol composition on growth characteristics of *Saccharomyces cerevisiae*. J Bacteriol 120:779–784
Van Cutsem J, Van Gerven F, Janssen PAJ (1987) The in vitro and in vivo antifungal activity of itraconazole. In: Fromtling RA (ed) Recent trends in the discovery, development and evaluation of antifungal agents. J R Prous, Barcelona, pp 177–192
Vanden Bossche H (1987) Itraconazole: a selective inhibitor of the cytochrome P-450 dependent ergosterol biosynthesis. In: Fromtling RA (ed) Recent trends in the discovery, development and evaluation of antifungal agents. J R Prous, Barcelona, pp 207–221

Vanden Bossche H, Willemsens G, Marichal P, Cools W, Lauwers W (1984) The molecular basis for the antifungal activities of N-substituted azole derivatives. Focus on R51211. In: Trinci APJ, Ryley JF (eds) Mode of action of antifungal agents. British Mycological Society Symposium 9. Cambridge University Press, Cambridge pp 321–341
Wojciechowski ZA, Goad LJ, Goodwin TW (1973) S-adenosyl-L-methionine-cycloartenol methyltransferase activity in cell free systems from *Trebouxia* sp. and *Scenedesmus obliquus*. Biochem J 136:405–412
Worthington PA (1982) Heterocyclic compounds. Br Patent Appl 2078719A

CHAPTER 2

Drug Discovery: A Biochemist's Approach

DAVID KERRIDGE and HUGO VANDEN BOSSCHE

A. Introduction

A complete exhaustive knowledge of all the different chemo-receptors of a certain definite parasite is what I should like to characterise as the therapeutic physiology of the parasite cell and this is the *sine quâ non* of any successful chemotherapeutic treatment. (PAUL EHRLICH 1913)

Antifungal chemotherapy is an essay in comparative biochemistry. It is the metabolic differences between plant and animal hosts and their fungal pathogens which provide us with selective targets for chemotherapeutic attack. Unfortunately, both fungi and their hosts are eukaryotic organisms, and the differences between them, with few exceptions (for example, chitin synthase and chitinase), result from variations upon a fundamental organisational theme, rather than from different themes as is the case with bacterial pathogens. The essence of chemotherapy is that the host, in this case humans, should be unaffected by the drug at the concentration required at the site of infection to eliminate the fungus. Unfortunately, it is unlikely that patient acceptibility will ever be predictable from studies of the mode of action of any antifungal drug in vitro or even from studies using animal models.

The ultimate aim of a biochemist interested in the development of new antifungal drugs is to have sufficient knowledge of the metabolism of both host and fungal pathogen to select the 'perfect' target or targets and from a knowledge of their 'molecular biology' to select or design a 'magic bullet' (EHRLICH 1913). Unfortunately, the complexities of the two organisms and of their interactions with each other are such that it might be impossible to attain this ideal. However, this should not preclude us from attempting a logical approach to target selection and drug design. The introduction of the 'first generation' of effective antifungal drugs resulted from a random screening of both natural compounds and the products of organic chemists. Studies on their mode of action then highlighted differences between the organisms. As a result, this approach has now been largely superseded by what can be classed as 'prepared mind' screening. The most important finding arising from such studies is that there is a wide range of suitable targets, but a limited number of mechanisms by which organisms can be or become less sensitive to chemotherapeutic agents (Table 1).

These mechanisms are equally important in mediating intrinsic resistance (i.e. low sensitivity) in the host and acquired resistance in the pathogen. Drug

Table 1. The biochemical basis of low sensitivity (resistance) to antifungal drugs

1. Target is absent from insensitive cells
2. Target is present in insensitive cells but modified
3. Target is present in insensitive cells but is no longer essential for growth
4. Target is present in insensitive cells but protected by a barrier (usually the plasma membrane)
5. Insensitive cells fail to metabolise the drug to an active derivative
6. Insensitive cells actively excrete the drug
7. Insensitive cells metabolise the drug to an inactive derivative
8. Insensitive cells overproduce a competing metabolite
9. Insensitive cells overproduce the target
10. Drug is sequestered internally

resistance in the pathogen must always be related to the drug concentration attainable at the site of infection during therapy rather than the concentration attainable in a test tube in the laboratory. Many of the fungal diseases to which humans are exposed are topical rather than systemic, and as a result it may be possible to achieve high local concentrations of the drug without adversely affecting the host, provided always that the drug is not absorbed through the skin or metabolised by it. Unfortunately this cannot always be guaranteed since the skin is a 'chemical conversion factory' that rivals the liver, and many of the body's crucial functions are considered by ROSENFELD (1988) to be only skin deep. The development of drug resistance in fungi causing superficial infections is not a frequent occurrence.

But what are the underlying clinical problems? There is a limited range of fungal species capable of causing diseases in humans, although many more affect plants and animals and are important economically. Fungal diseases of humans range from topical to systemic and the fungi from obligate to opportunistic pathogens (Table 2).

Table 2. Examples of human mycoses

Superficial mycoses	Deep mycoses
Dermatomycoses	Subcutaneous mycoses
Trichophyton spp	Blastomycosis
Microsporum spp.	Chromomycosis
Epidermophyton	Maduromycosis
Pityriasis	Sporotrichosis
Candidosis	Systemic mycoses
	Aspergillosis
	Candidosis
	Coccidioidomycosis
	Cryptococcosis
	Histoplasmosis
	Paracoccidioidomycosis
	Phycomycosis

There are distinct regional variations in the fungal diseases affecting humans, but even more important clinically are the changes in the relative importance of different pathogenic fungi which have occurred as a result of advances in medical practice and the nature of the diseases to which humans are exposed. Fungal infections occur frequently in immunocompromised patients whose defence mechanisms make only a minimal contribution to the elimination of the pathogen and in whom eradication of the fungus is essential. The search for an antifungal drug which is fungicidal in vivo is still the most important challenge.

The ideal drug is one which can be administered both prophylactically and therapeutically, has no adverse side effects on the host and is effective against all fungal infections. The sites of infection in humans are diverse, ranging from the skin to the meninges of the brain, from the vagina to muscle tissue. Is it reasonable to expect that one drug, even in different formulations, will be effective against all the fungal species responsible for these infections? *Candida albicans* is the most common fungal pathogen of humans, and for most patients suffering from candidosis the currently available drugs do an excellent job. Yet there are a number of reasons for continuing to use this organism as the model in the search for new antifungal drugs. The first is that there is always the possibility of drug resistance arising. In a limited number of patients suffering from candidosis the yeast strains isolated are somewhat less sensitive to the currently available drugs, and for immunocompromised patients it is important that as wide a range of drugs as possible is available to control the fungi which infect them. *C. albicans* is also the best studied fungal pathogen (ODDS 1988), and good animal models are available for testing new compounds (GUENTZEL et al. 1985; see also Chap. 5). Any compound developed in this way can then be used as a model for subsequent drug development. Of course, there are significant differences between *C. albicans* and other fungi. Therefore other dimorphic (e.g. *Histoplasma* spp. and *Blastomyces* spp.) and filamentous fungi (e.g. *Aspergillus* spp.) should not be neglected.

A number of possible approaches can be adopted by the biochemist in the search for the ideal drug; these range from the perfect to the pragmatic. At one extreme we can study the metabolism of both host and parasite in the laboratory, examine their interactions in vivo, select targets from these studies for detailed examination and finally design suitable chemotherapeutic drugs. At the other extreme, we can screen randomly for fungistatic or fungicidal agents and investigate thoroughly those which appear from initial in vivo studies to be effective. The latter approach to antifungal chemotherapy has been most effective in the past and responsible for the introduction of the majority of antifungal drugs in current use. It is interesting to speculate whether or not the logical scientific approach would have been more effective if as much money had been devoted to basic research as has been devoted to random screening.

There are a number of ways in which biochemical research has in the past contributed to and can contribute in the future to drug development. The most effective so far has been the chemical modification of an existing drug. This is best illustrated by the wide range of beta-lactam antibiotics active against bacteria (MORIN and GORMAN 1982) and azole derivatives against pathogenic fungi (VANDEN BOSSCHE 1985, 1988; VANDEN BOSSCHE et al. 1987b). It has not been true with the polyene macrolide antibiotics where amphotericin B is still, in spite of its toxicity, used for treating patients with systemic fungal infections (GRAYBILL 1988). There is, however, still considerable interest in the development of less toxic and more effective derivatives of amphotericin B (SCHAFFNER 1987; CHERON et al. 1988). This is essentially a matter for the chemist with the roles of the biochemist and the mycologist being restricted to testing these compounds and to guiding the chemist in the directions to be taken in modifying the parent compound. The value of these studies lies in the information to be gained concerning the nature of the cellular target(s) and their molecular interaction(s) with the drug. These studies are important for the biochemist in increasing the understanding of the mode of action of and mechanisms of resistance to existing drugs. It is possible that such information will hasten the development of more effective derivatives of existing drugs, since any advance in our knowledge of structure-function relationships will have a predictive value. It will not necessarily have a significant impact on the development of new drugs.

Our knowledge of the biochemistry of both humans and their fungal pathogens, although far from complete, is already sufficient to enable us to select potential targets for therapeutic attack. These targets can then be used to screen for selective inhibitors which may require further development, or after detailed studies on the target it might be possible to design new drugs. The *primary* role of the biochemist in the development of antifungal drugs is to *select* and *study potential targets*. There is always the danger of becoming too narrow in one's approach to such a subject, and it is essential to use information gained by studies on the chemotherapy of cancer and eukaryotic pathogens. Fungal infections are important in agriculture; in fact, the fungal diseases of plants are economically far more important than infections of humans, and studies on plant pathogens should not be ignored in the search for clinically useful drugs (TRINCI and RYLEY 1984). Fungal pathogens of humans are structurally and metabolically diverse, and it is unwise to restrict research to one organism. The discussion in this chapter will be primarily concerned with clnically important drugs. However, the approach adopted is relevant to the development of antifungal drugs to prevent and cure infections in other organisms.

B. Factors Affecting the Choice of Target

The target must be essential for fungal growth. It is not always necessary to kill the fungus since if growth is reduced, the delicate balance between host and pathogen may be altered sufficiently to enable the host's defense mechanisms to eliminate the fungus. There are additional complications in immunocompromised patients in whom it will be necessary to kill the pathogen in order to prevent relapses occurring after cessation of treatment. For a drug to be selective, the host must tolerate it at the concentration required at the site of infection to eliminate the fungus. Sensitivity to a particular drug may vary considerably from one organism to another, but the molecular mechanisms for this variation are restricted (Table 1). Ideally, low sensitivity (i.e. intrinsic resistance) in the host should be associated with the absence of the target, as with the penicillin-binding proteins in bacteria, which of course do not occur in humans. As we are dealing with two eukaryotic organisms, this will be uncommon as the basic patterns of metabolism are similar in plants, animals and fungi. It is more likely that the target(s) will be present in both organisms but differ in their affinities for the drug.

All eukaryotic organisms show significant intracellular compartmentalisation of metabolic function. One problem in drug development is choosing suitable targets within the cell which are readily accessible. Although there will be differences in drug transport into human and fungal cells, this is not an important factor in the selectivity of antimycotic drugs in current clinical use and may not be an important factor in drug design in the future. However, drug distribution in the intact animal does have a significant role to play in in vivo activity and selectivity. This is well illustrated by griseofulvin, an antibiotic shown to be a mitotic poison in tissue cutlure cells, yet which can be administered orally to humans for prolonged periods without serious side effects (DAVIES 1980).

I. The Cell Wall as a Barrier to Drug Uptake

Fungal cells, unlike those of humans, are bounded by a complex cell wall composed of glucan, mannan, chitin, proteins and lipids (for a review, see FLEET 1985). In *C. albicans* the structural polysaccharides are largely β-glucans, chitin and mannoproteins (SHEPHERD 1987). This structure provides a mechanical barrier around the cell, an osmotic protection for the protoplast, regulates secretion and uptake of large molecules and provides the interface with the host. The organisation of the cell wall of *C. albicans* is such that it excludes molecules of M_r much greater than 700 (COPE 1980a). It is not a metabolically inert structure, and the barrier function of the yeast cell wall can be modified both phenotypically and genotypically to exclude polyene macrolide antibiotics (GALE 1986) and synthetic azole derivatives (KERRIDGE et al. 1987). In exponentially growing cultures of *C. albicans*, passage of amphotericin B across the cell wall is the rate-limiting step in the interaction of the antibiotic with the plasma membrane (ELLUL et al. 1985), and alterations in cell wall β-glucans are responsible for the development of phenotypic resistance to amphotericin B (GALE 1986). The detailed structure of the cell wall is not known nor are the changes responsible for the yeast-mycelial transformation understood. Cytochemical studies demonstrated that mannoprotein constitutes a major part of the outer layer, but it also permeates the underlying glucan layers (FLEET 1985). It would appear from electron microscopical studies (SHEPHERD 1987) that the wall is a layered structure, but these layers represent quantitative rather than qualitative differences in the distribution of constituent macromolecular components.

The first task for the biochemist is to determine the molecular structure of the cell wall, explain the mechanisms by which drugs, in particular the polyene macrolide antibiotics and the azole derivatives, cross it to reach the plasma membrane and in addition how the azole drugs reach their primary target organelle, the endoplasmic reticulum.

Although the cell wall can provide a barrier to antifungal drugs, it is the plasma membrane which has the essential role in transporting drugs to their target site within the cell, but it can also prevent them reaching it. Potential targets occur outside the plasma membrane which can be exploited in drug development. In bacteria, for example, binding sites for beta-lactam antibiotics are plasma membrane proteins exposed to the exterior, and the penicillins and cephalosporins do not enter the cell (GALE et al. 1981). The question to be asked here is: are there similar systems in fungi to be exploited as 'external' targets for therapeutic attack? The great advantage of such targets is that the problems of transporting antifungal drugs across the plasma membrane are circumvented. This can influence drug design in that it need not mimic a cell metabolite in order to be transported illicitly into the cell and hence reduce the possibility of the selection of resistant strains, nor need it be a hydrophobic molecule able to diffuse across the bulk phase of the plasma membrane.

C. Potential Targets

I. External to the Plasma Membrane

1. Structural Polysaccharides

The cell wall polysaccharides comprise a rigid framework, and during cell wall growth, new polysaccharide molecules are synthesised and old ones partially degraded to allow their insertion (VILLANUEVA et al. 1976; FARKAS 1979; CABIB et al. 1988). The binding of a drug to the polysaccharide strands in a manner analogous to the binding of the glycopeptide antibiotics vancomycin and teichoplanin to bacterial peptidoglycan (REYNOLDS 1985) might prevent hydrolysis of cell wall polysaccharides and hence insertion of newly synthesised β-glucans or chitin into the growing cell wall. The problem is to find compounds which specifically interact with these structural polysaccharides. Such molecules will be relatively small (M_r less than 1000) since they must penetrate the wall to associate with the structural polysaccharides. β-Glucans and chitin are both absent in humans, and such inhibitors, if they could be found, would be expected to show a considerable degree of specificity. Since their potential targets are exterior to the plasma membrane, passage of such compounds across a lipid bilayer would not be a problem.

2. Cell Wall Associated Enzymes

There are a number of hydrolytic enzymes associated with the cell wall of *C. albicans*; these include phospholipases, proteases and β-glucanases. Proteases and phospholipases are involved in the establishment of fungal infections on mucous membranes (ODDS 1988), and glucanases (NOMBELA et al. 1988) are essential for cell wall biogenesis. Inhibition of any enzyme involved in the establishment of an infection would be ideal in prophylaxis. Since these targets are external to cell, there is no necessity to transport the drug across the plasma membrane, hence toxicity to humans may be minimised.

The cell wall located β-glucanases are involved not only in the growth of *C. albicans* but are also associated with organisational changes in the cell wall which result in the development of the phenotypic resistance to both polyene macrolide antibiotics and synthetic azole drugs, which occurs after cessation of growth (GALE 1986; GALE et al. 1980). Two cell wall associated β-glucanases have been demonstrated in *C. albicans*; these differ in molecular weight and in their reaction products. Enzyme 1 yields predominantly glucose whereas enzyme II gives laminaritetraose as the initial product. These enzymes are linked to other cell wall components though the precise nature of the linkage is not known (NOTARIO 1982).

The importance of these enzymes in cell growth, the absence of their substrate from mammalian cells and their location outside the plasma membrane make them ideal candidates for therapeutic attack. As yet they have not been exploited as potential targets, even though compounds exist which

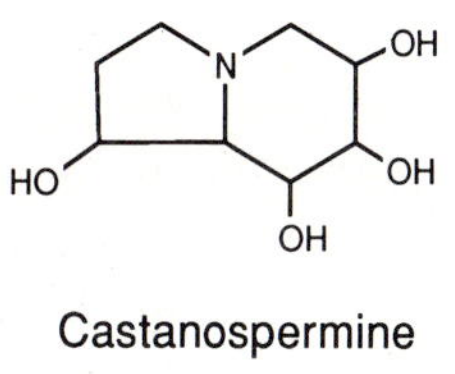

Castanospermine

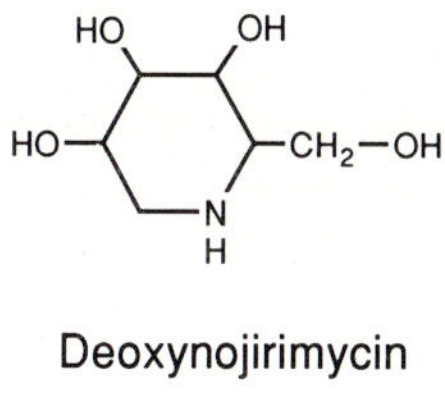

Deoxynojirimycin

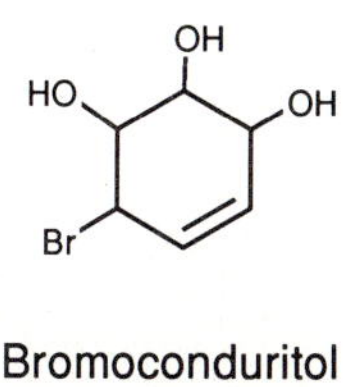

Bromoconduritol

Fig. 1. Structural formulae of oligosaccharide processing inhibitors specifically inhibit oligosaccharide processing in eukaryotic cells (FUHRMANN et al. 1985). These compounds (Fig. 1) inhibit glycosidases from a variety of sources including *Saccharomyces cerevisiae*, in which deoxynojirimycin inhibits both glucosidase 1 and 2 and bromoconduritol inhibits the α-glucosidase from the same organism. Castanospermine also inhibits the β-xylosidase from *Aspergillus* spp. These compounds have not been tested for their potential effects on cell wall β-glucosidases of *C. albicans*.

Oligosaccharide processing takes place within eukaryotic cells, and these inhibitors traverse the plasma membrane to reach their target enzymes although the mechanism is unknown. They are ideal models for the development of drugs capable of inhibiting cell wall synthesis. It should be possible to modify them to increase their affinity for the cell wall hydrolases and to reduce their affinity for the 'transport system' and hence their potential toxicity to the host. So far, the main purpose of studying these compounds has been to gain an insight into the enzymology of oligosaccharide processing, to assess their potential as antiviral drugs (TYMS and TAYLOR 1988) and their possible role in controlling diabetes (DIMITRIADIS et al. 1988). Unlike tunicamycin, an antibiotic affecting glycopeptide synthesis in eukaryotic cells, these compounds have a comparatively low toxicity for tissue culture cells. However, it is not clear whether this reuslts from a lower K_i value for the inhibitor or from failure of these drugs to reach their intracellular targets, clearly a feature that is worth further investigation.

Chitin is an important structural component of the fungal cell wall, and in the yeast form of *C. albicans* it is located at the site of the septum separating mother and daughter cells. In the mycelial form it is dispersed throughout the cell wall, but higher quantities are found at the septa and at the growing tip in a manner similar to the mycelial fungus *Aspergillus fumigatus* (MARICHAL et al. 1985; VANDEN BOSSCHE et al. 1988a). As with glucan synthesis the insertion of chitin into the cell wall involves hydrolysis of preexisting polysaccharide strands mediated by a chitinase located in the periplasmic space. Allosamidin (Fig. 2), a streptomycete antibiotic first isolated by SAKUDA et al. (1986), is a speciic competitive inhibitor of an insect

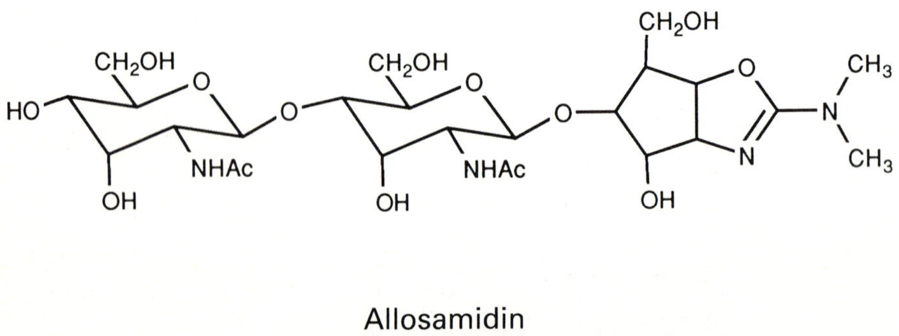

Fig. 2. Chemical structure of the chitinase inhibitor, allosamidin

chitinase with an IC_{50} value of about 0.4 μM (KOGA et al. 1987). This C-3 epimer of N-acetyl-β-D-glucosamine is also a potent inhibitor of the chitinase of *Neurospora crassa* with an IC_{50} value of 0.5 μM (GOODAY, personal communication). It is of interest to note that the same author found allosamidin to be a potent inhibitor of the chitinase of the filarial worm *Onchocerca gibsoni*, having an IC_{50} value of 200 pM (GOODAY et al. 1988). This compound has yet to be tested against human and plant pathogenic fungi. Allosamidin is obviously a good model for the development of antifungal drugs acting on a specific target outside the cell membrane. However, it might not be as effective in controlling phytopathogenic fungi since some plants produce chitinase in response to fungal infections (FINK et al. 1988; MAUCH et al. 1988; KOMBRINK et al. 1988), possibly as a protection against the fungus, and the use of chitinase inhibitors thus could antagonise the plant's own defence system and as a result prove ineffective.

3. Plasma Membrane Associated Targets

The function of the plasma membrane is to provide a selective barrier between the cell and its environment. It is involved in cell wall synthesis and is responsible for the selective uptake and excretion of low molecular weight materials. It comprises a lipid bilayer and associated hydrophobic proteins, many of which be exposed to the exterior of the cell. Any impairment of membrane function will affect cell growth and viability, and it is of interest to note that the plasma membrane of fungi is an important target for a number of antifungal drugs. A somewhat surprising feature, given the similarities between mammalian and fungal plasma membranes, and where the most significant difference resides, is in the nature of the membrane sterols, with ergosterol being the major sterol in fungi and cholesterol the major sterol in humans.

There are two types of interactions with the plasma membrane. The first is with the lipid bilayer, resulting in an impairment of barrier function and possibly indirect effects on the functioning of membrane proteins. The second involves specific interactions with plasma membrane associated proteins.

a) Impairment of Barrier Function

The polyene macrolide antibiotics interact with plasma membranes of sensitive fungi, causing impairment of function and cell death (KERRIDGE 1986, 1988). For amphotericin B, this is the primary event which occurs at the minimum growth inhibitory concentration (MIC) and is responsible for cessation of growth and ultimately cell death. Certain azole derivatives, for example, clotrimazole (IWATA et al. 1973), miconazole (COPE 1980b), propiconazole and penconazole (DAHMEN et al. 1988), also interact with lipid membranes, causing an impairment of barrier function. Fluconazole and fenetriazole (terbuconazole, tebuconazole) also possess the ability to interact directly with membranes; in *Saccharomycopsis lipolytica* this interaction induces a leakage of the cell contents as measured by increased conductivity (BERG et al. 1988). The interaction of miconazole with the plasma membrane of sensitive fungi might have a role to play in the elimination of the fungi when the drug is applied topically. This direct impairment of the barrier function of the plasma membrane does not occur with all azoles. Ketoconazole, itraconazole (VANDEN BOSSCHE et al. 1982) and flutriafol do not affect membranes directly; imazalil has a slight effect at 50 μg/ml (DAHMEN et al. 1988). Even for those derivatives with which disruptive interaction does occur, this is at concentrations in excess of those required to inhibit growth.

The mode of action of these compounds is considered in detail in Chap. 6. The polyene macrolide antibiotics interact directly with the lipid constituents of the bilayer, and the specificity of the interaction results from differences in the lipid (sterol) composition of the plasma membranes of host and pathogen. Although membrane sterols appear to play a primary role in the interaction of the polyenes with the membrane, other lipids may be involved, especially in so far as they affect membrane fluidity (BOLARD 1986; KERRIDGE 1988). The azoles do not interact directly with membrane lipids in a manner analogous to the polyene/sterol interaction, and unlike the polyene macrolides it is the presence of unsaturated fatty acids rather than sterols that is important in the disruptive interaction with artificial membranes and plasma membranes of sensitive cells (VANDEN BOSSCHE et al. 1982; BRASSEUR et al. 1983). The other feature of great importance is that although amphotericin B inserts into the outer leaf of the bilayer it does not penetrate to the interior of the cell, whereas the azole antimycotics cross the plasma membrane to reach their target organelle, the endoplasmic reticulum.

Studies on the mode of action of the polyene macrolide antibiotics have emphasised the differences between the plasma membranes of humans and their fungal pathogens and the importance of these differences in the mode of action of existing antifungal drugs. The major question is how can these differences be exploited in the search for new antifungal drugs? One major problem is that membrane composition can be manipulated both phenotypically and genotypically (KOH et al. 1977). Lipid fluidity is important in the functioning of the plasma membrane; genotypically induced changes in one lipid constituent may be compensated for by changes in other membrane lipids. Studies of the effect of lipid composition on membrane antibiotic interactions have been carried out in vitro rather than in vivo. The environment within the host is complex and will affect the composition of the fungal cell envelope and hence its interaction with antifungal drugs. However, we must consider how studies on the mode of action of polyene macrolide antibiotics and certain azoles have emphasised the importance of the plasma membrane as a target and how the results obtained in such studies can be used in the development of new drugs.

The first relevant feature is the complexity of the interactions. Despite all the efforts that have been put into examining the mode of action of these compounds, the precise molecular mechanisms whereby these drugs interact with the plasma membrane and impair the barrier function are still not understood. The specificity of interaction results from an association with the lipid constituents, but in neither case is it completely specific. The polyene macrolide antibiotics have been studied in some detail (BOLARD 1986); the membrane sterols play an important role in selectivity, and these compounds interact with polyene macrolides in vitro, but other factors, in particular lipid fluidity, are important. There are environmental conditions under which the presence of sterols, far from enhancing the destructive interaction of the polyenes with the plasma membranes, actually diminishes the effects (ARCHER 1976). Recent advances in the chemistry of amphotericin B have made it possible to study structure-function relationships (CHERON et al. 1988). We can now determine which changes will be most effective in the development of polyene derivatives. At present our understanding of the molecular mechanism of action of these compounds is insufficient to provide a basis for the development of novel drugs which interfere with plasma membrane function.

The fungistatic effects of nystatin and amphotericin B result from a dissipation of the plasma membrane proton gradient (PALACIOS and SERRANO 1978). However, other biological and physical changes occur in the presence of amphotericin B that are difficult to explain on the basis of a drug-induced proton leakage. It is possible that the polyene-membrane interaction is more complex than present hypotheses would suggest (KERRIDGE 1988).

The most important interaction of the synthetic azole drugs with the plasma membranes of sensitive cells is an indirect one resulting from an inhibition of sterol biosynthesis (see later). Some but not all of these compounds also interact directly with both artificial and cellular membranes, causing an impairment of the barrier function. Miconazole is one derivative that has been studied in some detail (VANDEN BOSSCHE et al. 1982; BRASSEUR et al. 1983). This compound inserts into the lipid bilayer, causing physical disruption and ion leakage. Membrane phospholipids are important, and in this study sterols were not involved. Computer modelling studies would suggest that the area occupied by the azole molecule within the bilayer is an important factor in determining the extent of disruption.

From our knowledge of the interactions of amphotericin B and miconazole with membranes, is it likely that novel antifungal drugs will be developed which impair the barrier function of the plasma membrane? First we must consider what molecular properties are essential for a disruptive interaction with lipid bilayers. The most important one is that the molecule should be, at least in part, hydrophobic in order to insert into the lipid bilayer. This can have a number of effects: it can interact directly with membrane proteins; it can interfere with the interactions between membrane lipids, thus affecting their fluidity; it can affect the lipid environment of membrane proteins and hence their function; interaction of the drug molecules within the membrane may result in the production of aqueous pores through which low molecular weight substances can leak. All these effects have been proposed for amphotericin B. It is possible that the multiplicity of interactions with the plasma membrane of sensitive fungi is the reason why this compound is such an effective antifungal drug. Solubility is always a problem with hydrophobic molecules, and amphotericin B is no exception. It has both hydrophobic and hydrophilic faces. The addition of charged groups onto the carbohydrate moiety increases its solubility without affecting its interaction with lipid bilayers, and thus molecules with the correct hydrophobic and hydrophilic properties are possible. The most important question concerns the low sensitivity of the host. Selectivity depends upon differences in the lipid composition of the plasma membrane. These are such that it is unlikely that drugs will ever be produced with which there are no adverse side effects on the host. As with amphotericin B, selectivity will depend upon quantitative rather than qualitative differences in the interactions with membrane targets. Developments are possible from modifications of existing drugs and random screening for new antibiotics rather than comparative studies of membrane structure and subsequent de novo design of drugs.

b) Inhibition of Plasma Membrane Associated Enzymes

There are a number of possibilities for the drug-induced inhibition of plasma membrane enzymes. The first is an indirect effect resulting from alterations in the lipid environment of the enzyme, and the specificity of such effects will reflect the relative affinities of the drug for membrane lipids rather than membrane proteins.

These 'indirect' effects may be of a fairly general occurrence since many clinically important antifungal drugs affect plasma membrane enzymes of *C. albicans* at concentrations equivalent to the MIC (SURARIT and SHEPHERD 1987). These generalised effects are not restricted to drugs normally thought to interact with lipid bilayers, and compounds, for example, echinocandin and papulacandin, normally considered as specific inhibitors of β-glucan synthase also affect other membrane enzymes. The question as to whether these compounds interact directly with the membrane enzymes or indirectly via an alteration of the lipid environment of the protein has not been resolved.

How important is it in the search for new and more effective antifungal drugs to aim for compounds conforming to the ideal of a 'magic bullet'? It could be more effective to search for drugs with a multiplicity of biological effects. This would be true if each effect arose from an interaction with a specific target rather than secondary results from the interaction with one primary target. Generalised effects on microbial membrane function are very useful in inhibiting fungal growth, but drugs exhibiting such effects show reduced selectivity.

If the aim is to select targets exposed to the exterior of the cell which can be inhibited without the drug entering the cell, then specific inhibition of membrane transport should be considered. Many transport processes in yeasts are energised by a proton gradient (EDDY 1982), and inhibition of nutrient uptake can result from an effect on either the plasma membrane ATPase or the specific permease. Where transport results from facilitated diffusion, then it is necessary for the drug to interact with a carrier protein. Miconazole inhibits both the mitochondrial (K_i 47 μM) and plasma membrane (K_i 5.3 μM) ATPase of *Schizosaccharomyces pombe* (DUFOUR et al. 1980) and the mitochondrial ATPase of *S. cerevisiae* (K_i 1 μM) (PORTILLO and GANCEDO 1984). The K_i values of miconazole for the plasma membrane and mitochondrial ATPases differ appreciably. If similar differences occur between fungal and mammalian ATPases, then this enzyme can be exploited as a target in the design of antifungal drugs. Of interest are the bafilomycins, a class of inhibitors of membrane ATPases from microorganisms, animal cells and plant cells (BOWMAN et al. 1988). The macrolide antibiotic bafilomycin A_1 does not affect the F_1F_0 ATPases from bacteria and mitochondria. The K^+-dependent ATPase from *Escherichia coli*, the Na^+,K^+-ATPase from ox brain and the Ca^{2+}-ATPase from sarcoplasmic reticulum are moderately sensitive to this antibiotic. In contrast, membrane ATPases from *Neurospora* vacuoles, chromaffin granules (from bovine adrenal medulla) and plant vacuoles are extremely sensitive. These results not only show that bafilomycin A_1 is an excellent candidate for the study of vacuolar ATPases but also that the differences among groups of ATPases might be greater than between ATPases from various organisms.

A more interesting possibility is the inhibition of specific transport processes in fungi. In an early paper on its mode of action, it was reported that miconazole had differential inhibitory effects on nutrient uptake in *C. albicans* (VANDEN BOSSCHE 1974), but the mechanism was not elucidated. It could be that these were secondary effects resulting from a depletion of membrane ergosterol and concomitant accumulation of methylated sterols. With *C. albicans* the difficulty is that it can utilise glucose and ammonium ions as carbon, nitrogen and energy sources and does not require a wide range of precursors for growth, and so inhibition of uptake of specific nutrients may not be effective in preventing growth. It is the exploitation of these systems leading to the accumulation of toxic compounds within the cell which has greater potential (see later).

Nucleic acid precursor analogues are effective growth inhibitors, and 5-fluorocytosine is used clinically to treat patients with fungal infections (SCHOLER 1980). The use of such analogues is not restricted to fungi but extends to tumours and a variety of other diseases (DE CLERCQ 1985). These compounds are often toxic to humans, and this seriously restricts their clinical use. However, recent studies (EL KOUNI et al. 1983, 1985; EL KOUNI and CHA 1987) have demonstrated that it is possible by using a nucleoside transport inhibitor to restrict their effect on the host. Schistosomes lack the ability to synthesise purines de novo and rely on salvage pathways for their purine requirements. As a result, purine analogues are effective inhibitors.

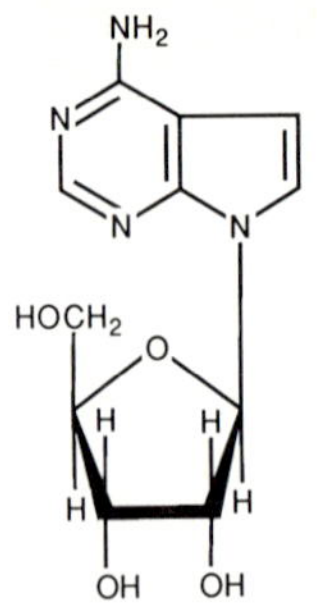

Tubercidin (7-Deazaadenosine)

Fig. 3. Chemical structure of tubercidin

7-Deazaadenosine (tubercidin, Fig. 3) is an effective inhibitor of *Schistosoma mansoni* but is also toxic to the host. However, the selectivity of this compound is improved by simultaneous administration of a specific nucleoside transport inhibitor, nitrobenzylthioinosine. This effectively blocks nucleoside transport into mammalian cells but is ineffective in preventing the uptake of tubercidin into *S. mansoni* and *S. japonicum*. The potential of this system may be restricted by the fact that the inhibitor is metabolised to 6-mercaptopurine, which is itself toxic.

This raises some very interesting possibilities with regard to the use of toxic drugs in chemotherapy.If these drugs are normally illicitly transported into cells by a pre-existing permease, then selective inhibition of the host's permeases by a non-penetrant inhibitor will be effective in achieving a therapeutic advantage, provided always that it is itself selective and non-toxic. This again emphasises the complexities of the problem and the difficulties in predicting whether a particular approach will be effective in developing suitable drugs for controlling fungal infections.

Another possible system for exploitation in the development of clinically useful antifungal drugs is the multiple drug transporter in mammalian cells. In the past one puzzling feature of drug resistance in tumour cells has been the emergence of multiple resistance to apparently unrelated drugs of natural product origin. Recent research (GOTTESMAN and PASTAN 1988a,b) has demonstrated that a multidrug transport protein (P-glycoprotein or P170 which is the product of the *MDR* 1 gene) in the plasma membrane is responsible for drug resistance in tumour cells. The human protein contains 1280 amino acids and has 12 predicted transmembrane domains. This protein is responsible for an energy (ATP)-dependent efflux of drugs, and resistant tumour cells accumulate far less drug than sensitive ones. Although the multidrug transporter has been studied extensively in tumour cells, studies of expression of *MDR* 1 mRNA in normal tissues have demonstrated substantial expression in a variety of tissues (e.g. liver, kidney, colon, jejunum and adrenal gland).

It is possible that the transporter serves to protect animals from toxic materials normally present in their diet. Whether this can be extended to include antifungal drugs remains to be seen. There is a need for more research on this protein and its potential role in eliminating antifungal agents. It does, however, raise the possibility of designing antifungal drugs whose selectivity depends upon their excretion from the host cells by this multidrug transporter system. There is a precedent for this in that decreased sensitivity to fenarimol associated with drug efflux has been reported in a strain of *Aspergillus nidulans* (DE WAARD and FUCHS 1982). However, the molecular basis of the efflux is not understood, and it is impossible to compare this system with the multidrug transporter in mammalian cells.

II. Internal Targets

1. Transport of Drugs into Sensitive Fungi

There are three mechanisms by which drugs can be transported into sensitive fungi: a) physical diffusion of hydrophobic compounds across the lipid bilayer, b) facilitated diffusion involving a protein carrier in the plasma membrane, c) active transport energised by dissipation of an ion gradient. The efficiency of the first method depends on the chemical structure and molecular volume of the individual compounds and their concentration gradient across the membrane. Differences in the lipid composition of fungal and mammalian membranes will be insufficient to affect significantly the uptake of different hydrophobic drugs. The transport mechanisms for compounds to which the bulk lipid phase of the plasma membrane is relatively impermeable show a higher degree of specificity and involve specific proteins within the cell membrane (EDDY 1982). Specific mechanisms for the uptake of antifungal drugs do not occur, but it is possible to exploit the normal nutrient transport systems for the illicit transport of drugs into fungi.

5-Fluorocytosine, and the polyoxins, nikkomycins and bacilysin are transported by the cytosine permease and the peptide permeases, respectively, into fungal cells (POLAK and GRENSON 1973; LICHLITER et al. 1976; YADAN et al. 1984; MÜLLER et al. 1981; RINGROSE 1985). Cytosine uptake is energised by dissipation of a proton gradient (FORET et al. 1978), but so far knowledge of its structure and mechanism has not led to the development of more effective pyrimidine analogues. There are two distinct peptide permeases in *C. albicans* effective in the uptake of the chitin synthase inhibitors (YADAN et al. 1984). Numerous derivatives of the polyoxins and nikkomycins have been synthesised and studied both for their transport into the cell and efficacy as growth inhibitors (EMMER et al. 1985; CASSONE 1986a), but no derivatives are used clinically. Where antifungal drugs are illicitly transported into sensitive fungi, the efficacy of these compounds is affected by nutrients in the environment and in particular the relative affinities of nutrient and drug for the carrier molecules. Any modification of a drug which increases its affinity for the transport system will enhance its antifungal activity, and this approach to drug development should be exploited.

Unfortunately, with the exception of 5-fluorocytosine, our knowledge of the transport of clinically important antifungal drugs into sensitive fungi is minimal. This is a matter of some concern since all antifungal drugs in current use, except amphotericin B, must cross the plasma membrane to reach their intracellular targets.

Griseofulvin has been used for some 3 decades (DAVIES 1980), and although EL-NAKEEB and LAMPEN (1965) provided evidence that selectivity in fungi was associated with a failure of the less sensitive cells to take up the drug, the mechanism by which this compound crosses the membrane is unknown. Since transport into sensitive cells is essential, one might expect that illicit transport rather than physical diffusion is involved. Griseofulvin has been an effective drug for treating patients with dermatophyte infections for many years, but is now being superseded by azole derivatives. However, an understanding of the mechanism by which it is transported into sensitive cells might aid in the development of new drugs.

The azole derivatives are now the most important group of antifungal drugs in current use, both clinically and in agriculture. These compounds cross the plasma membrane of sensitive organisms to reach their intracellular target on the endoplasmic reticulum. There have been few studies on the molecular mechanisms by which these compounds penetrate the cell envelope. The one feature that these drugs have in common is either an imidazole or a triazole group; they differ significantly in the remainder of the molecule (Fig. 4).

Transport across the cell envelope is apparently under genotypic control since strains of *C. albicans* have been isolated in which failure to cross either the cell wall (KERRIDGE et al. 1987) or the plasma membrane (RYLEY et al. 1984) is responsible for reduced sensitivity to miconazole. Phenotypic changes in the cell wall of *C. albicans* occuring after cessation of growth also prevent miconazole reaching the plasma membrane (GALE et al. 1980). This specificity of transport across the plasma membrane is supported by studies of Drouhet's group in the Pasteur Institute, who found that at low drug concentrations (less than 0.1 μg/ml) ketoconazole was actively transported into *C. albicans* with a K_m value of 50 nM and a V_{max} value of 1.4 μmol/min per 10^7 cells. At high concentrations (>0.1 μg/ml) the drug entered by non-saturable passive diffusion. It was not possible to remove radioactive drug from cells by adding excess unlabelled ketoconazole (BOIRON et al. 1987). Reduced sensitivity to fenarimol in *A. nidulans* results from an enhanced energy-dependent efflux of the drug from the cells (DE WAARD and FUCHS 1982). In this organism the ergosterol inhibitors enter the cell by simple diffusion, but in contrast to *C. albicans* it would appear that a specific (illicit?) transport system is responsible for their efflux.

This raises a number of questions for the biochemist which are of fundamental importance not only in enhancing our knowledge of membrane

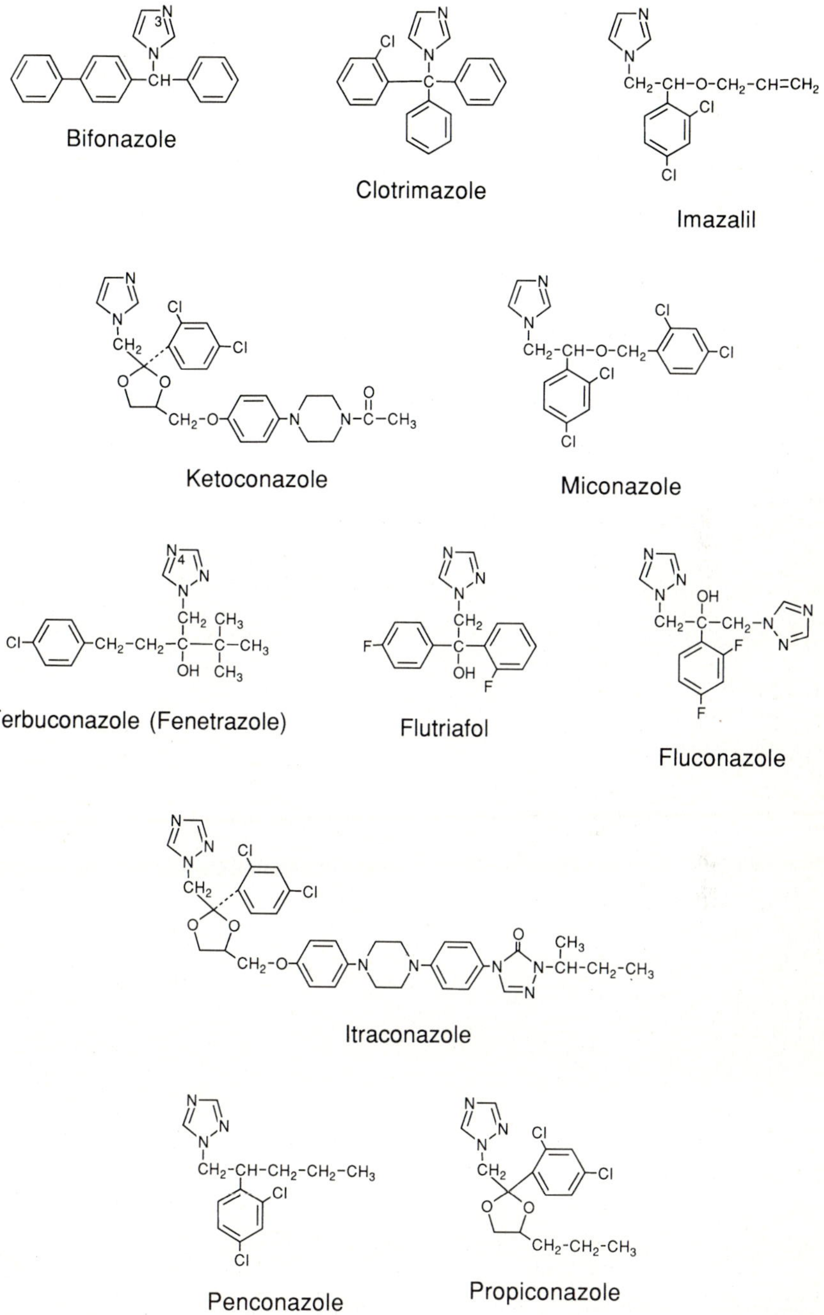

Fig. 4. Structures of imidazole and triazole antifungals of use in the chemotherapy of human mycoses and in plant protection

transport but also in developing new and more effective azole derivatives. The first question is, do all imidazoles and triazoles enter sensitive fungi by the same mechanism(s)? The evidence from certain less sensitive strains would suggest that this might be the case since they show a reduced drug uptake and are cross-resistant to other azole derivatives (RYLEY et al. 1984). Does this reduced uptake result from a decreased influx or from an increased efflux of the drug? Does the uptake of ketoconazole (at low concentrations) involve a protein carrier molecule in the plasma membrane? The structural differences between members of this group of drugs are such that it is unlikely that a single transport mechanism is responsible for their specific uptake (at low external concentrations) into sensitive cells.

If resistance results from a failure of the cells to take up the drug as in the case of *C. albicans* strains AD & KB (RYLEY et al. 1984), then the question to ask is, what change or changes in the membrane are responsible? Does it result from a change in the lipid composition of the plasma membrane affecting not only the diffusion of the drug across the bulk phase of the plasma membrane but also the environment of an 'azole permease'(?), or is there a specific defect in a permease protein? The evidence would appear to support the former hypothesis since in the two azole-resistant strains (AD & KB) the cellular phospholipid:sterol ratio is markedly lower than in sensitive permeable strains (HITCHCOCK et al. 1986).

In general, research has concentrated on the intracellular target and the mechanisms by which the imidazole and triazole drugs interact with it to prevent growth, rather than on the mechanism(s) by which they cross the plasma membrane to reach the endoplasmic reticulum. This lack of knowledge applies also to the allylamines, thiocarbamates and morpholine derivatives. In a number of cases it is probable that transport across the lipid bilayer is by diffusion, and uptake will depend upon the structure and size of the drug and the concentration gradient across the plasma membrane. Even with these drugs, knowledge of their interaction with membrane lipids and the molecular mechanisms by which they enter sensitive cells will be invaluable in the development of new antifungal agents. This is clearly an area of research in which the biochemist has a great deal to offer in the development of more effective antifungal drugs.

2. Plasma Membrane Proteins

a) Chitin Synthase

Chitin synthesis has been studied in great detail (CABIB et al. 1984; SHEPHERD 1987) since not only is it an ideal model for studying morphogenesis in yeast but also it has considerable potential as a target for antifungal drugs. It is competitively inhibited by polyoxins and nikkomycins, which are structural analogues of *N*-acetylglucosamine (MÜLLER et al. 1981; EMMER et al. 1985; CASSONE 1986b; HILENSKI et al. 1986) (Fig. 5). The organisation of chitin synthesis is also affected indirectly by azole drugs (BARUG et al. 1983; VANDEN BOSSCHE 1985; MARICHAL et al. 1985).

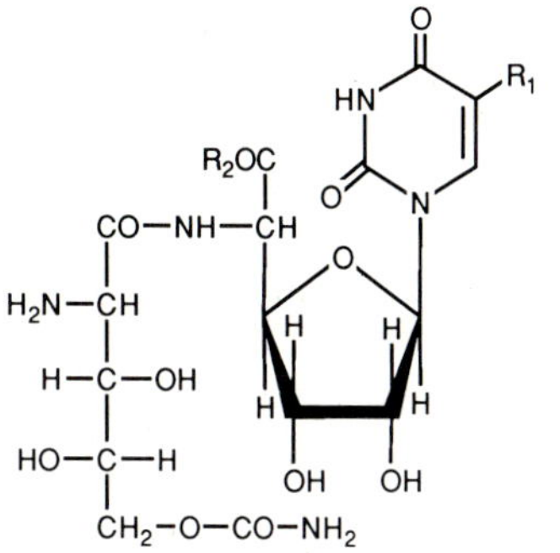

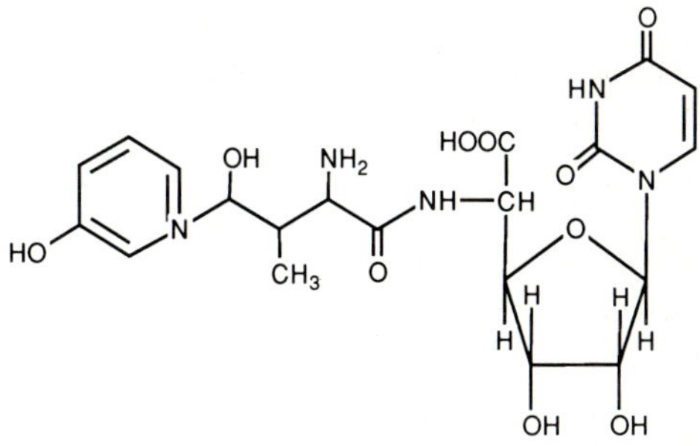

Nikkomycin Z

Polyoxin B: R_1= -CH_2OH
R_2= -OH

Polyoxin D: R_1= -COOH
R_2= -OH

Fig. 5. Structural formulae of chitin synthase inhibitors

Since chitin is absent from plants and mammals, chitin synthase is an ideal target for antifungal drugs. Recent studies have demonstrated that two distinct chitin synthases exist in *S. cerevisiae*, only one of which (CHS_2) is essential for yeast growth, but the role of the other enzyme (CHS_1) in cell growth and division is not understood (BULAWA et al. 1986; SBURLATI and CABIB 1986; ORLEAN 1987). The presence of two enzymes has not been demonstrated so far in *Candida* spp.

Chitin synthase of human pathogenic fungi is highly sensitive to polyoxins in cell-free systems (K_i values 0.4–1.2 μM) (CHIEW et al. 1980). However, growth is inhibited by these antibiotics only at high concentrations (BECKER et al. 1983). Polyoxin-induced inhibition of growth of *C. albicans* is highly dependent upon the composition of the medium (YADAN et al. 1984). These compounds are almost inactive in rich media containing peptides, but in liquid minimal media devoid of peptides, MIC values of 5–10 μg polyoxin/ml are obtained. *C. albicans* possesses a transport system for peptides, and since polyoxins possess a peptide backbone, these compounds can be accumulated by the same system. Thus, in media containing peptides, uptake of polyxins will be inhibited.

YADAN et al. (1984) observed that the activity of a closely related compound nikkomycin Z was much less sensitive to competition by peptides for the peptide transport system. The same researchers also demonstrated that *C. albicans* has two transport sytems for peptides and that polyoxin D and nikkomycin Z are not transported by the same peptide permease. They suggest that nikkomycins and their tripeptide derivatives should prove useful for the inhibition of both wild-type and dipeptide transport-deficient mutants of *C. albicans*. Microorganisms are able to change their peptide transport ability, and a nikkomycin-resistant mutant of *C. albicans* has been isolated with a decreased dipeptide uptake, although the uptake of trimethionine was markedly increased. This mutant apparently lacks the general peptide transport system present in the wild type but satisfies its nutritional requirements by developing a transport system more specific for oligopeptides. This latter system is less efficient in transporting nikkomycin Z. The development of such mutant strains casts doubts on the use of these inhibitors in the treatment of patients suffering from candidosis. Another possibility for the development of resistance to these compounds and for their failure to inhibit chitin synthesis both in vivo and in vitro is metabolic degradation by peptidases of both host and fungus. It should also be noted that the existence of two chitin synthases in *S. cerevisiae* now needs to be taken into account when screening for antifungal agents. Indeed, the enzyme measured in vitro may not be the one that is active in vivo (ORLEAN 1987).

Polyoxin B is used in Japan to control pear black spot caused by *Alternaria kikuchiana* and polyoxin D, to control rice sheath blight caused by *Pellicularia susukii* (DEKKER 1985), but apart from these, no other inhibitors of chitin synthase are used to control fungal infections. There is still considerable interest in this enzyme as a potential target and in the polyoxins and nikkomycins as models for specific antifungal drugs. It has been demonstrated that nikkomycin given intravenously prolongs the life of mice infected with *C. albicans*, but on cessation of therapy the mice die (BECKER et al. 1988). Chitin synthase is a plasma membrane enzyme with the active site, and hence the target for both polyoxins and nikkomycins, facing the interior of the cell. The product, chitin, is extruded through the membrane for insertion into the cell wall. Any antibiotic which interacts with the active centre of chitin synthase must cross the plasma membrane to reach its target. Polyoxins and nikkomycins are analogues of UDPGlcNAc and are transported into sensitive cells via peptide permeases (FURTER and RAST 1985) rather than nucleoside permeases, even though they can be considered as nucleotide analogues. Selectivity is usually associated with their affinity for the permease, not the synthase, since in insensitive fungi the IC_{50} for chitin synthase in vitro is several orders of magnitude less than the MIC for the fungus (GOODAY 1977). So for chitin synthase inhibitors, the problem is one of achieving a sufficiently high internal drug concentration, i.e. of enhancing uptake of UDPGlcNAc analogues into the cell. If advances are to be made in the development of chitin synthase inhibitors, these must come from studies of their uptake, rather than their interaction with the active centre of the enzyme, since the former is the limiting step.

Chitin synthase is membrane associated, and changes in the lipid environment affect its activity. This has been shown with polyene macrolide antibiotics: at concentrations in excess of the MIC, amphotericin B and nystatin inhibit the enzyme in *Mucor rouxii* (RAST and BARTNICKI-GARCIA 1981). These inhibitory effects apparently result from the interaction of the antibiotics with the lipids, altering the environment of the enzyme and hence its function. Clearly, one major function of the biochemist here is to study protein-lipid interactions, their role in modulating the activity of membrane-associated enzymes and their possible exploitation in drug development.

b) β-1,3-Glucan Synthase

This plasma membrane protein is responsible for the synthesis of cell wall β-glucans. As with chitin synthase the substrate (UDP-glucose) is produced internally, and the active centre is directed towards the interior of the cell, so drugs designed to interact with the active centre of the enzyme must cross the plasma membrane. β-Glucan synthase is under complex control from intracellular nucleotides (SHEMATEK et al. 1980; ORLEAN 1982; NOTARIO et al. 1982).

β-Glucan synthase is inhibited by papulacandin, echinocandin and aculeacin. As yet, none is used clinically, although derivatives of echinocandin, e.g. cilofungin (LY 121019), are currently being evaluated as potential antifungal drugs. Papulacandin B (Fig. 6) is an amphiphilic molecule in which the hydrophilic portion contains glucose and galactose residues and the hydrophobic portion, two unsaturated partially hydroxylated fatty acids; echinocandin and aculeacin are polypeptides.

Papulacandin B and echinocandin B (Fig. 6) acts as inhibitors of β-glucan synthesis in membrane fractions and in regenerating spheroplasts of *C. albicans*. In the spheroplasts, both antibiotics inhibited the incorporation of ^{14}C-labeled glucose into β-1,3- and β-1,6-glucan (SHEPHERD et al. 1984). In vivo and in vitro papulacandin B also inhibits the β-1,3-glucan synthase of *Geotrichum candidum* and *S. pombe* (DURAN et al. 1984). Attempts to show an in vitro effect on the corresponding enzymes of *S. cerevisiae* and *Saprolegnia monoica* were unsuccessful (DURAN et al. 1984). In vitro papulacandin B (concentrations up to 0.1 mg/ml) does not inhibit glucan synthesis in crude membrane extracts of *Paracoccidioides brasiliensis*. However, in vivo this antibiotic (2 μg/ml) affects the mycelial form of *P. brasiliensis* with the production of yeast-like structures at 23°C. The yeast-mycelium transition proceeds only to an incipient stage, whereas mycelium-yeast transition is not affected (SAN-BLAS 1985; SAN-BLAS and SAN-BLAS 1985). It should be noted that the yeast wall differs from the mycelial wall in *P. brasiliensis* by the presence of α-glucan in the former and β-glucan in the latter (SAN-BLAS 1985). It would be of interest to know whether papulacandin B binds preferentially to the α- or β-glucan synthase. Its narrow spectrum of activity restricts its value as a potential antifungal drug. It might be more useful as a model for the development of other inhibitors of cell wall synthesis in pathogenic fungi and as a tool to study the glucan synthases in different fungi.

This limitation also applies to the cyclic peptide antibiotics echinocandin and aculeacin. These are active against some species of yeasts but inactive against filamentous fungi. Echinocandin is fungicidal, causing lysis of

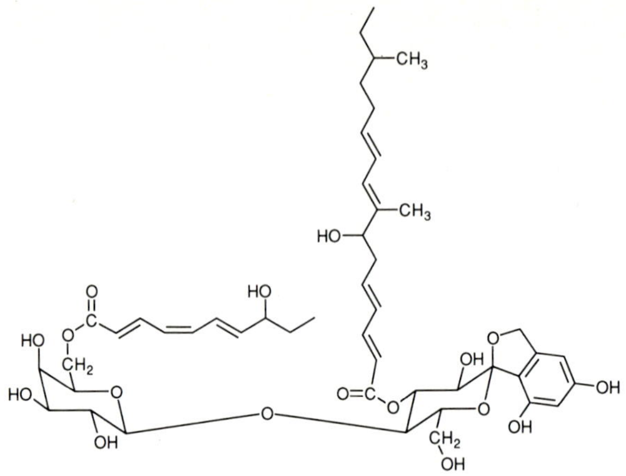

Papulacandin B

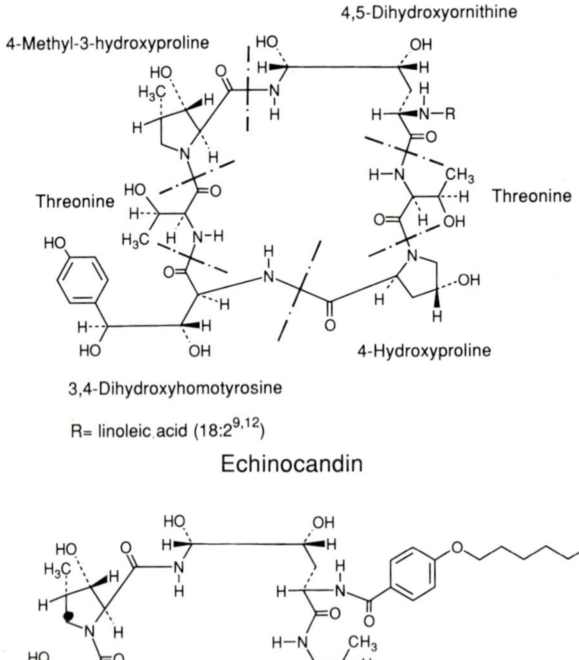

Echinocandin

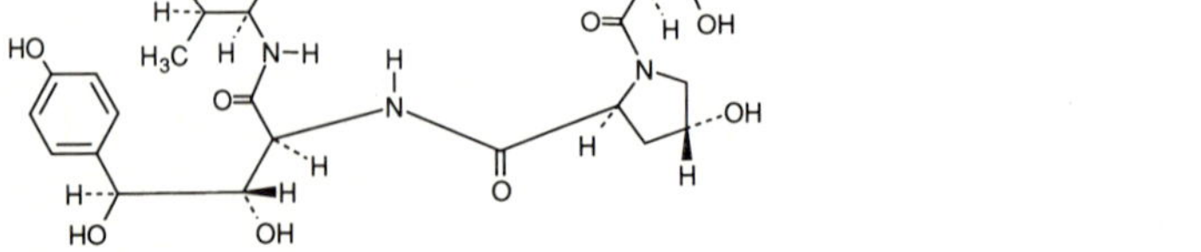

LY121019 - Cilofungin

Fig. 6. Structural formulae of glucan synthase inhibitors exponentially growing cells of *C. albicans* (CASSONE et al. 1981), and inhibits β-1,3-glucan synthase both in vitro and in vivo (SAWISTOWSKA-SCHRODER et al. 1984). The precise mechanisms of the inhibitory interaction have yet to be elucidated. Of greater interest is the semisynthetic antibiotic LY121019 (cilofungin). This compound is derived from echinocandin (Fig. 6) and non-competitively inhibits β-1,3-glucan synthases of both *C. albicans* and *Neurospora crassa*; the apparent K_i values are 2.5 μM and 16 μM, respectively (GORDEE et al. 1984; TAFT and SELINTRENNIKOFF 1988; TAFT et al. 1988; MÜLLER and SCHEIDECKER 1988). Incubation of *C. albicans* with cilofungin results in a number of morphological changes in the cell-envelope. The glucan layer becomes dispersed and loses its normal texture. The cytoplasmic membrane is ruptured, resulting in the release of cytoplasmic material and cell death. Cilofungin is active in vivo as well as in vitro against *C. albicans* isolates and is at least 20-fold less toxic than amphotericin B (GORDEE et al. 1984). The former has a very narrow spectrum of activity, with isolates of *Candida glabrata* being less susceptible than to amphotericin B; *Candida parapsilosis* is relatively insensitive, and *Cryptococcus neoformans* is resistant (HALL et al. 1988). This high degree of selectivity would restrict its potential role in antifungal therapy to the treatment of patients suffering from candidosis due to *C. albicans*.

If these inhibitors of glucan synthesis are to interact directly with the active centre of the enzyme they must enter the cell. There are no published data on their uptake or on their interaction with lipid bilayers. In their paper SURARIT and SHEPHERD (1987) report that echinocandin and papulacandin, like amphotericin B and miconazole, affect a number of other membrane enzymes including ATPase and adenyl cyclase at their MIC. This occurs presumably by modifying the lipid environment of these membrane proteins, since it is difficult to visualise how one antibiotic can have specific inhibitory effects on such diverse enzymes. It does raise an important question concerning the specificity of interaction of these antifungals with the membrane-associated β-glucan synthase. The assumption in the past has been that these antibiotics specifically inhibit this enzyme, and inhibition of cell wall synthesis results in cell lysis. If these compounds also affect other membrane-associated proteins then the importance of their interaction with β-glucan synthase must be reassessed. It could be, for example, that passage of these complex molecules across the plasma membrane is not essential,and their interaction with the lipid bilayer alters the environment of the membrane-associated enzymes sufficiently to affect their functioning without the necessity of interacting with their inwardly directed active centre.

c) Mannoprotein Synthesis

Although mannoprotein synthesis is not strictly a plasma membrane-associated function, it is convenient to discuss it at this stage since the final stage of the synthesis and export of the mannoproteins across the plasma membrane before inclusion into the cell wall is a fusion of intracellular vesicles with the membrane. Mannoprotein synthesis is complex (Fig. 7), involving the coordinated synthesis of both protein and polysaccharide moieties, and occurs in association with intracellular membranes (PARODI 1981; ELBEIN 1981; SCHEKMAN 1982, 1985). Lipid intermediates are involved in transferring the polysaccharide to the protein, and nucleoside diphosphate derivatives of *N*-acetyl glucosamine, mannose and glucose serve as precursors. The complexity of this synthesis is analogous to the synthesis of bacterial peptidoglycan, and it is surprising that given the number of possible targets (i.e. enzymatic steps), there are no antifungal drugs in clinical use which affect the synthesis of this cell wall component.

Enzymes involved in the biosynthesis of polysaccharide constituents of the fungal cell wall are ideal targets for therapeutic attack, yet no antifungal drugs which specifically inhibit polysaccharide synthesis are used clinically. If these systems are to be studied as potential targets for the next generation of antifungal drugs, we must consider possible reasons for this. There are antibiotics which inhibit the formation of all polysaccharide constituents of the fungal cell wall and which can act as models for future antimycotic drugs. However, certain glucan synthase inhibitors also inhibit other membrane-associated enzymes at concentrations equivalent to the MIC (SURARIT and SHEPHERD 1987). Before these compounds can be used as models, it is important to answer the question, Do these compounds act directly on the membrane-associated enzyme or indirectly by altering its lipid environment? If the effects of glucan synthase inhibitors are indirect, then inhibition could occur without these antibiotics entering the cell. For the development of drugs inhibiting cell wall synthesis, it is important to determine the importance of membrane lipids in modulating enzyme function. How can this be done, and what will be the potential use of the information in the drug design? There are obvious experimental approaches which can be adopted for such studies; the first is to manipulate the membrane lipids of fungi either phenotypically using controlled environmental conditions in a chemostat or genotypically and then to examine the role of lipid composition in modulating antibiotic activity both in vivo and in vitro using reconstituted membrane vesicles. It is possible with the techniques of molecular genetics to clone the genes for the synthases and determine their nucleotide sequence. From these data, the amino acid sequence of the enzyme can be obtained, and computer analysis will give some indication of the organisation of the peptide chain within the lipid bilayer. Ideally, X-ray crystallographic analysis is required to give a complete three-dimensional picture of the protein, but unless the protein can be crystallised, this cannot be done. Site-directed mutations within the peptide sequences spanning the lipid bilayer can be used to assess the relative importance of individual amino acids in the protein-lipid interaction and the role of such interactions in modulating both enzyme activity and drug action. This information is required if specific membrane enzymes are to be exploited as targets in the de novo design of selective antimycotic drugs.

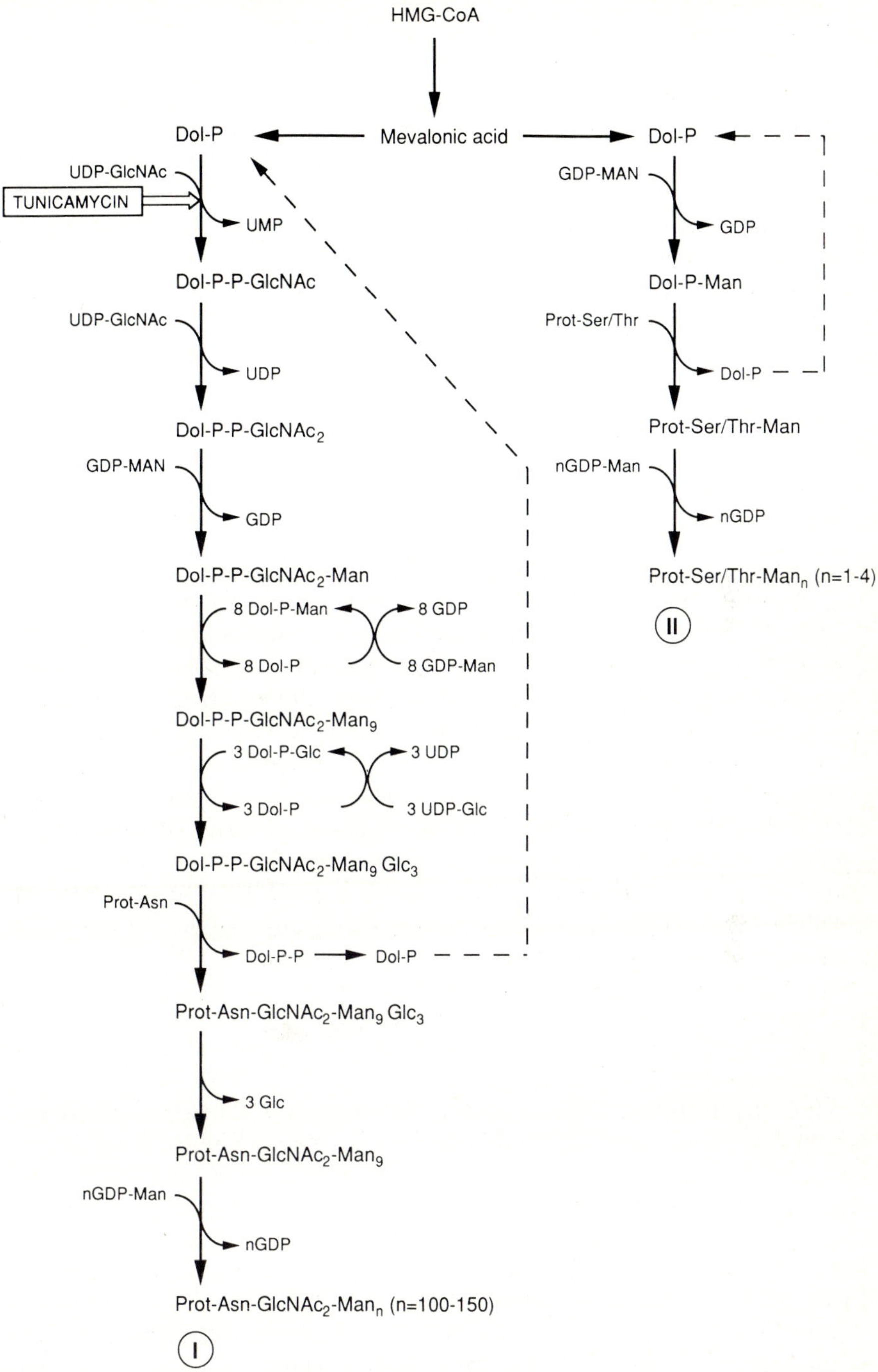

Fig. 7. The lipid-linked pathway for the synthesis of saccharide moieties of mannoprotein. (*I*) Biosynthesis of the asparagine-linked and (*II*) of the serine/threonine-linked saccharides. *Dol*, dolychol (a polyprenol containing 14–18 isoprene units); *P*, phosphate; *GlcNAc*, *N*-acetylglucosamine; *Man*, mannose; *Glc*, glucose; *Prot*, protein; ⇒ tunicamycin blocks the first step in the pathway; *HMG-CoA*, hydroxy methyl glutaryl-coenzyme A. The schematic representations are based on those of Elbein (1981) and Parodi (1981)

Membrane-associated proteins carry out functions in fungi which do not occur in mammalian cells. These proteins are ideal as potential targets for antifungal drugs. However, the complexities of protein-lipid interactions are such that design of specific inhibitors may not be a fruitful line of research, and a more pragmatic approach should be adopted. Assay systems for many membrane functions are already available, and these can be used to test both natural products and synthetic chemicals for their efficiency as inhibitors. The importance of the plasma membrane in antifungal chemotherapy cannot be overemphasised; not only are many of its constituent macromolecules specific targets for antifungal drugs, but also it is responsible for the uptake of drugs with intracellular targets. For the biochemist the plasma membrane is potentially one of the most productive areas of research.

3. Pathways of Intermediary Metabolism

Here there is a wealth of possible targets. Any enzymic reaction either anabolic or catabolic which is essential for fungal growth is a possible target for therapeutic attack. There are, however, a number of constraints. The drug must be able to penetrate the cell envelope to reach the target enzyme, and possible mechanisms for drug uptake have already been considered in this chapter. Ideally, the target enzyme should be absent from the host, and here a detailed knowledge of the metabolic pathways in both host and pathogen is invaluable. If, however, the target enzyme is present within the host, it should have a significantly lower affinity for the drug than the fungal enzyme. At present, it is impossible to predict the relative affinities of antifungal drugs for their target enzymes, and this information can only be obtained experimentally, but as our knowledge of the relationships between protein structure and function increases, this may become possible in the future.

Let us first consider the present and examine the pathways of intermediary metabolism which already provide targets for economically important antifungal drugs. The most important one is that involved in sterol biosynthesis (Fig. 8).

It is surprising that allylamines, thiocarbamate (e.g. tolnaftate), azole and morpholine (e.g. amorolfine) derivatives (see Chap. 6) all inhibit enzymes involved in sterol biosynthesis. Allylamines (naftifine and terbinafine) and thiocarbamates inhibit squalene epoxidase, although the precise molecular mechanism is not understood (Ryder 1984, 1985; Petranyi et al. 1984; Ryder and Dupont 1985; Ryder et al. 1986; Barrett-Bee et al. 1986; Stütz 1987). Synthetic azole derivatives interact with cytochrome P-450-mediated sterol 14α-demethylase. These drugs bind via the N(3) of the imidazole ring or the N(4) of the triazole ring to the sixth coordination position of the haem iron of cytochrome P-450. Selectivity results from the different affinities of the drugs for the fungal and mammalian enzymes, reflecting both the structure of the drug and protein moiety of the enzyme (Vanden Bossche 1985, 1988; Vanden Bossche et al. 1987a, 1988b; Yoshida and Aoyama 1986,

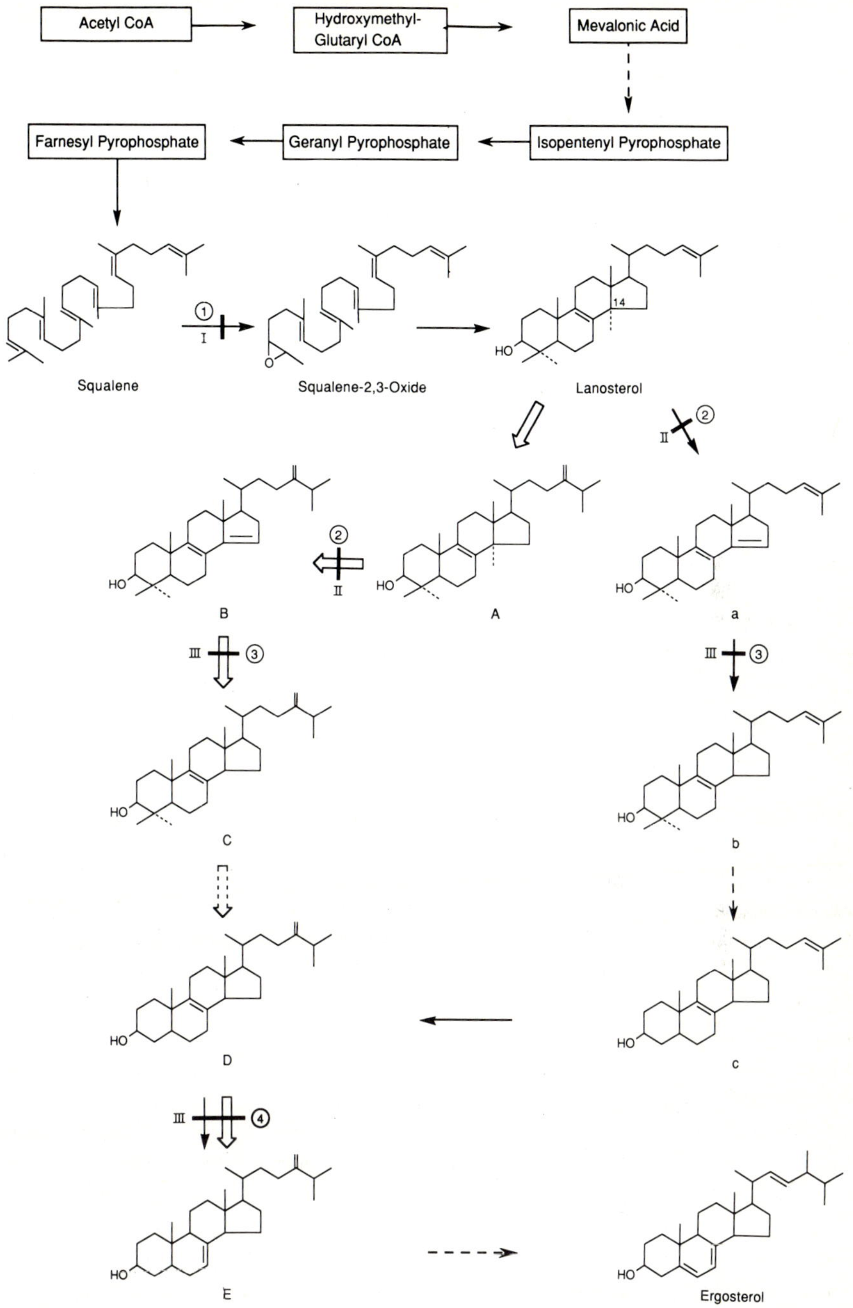

Fig. 8. Inhibition of ergosterol biosynthesis by allylamines and thiocarbamates (*I*), imidazole, triazole, pyrimidines and pyridine antifungals (*II*) and morpholines (*III*). *1*, squalene epoxidase; *2*, 14α-demethylase; *3*, Δ^{14}-reductase; *4*, $\Delta^{8} \rightarrow \Delta^{7}$-isomerase; *A*, 24-methylene dihydrolanosterol; *B*, 4,4-dimethyl-$\Delta^{8,14,24(28)}$-ergostatrienol; *C*, 4,4-dimethyl-$\Delta^{8,24(28)}$-ergostadienol; *D*, fecosterol; *E*, episterol; *a*, 4,4-dimethyl-$\Delta^{8,14,24(25)}$-cholestatrienol; *b*, $\Delta^{8,24}$-cholestdienol; *c*, zymosterol; ⇒ possible pathway in fungal cells; → possible pathway in *Saccharomyces cerevisiae*; – – – → / = = = ⇒ reactions requiring several steps; ▬ sites of inhibition

1987; YOSHIDA 1988). Some of the azole drugs also inhibit at higher concentrations other cytochrome P-450-mediated reactions in plants and animals. It is possible that these systems can be exploited in the development of drugs for the therapy of steroid-mediated diseases or as plant growth regulators (SANTEN et al. 1983; JANSSEN and VANDEN BOSSCHE 1987; VANDEN BOSSCHE and JANSSEN 1987; VANDEN BOSSCHE et al. 1985, 1987b; MASON et al. 1987; LÜRSSEN 1988). The morpholine derivatives inhibit sterol biosynthesis at a stage subsequent to the C14-demethylation step (for reviews, see KERKENAAR 1987; MERCER 1988).

The important question here is, What are the specific features of this anabolic pathway that make it suitable as a target for so many antifungal drugs? We can only speculate on possible answers. Ergosterol is essential for fungal growth and has a multiplicity of roles to play in fungi. It is required for initiation of cell proliferation, and for this function it cannot be replaced by other sterols. The quantities required for this are less than 5 fg/cell. Ergosterol controls the fluidity of certain critical domains, a factor of importance in the activity of a number of membrane enzymes. Higher amounts of ergosterol are required to bring rather more of the membrane into the proper physicochemical state. Finally, it has a bulk function, a role that can be filled by a number of sterols (RODRIGUEZ et al. 1985; VANDEN BOSSCHE 1988; NES and DHANUKA 1988). Cholesterol, not ergosterol, is the major sterol constituent of mammalian membranes (BLOCH 1983), and although many enzymes which are inhibited by antimycotic drugs occur both in fungal and mammalian cells, they are sufficiently diverse to have different binding affinities for individual drugs. The relative binding efficiencies for a specific cytochrome P-450 also vary for different azoles, for example, itraconazole shows high selectivity whereas bifonazole is much less selective (VANDEN BOSSCHE et al. 1987b). Many enzymes involved in sterol biosynthesis are membrane associated. Is this an important feature in selectivity? We have already seen the importance of the plasma membrane enzymes in mediating the action of antifungal drugs, and now we have a further example of the importance of membrane-associated enzymes as specific targets for antimycotic drugs.

Inhibitors of sterol biosynthesis have a major role as antifungal agents both in clinical and agricultural practice, but there are other pathways of lipid biosynthesis affected by antimycotic agents. Early stages in the synthesis of both fatty acids and sterols are inhibited by cerulenin (VANCE et al. 1972); unfortunately, this compound is unstable and of little potential commercial value. Validamycin A (TRINCI 1984; YAMAMOTO 1985) is widely used in Japan to control rice sheath blight caused by *Rhizoctonia solani*. The antibiotic induces a reduction in the endogenous inositol content of *Rhizoctonia cerealis*, as a result of which there is a stimulation of hyphal branching and a decreased hyphal extension. The inhibition of hyphal extension is associated with a decrease in the β-1,3-glucomannan fraction of the cell wall. Internode length varies with inositol content, and phospholipids play a role in branching.

Although such an antibiotic may have some use in the control of fungal infections of plants, as the invasive organisms are essentially mycelial, it is doubtful whether this compound will be equally useful in controlling fungal pathogens of humans, where the yeast form predominates.

But what of other anabolic pathways currently being exploited in the search for new antimicrobial drugs? Polyamines are essential metabolites in microorganisms. Their importance in cell growth and multiplication has been

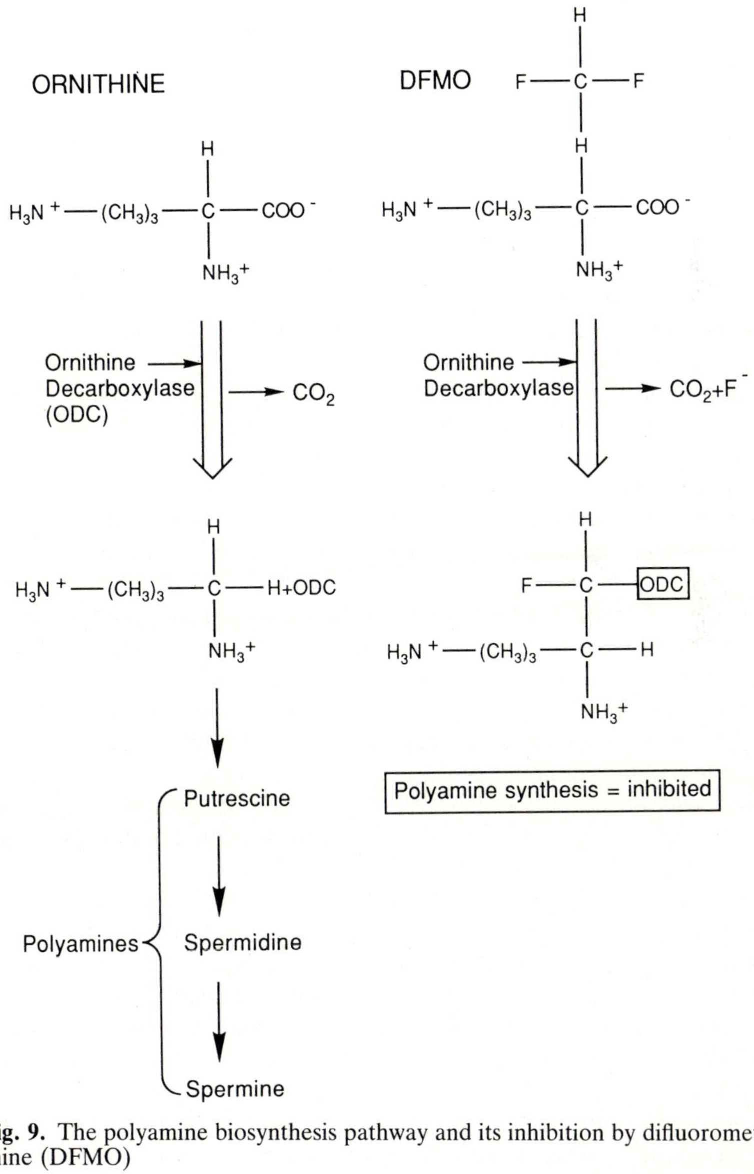

Fig. 9. The polyamine biosynthesis pathway and its inhibition by difluoromethylornithine (DFMO)

highlighted by studies of inhibition of their synthesis by catalytically activated irreversible inhibitors (BACCHI 1981), but their precise function in cell growth is still not understood. The first inhibitor developed was DL-α-difluoromethylornithine (DFMO), a potent inhibitor of ornithine decarboxylase (ODC) and hence putrescine synthesis (MAMONT et al. 1978). The mechanism of action of these compounds is well understood; the enzyme recognises DFMO as a 'substrate', and in the presence of pyridoxal phosphate, the decarboxylation product generates an electrophilic amine. This amine is able to form a covalent bond and alkylate the enzyme at its active centre (Fig. 9).

Polyamine metabolism offers realistic targets for antimicrobial chemotherapy, in particular for patients suffering from protozoal diseases (WANG 1984; MCCANN et al. 1981, 1986; TYMS et al. 1988). DFMO is active against *Plasmodium* and African but not American trypanosomiasis. Its role as an antifungal agent has not been examined so extensively, but DFMO is used therapeutically for *Pneumocystis carinii* pneumonia (MCCANN et al. 1986) [recent studies of EDMAN et al. (1988) showed *P. carinii* to be a member of the fungi], and it has been used as a spray to protect *Phaseolus vulgaris* plants against the bean rust fungus, *Uromyces phaseoli* (RAJAM et al. 1985). Since it shows considerable selectivity with different protozoa, it would be interesting to see whether similar variations occur in the fungi. Polyamine synthesis in a number of *Candida*, *Trichophyton* and *Microsporum* species is inhibited by DFMO in vitro (PFALLER et al. 1987; BOYLE et al. 1988). Toxicity tests have been carried out with these compounds, and the side effects are predictable on the basis of its mode of action as an inhibitor of polyamine synthesis. DFMO is considered to be safe and well tolerated by humans. The side effects that do occur are reversible, and inhibitors of polyamine synthesis might prove suitable for future development as antimycotic drugs.

One other pathway of intermediary metabolism with considerable potential as a target for antimycotic drugs is the synthesis of chitin precursors. Bacilysin is active against both bacteria and *C. albicans* (KENIG and ABRAHAM 1976). It is taken up by a peptide permease into sensitive cells where it is hydrolysed by intracellular aminopeptidases to anticapsin and L-alanine. Anticapsin is a potent inhibitor of L-glutamine:D-fructose-6-phosphate amino transferase and hence chitin synthesis. Studies on the synthesis of chitin precursors have been extended by BOROWSKI and his collaborators (CHMARA et al. 1986), and they are currently investigating fumaroyl diaminopropanoic acid derivatives, a novel group of glutamine analogues, as specific inhibitors of glucosamine-6-phosphate synthase (Fig. 10). Glucosamine is important in the synthesis of mammalian glycopeptides, and toxicity problems could arise if inhibitors of its synthesis were ever used therapeutically. Bacilysin does, however, introduce a novel concept in drug design. Here we have a non-toxic compound transported into sensitive cells by a specific permease. Once inside the cell it is hydrolysed to give a toxic warhead which interacts with a target enzyme within the cell, so inhibiting growth (RINGROSE 1985). At the same time as the studies on bacilysin, independent studies were being carried out

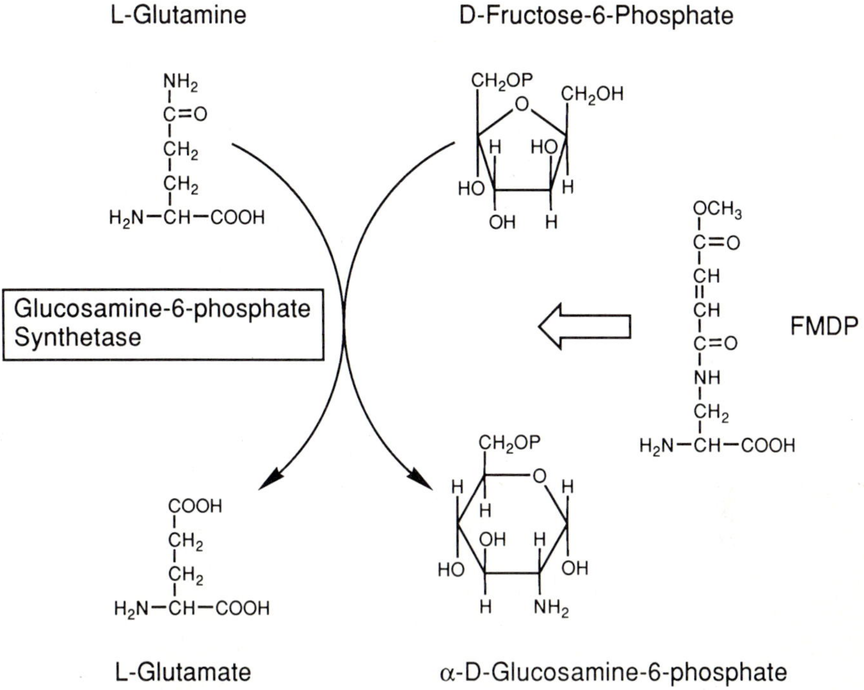

Fig. 10. Inactivation of glucosamine-6-phosphate synthase by N^3-(4-methoxy-fumaroyl)-L-2,3-diaminopropanoic acid (FMDP)

on phosphonopeptides (e.g. alafosfalin) by scientists working at Roche. These compounds are transported into cells by a peptide permease and once inside the cell are hydrolysed by intracellular amino peptidases to release the toxic warhead (see RINGROSE 1985). Unfortunately, there are practical problems in using these compounds as chemotherapeutic agents, in particular the influence of the environment on their transport into cells and their breakdown by the host. This approach has not been used successfully in the de novo development of new antifungal drugs but is clearly worth further investigation.

Drug metabolism is important in controlling fungal infections. 5-Fluorocytosine is a taken up by sensitive fungi and deaminated to 5-fluorouracil; this latter compound is then metabolised by the pyrimidine salvage pathway to 5-fluorouridine triphosphate and 5-fluorodeoxyuridylate. The former is a precursor of aberrant RNA and the latter, a potent inhibitor of thymidylate synthase (Chap. 6). Selectivity results from the fact that humans lack a cytosine deaminase responsible for converting cytosine to uracil; 5-fluorocytosine is itself non-toxic. So we have two examples of non-toxic compounds being specifically taken up into sensitive cells and subsequently metabolised to toxic derivatives by either intracellular peptidases or a specific cytosine deaminase. The selectivity of 5-fluorocytosine results from the failure of the host to metabolise the drug to an 'active derivative' and provides us with a model for subsequent drug development.

So far, differences between pathogenic fungi and their mammalian hosts have been highlighted by studies of antifungal drugs, and the question to be asked by the biochemist is, Are there other pathways that might provide additional selective targets? One major difference between humans and fungi is that humans have lost the ability to synthesise a number of amino acids, and as a result these compounds are essential constituents of their diet. *C.albicans* and many other fungi have the inherent ability to synthesise all their amino acid requirements from glucose and ammonium salts, although they can, of course, utilise these compounds if they are provided in the growth medium. Here are obvious targets to be exploited in the development of new antifungal drugs. Either we can develop drugs which will prevent the synthesis of specific amino acids and hopefully prevent or reduce the growth of the pathogen, or we can utilise the metabolic steps to synthesise amino acid analogues capable of inhibiting fungal growth. 5-Fluorocytosine is an excellent model for such a system. It is surprising that given the success of 5-fluorocytosine as an antifungal drug and the inability of humans to synthesise certain amino acids, we do not have antifungal drugs which interfere with amino acid biosynthesis or exploit these pathways to produce toxic derivatives. There is a clear need for a comprehensive study of amino acid biosynthesis in fungi and their hosts. Any differences detected can then be exploited in the development of either specific enzyme inhibitors or metabolite analogues which can be 'utilised' by the pathogen but not by the host.

4. Macromolecular Synthesis

Even though there are innumerable compounds which inhibit macromolecular synthesis in fungi (RYLEY et al. 1981), these with the exception of 5-fluorocytosine have not been exploited in the treatment of patients suffering from fungal infections. In certain cases it is clear that failure of the cells to transport the drug across the plasma membrane is responsible for the low sensitivity, and in others the drug is too toxic to be effective as a selective agent. It is important to consider possible reasons for this lack of selectivity and assess the potential value of studying these systems in the search for new chemotherapeutic agents.

Proteins and nucleic acids are complex molecules, and the mechanisms for their synthesis have been highly conserved throughout evolution. There are differences between the mechanisms of macromolecular synthesis in the three different types of organisms, i.e. eubacteria, archaebacteria and eukaryotic organisms. These are highlighted by their different sensitivities to a number of antibiotics, but within each group there are few significant differences. Where selectivity occurs in vivo, it is often associated with a failure of the cell to take up the drug. If the mechanisms of protein and nucleic acid synthesis are highly conserved, as appears to be the case, then attempts to exploit what will after all be small differences between fungi and humans in the search for novel antifungal drugs may not be productive, and research should be centred on other potentially more useful targets.

III. Miscellaneous Targets

We have considered possible targets within the fungal cell and attempted to assess their potential value in the search for novel antifungal drugs. There are other approaches to the prevention and cure of fungal diseases. The establishment of an infection involves a complex interaction between the host and parasite. It is not merely a matter of two cell types sharing a common environment. SMITH (1985) outlined the stages involved in development of microbial diseases:

1. Colonisation by the pathogen of the mucous surfaces of the respiratory, alimentary or urogenital tract.
2. Penetration of these surfaces by the pathogen.
3. Multiplication of the pathogen in the environment.
4. Pathogen should resist the host's defense mechanisms.
5. Pathogen should damage the host's tissues.

In spite of the increasing importance of fungal infections, studies on fungal pathogenicity are still in their infancy, and those that have been carried out have concentrated on four aspects: adhesion, determinants of growth and morphology in vivo, role of exocellular enzymes in the establishment of infections, and finally, interference with the host's defense mechanisms. Although cell penetration by hyphal forms of *C. albicans* occurs, it has not been extensively studied. Any drug which interferes with the establishment of infection (provided it is non-toxic to the host) will be ideal for prophylactic administration to patients at risk from fungal infections.

1. Drugs Preventing Adhesion

There is considerable interest in the nature of the surface constituents of *C. albicans* responsible for adhesion to epithelial cells and to plastic (important in denture stomatitis). The evidence suggests that surface mannoproteins are involved, but there have been no reports of inhibitors which specifically inhibit the synthesis of these surface components or which prevent the yeast adhering to mammalian cell surfaces. However, if the interactions between host and parasite were understood, it might be possible to design antimycotic agents, possibly peptides or oligosaccharides, to interfere with the early stages of the establishment of the infection.

Studies with bacteria have emphasised the difficulties associated with the development of drugs capable of preventing adhesion (SMITH 1985). The complexity of the interaction in vivo is such that drugs developed and tested in vitro or in animal models may be ineffective. Research into the development of drugs preventing adhesion may also prove to be counterproductive as adhesion to mammalian cells is advantageous to the host in promoting phagocytosis.

2. Dimorphism

One fruitful line of research relates to fungal morphology in vivo. In most dimorphic pathogenic fungi, it is usually the yeast form which exists in the host. *C. albicans* is different in that both yeast and mycelial forms occur together, and the relative importance of the two morphological forms in the establishment of infection is uncertain (Odds 1988). Yeast-mycelial transitions have been studied in vitro for a variety of dimorphic fungi (Patiño et al. 1984; San-Blas 1985; San-Blas and San-Blas 1983; Kobayashi et al. 1985; Odds 1986; Lombardi et al. 1988). These changes can be readily induced in the laboratory, although the relevance of such studies to the infectious state is still obscure. Here is an area of great potential importance in the development of antifungal drugs.

Fungal morphology is closely related to the synthesis and organisation of the cell wall. We have already discussed the inhibition of synthesis of specific macromolecular constitutents, but there may be more subtle effects involving the synthesis and organisation of individual wall components in both the yeast and mycelial phases. It is inappropriate at this stage to indulge in a critical survey of the literature on fungal dimorphism since it deserves a book to itself (see, for example, Szaniszlo 1985), but the importance of yeast-mycelial dimorphism in fungal infections cannot be overemphasised, and any advances in the understanding of the molecular biology of this process will have a major impact on the treatment of patients with mycotic infections.

3. The Cytoskeleton

One cellular structure which has not been considered as a possible target in spite of its relevance to structural dimorphism is the cystoskeleton. Griseofulvin is an antibiotic which interacts specifically with tubulin (Sloboda et al. 1982) and acts as a mitotic poison. It may alter the function of intact microtubules rather than cause their disaggregation (Wilson 1975), and Langcake et al. (1983) have suggested that it affects a process vital to the sliding of microtubules, which is essential for chromosome separation. The effect of griseofulvin on microtubules differs from that of compounds such as carbendazim, which prevent mitosis by binding to tubulin subunits of the mitotic spindle, and cross-resistance to these drugs does not occur (Dekker 1984). Griseofulvin causes major growth abnormalities in sensitive fungi and has been referred to as a 'curling factor' (Brian et al. 1946). It is inactive against *C. albicans*. Selectivity arises from its failure to enter resistant organisms since griseofulvin interacts with tubulins from a variety of sources ranging from humans to dermatophytic fungi (Kerridge 1986). Extensive chemical modification of griseofulvin has not resulted in the replacement of the parent compound in therapy (Crosse et al. 1964), although the drug itself is now being superseded by other compounds. Benzimidazole derivatives are used widely as systemic fungicides and like griseofulvin cause abnormal nuclear division in sensitive fungi. These compounds, like griseofulvin, react specifically with β-tubulin, and resistance to benzimidazole derivatives in certain strains of fungi is associated with changes in this protein (BURLAND and GULL 1984).

There are other compounds (e.g. cytochalasins A and E) which interact with cytoskeletal actin and as a result cause enhanced branching in the mycelia of *Achlya bisexualis* (HAROLD and HAROLD 1986) and *Aspergillus fumigatus* (VANDEN BOSSCHE, unpublished results), possibly as a result of disorganised chitin synthesis (NOVICK and BOTSTEIN 1985). The questions to be answered are, Are there differences between the cytoskeletal components of humans and pathogenic fungi to be exploited in the search for antifungal drugs, or will the selectivity of such drugs result from differences in their transport into cells? In this context it is interesting to note that after 3 decades as an oral antimycotic for treating patients suffering from dermatophytic infections, the mechanism by which griseofulvin enters sensitive cells is still unknown.

4. Exocellular Compounds Involved in Disease

Fungal toxins are important in food spoilage, but there is little evidence for any role in the development of infection. It is unlikely from the studies carried out so far that these compounds, in spite of their importance in food or as food contaminants, have a 'short-term role' in the establishment of infections. Nevertheless, it is important to assess their role and if they prove to be involved, to analyse their path of biosynthesis and investigate the possibility of inhibiting this process.

IV. Which Target?

The success of the beta-lactam antibiotics in treating patients with bacterial infections has conditioned many biochemists to thinking that the ideal antifungal drugs are inhibitors of cell wall synthesis. In this chapter we have endeavoured to emphasise the fact that this is not necessarily true, and one should not have preconceived ideas in the search for the 'perfect' target. All metabolic processes, provided they are essential for fungal growth, are possible targets. The only constraints are that the target be accessible to the drug and that at therapeutic concentrations it has no serious adverse effects on humans. In a patient suffering from a systemic infection, it may be sufficient merely to reduce the growth rate of the fungus, thus allowing the host's defence mechanisms to eliminate the pathogen. For immunocompromised patients, however, fungicidal drugs are clearly desirable if one wishes to avoid a recurrence of the infection after cessation of therapy.

Not all metabolic systems have the same potential as targets for therapeutic attack. There are complex systems in eukaryotic cells whose structures have been highly conserved during evolution. It may be difficult to select or develop suitable drugs which distinguish between such structures in humans and pathogenic fungi. This might explain the fact that there are no antifungal agents in clinical use which inhibit DNA replication, transcription or translation, even though there are many compounds which inhibit these processes in eukaryotic cells. If this is so, then attempts to develop inhibitors of nucleic acid or protein synthesis as clinically useful drugs may be doomed before studies are started. We have emphasised the importance of accessibility of the fungal target to the drug. The mechanisms of drug transport across the fungal plasma membrane are in many cases still not understood, although studies on multiple drug resistance in tumour cells are at a very exciting stage. In these cells resistance results from a transport protein in the membrane that actively excretes drugs from the cell. This is an area of research which could well pay dividends both in our understanding of drug transport and drug development.

So far we have considered the long-term approach involving basic biochemical research and have suggested the directions it might take. The biochemist must also be receptive to chance observations, however trivial, which might prove to be the lead required in the search for antifungal drugs. Unfortunately, there is no guarantee that the logical scientific approach we are advocating will be successful in providing us with the antifungal drugs we require in the immediate future, and possible short-term solutions cannot be neglected.

D. Short-Term Solutions to Antifungal Therapy

I. Combination Therapy

Combined drug therapy is of particular importance in bacterial infections but has not been extensively exploited for treating patients with mycoses. However, combinations of 5-fluorocytosine with amphotericin B have been used in, for example, the treatment of patients with chronic pulmonary aspergillosis (DUPONT and DROUHET 1988) or with cryptococcal meningitis (GRAYBILL et al. 1986; POLAK 1988). The literature is confusing, and there are conflicting reports of the interactions between antimycotic drugs both in vitro and in vivo. Difficulties have arisen in the interpretation of data largely due to variations in the techniques used for studying these complex systems. In spite of technical difficulties, this is an important area of research and one likely to produce results in a relatively short time. One particular line of study relates to the effects of amphotericin B on the uptake of other drugs. Amphotericin B (at concentrations lower than the MIC) can enhance the uptake of normally non-penetrating (and hence ineffective) compounds (MEDOFF 1988; KERRIDGE 1988). The mechanism by which this is achieved is not understood, and it is interesting to speculate how a drug whose primary effect is to dissipate the plasma membrane proton gradient can enhance the ability of the fungi to take up other drugs.

II. Drug Formulation

Although this is largely a matter for the pharmacist, the biochemist has a significant part to play in developing liposomal vesicles for targetted drug delivery. The activity of polyene macrolide antibiotics can be increased and their toxicity reduced by encapsulating them in liposomes (New et al. 1981; Taylor et al. 1982; Graybill et al. 1982; Lopez-Berestein et al. 1985; see also Chap. 10). Liposomes can also be targetted to particular organisms by labelling their surface layers with monoclonal antibodies (Barbet et al. 1981). This is the development of an old idea rather than the initiation of a novel approach to antifungal therapy.

Combined therapy and improvements in drug formulation are possible short-term panaceas and although worthy of study should not preclude the development of a longer term strategy.

E. Long-Term Developments

So far we have emphasised our belief that chemotherapy is an essay in comparative biochemisty and endeavoured to assess what has been gained from studies on the mode of action of antifungal drugs. We consider that the fundamental role of the biochemist is to study the metabolism of both host and fungal parasite and from the information gained select potential targets. Once possible targets have been identified the next problem is to select or design drugs which affect their functioning.

There have been significant advances in our understanding of the biochemisty of the growth and development of both fungal and mammalian cells. These have arisen as a result of major developments in investigative techniques. We have seen an explosion in our knowledge of molecular genetics resulting from the ability to clone genes, sequence DNA and indulge in site-directed mutations. From these and X-ray crystallographic studies the three-dimensional structure of target proteins and the nature of the active centre can be determined. Computer simulations can be used to study the molecular mechanisms of the interaction of existing drugs with these sites. This information could be used either to modify old drugs or to design new ones.

There have been major advances in the development of physical techniques for following drug metabolism by non-invasive procedures (NMR), for determining three-dimensional structures of cellular constituents (X-ray crystallography) and for studying the specific interactions of drugs with their targets (spectrophotometry). These have been used successfully to follow the metabolism of 5-fluorocytosine in *Candida* strains (Di Vito et al. 1986;

VIALANEIX et al. 1986) and to analyse the interactions of polyene macrolide antibiotics (BOLARD 1986) and synthetic azole drugs (YOSHIDA and AOYAMA 1986; VANDEN BOSSCHE et al. 1988b) with their specific cellular targets. These studies in conjunction with a potential rational design (RINGROSE 1985) of new antimycotic drugs might help in the future to provide the clinicians with the 'magic bullets' they require to counter any possible upsurge in fungal infections with equanimity.

References

Archer DB (1976) Effect of the lipid composition of *Mycoplasma mycoides* subspecies *capri* and phosphatidyl choline vesicles upon the action of polyene antibiotics. Biochim Biophys Acta 436:68–78

Bacchi CJ (1981) Content, synthesis, and function of polyamines in trypanosomatids: relationship to chemotherapy. J Protozool 28:20–27

Barbet J, Machy P, Leserman LD (1981) Monoclonal antibody covalently coupled to liposomes: specific targetting to cells. J Supramol Struct Cell Biochem 16:243–258

Barrett-Bee KJ, Lane AC, Turner RW (1986) The mode of antifungal action of tolnaftate. J Med Vet Mycol 24:155–160

Barug D, Samson RA, Kerkenaar A (1983) Microscopic studies of *Candida albicans* and *Torulopsis glabrata* after in vitro treatment with bifonazole. Arzneim Forsch 33:528–537

Becker JM, Covert NL, Shenbagamurthi P, Steinfeld AS, Naider F (1983) Polyoxin D inhibits growth of zoopathogenic fungi. Antimicrob Agents Chemother 23: 926–929

Becker JM, Marcus S, Tullock J, Miller D, Kramer E, Khare RK, Naider F (1988) Use of the chitin synthesis inhibitor nikkomycin to treat disseminated candidosis in mice. J Infect Dis 117:212–214

Berg D, Büchel K-H, Kramer W, Plempel M, Scheinpflug H (1988) Mechanistic studies as a tool for the development of new compounds. In: Berg D, Plempel M (eds) Sterol biosynthesis inhibitors. Pharmaceutical and agrochemical aspects. Ellis Horwood, Chichester, pp 169–184

Bloch KE (1983) Sterol structure and membrane function. Crit Rev Biochem 14: 47–92

Bolard J (1986) How do the polyene macrolide antibiotics affect the cellular membrane properties? Biochim Biophys Acta 864:257–302

Boiron P, Drouhet E, Dupont B, Improvisi L (1987) Entry of ketoconazole into *Candida albicans*. Antimicrob Agents Chemother 31:244–248

Bowman EJ, Siebers A, Altendorf K (1988) Bafilomycins: a class of inhibitors of membrane ATPases from microorganisms, animal cells and plant cells. Proc Natl Acad Sci USA 85:7972–7976

Boyle SM, Sriranganathan N, Cordes D (1988) Susceptibility of *Microsporum* and *Trichophyton* species to suicide inhibitors of polyamine biosynthesis. J Med Vet Mycol 26:227–235

Brasseur R, Vandenbosch C, Vanden Bossche H, Ruysschaert JM (1983) Mode of insertion of miconazole, ketoconazole and deacylated ketoconazole in lipid bilayers a conformational analysis. Biochem Pharmacol 32:2175–2180

Brian PW, Curtis PW, Fleming HG (1946) A substance causing abnormal development of fungal hyphae produced by *Penicillium griseo-fulvin* Dierckx. Trans Br Mycol Soc 32:30–33

Bulawa CE, Sleter M, Cabib E, Au-Young J, Sburlati A, Adair WL, Robins PW (1986) The *S. cerevisiae* structural gene for chitin synthase is not required for chitin synthesis in vivo. Cell 46:213–225

Burland TG, Gull K (1984) Molecular and cellular aspects of the interaction of benzimidazole fungicides with tubulin and microtubules. In: Trinci APJ, Ryley JF (eds) Mode of action of antifungal agents. Cambridge University Press, Cambridge, pp 299–230

Cabib E, Kang MS, Bowers B, Elango N, Mattia E, Slater ML, Au Young J (1984) Chitin synthesis in yeast, a vectorial process in the plasma membrane. In: Nombela C (ed) Microbial cell wall synthesis and autolysis. Elsevier, Amsterdam, pp 91–100

Cabib E, Bowers B, Sburlati A, Silverman SJ (1988) Fungal cell wall synthesis: the construction of a biological structure. Microbiol Sci. 5:370–375

Cassone A (1986a) Chitin synthesis, dimorphism and virulence in the pathogenic fungus *Candida albicans*. In: Mazzarelli A, Jeanimur C, Gooday GW (eds) Chitin in nature and technology. Plenum, New York, pp 71–78

Cassone A (1986b) Cell wall of pathogenic yeasts and implications for antimycotic therapy. Drugs Expt Clin Res 12:635–648

Cassone A, Mason RE, Kerridge D (1981) Lysis of growing yeast form cells of *Candida albicans* by echinocandin: a cytological study. Sabouraudia 19:97–110.

Cheron M, Cybulska B, Mazerski J, Grzybowska J, Czerwinski A, Borowski E (1988) Quantitative structure-activity relationships in amphotericin B derivatives. Biochem Pharmacol 37:827–836

Chiew YY, Shepherd MG, Sullivan PA (1980) Regulation of chitin synthesis during germ-tube formation in *Candida albicans*. Arch Microbiol 125:97–104

Chmara H, Andruszkiewicz R, Borowski E (1986) Inactivation of glucosamine-6-phosphate synthetase from *Salmonella typhimurium* LT2 by fumaroyl diaminopropanoic acid derivatives, a novel group of glutamine analogs. Biochim Biophys Acta 870:357–366

Cope JE (1980a) The porosity of the cell wall of *Candida albicans*. J. Gen Microbiol 119:253–255

Cope JE (1980b) Mode of action of miconazole on *Candida albicans*: effect on growth viability and K^+ release. J Gen Microbiol 119:245–251

Crosse R, McWilliam R, Rhodes A (1964) Some relations between chemical structure and antifungal effects of griseofulvin analogues. J Gen Microbiol 34:51–65

Davies RR (1980) Griseofulvin. In: Speller DCE (ed) Antifungal Chemotherapy. Wiley, Chichester, pp 149–182

Dahmen H, Hock HC, Staub T (1988) Differential effects of sterol inhibitors on growth, cell membrane permeability and ultrastructure of two target fungi. Phytopathology 78:1033–1042

De Clercq E (1985) Antiviral agents. Symp Soc Gen Microbiol 38:155–184

Dekker J (1984) Development of resistance to antifungal agents. In: Trinci APJ, Ryley JF (eds) Mode of action of antifungal drugs. Cambridge University Press, Cambridge, pp 89–111

Dekker J (1985) The development of resistance to fungicides. In: Hutson DH, Roberts TR (eds) Progress in pesticide biochemistry and toxicology. Wiley, Chichester, 4:165–218

De Waard MA, Fuchs A (1982) Resistance to ergosterol biosynthesis inhibitors. II Genetic and physiological aspects. In: Dekker J, Georgopoulos SG (eds) Fungicide resistance and crop protection. Pudoc Centre for Agricultural Publishing and Documentation, Wageningen, pp 87–100

Dimitriadis G, Hatziagelaki E, Ladias S, Linos A, Hillebrand I, Raptis S (1988) Effects of prolonged administration of two new alpha-glucosidase inhibitors on blood glucose control, insulin requirements and breath hydrogen excretion in patients with insulin-dependent diabetes mellitus. Eur J Clin Invest 18:33–38

Di Vito M, Podo F, Torosantucci A, Carpinelli G, Whelan WL, Kerridge D, Cassone A (1986) A ^{19}F nuclear magnetic resonance study of uptake and metabolism of 5-fluorocytosine in susceptible and resistant strains of *Candida albicans*. Antimicrob Agents Chemother 23:303–308

Dufour J-P, Boutry M, Goffeau A (1980) Plasma membrane ATPase of yeast. Comparative inhibition studies of the purified and membrane bound enzymes. J Biol Chem 255:5735–5741

Dupont B, Drouhet E (1988) The treatment of aspergillosis with azole derivatives. In: Vanden Bossche H, Mackenzie DWR, Cauwenbergh G (eds) *Aspergillus* and aspergillosis. Plenum, New York, pp 243–251

Duran A, Varona R, Perez P, Garcia-Acha I (1984) Biosynthesis of fungal wall β-glucan and its inhibition by antifungal agents. In: Nombela C (ed) Microbial cell wall synthesis and autolysis. Elsevier, Amsterdam, pp 297–306

Eddy AA (1982) Mechanisms of solute transport in selected eukaryotic microorganisms. Adv Microb Physiol 23:2–78

Edman JC, Kovacs JA, Masur H, Santi DV, Elwood HJ, Sogin ML (1988) Ribosomal RNA sequence shows *Pneumocystis carinii* to be a member of the fungi. Nature 334:519–522

Ehrlich P (1913) Address on pathology in chemotherapeutics: scientific principles, methods and results. Lancet ii:445–451

Elbein AD (1981) The tunicamycins – useful tools for studies on glycoproteins. TIBS 6:219–221

El Kouni MH, Cha S (1987) Metabolism of adenosine analogues by *Schistosoma mansoni* and the effect of nucleoside transport inhibitors. Biochem Pharmacol 36:1099–1106

El Kouni MH, Diop D, Cha S (1983) Combination therapy of schistosomiasis by tubercidin and nitrobenzylthioinosine 5′-monophosphate. Proc Natl Acad Sci USA 80:6667–6670

El Kouni MH, Knopf PM, Cha A (1985) Combination therapy of *Schistosoma japonicum* by tubercidin and nitrobenzylthioinosine 5′-monophosphate. Biochem Pharmacol 34:3921–3923

Ellul H, Beezer AE, Brain APR, Miles RJ, Sivayogan SR (1985) The effect of chemical modification of *Saccharomyces cerevisiae* on electrophoretic mobility, cell wall structure and amphotericin B uptake. Biochim Biophys Acta 845: 151–157

El-Nakeeb MA, Lampen JO (1965) Uptake of ^{3}H-griseofulvin by microorganisms and its correlation with sensitivity to griseofulvin. J Gen Microbiol 39:285–293

Emmer G, Ryder NS, Grassberger MA (1985) Synthesis of new polyoxin derivatives and their activity against chitin synthase from *Candida albicans*. J Med Chem 28:278–281

Farkas V (1979) Biosynthesis of cell walls of fungi. Microbiol Rev 43:117–144

Fink W, Liefland M, Mendgen K (1988) Chitinases and β-1-3-glucanases in the apoplastic compartment of oat leaves (*Avena sativa*). Plant Physiol 88:270–275

Fleet G (1985) Composition and structure of the yeast cell wall. In: McGinnis MR (ed) Current topics in medical mycology. Springer, Berlin Heidelberg New York, 1:24–56

Forêt M, Schmidt R, Reichert W (1978) On the mechanism of substrate binding to the purine-transport system of *Saccharomyces cerevisiae*. Eur J Biochem 82:33–43

Fuhrmann U, Bause E, Ploegh M (1985) Inhibitors of oligosaccharide processing. Biochim Biophys Acta 825:95–110

Furter R, Rast DM (1985) A comparison of the chitin synthase EC 2.4.1.16. Inhibitory and antifungal efficacy of nucleoside-peptide antibiotics: structure activity relationships. FEMS Lett 28:205–212

Gale EF (1986) Nature and development of phenotypic resistance to amphotericin B in *Candida albicans*. Adv Microbiol Physiol 27:278–320

Gale EF, Johnson AM, Kerridge D, Wayman FJ (1980) Phenotypic resistance to miconazole and amphotericin B in *Candida albicans*. J Gen Microbiol 117: 525–528

Gale EF, Cundliffe E, Reynolds PE, Richmond MH, Waring MJ (1981) The molecular basis of antibiotic action, 2nd edn Wiley, New York

Gooday GW (1977) Biosynthesis of the fungal wall. Mechanisms and implications. J Gen Microbiol 99:1–11

Gooday GW, Brydon LJ, Chappel LH (1988) Chitinase in *Onchocerca* and its inhibition by alllosamidin. Trop Med Parasitol 39:76

Gordee RS, Zeckner DJ, Ellis LF, Thakkar AL, Howard LC (1984) In vitro and in vivo anti-*Candida* activity of LY121019. J Antibiot 37:1054–1064
Gottesman MM, Pastan I (1988a) The multidrug transporter, a double edged sword. J Biol Chem 263:12163–12166
Gottesman MM, Pastan I (1988b) Resistance to multiple chemotherapeutic agents in human cancer cells. TIPS 9:54–58
Graybill JR (1988) A history of the treatment of aspergillosis. In: Vanden Bossche H, Mackenzie DWR, Cauwenbergh G (eds) *Aspergillus* and aspergillosis. Plenum, New York, pp 229–242
Graybill JR, Craven PC, Taylor RL, Williams DM, Magee WE (1982) Treatment of murine cryptococcosis with liposomes associated with amphotericin B. J Infect Dis 145:748–752
Graybill JR, Stevens D, Galgiani J, Dismukes W (1986) Recent developments in the treatment of fungal meningitis. In: Iwata K, Vanden Bossche H (eds) In vitro and in vivo evaluations of antifungal agents. Elsevier, Amsterdam, pp 259–270
Guentzel MN, Cole GT, Pope LM (1985) Animal models for candidiasis. In McGinnis MR (ed) Current topics in medical mycology. Springer, Berlin Heidelberg New York, 1:57–116
Hall GS, Myles C, Pratt KJ, Washington JA (1988) Cilofungin (LY121019), an antifungal agent with specific activity against *Candida albicans* and *Candida tropicalis*. Antimicrob Agents Chemother 32:1331–1335
Harold RL, Harold FM (1986) Ionophores and cytochalasin modulate branching in *Achlya bisexualis*. J Gen Microbiol 132:213–219
Hilenski LL, Naider F, Becker JM (1986) Polyoxin D inhibits colloidal gold-wheat germ agglutinin labelling of chitin in dimorphic forms of *Candida albicans*. J Gen Microbiol 132:1441–1451
Hitchcock CA, Barrett-Bee KJ, Russell NJ (1986) The lipid composition of azole sensitive and azole resistant strains of *Candida albicans*. J Gen Microbiol 132:2421–2431
Iwata K, Yamaguchi H, Hiratani T (1973) Mode of action of clotrimazole. Sabouraudia 11:158–166
Janssen PAJ, Vanden Bossche H (1987) Mode of action of cytochrome P-450 monooxygenase inhibitors. Focus on azole derivatives. Arch Pharm Chem Sci Ed 15:23–40
Kenig M. Abraham EP (1976) Antimicrobial activities and antagonists of bacilysin and anticapsin. J Gen Microbiol 94:37–46
Kerkenaar A (1987) The mode of action of dimethylmorphilines. In: Fromtling RA (ed) Recent trends in the discovery, development and evaluation of antifungal agents. JR Prous, Barcelona, pp 523–542
Kerridge D (1986) Mode of action of clinically important antifungal drugs. Adv Microbiol Physiol 27:1–72
Kerridge D (1988) Polyene macrolide antibiotics. In: Vanden Bossche H, Mackenzie DWR, Cauwenbergh G (eds) *Aspergillus* and aspergillosis. Plenum, New York, pp 147–160
Kerridge D, Nicholas RO, Wayman FJ (1987) Resistance to clinically important antimycotic drugs in *Candida* spp. Ann 1st Supr Sanita 23:827–834
Kobayashi GS, Medoff G, Maresca B, Sacco M, Kumar BV (1985) Studies on the phase transition in the dimorphic pathogen *Histoplasma capsulatum*. In: Szaniszlo PJ (ed) Fungal dimorphism, with emphasis on fungi pathogenic for humans. Plenum, New York, pp 69–91
Koga D, Isogai A, Sakuda S, Matsumoato S, Suzuki A, Kimura S, Ide A (1987) Specific inhibition of *Bombyx mori* chitinase by allosamidin. Agric Biol Chem 51:471–476
Koh TY, Marriott MS, Taylor J, Gale EF (1977) Growth characteristics and polyene sensitivity of a fatty acid auxotroph of *Candida albicans*. J Gen Microbiol 102: 105–110
Kombrink E, Schroder M, Hahlbrock K (1988) Several 'pathogenesis-related' proteins

in potato are 1,3-β-glucanases and chitinases. Proc Natl Acad Sci USA 85: 782–786

Langcake P, Kuhn PJ, Wade M (1983) The mode of action of systemic fungicides. In: Hutson DH, Roberts TR (eds) Progress in pesticide biochemistry and toxicology. Wiley, Chichester, 3:1–109

Lichliter WD, Naider F, Becker JM (1976) Basis for the design of anticandidal agents from studies of peptide utilization in *Candida albicans*. Antimicrob Agents Chemother 10:483–490

Lombardi G, Padhye AA, Ajello L (1988) In vitro conversion of African isolates of *Blastomyces dermatitidis* to their yeast form. Mycoses 31:447–450

Lopez-Berestein G, Fainstein V, Hopfer R, Mehta K, Sullivan MP, Keating M, Rosenblum MG, Mehta R, Luna M, Hersh E, Reuben J, Juliano RL, Bodey GP (1985) Liposomal amphotericin B for the treatment of systemic fungal infections in patients with cancer: a preliminary study. J Infect Dis 151:704–710

Lürssen K (1988) Triazole plant growth regulators: effects and mode of action. In: Berg D, Plempel M (eds) Sterol biosynthesis inhibitors. Pharmaceutical and agrochemical aspects. Ellis Horwood, Chichester, pp 305–331

Mamont PS, Duchesne M-C, Grove J, Bey P (1978) Anti-proliferative properties of DL-α-difluoromethylornithine in cultured cells. A consequence of the irreversible inhibition of ornithine decarboxylase. Biochim Biophys Res Commun 81:58–66

Marichal P, Gorrens J, Vanden Bossche H (1985) The action of itraconazole and ketoconazole on growth and sterol synthesis in *Aspergillus fumigatus* and *Aspergillus niger*. J Med Vet Mycol 23:13–21

Mason JI, Carr BR, Murray BA (1987) Imidazole antimycotics: selective inhibitors of steroid aromatization and progesterone hydroxylation. Steroids 50:180–189

Mauch F, Mauch-Mani B, Boller T (1988) Antifungal hydrolases in pea tissue II. Inhibition of fungal growth by combinations of chitinases and β-1-3-glucanase. Plant Physiol 88:936–942

McCann PP, Bacchi CJ, Hanson CJ, Cain GD, Nathan HC, Hutner SH, Sjoerdsma A (1981) Effect on parasitic protozoa of α-difluromethylornithine, an inhibitor of ornithine decarboxylase. In: Caldara CM, Zappia V, Bachrach U (eds) Advances in polyamine research. Raven, New York, 3:97–110

McCann PP, Bacchi CJ, Clarkson AB, Bey P, Sjoerdsma A, Schecter PJ, Walzer PD, Barlow JLR (1986) Inhibition of polyamine synthesis by α-difluoromethylornithine in African trypanosomes and *Pneumocystis carinii* as a basis of chemotherapy: biochemical and clinical aspects. Am J Trop Med Hyg 35:1153–1156

Medoff G (1988) The mechanism of action of amphotericin B. In: Vanden Bossche H, Mackenzie DWR, Cauwenbergh G (eds) *Aspergillus* and aspergillosis. Plenum, New York, pp 161–164

Mercer EI (1988) The mode of action of morpholines. In: Berg D, Plempel M (eds) Sterol biosynthesis inhibitors. Pharmaceutical and agrochemical aspects. Ellis Horwood, Chichester, pp 120–150

Morin RB, Gorman M (eds) (1982) Chemistry and biology of β-lactam antibiotics. Academic, New York

Müller H, Furter R, Zahner H, Rast DM (1981) Metabolic products of microorganisms, Inhibition of chitosomal chitin synthetase and growth of *Mucor rouxii* by nikkomycin Z, nikkomycin X and polyoxin A; a comparison. Arch Microbiol 130:195–197

Müller J, Scheidecker I (1988) Immunoelectronmicroscopic studies on the influence of an echinocandin B analog on the cell wall antigenicity of *Candida albicans*. Proc Xth Congress of the Int Soc Hum An Mycol, p 152

Nes WR, Dhanuka IC (1988) Inhibition of sterol synthesis by Δ5-sterol in a sterol auxotroph of yeast defective in oxidosqualene cyclase and cytochrome P-450. J Biol Chem 263:11844–11850

New RRC, Chance ML, Heath S (1981) Antileishmanial activity of amphotericin and other antifungal agents entrapped in liposomes. J Antimicrob Chemother 8: 371–382

Nombela C, Molina M, Cenamor R, Sanchez M (1988) Yeast β-glucanases: a complex sytem of secreted enzymes. Microbiol Sci 5:328–332

Notario V (1982) β-glucanases from *Candida albicans*: purification characterisation and nature of their attachment to cell wall components. J Gen Microbiol 128: 747–759

Notario V, Kawai H, Cabib E (1982) Interaction between yeast β (1–3) glucan synthetase and activating phosphorylated compounds. A kinetic study. J Biol Chem 257:1902–1905

Novick P, Botstein D (1985) Phenotypic analysis of temperature-sensitive yeast actin mutants. Cell 40:405–416

Odds FC (1986) Morphogenesis in *Candida albicans*. CRC Crit Rev Microbiol 12: 45–93

Odds FC (1988) Candida and candidosis, 2nd edn Baillière Tindall, London

Orlean PAB (1982) (1,3)-β-D-Glucan synthase from budding and filamentous cultures of the dimorphic fungus *Candida albicans*. Eur J Biochem 127:397–403

Orlean PAB (1987) Two chitin synthases in *Saccharomyces cerevisiae*. J Biol Chem 262:5732–5739

Palacios J, Serrano R (1978) Proton permeability induced by polyene antibiotics. A plausible mechanism for their inhibition of maltose fermentation in yeast. FEBS Lett 91:198–201

Parodi AJ (1981) Biosynthetic mechanisms for cell envelope polysaccharides. In: Arnold WN (ed) Yeast cell envelopes: biochemistry, biophysics and ultrastructure. CRC Press, Boca Raton, II:47–64

Patiño MM, Burgos LC, Restrepo A (1984) Effect of temperature on the mycelium to yeast transformation of *Paracoccidioides brasiliensis*. J Med Vet Mycol 22: 509–511

Petranyi G, Ryder NS, Stütz A (1984) Allylamine derivatives: new class of synthetic antifungal agents inhibiting fungal squalene epoxidase. Science 224:1239–1241

Pfaller MA, Gerarden T, Riley J (1987) Growth inhibition of pathogenic yeast isolates by α-difluoromethylornithine: an inhibitor of ornithine decarboxylase. Mycopathologia 98:3–8

Pfaller MA, Riley J, Gerarden T (1988) Polyamine depletion and growth inhibition in *Candida albicans* and *Candida tropicalis* by α-difluormethylornithine and cyclohexylamine. J Med Vet Mycol 26:119–126

Polak A-M (1988) Combination therapy with antifungal drugs. Mycoses 31 (Suppl 2):45–53

Polak A-M, Grenson M (1973) Evidence for a common transport system for cytosine, adenine and hypoxanthine in *Saccharomyces cerevisiae* and *Candida albicans*. Eur J Biochem 32:276–282

Portillo F, Gancedo C (1984) Mode of action of miconazole on yeasts: inhibition of the mitochondrial ATPase. Eur J Biochem 143:273–276

Rajam MV, Weistein LH, Galston AW (1985) Prevention of a plant disease by specific inhibition of fungal polyamine biosynthesis. Proc Natl Acad Sci USA 82: 6874–6878

Rast DM, Bartnicki-Garcia S (1981) Effects of amphotericin B, nystatin and other polyene antibiotics on chitin synthase. Proc Natl Acad Sci USA 78:1233–1236

Reynolds PE (1985) Inhibitors of bacterial cell wall synthesis. Symp Soc Gen Microbiol 38:13–40

Ringrose PS (1985) Warhead delivery and suicide substrates as concepts in antimicrobial drug design. Symp Soc Gen Microbiol 38:219–266

Rodriguez RJ, Low C, Bottema CDK, Parks LW (1985) Multiple functions for sterols in *Saccharomyces cerevisiae*. Biochim Biophys Acta 837:336–343

Rosenfeld A (1988) Some of a body's crucial functions are only skin deep. Smithsonian (May): 159–180

Ryder NS (1984) Selective inhibition of squalene epoxidation by allylamine antimycotic agents. In: Nombela C (ed) Microbial cell wall synthesis and autolysis. Elsevier, Amsterdam, pp 313–321

Ryder NS (1985) Specific inhibition of fungal sterol biosynthesis by SF-86-327, a new allylamine antimycotic agent. Antimicrob Agents Chemother 17:252–256
Ryder NS, Dupont MC (1985) Inhibition of squalene epoxidase by allylamine antimycotic compounds. Biochem J 230:765–770
Ryder NS, Dupont MC, Frank I (1986) Ergosterol biosynthesis inhibition by the thiocarbamate antifungal agents tolnaftate and tolciclate. Antimicrob Agents Chemother 29:858–860
Ryley JF, Wilson RG, Gravestock MB, Poyser JP (1981) Experimental approaches to antifungal chemotherapy. Adv Pharmacol Chemother 18:49–176
Ryley JF, Wilson RG, Barrett-Bee KJ (1984) Azole resistance in *Candida albicans*. Sabouraudia: J Med Vet Mycol 22:53–63
Sakuda S, Isogai A, Matsumoto S, Suzuki A, Koseki K (1986) The structure of allosamidin, a novel insect chitinase inhibitor, produced by *Streptomyces* sp. Tetrahedron Lett 27:2475–2478
San-Blas F, San-Blas G (1985) *Paracoccidioides brasiliensis*. In: Szaniszlo PJ (ed) Fungal dimorphism with emphasis on fungi pathogenic for humans. Plenum, New York, pp 93–120
San-Blas G (1985) *Paracoccidioides brasiliensis*: cell wall glucans, pathogenicity and dimorphism. In: McGinnis MR (ed) Current topics in medical mycology. Springer, New York, 1:235–257
San-Blas G, San-Blas F (1983) Molecular aspects of fungal dimorphism. CRC Crit Rev Microbiol 11:101–127
Santen RJ, Vanden Bossche H, Symoens J, Brugmans J, DeCoster R (1983) Site of action of low dose ketoconazole on androgen biosynthesis in men. J Clin Endocrinol Metab 57:732–736
Sawistowska-Schröder ET, Kerridge D, Perry H (1984) Echinocandin inhibition of 1,3-β-D-glucan synthase from *Candida albicans*. FEBS Lett 173:134–138
Sburlati A, Cabib E (1986) Chitin synthase 2, a presumptive participant in septum formation in *S. cerevisiae*. J Biol Chem 261:15147–15152
Schaffner CP (1987) Amphotericin B derivatives. In: Fromtling RA (ed) Recent trends in the discovery, development and evaluation of antifungal agents. JR Prous, Barcelona, pp 595–618
Schekman R (1982) The secretory pathway in yeast. TIBS 7:243–246
Schekman R (1985) Protein localization and membrane traffic in yeast. Ann Rev Cell Biol 1:115–143
Scholer HJ (1980) Flucytosine. In: Speller DCE (ed) Antifungal chemotherapy. Wiley, Chichester, pp 35–106
Shematek EM, Bratz JA, Cabib E (1980) Biosynthesis of the yeast cell wall. I Preparation and properties of β-(1–3) glucan synthetase. J Biol Chem 255: 888–894
Shepherd MG (1987) Cell envelope of *Candida albicans*. CRC Crit Rev Microbiol 15:7–26
Shepherd MG, Suratti R, Gopal PK, Sullivan PA (1984) Cell wall metabolism of *C. albicans* β-(1–3) and β-(1–6) glucan synthesis. In: Nombela C (ed) Microbial cell wall synthesis and autolysis. Elsevier, Amsterdam, pp 73–83
Sloboda RD, Van Blaricom G, Creasey WA, Rosenbaum JL, Malewista SE (1982) Griseofulvin: association with tubulin and inhibition of in vitro microtubule assembly. Biochem Biophys Res Commun 105:882–888
Smith H (1985) The chemotherapeutic potential of inhibition or circumvention of the determinants of microbial pathogenicity. Symp Soc Gen Microbiol 38:363–393
Stütz A (1987) Allylamine derivatives – a new class of active substances in antifungal chemotherapy. Angew Chem int Ed Engl 26:120–128
Surarit R, Shepherd MG (1987) The effects of azole and polyene antifungals on the plasma membrane enzymes of *Candida albicans*. J Med Vet Mycol 22:403–413
Szaniszlo PJ (1985) Fungal dimorphism with emphasis on fungi pathogenic for humans. Plenum, New York
Taft CS, Selitrennikoff CP (1988) LY121019 inhibits *Neurospora crassa* growth and (1–3)-β-D-glucan synthase. J Antibiot 51:697–701

Taft CS, Stark T, Selitrennikoff CP (1988) Cilofungin (LY121019) inhibits *Candida albicans* (1–3)-β-D-glucan synthase activity. Antimicrob Agents Chemother 32: 1901–1903.

Taylor RL, Williams DM, Craven PC, Graybill JR, Drutz DJ, Magee WE (1982) Amphotericin B in liposomes: a novel therapy for histoplasmosis. Am Rev Resp Dis 125:610–611

Trinci APJ (1984) Antifungal agents which affect hyphal extension and hyphal branching. In: Trinci APJ, Ryley JF (eds) Mode of action of antifungal agents. Cambridge University Press, Cambridge, pp 113–134

Trinci APJ, Ryley JF (eds) (1984) Mode of action of antifungal agents. Symp Br Mycol Soc 9. Cambridge University Press, Cambridge

Tyms AS, Taylor DL (1988) Activity of glucosidase inhibitors against HIV infections. J Antimicrob Chemother 22:271–274

Tyms AS, Williamson JD, Bacchi CJ (1988) Polyamine inhibitors in antimicrobial chemotherapy. J Antimicrob Chemother 22:403–427

Vance D, Goldberg I, Mitsuhashi O, Bloch K (1972) Inhibition of fatty acid synthesis by the antibiotic cerulenin. Biochem Biophys Res Comm 48:649–656

Vanden Bossche H (1974) Biochemical effects of miconazole on fungi 1. Effects on the uptake and/or utilisation of purines, pyrimidines, amino acids and glucose by *Candida albicans*. Biochem Pharmacol 26:887–899

Vanden Bossche H (1985) Biochemical targets for antifungal azole derivatives: hypothesis on the mode of action. In: McGinnis MK (ed) Current topics in medical mycology. Springer, Berlin Heidelberg New York, 1:313–351

Vanden Bossche H (1988) Mode of action of pyridine, pyrimidine and azole antifungals. In: Berg D, Plempel M (eds) Sterol biosynthesis inhibitors. Pharmaceutical and agrochemical aspects. Ellis Horwood, Chichester, pp 79–119

Vanden Bossche H, Janssen PAJ (1987) Biological activities of cytochrome P-450. In: Benford DJ, Bridges JW, Gibson GG (eds) Drug metabolism – from molecules to man. Taylor and Francis, London, pp 244–262

Vanden Bossche H, Ruysschaert JM, Defrise-Quertain F, Willemsens G, Cornelissen F, Marichal P, Cools W, Van Cutsem J (1982) The interaction of miconazole and ketoconazole with lipids. Biochem Pharmacol 32:2175–2180

Vanden Bossche H, Lauwers W, Willemsens G, Cools W (1985) The cytochrome P-450 dependent C17,20-lyase in subcellular fractions of the rat testis: differences in sensitivity to ketoconazole and itraconazole. In: Boobis AR, Caldwell J, De Matteis F, Elcombe CR (eds) Microsomes and drug oxidations. Taylor & Francis, London, pp 63–73

Vanden Bossche H, Marichal P, Gorrens J, Bellens D, Berhoeven H, Coene M-C, Lauwers W, Janssen PAJ (1987a) Interaction of azole derivatives with cytochrome P-450 isozymes in yeast, fungi, plants, and mammalian cells. Pestic Sci 21:289–306

Vanden Bossche H, Willemsens G, Marichal P (1987b) Anti-*Candida* drugs – the biochemical basis for their action. CRC Crit Rev Microbiol 15:57–72

Vanden Bossche H, Marichal P, Geerts H, Janssen PAJ (1988a) The molecular basis for itraconazole's activity against *Aspergillus fumigatus*. In: Vanden Bossche H,Mackenzie DWR, Cauwenbergh G (eds) *Aspergillus* and aspergillosis. Plenum, New York pp 171–197

Vanden Bossche H, Marichal P, Gorrens J, Geerts H, Janssen PAJ (1988b) Mode of action studies – basis for the search for new antifungals. Ann N Y Acad Sci 544:191–207

Vialaneix JP, Chamini N, Malet-Martino MC, Martino R, Michel G, Lepargneur JP (1986) Noninvasive and quantitative ^{19}F nuclear magnetic resonance study of flucytosine metabolism in *Candida* strains. Antimicrob Agents Chemother 30:756–762

Villaneuva JR, Notario V, Santos T, Villa TG (1976) β Glucanases in nature. Biochemistry and function of β-glucanases in yeast. In: Peberdy JF, Rose AH, Rogers HJ, Cocking EC (eds) Microbial and plant protoplasts. Academic, London, pp 323–355

Wang CC (1984) Parasite enzymes as potential targets for antiparasitic chemotherapy. J Med Chem 27:1–9

Wilson L (1975) Action of drugs on microtubules. Life Sciences 17:303–310

Yadan J-C, Gonneau M, Sarthou P, Le Goffic F (1984) Sensitivity to nikkomycin Z in *Candida albicans*: role of peptide permeases. J Bacteriol 160:884–888

Yamamoto H (1985) Development of validamycin, its controlling effect on rice sheath blight. Jap Pest Inform 47:17–22

Yoshida Y (1988) Cytochrome P450 of fungi: primary target for azole antifungal agents. In: McGinnis MR (ed) Current topics in medical mycology. Springer Berlin Heidelberg New York, 2:388–418

Yoshida Y, Aoyama Y (1986) Interaction of azole fungicides with yeast cytochrome P-450 which catalyzes lanosterol 14 α-demethylation. In: Iwata K, Vanden Bossche H (eds) In vitro and in vivo evaluation of antifungal agents. Elsevier, Amsterdam, pp 123–134

Yoshida Y, Aoyama Y (1987) Interaction of azole antifungal agents with cytochrome P-450 14DM purified from *Saccharomyces cerevisiae* microsomes. Biochem Pharmacol 36:229–235

CHAPTER 3

Drug Discovery: Nature's Approach

MANUEL DEBONO and ROBERT S. GORDEE

A. Introduction

The emergence of immune deficiency diseases, such as AIDS or those that arise from the use of antitumor and organ transplantation regimens, has resulted in major increases in serious fungal infections. Amphotericin B remains the standard treatment of systemic mycoses, but its use is limited by severe toxic properties which make it imperative that safer and more effective therapies be found. Natural products, especially antibiotics from fermentation sources, have played a key role in the search for therapeutically useful drugs. Microorganisms such as the actinomycetes, isolated and cultured from the soil, have provided many useful antimicrobial agents with a wide spectrum of action. However, only a small number of antifungal agents have been discovered using these techniques. This is attributed to the difficulty of finding compounds that are selectively toxic to the eukaryotic fungal cell without causing damage to mammalian cells. Herein we will cover some of the current research in the discovery and evaluation of new antifungal agents from natural sources, and also the current methodology used in their biological evaluation as potential clinical candidates. In addition, a survey of recent natural products with antimycotic activity obtained from both soil screening and marine sources is included. Though not covered in this report, there has been recent interest in higher plants as sources of new structural prototypes for antifungal agents (CLARK et al. 1987). Although the soil screen remains a major route for the discovery of new antifungal agents, intensive efforts have been undertaken to develop new methods for screening based upon mode of action. These mechanism-based tests may provide important alternatives to the more direct but capricious screen based on broth or agar dilution.

Although unmodified natural products have provided few therapeutically useful agents, a number of these have been valuable tools for the study of important biochemical functions in the fungal cell. Biochemical targets such as the fungal cell wall have been identified for use in discovering new antifungal agents. Natural products with antimycotic activity provide valuable structure-activity relationships as a basis for rational syntheses of new analogues or derivatives This point is illustrated by the conversion of echinocandin B (ECB) (1) to cilofungin (2), a new semisynthetic anti-*Candida* agent, currently undergoing clinical evaluation (DEBONO et al. 1989). Other examples include modification of the papulacandins and the chitin synthase inhibitors, polyoxin and nikkomycin (TRAXLER et al. 1987; SHENBAGAMURTHI et al. 1983; SMITH et al. 1986; FIANDOR et al. 1987).

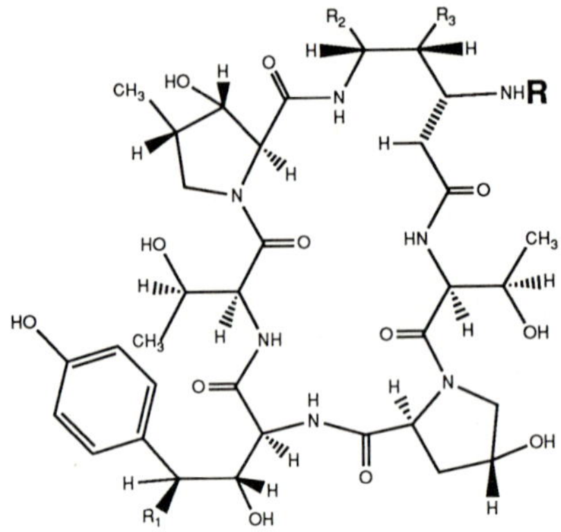

	Echinocandin	R	R_1	R_2	R_3
1:	B	Linoleoyl	OH	OH	OH
	C	Linoleoyl	H	OH	OH
	D	Linoleoyl	H	H	H
2:	Cilofungin	n-Octyloxybenzoyl	OH	OH	OH
3:	Aculeacin A	Palmitoyl	OH	OH	OH

B. Sources of Samples for Screening

I. Soil

Since Alexander Fleming's serendipitous discovery of penicillin, microbiologists have been involved with the systematic search for antibiotic-producing organisms (ABRAHAM 1983). The work of WAKSMAN (1937, 1941, 1947) and others showed the actinomycetes and other microorganisms to be excellent sources of substances with interesting biological activities (NOLAN and CROSS 1988). The need to isolate and screen antibiotic-producing organisms from a vast population for novel biological activities requires highly systematized methods designed to minimize rediscovery. The design of such a process varies with the focus and priorities of a given research group. For the purpose of the present discussion a simplified form of the screening or 'discovery' process is presented in Fig. 1. This scheme does not include steps required for cross-checking observations and repetition of certain tests, which add substantially to the labor-intensive nature of this process.

CULTURE ISOLATION FROM SOIL SAMPLE (SELECTIVE CONDITIONS)

↓

FERMENTATION (MEDIA AND INCUBATION VARIATION)

↓

ISOLATION OF FERMENTATION SAMPLES

↓ samples include whole broths, filtrates, mycelial extracts, etc.

IN VITRO AND IN VIVO SCREENING OF FERMENTATION SAMPLES

↓ samples screened for antifungal, antibacterial, antitumor, antiviral, selected enzyme inhibition, etc.

SAMPLES WITH NOVEL ANTIBIOTIC ACTIVITY

↓ direct comparison with antibiotic standards by chromatographic, physical or chemical means

ISOLATION AND STRUCTURE DETERMINATION OF NOVEL AGENTS

↓

ADVANCED BIOLOGICAL EVALUATION OF NOVEL AGENTS

mode of action, toxicology,

animal models, pharmacokinetics, etc.

Fig. 1. General method for screening soil samples for discovery of biologically active agents

The discovery procedure based on the soil screen has at least seven basic parts (Berdy 1985). A suspension of a soil sample, chosen from collections representing a wide variety of geographic and environmental locales, is used to seed agar plates from which single colonies of microorganisms are isolated for study as potential antibiotic producers. Single colonies are selected from inoculated plates and regrown to test for production of biologically interesting products. Media choice and culture conditions provide a wider range of options that broaden or restrict the numbers and types of organisms isolated. These factors aid in minimizing the rediscovery rate of antimicrobial agents.

Screening procedures have become increasingly more complex. Introduction of a variety of selective pressures such as antibiotic resistance, soil pretreatment by dry heat, selective growth media, and variable incubation periods limit the repetitive isolation of the same culture types (IWAI and OMURA 1982). Selective pressures increase isolation of organisms which could not otherwise grow. Some laboratories concentrate their efforts on taxonomically defined rare actinomycetes such as *Actinoplanes*, *Actinomadura*, and *Micromonospora*. However, it has often been the case that these organisms have produced structural types available from more common, robust organisms.

The primary test for antimicrobial activity is a direct lethal effect on the test organism (WAKSMAN and LECHEVALIER 1962). An agar diffusion-based test using *Candida albicans* and *Aspergillus* sp. is commonly used for antifungal screening. A solution of a test compound or fermentation broth is dispersed into agar wells. After 24–48 h incubation the zone of inhibition is measured (12-mm zone minimum) as an indication of antifungal activity. *Neurospora* and *Saccharomyces* species are also used as test organisms for antifungal screening. Current trends in screening for bioactive natural products include more selective tests based on an essential enzymatic target or use of hypersensitive organisms (OKAMI and HOTTA 1988). These methods facilitate the discovery of antibiotics produced at low levels, increase the numbers of cultures examined, and focus discovery on specific modes of action. They have begun to revolutionize antibacterial screening and have recently begun to be utilized in the antifungal field.

A successful screening program is predicated on the ability to identify new, biologically active, natural products while eliminating rediscovery of known compounds. Chromatographic behavior serves as an important 'fingerprint' for dereplication. Comparisons with known compounds can be facilitated by automated techniques involving robotics, microtiter methods, and liquid chromatography (LC)-mass spectrometry. Such techniques have been reported in the identification of fermentation products having antitumor activity (HOOK et al. 1987).

New antibiotics with interesting properties become candidates for isolation and purification. Advances in isolation techniques such as high pressure liquid chromatography (HPLC), coupled with major advances in mass spectrometry, NMR, and X-ray crystallography have resulted in increased efficency in purification of complex mixtures and structure determination. As a result, increasingly complex molecules have been isolated. These same techniques have allowed rational structural modification to be performed with greater ease.

Table 1. Recently discovered antifungal antibiotics

Name Producing organism	Structure	Reference
Mulundocandin *Aspergillus sydowi*	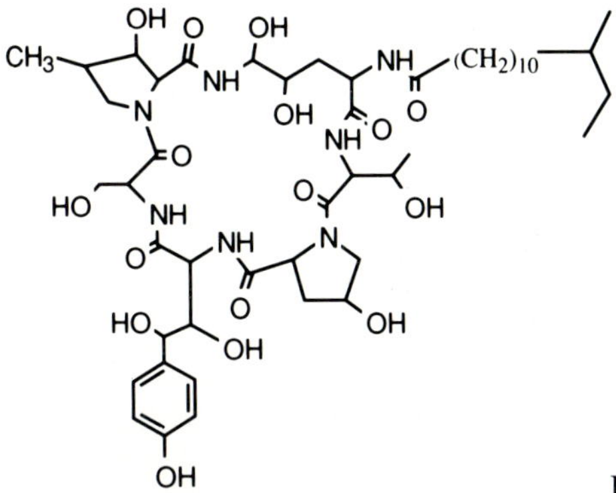	Roy et al. (1987b)
L-671,329 *Zalerion arboricola*	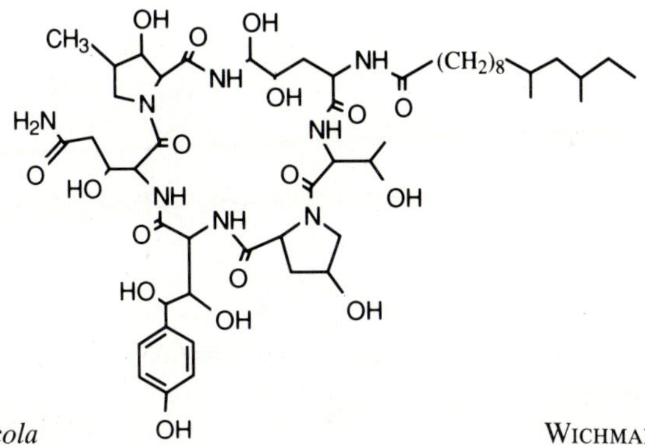	Wichmann et al. (1989)
Fumifungin *Aspergillus fumigatus* Y-83,0405	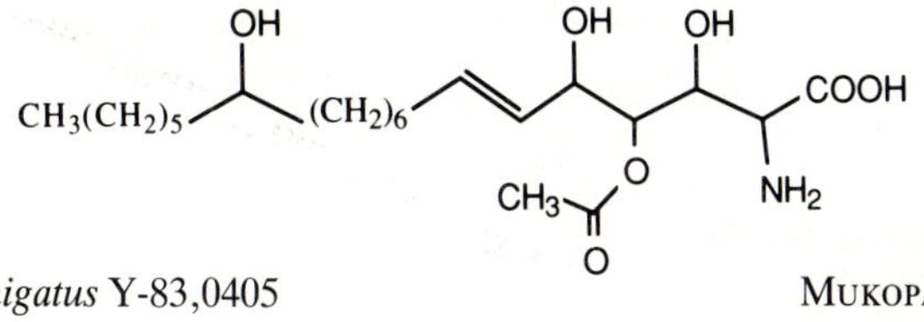	Mukopadhyay (1987b)

Table 1. (continued)

Name Producing organism	Structure	Reference
Catacandins *Lysobacter gummosus*	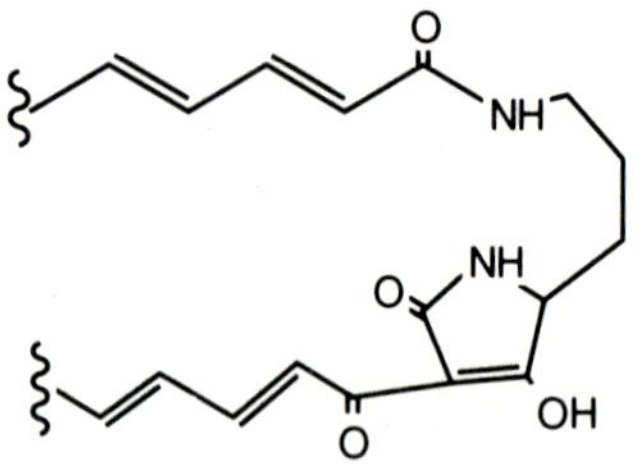 (Partial structure)	MEYERS et al. (1985)
Iturins *Bacillus subtilis*	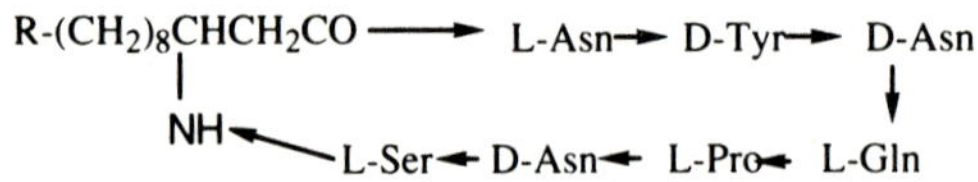	BESSON and MICHEL (1987)
Arginomycin *Streptomyces arginensis* NRRL 15941	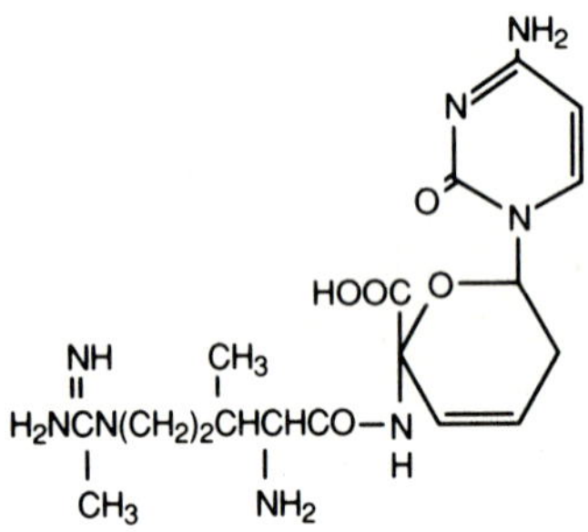	ARGOUDELIS et al. (1987)
Neoenactin B_1 *Streptoverticillium olivoreticuli* subsp. neoenacticus	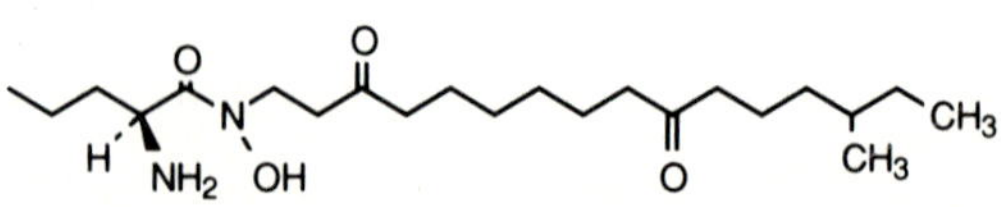	ROY et al. (1987a)

Table 1. (continued)

Name Producing organism	Structure	Reference
Neopeptin A *Streptomyces* sp. K-710	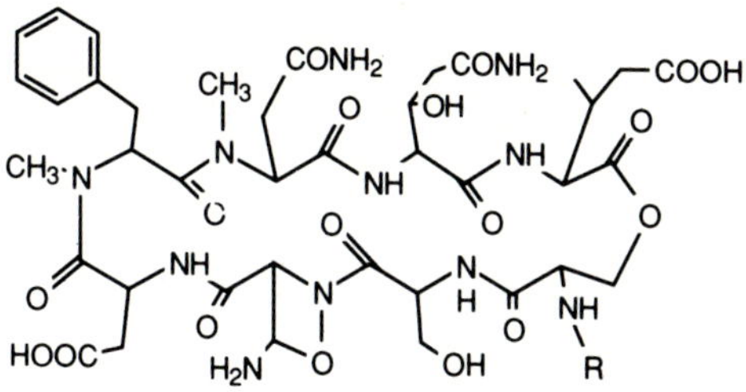 R = 12-Methyltridecanoyl	UBUKATA et al. (1984)
Leptomycin *Streptomyces* sp. ATS1287	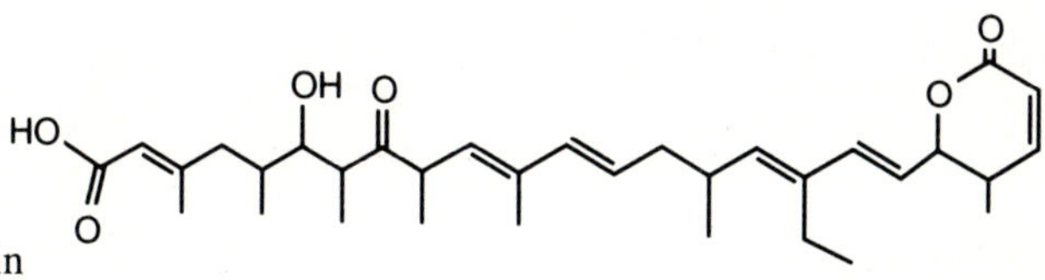	HAMAMOTO et al. (1983)
Chaetiacandin *Monochaetia dimorphospora*	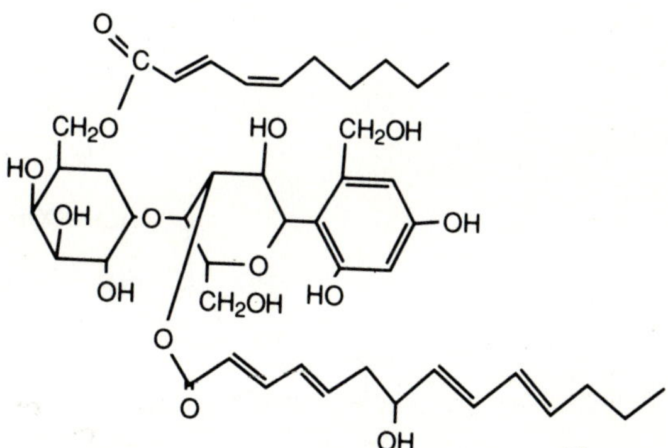	KOMORI et al. (1985) KOMORI and ITOH (1985)

Table 1. (continued)

Name Producing organism	Structure	Reference
Halomonilicins *Monolinia fructicola*	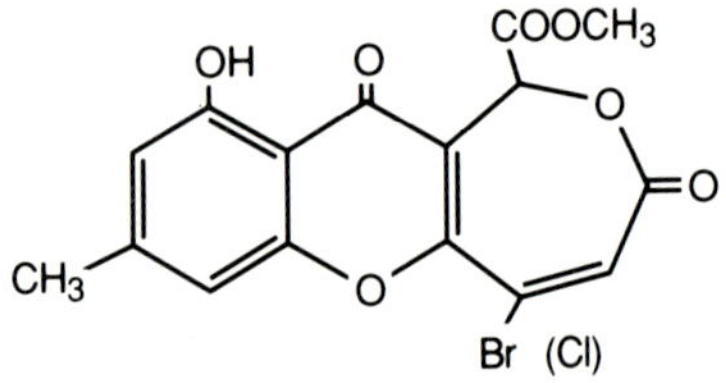	KACHI et al. (1986) SASSA et al. (1985)
Glidobactin A *Polyangium brachysporum*	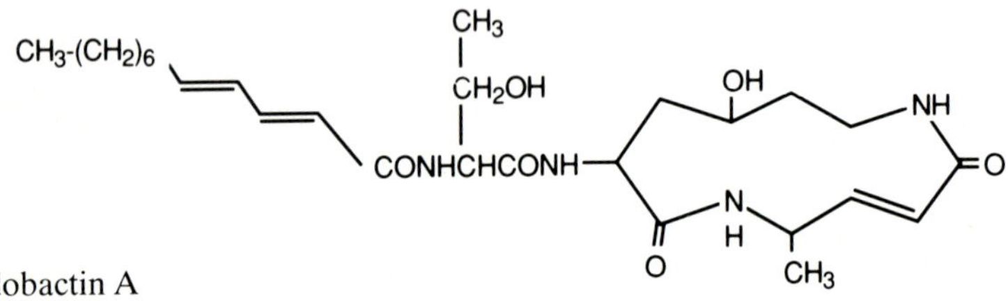	OKA et al. (1988a,b)
SCH 37137 *Micromonospora* sp.	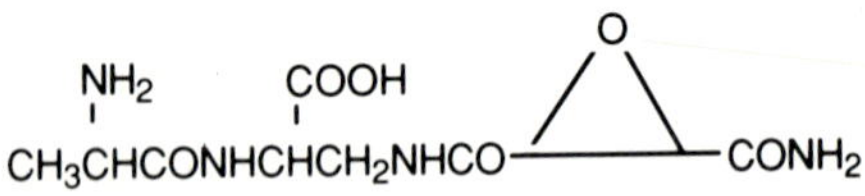	COOPER et al. (1988)
Benanomicin A unidentified actinomycete Pradimicin A *Actinomadura hibisca*	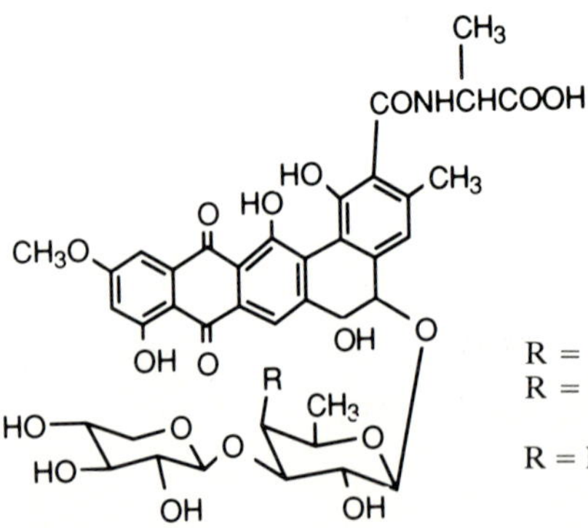 R = OH : Benanomicin A R = NH_2: Benanomicin B R = $NHCH_3$: Pradimicin A	TAKEUCHI et al. (1988) OKI et al. (1988)

Table 1. (continued)

Name Producing organism	Structure	Reference
Galbonolide A *Streptomyces galbus*	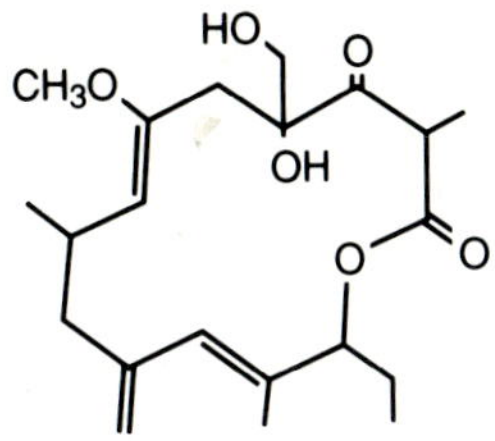	FAUTH et al. (1986)
SCH 38516 *Actinomadura vulgaris*	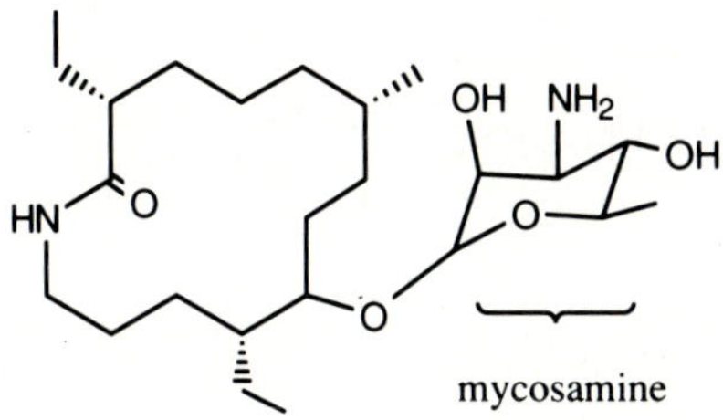	HEGDE et al. (1988)
Clavamycins *Streptomyces hygroscopicus*	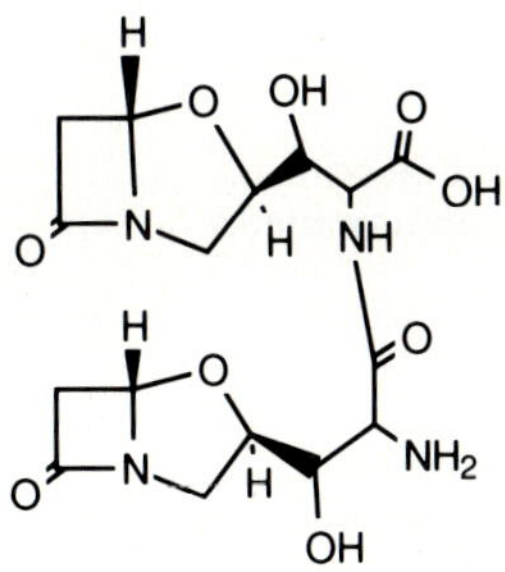	KING et al. (1986)

Table 1. (continued)

Name Producing organism	Structure	Reference
Aranorosin *Pseudoarachniotus roseus*	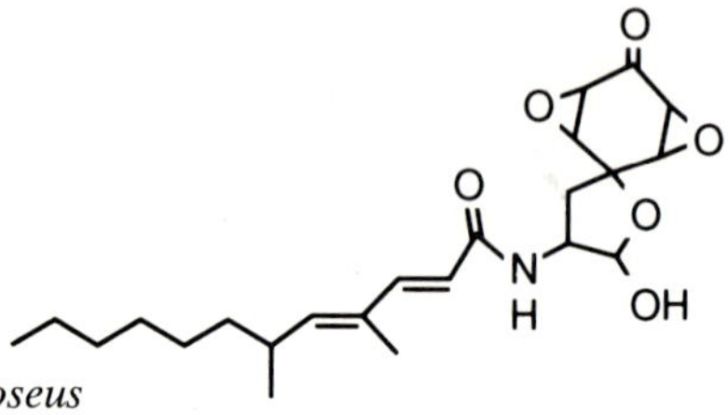	ROY et al. (1988)
Octacosamicin *Amycolatopsis azurea*	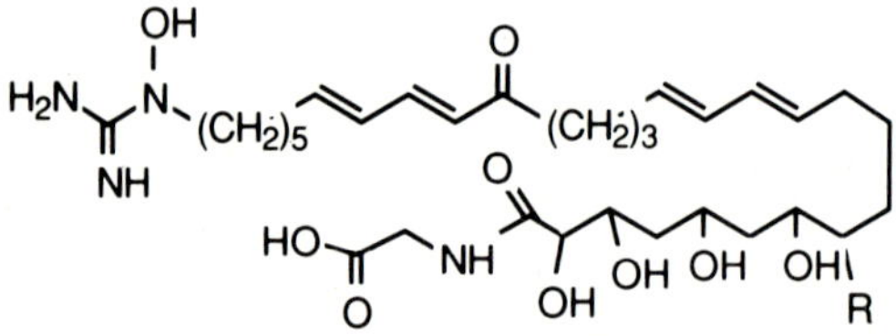 A: R = H B: R = CH_3	DOBASHI et al. (1988)
Globopeptin *Streptomyces* sp. MA-23	Lipopeptide of unknown structure	TANAKA et al. (1987)
Fengycin *Bacillus subtilis* F-29-3	Lipopeptide of undetermined structure	VANITTANAKOM et al. (1986)
LI-FO3 *Bacillus polymyxa*	Lipopeptide of undetermined structure	KURUSU et al. (1987)
Xylocandins *Pseudomonas cepacia*	Lipopeptide of undetermined structure	BISACCHI et al. (1987)

Despite the limitations of classic soil screening, antifungal compounds continue to be reported. Recently reported natural products with antifungal activity are listed in Table 1. These products are produced by diverse microorganisms and include a wide variety of structural types such as macrolactones, lipopeptides, and peptides.

One group of anti-*Candida* lipopeptides includes mulundocandin (4), L-671-329 (see Table 1), ECB (1) and aculeacin A (3) (Mukhopadhyay et al. 1987a; Benz et al. 1974; Keller-Juslen et al. 1976; Satoi et al. 1977;

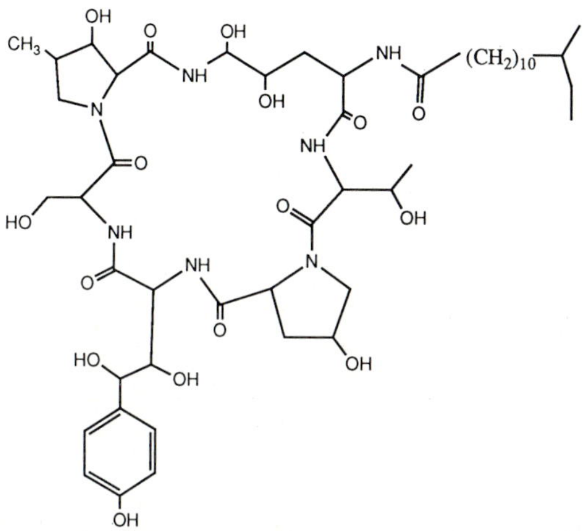

4: Mulundocandin

Schwartz et al. 1989). ECB, which is produced by *Aspergillus nidulans*, is an important antifungal lead and will be discussed in detail below.

The new antifungal antibiotics benanomicin A and B and pradimicin A (see Table 1) possess a benzo-[*a*]napthacene quinone linked to a diglycoside and an alanine group (Takeuchi et al. 1988; Oki et al. 1988). These compounds have only moderate in vitro activity but are effective against *C. albicans* and *Aspergillus fumigatus* infections and show low toxicity.

The structural variation among the compounds with antimycotic activity listed in Table 1 demonstrates the wide latitude found. While the polyenes are frequently encountered, they are usually eliminated from consideration because of their high toxicity.

II. Marine Organisms

The increased demand for new antimycotic agents has prompted the investigation of unconventional sources for new leads. Organisms from the marine environment, such as blue-green algae, are expected to play an increasingly important role. Marine sources have produced many diverse structures which have been tested broadly against bacteria, fungi, viruses, and tumor cells. A recent review of new antifungal agents obtained from marine invertebrates reveals that these sources are rich in unusual structures (FUSETANI 1988). The collection of marine organisms for this purpose is labor intensive and often hampered by the cost of collection and the uncertainty of supplies of organisms. These factors have increased interest in finding marine organisms which can be cultured.

Studies on the culturable blue-green alga *Hapalosiphon fontanalis* resulted in the isolation of an extensive series of indole alkaloids with antibacterial and antimycotic activity (MOORE et al. 1984, 1987a,b; SCHWARTZ et al. 1987). *H. fontanalis* collected in the Marshall Islands was cultured in large, illuminated, glass vessels. The lipophilic extracts of the cultured alga showed antialgal and antimycotic activities. The structure of hapalindole A (5) reveals an unusual

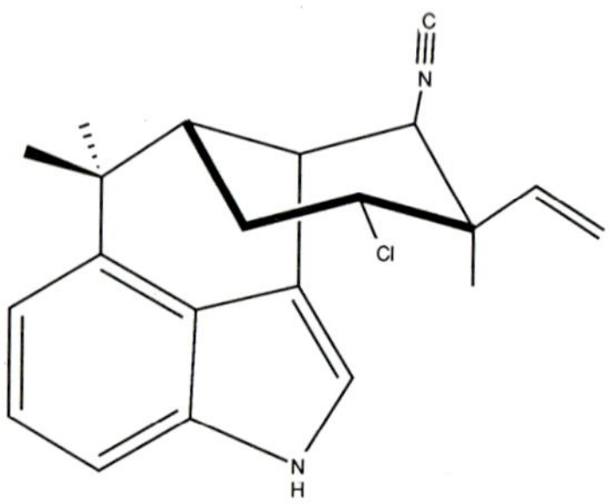

5: Hapalindole A

structure which includes a fused indole-bicyclooctane system bearing chloro and isonitrile substitutents.

Sponges, tunicates, and other marine animals have also yielded a number of interesting new structures. Several soft-bodied sponges have been found whose crude extracts are active against *C. albicans*. Sponges of the genus

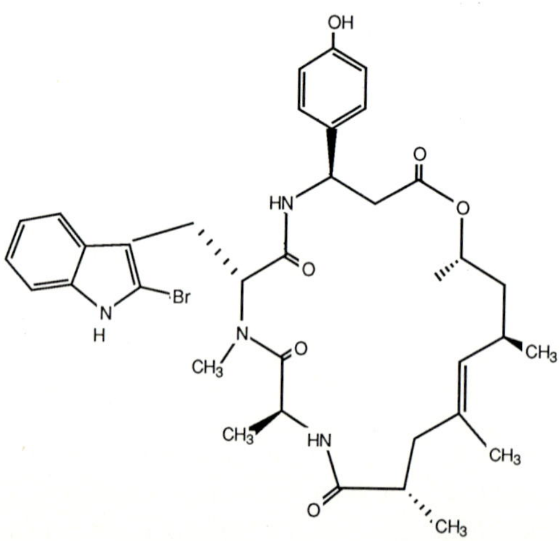

6: Jasplakinolide

Jaspis yielded the cyclodepsipeptide jasplakinolide (6) which had a minimum inhibitory concentration (MIC) of 25 μg/ml against *C. albicans* and had topical anti-*Candida* activity comparable with miconazole in a murine vaginal model (Zabriskie et al. 1986; Crews et al. 1986). This antibiotic has recently been totally synthesized (Grieco et al. 1988). Other novel cyclodepsipeptides, the geodiamolides A and B (7 and 8, respectively), were isolated from the marine sponge *Geodia* sp. collected in Trinidad (Chan et al. 1987). The geodiamolides, which are structurally related to the jasplakinolides, were active against *C. albicans* but were devoid of antibacterial activity.

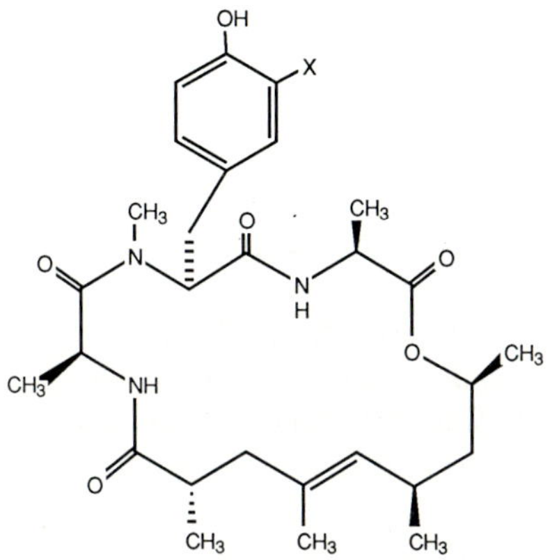

7: Geodiamolide A X = I

8: Geodiamolide B X = Br

Extracts of the egg masses from the nudibranch *Hexabranchus sanguineus* yielded ulapualide A (9) (Roesener and Scheuer 1986). In addition to good inhibition of L1210 leukemia cells (IC_{50} 0.01–0.03 μg/ml), these natural products inhibited the growth of *C. albicans*. Two related macrolides are kabiramide C, (10), isolated by *Matsunaga* et al. (1986) from egg masses of an unidentified nudibranch collected in Okinawa, and halichondramide, which

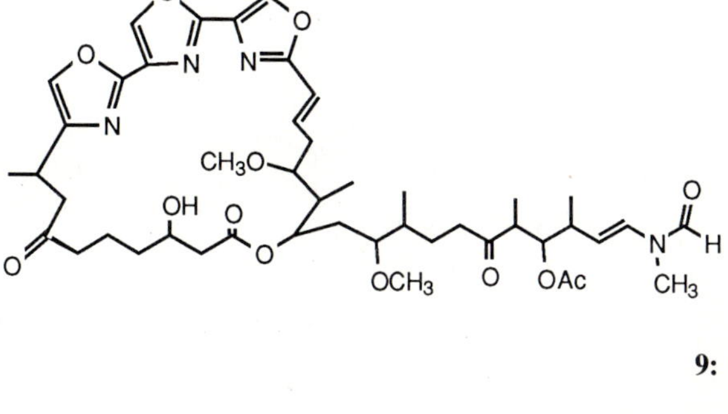

9: Ulapualide A

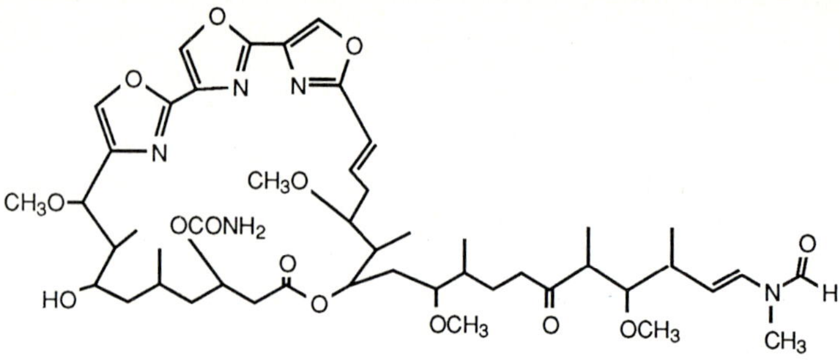

10: Kabiramide C

was isolated from a sponge, *Halichondria* sp., collected in Palau (KERNAN and FAULKNER 1987). These three complex macrolides have the same three contiguous isoxazole rings as a distinguishing feature.

In separate studies a group of secondary metabolites with cytotoxic and antimycotic activity, the scytophycins (scytophycin B, 11), were isolated from the cultured cyanophyte *Scytonema pseudohomanni* (MOORE et al. 1986; ISHIBASHI et al. 1986). These compounds are related to swinholide (12) which was isolated from a Red Sea sponge that is symbiotically associated with a unicellular blue-green alga (CARMELY and KASHMAN 1985).

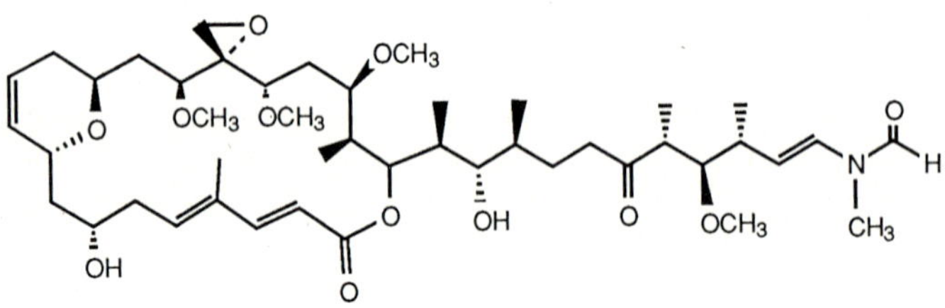

11: Scytophycin B

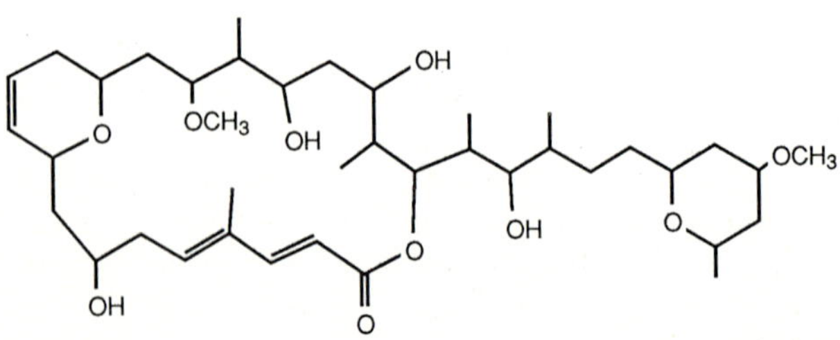

12: Swinholide A

C. The Fungal Cell Wall as an Antifungal Target

I. Biomolecular Composition and Approaches to Screening for Inhibition of Cell Wall Biosynthesis

In the past, lack of knowledge of fungal cell wall biosynthesis has prevented the identification of suitable targets for antimycotics. In a discussion of appropriate cellular targets for pathogenic fungi, CASSONE (1986) stated that "we are dealing with a eukaryotic pathogen in a eukaryotic host and from a structural point of view the two do not greatly differ from each other." Because of this characteristic, antifungal agents must possess a high degree of selectivity to differentiate safely the host from the pathogen. Amphotericin B attacks the fungal cell membrane by complexing with its key sterol components and shows toxicity because it fails to discriminate sufficently between the cytoplasmic membranes of the host and pathogen (KERRIDGE 1986).

On the other hand, the highly organized cell wall is responsible for cellular morphology and controls many processes critical to fungal viability. The presence of a cell wall differentiates fungal cells from mammalian cells and presents an 'ideal' target for therapy (CASSONE 1986). Fungal cell walls contain chitin, glucan, and mannan as well as a group of associated proteins (SULLIVAN et al. 1983; ELORZA et al. 1985; PASTOR et al. 1984; MURGUI et al. 1986; CABIB et al. 1988). Cell-wall regeneration in protoplasts of *C. albicans* has been reported to include the formation of a chitin microfibrillar layer on the cell membrane. This structure allows the incorporation of a variety of protein molecules utilizing noncovalent bonds and the deposition of glucan and covalently bonded mannoproteins (ELORZA et al. 1987). Chitin and glucan in the cell wall of *C. albicans* are covalently linked through the 1-position of β-(1,6) glucan and the 6-position of a *N*-acetylglucosamine on chitin (SURARIT et al. 1988).

Two important groups of antifungals have been discovered whose mode of action is one of inhibition of biomolecular synthesis: the glucan synthase inhibitors (ECB (1), aculeacin A (3), and papulacandin B (13)) and chitin synthase inhibitors (the polyoxins (14) and nikkomycins (15)) (BAGULEY et al. 1979; MIZOGUCHI et al. 1977; CASSONE et al. 1981; BECKER et al. 1983; FIEDLER et al. 1982). These natural antifungal leads are discussed in the following sections. Although most of these compounds have yet to find clinical utility, they have provided important structural information for chemical modification and serve as valuable tools in the development of rational screens for antifungal agents.

A number of groups have incorporated mode of action parameters as part of their screening program. *Neurospora crassa* protoplasts have been utilized for the study of cell-wall biosynthesis and as a selective screen for agents that specifically inhibit cell-wall development (SELITRENNIKOFF 1983). A strain of temperature-sensitive mutants of this organism, osmotic-1 (*os*-1), was developed which forms protoplasts when cultured under special conditions.

These protoplasts maintain growth and division at 37°C. Shifting the incubation temperature from 37° to 22°C causes the *os*-1 mutants to regenerate cell walls. Incubation of these mutants with test drugs at 22°C permits testing for inhibition of fungal cell-wall regeneration. This system is used in the detection of antifungal drugs which inhibit cell-wall synthesis. It has recently been modified to focus on compounds which promote protoplast formation and can more readily be incorporated into a large throughput screen (KIRSCH and LAI 1986). Tests for cell-wall synthesis inhibition by observation of morphological changes and glucan synthase inhibition were employed in the discovery of the antifungal agents cystargin and neopeptin (URAMOTO et al. 1988; UBUKATA et al. 1984).

II. Inhibition of β-(1,3)-Glucan Synthesis

The lipopeptides (ECB) (1), aculeacin A (3), mulundocandin (4), and L-671, 329 (see Table 1) have selective activity against *C. albicans* (MUKHOPADHYAY et al. 1987a; BENZ et al. 1974; SATOI et al. 1977; FROMTLING and ABRUZZO 1989). Mode of action studies with aculeacin A, ECB, and the semisynthetic ECB analogue cilofungin (LY121019) have shown that they inhibit cell-wall synthesis (see below) (MIZOGUCHI et al. 1977; CASSONE et al. 1981; TAFT and SELTRENNIKOFF 1988; TAFT et al. 1988; GORDEE et al. 1988). This mode of action has also been reported for the glycolipid papulacandin B (13) (ELORZA et al. 1987). These cell wall-active antibiotics have provided the basis for structure modification studies with the goal of discovering new analogues with improved properties. Some of these studies will be described in this section.

Aculeacin A, which has the same cyclic peptide as ECB, inhibited the synthesis of β-1,3-glucan in *Saccharomyces cerevesiae* and *C. albicans* (YAMAGUCHI et al. 1985); synthesis of mannan and chitin were not affected. Morphological changes in intact *C. albicans* cells were consistent with inhibition of β-glucan synthesis, with concomitant deformation and weakening of the emerging cell wall. Similiar observations were reported for ECB and papulacandin B, demonstrating the importance of the β-1,3-glucan linkage in the assembly of the fungal cell wall (BAGULEY et al. 1979; SAWISTOWSKA-SCHRÖDER et al. 1984).

ECB, because of its excellent anti-*Candida* activity and specific cell-wall inhibition, represents an important antifungal lead. However, it causes red blood cell hemolysis (DEBONO et al. 1988b). Modification of the molecule was undertaken to synthesize an active analogue with decreased toxicity. The lipopeptides have chemical structures comprised of a complex peptide which is acylated with a fatty acid acyl group usually located at its N-terminus. The biological activity and toxicity of the lipopeptides are strongly influenced by the nature of the fatty acid acyl group. Modification of this group presented an opportunity to synthesize analogues with reduced toxicity (LAKEY and LEA 1986; DEBONO et al. 1988a). The chemical variation of the N-terminal acyl group of ECB was accomplished in a stepwise manner as shown in Fig. 2.

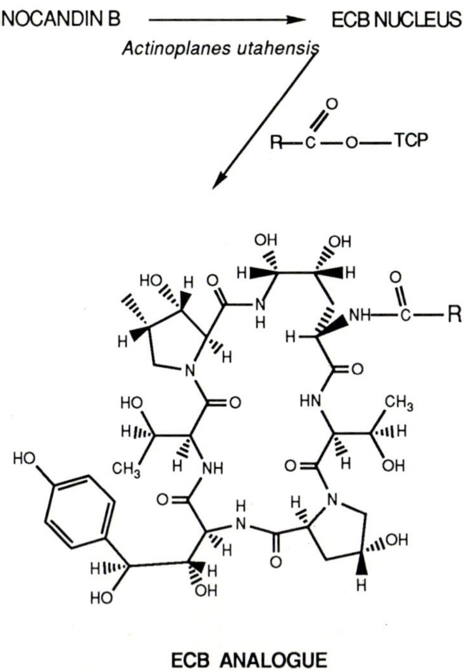

Fig. 2. Synthesis of ECB analogues TCP = 2,4,5-trichlorophenyl

First, the linoleoyl group of ECB was removed by enzymatic deacylation in a fermentation with *Actinoplanes utahensis* to produce the deacylated peptide (ECB nucleus) (Boeck et al. 1989). The ECB nucleus lacked anti-*Candida* activity. Activity was restored by reintroduction of the acyl group. Reconstitution of antifungal activity was strongly influenced by the lipophilicity of the new side chain (Debono et al. 1988b, 1989). A variety of synthetic side chains were attached at the N-terminus of the ECB nucleus by chemical acylation to give a series of ECB analogues bearing modified acyl groups (Debono et al. 1989). Table 2 shows the structure of a representative number of the ECB analogues synthesized by this scheme with their MIC, ED_{50}, and LF_0 values. It was possible to introduce a wide range of side chains which gave analogues having excellent in vitro and in vivo anti-*Candida* activity. Each subseries had its own optimum side chain with a number of series showing increases in activity as the alkyl portion of thc side chain was increased. Comparison of these analogues required determination of their hemolytic potential by the erythyrocyte fragility assay relative to the parent ECB molecule. Analogues with the best activity and minimal hemolytic potential were chosen for toxicity studies in animals. Comparative toxicity studies of cilofungin and two others bearing the tridecanoyl and the p-(dodecanamido)-benzoyl side chains were conducted in the beagle dog using a daily dose of 100 mg/kg for 5 days. ECB showed hemolysis and elevations in SGPT

Table 2. Evaluation data for echinocandin B analogues

	Activity against *Candida albicans*			Efficacy factor
	MIC[a] (μg/ml)	ED_{50}[b] (mg/ml)	LF_0[c] (μg/ml)	ED_{50}/LF_0
Fatty acid acyl ECB analogues $CH_3(CH_2)_nCO$-				
Chain length				
C-12	1.25	62.0	50	1.24
C-13	0.625	34.0	50	0.68
C-14	0.312	30.0	10	3.0
C-15	0.312	22.0	5	4.4
C-16	0.312	15.0	5	3.0
C-17	0.625	9.0	5	1.8
C-18	0.625	7.5	<5	1.3
C-19	2.5	8.5	<5	1.7
C-20	5.0	40.0	<5	8.0
C-22	5.0	50.0	5	10.0
Linoleoyl (ECB)	0.312	28.0	10	2.8
Alkoxybenzoyl ECB analogues *p*-R′O-C_6H_4-C(=O)-				
R′				
n-Hexyl	1.25	28.0	50	0.56
n-Octyl (cilofungin)	0.156	7.6	50	0.15
n-Decyl	0.156	8.0	10	0.80
n-Dodecyl	0.312	4.0	10	0.4
n-Tetradecyl	2.5	3.0	5	0.6
p-Amidobenzoyl ECB analogues *p*-R′-NH-C_6H_4-C(=O)-				
R′				
n-Heptanoyl	>20	>40	50	>0.8
n-Decanoyl	0.625	26.0	50	0.52
n-Dodecanoyl	0.625	15.0	25	0.6
n-Tetradecanoyl	1.25	11.0	10	1.1
n-Hexadecanoyl	0.312	7.0	10	0.7

[a] MIC, minimum inhibitory concentration.
[b] ED_{50}, effective dose for 50% of population.
[c] LF_0 is the highest concentration of test compound that could be added to a suspension of red blood cells without shifting the 50% lysis point from that of the 0.37% saline control. A minimal value for the ratio of ED_{50} to LF_0 is an indicator of a favorable therapeutic index (Debono et al. 1988b).

and BUN levels as well as decreased body weight. Cilofungin, a 4-octyloxybenzoyl ECB analogue, with the exception of a slight elevation in SGPT, showed the lowest toxicity and retained potent anti-*Candida* activity (DEBONO et al. 1988b).

The papulacandins are cell wall-active antifungal agents which were isolated from *Papularia sphaerosperma* (TRAXLER et al. 1977, 1980). The main member of this family is papulacandin B (13), which like the others, contains a spirocyclic diglycoside composed of modified glucose and galactose groups. This diglycoside is O-acylated with a long-chain and a short-chain unsaturated

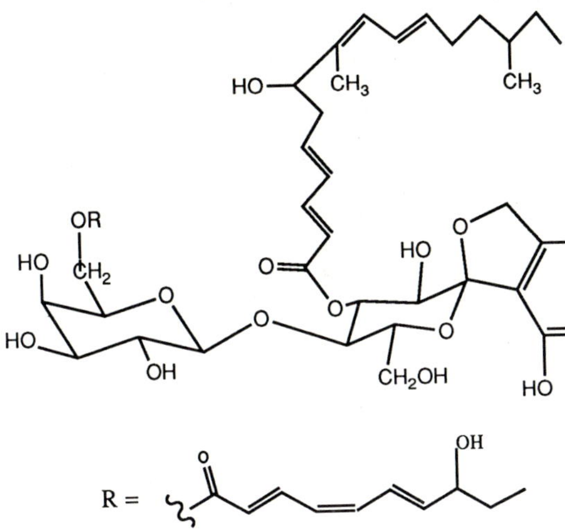

13: Papulacandin B

fatty acid. The papulacandins have in vitro activity primarily against *C. albicans* and have been shown to inhibit glucan synthesis in yeast spheroplasts but were less effective in experimental murine infections. An extensive structure modification effort was undertaken to improve in vivo activity by modification of the aromatic and carbohydrate moieties (TRAXLER et al. 1987). This study revealed that the double bonds in the fatty acid groups and the galactose moiety are essential for biological activity. The modifications resulted in little improvement in in vivo activity and without broadening of the antimicrobial spectrum. The inhibition of β-glucan synthase by these compounds was measured using *C. albicans* spheroplasts (BAGULEY et al. 1979). Glucan synthesis inhibition correlated well with in vitro activity for most of the derivatives, with the exception of the analogue with saturated fatty acid side chains. The latter compound retained its enzyme inhibition properties which did not correlate with in vitro antifungal activity.

III. Inhibitors of Chitin Synthase

Chitin, a polysaccharide composed of β-(1,4)-linked *N*-acetyl glucosamine units (GlcNAc), is an important component of the cell wall of most fungi and has been the subject of a thorough review (CABIB 1987). Chitin biosynthesis, utilizing the uridine diphosphonucleotide of GlcNAc, is controlled by chitin synthase and is represented in the following equation:

$$2n \text{ UDP-GlcNAc} \rightarrow 2n \text{ UDP} + [\text{GlcNAc-}\beta\text{-(1-4)GlcNAc}]_n\text{-}$$

Like the β-glucans, the synthesis of this cell wall biopolymer provides a possible target for antimycotic agents. There is now evidence for two chitin synthase enzymes (ORLEAN 1987). The structural gene for chitin synthase 2 has been cloned (SILVERMAN et al. 1988). Techniques for isolating specific *C. albicans* mutants by directed alteration of the genome have been reported (KELLY et al. 1988). The technology for cloning fungal genes that encode biosynthetic enzymes which are subsequently expressed by transformation is established. A phytoalexin-detoxification gene was cloned from *Nectria haematococca* and expressed in *A. nidulans* (WELTRING et al. 1988). The expression of genes for fungal enzymes should make them available in suitable quantity for use in antifungal screening.

The discovery and chemical modification of the naturally occurring chitin synthase inhibitors have played an important role in the study of the potential of chitin biosynthesis as an antifungal target. The polyoxins (14) and nikkomycins (15), a group of peptidyl nucleoside antibiotics produced by *Streptomyces cacoai* and *S. tendae*, respectively, inhibit the chitin synthase of several fungi (ISONO et al. 1969; BORMANN et al. 1985). Structure-activity relationships showed that free carboxyl and amino groups in the peptide

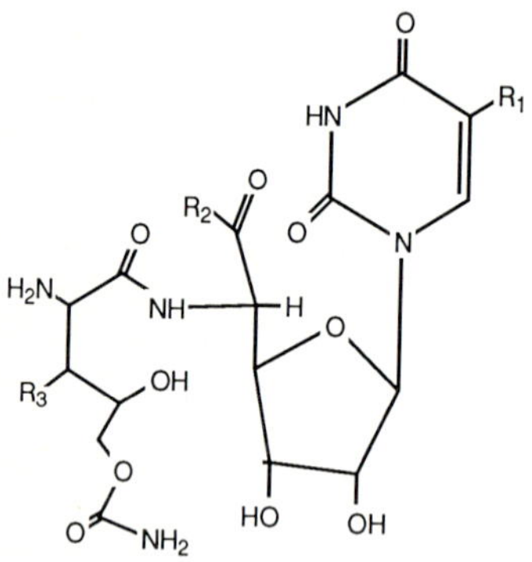

	R_1	R_2	R_3
Polyoxin A :	CH_2OH	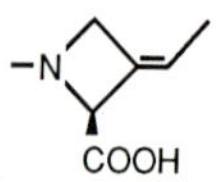	OH
Polyoxin D :	COOH	OH	OH
Polyoxin L :	H	OH	OH

14: Polyoxins

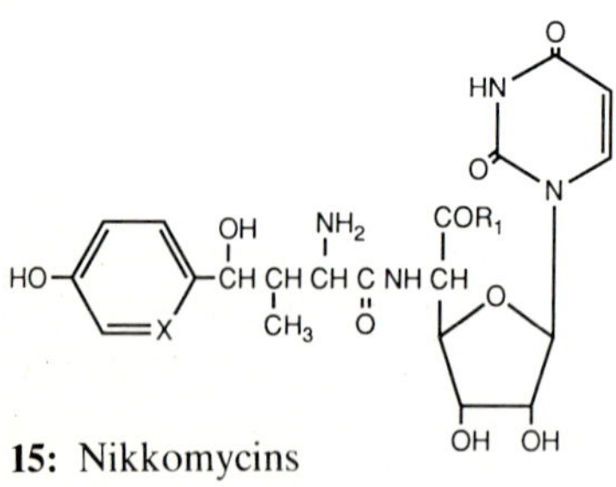

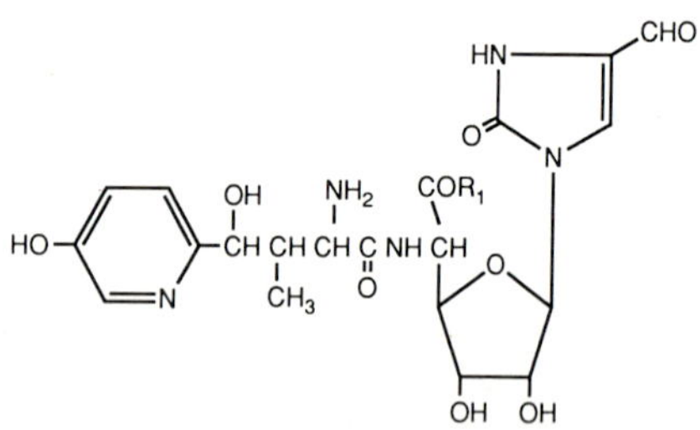

15: Nikkomycins

Nikkomycin Z : R_1 = OH X = N

Nikkomycin J : R_1 = $-NH\text{-}CH(COOH)\text{-}CH_2CH_2COOH$ X = N

Nikkomycin B_Z : R_1 = OH, X = C

Nikkomycin X : R_1 = OH

portion of these molecules are necessary for chitin synthase inhibition (Hori et al. 1971; Isono et al. 1971). These natural antibiotics, however, have poor activity against the whole cell (Isono et al. 1967; Boehm and Kingsbury 1986). New members of the nikkomycin group have been obtained from mutants of *S. tendae*, as well as by mutasynthesis (Delzer et al. 1984). Several new analogues of nikkomycin have been isolated with variations in the heterocyclic base as well as in the peptidyl portion of the nikkomycin molecule. However, none was more effective than the most active compounds in this group. The lack of efficacy was attributed to the difficulty of drug transport into the fungal cell and intracellular hydrolysis of the peptide bond (Naider et al. 1983; Shenbagamurthi et al. 1983). Chemical modification of the polyoxins was undertaken to resolve these problems (Emmer et al. 1985; Shenbagamurthi et al. 1986; Fiandor et al. 1987).

Smith et al. (1986) prepared two hydrophobic polyoxins (16) and (17) by increasing the number of carbon atoms at the N-terminal amino acid. These compounds inhibited chitin synthase from *C. albicans* and resisted intracellular degradation, but were ineffective against *C. albicans* at concentrations as high as 2 mM.

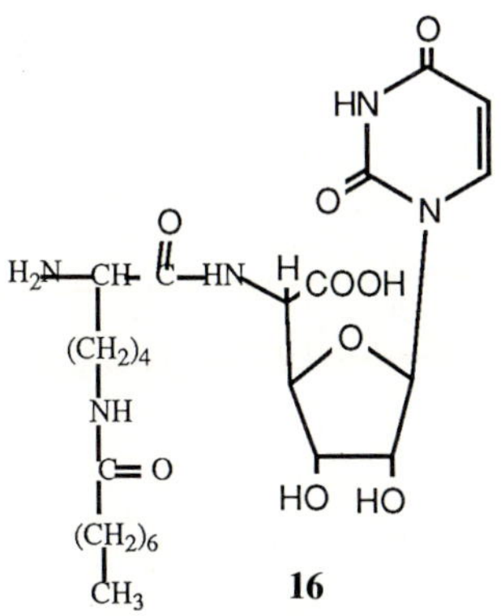

16

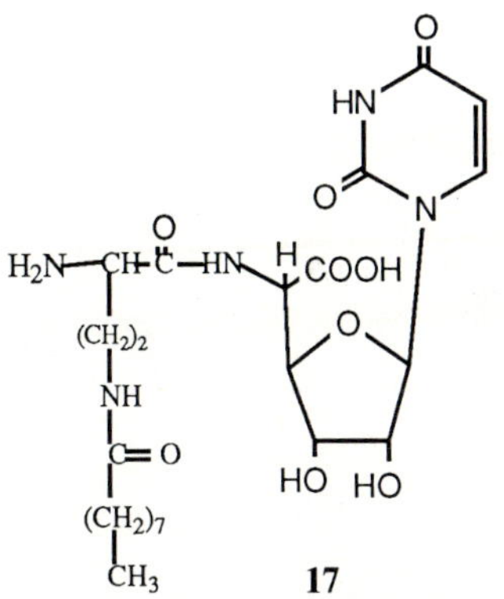

17

A number of polyoxin derivatives bearing large hydrophobic groups represented in structure 18 retained their chitin synthase activity and, like Smith's preparations (16 and 17), had increased stability against fungal peptidase (Khare et al. 1988). However, these derivatives were less active than polyoxin D against *C. albicans*.

Naider et al. (1983) attempted to make the polyoxin molecule more 'peptide-like' by the attachment of an amino acid to the N-terminus of the polyoxin molecule (see structure 19) to improve drug transport. This scheme required that intracellular peptidases remove the additional amino acid and release the active polyoxin from the 'prodrug' within the fungal cell. The prodrugs inhibited cell growth, affected cell morphology, and were hydrolyzed only intracellularly by *C. albicans*. The N-leucyl-norleucyl-uracil polyoxin C appeared to gain entrance into the cell by the desired peptide transport system. However, failure to kill *C. albicans* was attributed to a high degree of intracellular hydrolysis.

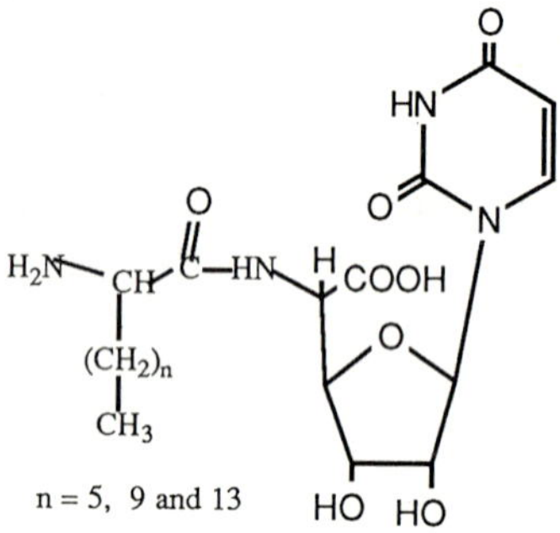

18

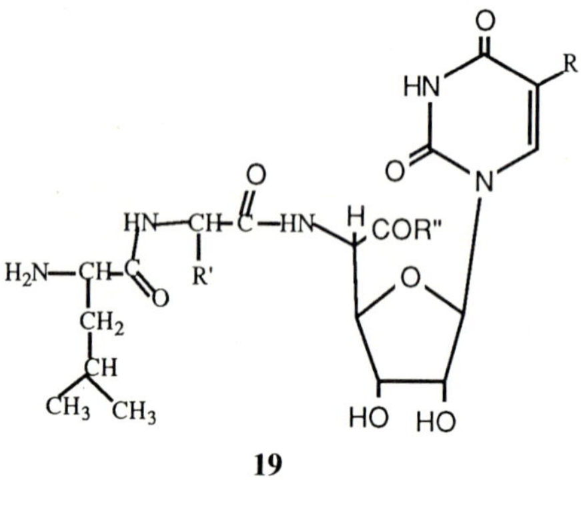

19

R = COOH; H

R' = 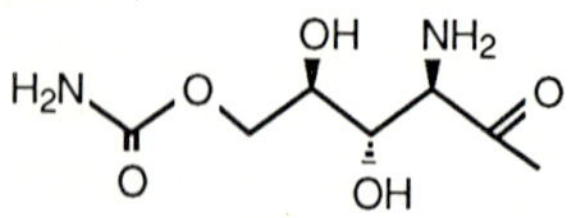

; CH_3-$(CH_2)_3$-

R" = OH; -NH-CH(COOH)-$(CH_2)_3$-CH_3

A recent preliminary study by BECKER et al. (1988) showed that nikkomycin could be used in experimental fungal infections in mice to prolong survival. However, cessation of treatment resulted in reestablishment of the infection and death of the animals.

D. Biological Evaluation of Antifungal Agents

Once a natural product has been identified as a novel compound, then its in vitro antifungal activity and in vivo effectiveness are evaluated. The methodology for successful evaluation of a new agent is essentially the same for natural and synthetic products. The following methods are widely used. The antifungal spectrum of a new compound is determined by using the microdilution microtiter test procedure (SHADOMY et al. 1985). The selected test organisms are the clinically important fungal pathogens, *C. albicans*, *Aspergillus fumigatus*, and *Trichophyton mentagrophytes*. The fungal growth media used are Sabouraud and RPMI tissue culture medium supplemented with 10% fetal calf serum. Amphotericin B is a positive control agent for *C. albicans* and *A. fumigatus*, and tolnaftate is a positive control agent for *T. mentagrophytes*. MIC values for these control agents are 0.78, 1.25, and 0.078 μg/ml, respectively. In order to determine the complete antifungal spectrum of new compounds, MIC determinations are made using an agar dilution test against the fungal pathogens *Histoplasma capsulatum*, *Cryptococcus neoformans*, and *Blastomyces dermatitidis* (TURNER et al. 1978). The MIC range for the positive control amphotericin B is 0.039–0.156 μg/ml for these organisms.

Compounds with an MIC of ≤5.0 μg/ml against *C. albicans* are selected for in vivo testing. When possible, the same fungal isolate used for in vitro studies is utilized for in vivo testing. A 7-day mouse protection test using immunocompromised animals has been developed which determines the correlation between the in vitro antifungal activity and in vivo efficacy (GORDEE and MATTHEWS 1970). Mice are X-irradiated with a uniform body exposure of 400 R 24 h before inoculation. X-irradiation as a means of immunocompromising mice offers the following advantages: (1) one can reduce the infective inoculum by approximately one $\log_{10}$, (2) it decreases individual animal variation to infection, (3) it produces less stress on the test animal and eliminates the possibility of drug interaction with the test compound because there are no injections of immunosuppressant drugs, and (4) infections are more disseminated and less localized (GORDEE and SIMPSON 1967). Test compounds are administered subcutaneously, intraperitoneally, intravenously, or orally by gavage. The average survival time of treated compared with untreated mice is then determined. Once a compound reproducibly increases the average survival time, the ED_{50} (mg/kg) can be estimated from dose titrations of the test compound, using amphotericin B as a positive control (ED_{50} values in the range of 2-4 mg/kg by intraperitoneal administra-

Table 3. Target organs for fungal pathogens

Fungus	Target organs
Candida albicans	Kidney
Aspergillus fumigatus	Lung
	Liver
	Spleen
Cryptococcus neoformans	Brain
Histoplasma capsulatum	Liver
	Spleen
Blastomyces dermatitidis	Liver
	Spleen

tion). ED_{50} values for other susceptible pathogenic fungi are also determined. A major hurdle in establishing a significant antifungal lead is the demonstration of a correlation between in vitro and in vivo activity. There is greater utilization of defined antifungal growth media as opposed to the complex Sabouraud and brain heart infusion media. Members of the azole class of synthetic antifungals do not consistently show a correlation between in vivo efficacy and in vitro activity in complex media, such as Sabouraud or brain heart infusion (Polak and Dixon 1987; see also Chapter 4).

Once in vitro active compounds are shown to have in vivo antifungal activity, unequivocal in vivo efficacy in animal models should be established. The ED_{50} model described above is based on prevention of mortality of infected animals. Another key measure of efficacy is the reduction of a fungal pathogen from target organs (Gordee and Matthews 1968). These target organs are listed in Table 3. Such studies can be carried out in normal or immunocompromised animals. The techniques for the determination of the efficacy by which an antifungal compound significantly reduces the recovery of a fungal pathogen compared with clinically used antifungal agents are well established (Gordee et al. 1984). Development of animal models for evaluating the efficacy of promising antifungal agents continues to be a challenge. There is an increasing number of models available for the evaluation of efficacy and safety (Odds 1979; see also Chap. 5). The criteria utilized for animal models of superficial, localized, or disseminated mycotic infections include the following: (1) selection of a virulent organism that is susceptible to the antifungal agents under study; (2) treatment of animals with a clinically used antifungal agent as a positive control at a dose that is efficacious in humans; (3) criteria of efficacy that are neither too rigid nor too permissive; (4) reproducibility of both the severity of infection and performance of the positive control, and (5) statistical verification of efficacy.

Animal models are used for determining dose regimens of antifungal agents for maximum effectiveness. Clearly, information about the pharmacokinetic properties of an agent can greatly facilitate obtaining the desired correlation of in vivo with in vitro activity. Once this correlation has been satisfactorily established, the key parameters of an antifungal compound listed below need to be determined.

Stability and Incubation Temperature. Chemical stability is essential under the conditions of biological testing. For example, should a greater than four fold increase in the MIC against *C. albicans* occur between 24 and 48 h while there is abundant growth in the untreated controls, the agent may be unstable under the experimental conditions. If variation in susceptibility occurs during a prescribed time period, a microbiological or chemical assay of the compound should be performed. Fungal cultures are most commonly incubated at 37°C. However, some of the faster growing fungi, such as *C. albicans* and *S. cerevisiae*, are incubated at 30°C. When the activity of an antifungal agent is being evaluated, the incubation time must be of sufficient duration to ensure outgrowth of control cultures.

Fungicidal Action. It is important to determine whether the antifungal action is fungistatic (suppression of growth) or fungicidal (lethal to the fungal pathogen). The limitation of fungistatic agents is that once the fungal pathogen is not longer exposed to the agent, growth will continue, or resistance can develop. Ideally, the concentration of antifungal agent required to kill an organism should be in the range of four fold the concentration which inhibits growth and reproduction (Gordee et al. 1988).

Susceptibility of Fungal Isolates and Inoculum Studies. Once the activity of a compound is established against test organisms, the antifungal activity against a number of clinical isolates of pathogenic fungi is determined. MIC_{50} and the MIC_{90} values are obtained for approximately 25 isolates of each fungal organism, and the percentage of isolates susceptible is related to the concentration of antifungal agent required for MIC. The shift in MIC using varying inocula is a useful parameter for antifungal testing. Agents that show a greater than four fold increase in MIC with increasing inocula size (e.g., 1×10^3 to 1×10^6 viable cells) are generally fungistatic and have potential for resistance development.

Mode of Action Studies. A well-defined understanding of the mode of the antifungal action is very useful information that can be utilized throughout the evaluation of a promising antifungal agent. The increasing body of knowledge about the metabolic pathways and physiological processes of fungi coupled with contemporary biochemical techniques provides a basis for carrying out meaningful mode of action studies. Developing parameters based on the mode of action of antifungal compounds is an effective approach for structure-activity studies and discovering novel antifungal compounds. Although there are a number of targets for the action of antifungal agents, a starting point for mode of action studies is the determination of the effect of an agent on the macromolecular biosynthesis of DNA, RNA, and proteins

(GORDEE et al. 1988). The cell membrane is a target for the azole, allylamine, and polyene antifungal agents and should be included in more detailed studies of the site of action (MARRIOTT 1980). The fungal cell wall is a highly desirable target for antifungal agents and should be investigated. The procedures for determining the effect of agents on the biosynthesis of glucan, mannan, and chitin cell wall components have been applied to the mode of action studies of cilofungin (GORDEE et al. 1988).

Resistance Development. Clinically used antifungal agents, with the exception of 5-fluorocytosine, engender resistance relatively infrequently (KERRIDGE et al. 1988). However, as more useful antifungal agents are developed, there is an increased potential for resistance development and cross-resistance with other agents. The results of studies should reflect the potential of an agent to cause development of resistance in the clinical rather than the in vitro laboratory situation. One approach is to compare the resistance development of antifungal agents with agents known to develop resistance. Determination of changes in susceptibility by pathogenic fungi exposed to subinhibitory concentrations of antifungal agents for prolonged periods can provide insight regarding the potential for resistance development (GORDEE et al. 1984). A rapid increase in resistance following 1 or 2 serial transfers may indicate a high potential. Should an antifungal agent fail in the treatment of fungal infections in animals caused by a susceptible organism, the fungus should be isolated and the susceptibility compared with the culture used in the original inoculation.

Considerable progress continues to be made in the preclinical evaluation process of promising antifungal agents. The comparative evaluation of new antifungal agents with clinically effective agents offers the best approach for assessing the therapeutic potential. Another important trend is utilization of expanded information on mode of action, metabolism, excretion, distribution in the body, and the peak/duration of blood levels of new antifungal agents in the preclinical evaluation process. Clearly, evaluation of the clinical potential of a new chemical class of antifungal agents offers a greater challenge than the comparative testing of agents in the same chemical class. A positive control agent provides a useful standardized response in antifungal testing; however, novel agents should not be expected to perform in the same manner as a positive control. The individuality of a novel compound should be recognized and assessed by appropriate testing procedures to avoid missing or underestimating the potential usefulness of new antifungal agents. The procedures and experimental approaches discussed in this section contribute to increased effectiveness in the evaluation of antifungal activity.

E. Conclusion

The discovery of a safe and effective antifungal agent has been an important goal for many years. However, the emergence of diseases such as AIDS, as well as the increasing numbers of immunocompromised patients, has made finding such an agent a high priority. Although advances in antifungal chemotherapy continue to be made in the field of synthetic agents, such as the azoles and allylamines, natural sources continue to provide important leads. The synthesis of cilofungin using semisynthetic procedures illustrates how natural products can serve as sources of leads for new therapeutic agents. Screening by traditional methods, such as the soil screen, remains the main source of antifungal leads. Newer sources, such as marine organisms and the blue-green algae, may provide an even greater range of new molecular structures. However, the increased understanding of fungal cell wall biosynthesis and its biomolecular composition is expected to help define new antifungal targets. The use of rapid screens based on fungal protoplast regeneration and targeted enzymes should facilitate discovery of safe and effective agents. As more clinically useful antifungal compounds are developed, the experience gained should increase the effectiveness by which promising new antifungal agents are evaluated in the laboratory.

Acknowledgements. We wish to acknowledge the efforts of Ms. Louise Crandall for her assistance in preparation and revision of this manuscript and Mrs. Verne K. Newton for secretarial assistance.

References

Abraham EP (1983) History of β-lactam antibiotics. In: Demain AL, Solomon NA (eds) Antibiotics containing the β-lactam structure. Part I, Chapter 1. Springer, Berlin Heidelberg New York, pp 1–13

Argoudelis AD, Baczynskyj L, Kuo MT, Laborde AL, Sebek OK, Truesdell SE, Shilladay FB (1987) Arginomycin: production, isolation, characterization and structure. J Antibiot 40:750–760

Baguley BC, Römmele G, Gruner J, Wehrli W (1979) Papulacandin B: an inhibitor of glucan synthesis in yeast spheroplasts. Eur J Biochem 97:345–351

Becker JM, Covert NL, Shenbagamurthi P, Steinfeld AS, Naider F (1983) Polyoxin D inhibits the growth of zoopathogenic fungi. Antimicrob Agents Chemother 23:926–929

Becker JM, Marcus S, Tullock J, Miller D, Krainer E, Khare RK, Naider F (1988) Use of the chitin-synthesis inhibitor nikkomycin to treat disseminated candidiasis in mice. J Infect Dis 157:212–214

Benz F, Knüsel F, Nüesch J, Treichler H, Voser W, Nyfeler R, Keller-Schierlein W (1974) Stoffwechselprodukte von Microorganismen. 143. Echinocandin B, ein neuartiges Polypeptid-Antibiotikum aus *Aspergillus nidulans* var *echinulatus:* Isolierung und Bausteine. Helv Chim Acta 57:2459–2477

Berdy J (1985) Screening, classification and identification of microbial products. In: Verrall MS (ed) Discovery and isolation of microbial products, Chapter 1. Ellis Horwood, Chichester, pp 9–31

Besson F, Michel G (1987) Isolation and characterization of new iturins: iturin D and iturin E. J Antibiot 40:437–442

Bisacchi GS, Hockstein DR, Koster WH, Parker WL, Rathnum ML, Unger SE (1987) Xylocandin: a new complex of antifungal peptides. II. Structural studies and chemical modifications. J. Antibiot 40:1520–1529

Boeck LD, Fukuda DS, Abbott BJ, Debono M (1989) Deacylation of echinocandin B by *Actinoplanes utahensis*. J Antibiot 42:382–388

Boehm JC, Kingsbury WD (1986) Rapid and convenient synthesis of polyoxin peptides containing N-methylated peptide bonds. J Org Chem 51:2307–2314

Bormann C, Huhn W, Zähner H, Rathmann R, Hahn H, König WA (1985) Metabolic

products of microorganisms. 228 new nikkomycins produced by mutants of *Streptomyces tendae*. J Antibiot 38:9–16
Cabib E (1987) The synthesis and degradation of chitin. Adv Enzymol 59:59–101
Cabib E, Bowers B, Sburlati A, Silverman SJ (1988) Fungal cell wall synthesis: the construction of a biological structure. Microbiol Sci 5:370–375
Carmely S, Kashman Y (1985) Structure of swinholide A, a new macrolide from the marine sponge *Theonella swinhoei*. Tetrahedron Lett 26:511–514
Cassone A (1986) Cell wall of pathogenic yeasts and implication for antimycotic therapy. Drugs Expt Clin Res 12:635–643
Cassone A, Mason RE, Kerridge D (1981) Lysis of growing yeast-form cells of *Candida albicans* by echinocandin: a cytological study. Sabouraudia 19:97–110
Chan WR, Tinto WF, Manchand PS, Todaro LJ (1987) Stereostructures of geodiamolides A and B, novel cyclodepsipeptides from the marine sponge *Geodia* sp. J Org Chem 52:3091–3093
Clark AM, Watson ES, Ashfaq MK, Hufford CD (1987) In vivo efficacy of antifungal oxoaporphine alkaloids in experimental disseminated candidiasis. Pharm Res 4:495–498
Cooper R, Horan AC, Gentile F, Gullo V, Loebenberg D, Marquez J, Patel M, Puar MS, Truumees I (1988) Sch 37137, a novel antifungal compound produced by a *Micromonospora* sp. J Antibiot 41:13–19
Crews P, Manes LV, Boehler M (1986) Jasplakinolide, a cyclodepsipeptide from the marine sponge, *Jaspis* sp. Tetrahedron Lett 27:2797–2800
Debono M, Abbott BJ, Molloy RM, Fukuda DS, Hunt AH, Daupert VM, Counter FT, Ott JL, Carrell CB, Howard LC, Boeck LD, Hamill RL (1988a) Enzymatic and chemical modifications of lipopeptide antibiotic A21978C: The synthesis and evaluation of daptomycin (LY146032). J Antibiot 41:1093–1105
Debono M, Abbott BJ, Turner JR, Howard LC, Gordee RS, Hunt AS, Barnhart M, Molloy RM, Willard KE, Fukuda DS, Butler TF, Zeckner DJ (1988b) Synthesis and evaluation of LY121019, a member of a series of semi-synthetic analogues of the antifungal lipopeptide echinocandin B. Ann NY Acad Sci 544:152–167
Debono M, Abbott BJ, Fukuda DS, Barnhart M, Willard KE, Molloy RM, Michel KH, Turner JR, Butler TF, Hunt AH (1989) Synthesis of new analogs of echinocandin B by enzymatic deacylation and chemical reacylation of the echinocandin B peptide: synthesis of the antifungal agent cilofungin (LY121019). J Antibiot 42:389–397
Delzer J, Fiedler H, Müller H, Zähner H, Rathmann R, Ernst K, König WA (1984) New nikkomycins by mutasynthesis and directed fermentation. J Antibiot 37: 80–82
Dobashi K, Naganawa H, Takahashi Y, Takita T, Takeuchi T (1988) Novel antifungal antibiotics octa-cosamicins A and B. II. The structure elucidation using various NMR spectroscopic methods. J Antibiot 41:1533–1541
Elorza MV, Murgui A, Sentandreu R (1985) Dimorphism in *Candida albicans*: contribution of mannoproteins to the architecture of yeast and mycelial cell walls. J Gen Microbiol 131:2209–2216
Elorza MV, Murgui A, Rico H, Miragall F, Sentandreu R (1987) Formation of a new cell wall by protoplasts of *Candida albicans*: effect of papulacandin B, tunicamycin and nikkomycin. J Gen Microbiol 133:2315–2325
Emmer G, Ryder NS, Grassberger MA (1985) Synthesis of new polyoxin derivatives and their activity against chitin synthase from *Candida albicans*. J Med Chem 28:278–281
Fauth U, Zähner H, Mühlenfeld A, Achenbach H (1986) Galbonolides A and B – two non-glycosidic antifungal macrolides. J Antibiot 39:1760–1764
Fiandor J, Garciá-López M-T, De las Heras FG, Méndez-Castrillón PP (1987) Synthesis of modified polyoxins by reaction of uridine-5'-aldehyde with trimethylsilylcyanide and amino acids. Synthesis 978–981
Fiedler HP, Kurth R, Langharig J, Delzer J, Zähner H (1982) Nikkomycins: microbial inhibitors of chitin synthase. J Chem Tech Biotechnol 32:271–280

Fromtling RA, Abruzzo GK (1989) L-671,329, a new antifungal agent. III. In vitro activity, toxicity and efficacy in comparison to aculeacin. J Antibiot 42:174–178
Fusetani N (1988) Antifungal substances from marine invertebrates. Ann NY Acad Sci 544:113–127
Gordee RS, Matthews TR (1968) Reliable technique for plating pathogenic fungi from organ homogenates. Appl Microbiol 16:1610
Gordee RS, Matthews TR (1970) Evaluation of systemic antifungal agents in X-irradiated mice. Appl Microbiol 20:624–629
Gordee RS, Simpson PJ (1967) Relationships of x irradiation to the enhancement of *Candida albicans* infections. J Bacteriol 94:6–12
Gordee RS, Zeckner DJ, Ellis LF, Thakkar AL, Howard LC (1984) In vitro and in vivo anti-*Candida* activity and toxicology of LY121019. J Antibiot 37:1054–1065
Gordee RS, Zeckner DJ, Howard LC, Alborn WE, Debono M (1988) Anti-*Candida* activity and toxicology of LY121019, a novel semisynthetic polypeptide antifungal antibiotic. Ann NY Acad Sci 544:294–309
Grieco PA, Hon YS, Perez-Medrano A (1988) A convergent, enantiospecific total synthesis of the novel cyclodepsipeptide (+)-jasplakinolide (jaspamide). J Am Chem Soc 110:1630–1631
Hamamoto T, Seto H, Beppu T (1983) Leptomycins A and B, new antifungal antibiotics II. Structure elucidation. J Antibiot 36:646–650
Hegde V, Patel M, Gunnarsson I, Horan A, Marquez J, Puar M, Gullo V (1988) Two novel macrolactam antifungal antibiotics, Sch 38518 and Sch 39185, produced by *Actinomadura vulgaris* sp. nov.: fermentation, isolation, structure, and biological properties. 28th Intersci Conf Antimicrob Agents Chemother, Los Angeles CA, Abstr 306
Hook DJ, More CF, Yacobucci JJ, Dubay G, O'Connor S (1987) Integrated biological-physicochemical system for the identification of antitumor compounds in fermentation broths. J Chromatogr 385:99–108
Hori M, Kakiki K, Suzuki S, Misato T (1971) Studies on the mode of action of polyoxins. III. Relation of polyoxin structure to chitin synthetase inhibition. Agric Biol Chem 35:1280–1291
Ishibashi M, Moore RE, Patterson GML, Xu C, Clardy J (1986) Scytophycins, cytotoxic and antimycotic agents from the cyanophyte *Scytonema pseudohofmanni*. J Org Chem 51:5300–5306
Isono K, Nagatsu J, Kobinata K, Sasaki K, Suzuki S (1967) Studies on polyoxins, antifungal antibiotics. V. Isolation and characterization of polyoxins C, D, E, F, G, H and I. Agric Biol Chem 31:190–199
Isono K, Asahi K, Suzuki S (1969) Studies on polyoxins, antifungal antibiotics. XIII. The structure of polyoxins. J Am Chem Soc 91:7490–7505
Isono, K, Azuma T, Suzuki S (1971) Polyoxin analogs. 1. Synthesis of aminoacyl derivatives of 5′-amino-5′-deoxyuridine. Chem Pharm Bull 19:505–512
Iwai Y, Omura S (1982) Culture conditions for screening of new antibiotics. J Antibiot 35:123–141
Kachi H, Hattori H, Sassa T (1986) A new antifungal substance, bromomonilicin, and its precursor produced by *Monilinia fructicola*. J Antibiot 39:164–166
Keller-Juslén C, Kuhn M, Loosli HR, Petcher TJ, Weber HP, von Wartburg A (1976) Struktur des cyclopeptid-antibiotikums SL 7801 (= echinocandin B). Tetrahedron Lett 4147–4150
Kelly R, Miller SM, Kurtz MB, Kirsch DR (1988) One-step gene disruption by cotransformation to isolate double auxotrophs in *Candida albicans*. Mol Gen Genet 214:24–31
Kernan MR, Faulkner DJ (1987) Halichondramide, an antifungal macrolide from the sponge *Halichondria* sp. Tetrahedron Lett 28:2809–2812
Kerridge D (1986) Mode of action of clinically important antifungal drugs. In: Rose AH, Tempest DW (eds) Adv microbial physiology, vol 27. Academic, New York, pp 1–64

Kerridge D, Fasoli M, Wayman FJ (1988) Drug resistance in *Candida albicans* and *Candida glabrata*. Ann NY Acad Sci 544:245–259

Khare RK, Becker JM, Naider FR (1988) Synthesis and anticandidal properties of polyoxin L analogues containing α-amino fatty acids. J Med Chem 31:650–656

King HD, Langhärig J, Sanglier JJ (1986) Clavamycins, new clavam antibiotics from two variants of *Streptomyces hygroscopicus*. I Taxonomy of the producing organisms, fermentation, and biological activities. J Antibiot 39:510–515

Kirsch DR, Lai MH (1986) A modified screen for the detection of cell wall-acting antifungal compounds. J Antibiot 39:1620–1622

Komori T, Itoh Y (1985) Chaetiacandin, a novel papulacandin. II. Structure determination. J Antibiot 38:544–546

Komori T, Yamashita M, Tsurumi Y, Kohsaka M (1985) Chaetiacandin, a novel papulacandin. I. Fermentation, isolation and characterization. J Antibiot 38: 455–459

Kurusu K, Ohba K, Arai T, Fukushima (1987) New peptide antibiotics, LI-FO3, FO4, FO5, FO7 and FO8, produced by *Bacillus polymyxa*. J Antibiot 40:1506–1514

Lakey JH, Lea EJA (1986) The role of acyl chain character and other determinants on the bilayer activity of A21978C, an acidic lipopeptide antibiotic. Biochim Biophys Acta 859:219–226

Marriott MS (1980) Inhibition of sterol biosynthesis in *Candida albicans* by imidazole-containing antifungals. J Gen Microbiol 117:253–255

Matsunaga S, Fusetani N, Hashimoto K, Koseki K, Noma M (1986) Bioactive marine metabolites. Part 13. Kabiramide C, a novel antifungal macrolide from nudibranch egg masses. J Am Chem Soc 108:847–849

Meyers E, Cooper R, Dean L, Johnson JH, Slusarchyk DS, Trejo WH, Singh PD (1985) Catacandins, novel anticandidal antibiotics of bacterial origin. J Antibiot 38:1642–1648

Mizoguchi J, Saito T, Mizuno K, Hayano K (1977) On the mode of action of a new antifungal antibiotic, aculeacin A: inhibition of cell wall synthesis in *Saccharomyces cerevesiae*. J Antibiot 30:308–313

Moore RE, Cheuk C, Patterson GML (1984) Hapaloindoles: new alkaloids from the blue-green alga *Hapalosiphon fontinalis* J Am Chem Soc 106:6456–6457

Moore RE, Patterson GML, Mynderse JS, Barchi J Jr, Norton TR, Furusawa E, Furusawa S (1986) Toxins from cyanophytes belonging to the *Scytonemataceae*. Pure Appl Chem 58:263–271

Moore RE, Cheuk C, Yang XQG, Patterson GML, Bonjouklian R, Smitka TA, Mynderse JS, Foster RS, Jones ND, Swartzendruber JK, Deeter JB (1987a) Hapaloindoles, antibacterial and antimycotic alkaloids from the cyanophyte *Hapalosiphon fontinalis*. J Org Chem 52:1036–1043

Moore RE, Yang XQG, Patterson GML (1987b) Fontonamide and anhydrohapaloxindole A, two new alkaloids from the blue-green alga *Hapalosiphon fontinalis*. J Org Chem 52:3773–3777

Mukhopadhyay T, Ganguli BN, Fehlhaber HW, Kogler H, Vertesy L (1987a) Mulundocandin, a new lipopeptide antibiotic II. Structure elucidation. J Antibiot 40:281–289

Mukhopadhyay T, Roy K, Coutinho L, Rupp RH, Ganguli BN, Fehlhaber HW (1987b) Fumifungin, a new antifungal antibiotic from *Aspergillus fumigatus* fresenius 1863. J Antibiot 40:1050–1052

Murgui A, Elorza MV, Sentandreu R (1986) Tunicamycin and papulacandin B inhibit incorporation of specific mannoproteins into the wall of *Candida albicans* regenerating protoplasts. Biochim Biophys Acta 884:550–558

Naider F, Shenbagamurthi P, Steinfeld AS, Smith HA, Boney C, Becker JM (1983) Synthesis and biological activity of tripeptidyl polyoxins as antifungal agents. Antimicrob Agents Chemother 24:787–796

Nolan RD, Cross T (1988) Isolation and screening of actinomycetes. In: Goodfellow M, Williams ST, Mordaski M (eds) Actinomyctes in biotechnology. Academic, London, pp 1–32

Odds FC (1979) Candida and candidosis, 1st edn. Leicester University Press, Leicester
Oka M, Nishiyama Y, Ohta S, Kamei H, Konishi M, Miyaki T, Oki T, Kawaguchi H (1988a) Glidobactins A, B and C, new antitumor antibiotics 1. Production, isolation, chemical properties and biological activity. J Antibiot 41:1331–1337
Oka M, Yaginuma K, Numata K, Konishi M, Oki T, Kawaguchi H (1988b) Glidobactins A, B, and C, new antitumor antibiotics. II. Structure elucidation. J Antibiot 41:1338–1350
Okami Y, Hotta K (1988) Search and discovery of new antibiotics. In: Goodfellow M, Williams ST, Mordaski M (eds) Actinomycetes in biotechnology. Academic, London, pp 33–67
Oki T, Konishi M, Tomatsu K, Tomita K, Saitoh K, Tsunakawa M, Nishio M, Miyaki T, Kawaguchi H (1988) Pradimicin, a novel class of potent antifungal antibiotics. J Antibiot 41:1701–1704
Orlean P (1987) Two chitin synthases in *Saccharomyces cerevisiae*. J Biol Chem 262:5732–5739
Pastor FIJ, Valentin E, Herrero E, Sentandreu R (1984) Structure of the *Saccharomyces cervisiae* cell wall. Mannoproteins released by zymolyase and their contribution to wall architecture. Biochim Biophys Acta 802:292–300
Polak A, Dixon DM (1987) In vitro/in vivo correlation of antifungal susceptibility testing using 5-fluorocytosine and ketoconazole as examples of two extremes. In: Fromtling RA (ed) Recent trends in the discovery, development and evaluation of antifungal agents. J R Prous, Barcelona, 45–59
Roesener JA, Scheuer PJ (1986) Ulapualide A and B, extraordinary antitumor macrolides from nudibranch egg masses. J Am Chem Soc 108:846–847
Roy SK, Inouye Y, Nakamura S, Furukawa J, Okuda S (1987a) Isolation, structural elucidation and biological properties of neoenactins B1, B2, M1 and M2, neoenactin congeners. J Antibiot 40:266–274
Roy K, Mukhopadhyay T, Reddy GCS, Desikan KR, Ganguli BN (1987b) Mulundocandin, a new lipopeptide antibiotic I. Taxonomy, fermentation, isolation and characterization. J Antibiot 40:275–280
Roy K, Mukhopadhyay T, Reddy GCS, Desikan KR, Rupp RH, Ganguli BN (1988) Aranorosin, a novel antibiotic from *Pseudoarachniotus roseus*. I. Taxonomy, fermentation, isolation, chemical and biological properties. J Antibiot 41:1780–1784
Sassa T, Kachi H, Nukina M, Suzukiy Y (1985) Chloromonilicin, a new antifungal metabolite produced by *Monilina fructicola*. J Antibiot 38:439–441
Satoi S, Yagi A, Asano K, Mizuno K, Watanabe T (1977) Studies on aculeacin. II. Isolation and characterization of aculeacin B, C, D, E, F and G. J. Antibiot 30:303–307
Sawistowska-Schröder ET, Kerridge D, Perry H (1984) Echinocandin inhibition of 1,3-β-D-glucan synthase from *Candida albicans*. FEBS Lett 173:134–138
Schwartz RE, Hirsch CF, Springer JP, Pettibone DJ, Zink DL (1987) Unusual cycloproprane-containing hapalindolinones from a cultured cyanobacterium. J Org Chem 52:3704–3706
Schwartz RE, Giacobbe RA, Bland JA, Monaghan RL (1989) L-671,329, a new antifungal agent. I. Fermentation and isolation. J Antibiot 42:163–167
Scott VR, Boehme R, Matthews TR (1988) New class of antifungal agents: jasplakinolide, a cyclodepsipeptide from the marine sponge, *Jaspis* species. Antimicrob Agents Chemother 32:1154–1157
Selitrennikoff CP (1983) Use of a temperature-sensitive, protoplast-forming *Neurospora crassa* strain for the detection of antifungal antibiotics. Antimicrob Agents Chemother 23:757–765
Shadomy S, Espinel-Ingroff S, Cartwright RY (1985) Laboratory studies with antifungal agents: susceptibility tests and bioassays. In: Lenteet EH, Balows AS, Hausler WJ, Shadomy HJ (eds) Manual of clinical microbiology, 4th edn. American Society for Microbiology, Washington DC, pp 991–999
Shenbagamurthi P, Smith HA, Becker JM, Steinfeld A, Naider F (1983) Design of anticandidal agents: synthesis and biological properties of analogues of polyoxin L. J Med Chem 26:1518–1522

Shenbagamurthi P, Smith HA, Becker JM, Naider F (1986) Synthesis and biological properties of chitin synthetase inhibitors resistant to cellular peptidases. J Med Chem 29:802–809

Silverman SJ, Sburlati A, Slater ML, Cabib E (1988) Chitin synthase 2 is essential for septum formation and cell division in *Saccharomyces cerevisiae*. Proc Natl Acad Sci USA 85:4735–4739

Smith HA, Shenbagamurthi P, Naider FR, Kundu B, Becker JM (1986) Hydrophobic polyoxins are resistant to intracellular degradation in *Candida albicans*. Antimicrob Agents Chemother 29:33–39

Sullivan PA, Yin CY, Molloy C, Templeton MD, Shepherd MG (1983) An analysis of the metabolism and cell wall composition of *Candida albicans* germ-tube formation. Can J Microbiol 29:1514–1525

Surarit R, Gopal PK, Shepherd MG (1988) Evidence for a glycosidic linkage between chitin and glucan in the cell wall of *Candida albicans*. J Gen Microbiol 134: 1723–1730

Taft CS, Selitrennikoff CP (1988) LY121019 inhibits *Neurospora crassa* growth and (1–3)-β-D-glucan synthase. J Antibiot 41:697–701

Taft CS, Stark T, Selitrennikoff CP (1988) Cilofungin (LY121019) inhibits *Candida albicans* (1–3)-β-D-glucan synthase activity. Antimicrob Agents Chemother 32: 1901–1903

Takeuchi T, Hara T, Naganawa H, Okada M, Hamada M, Umezawa H, Gomi S, Sezaki M, Kondo S (1988) New antifungal antibiotics, Benanomicins A and B from an *Actinomycete*. J Antibiot 41:807–811

Tanaka Y, Hirata K, Takahashi Y, Iwai Y, Omura S (1987) Globopeptin, a new antifungal peptide antibiotic. J Antibiot 40:242–244

Traxler P, Fritz H, Richter WJ (1977) Zur Struktur von Papulacandin B, einem neuen antifungischen Antibiotikum. Helv Chim Acta 60:578–584

Traxler P, Fritz H, Fuhrer H, Richter WJ (1980) Papulacandins, a new family of antibiotics with antifungal activity. Structures of papulacandins A, B, C and D. J Antibiot 33:967–978

Traxler P, Tosch W, Zak O (1987) Papulacandins – synthesis and biological activity of papulacandin B derivatives. J Antibiot 40:1146–1164

Turner JR, Butler TF, Gordee RS, Thakkar AL (1978)A32390A, a new biologically active metabolite III. In vitro and in vivo antifungal activity. J Antibiot 31:33–37

Ubukata M, Uramoto M, Isono K (1984) The structure of neopeptins, inhibitors of fungal cell wall biosynthesis. Tetrahedron Lett 25:423–426

Uramoto M, Itoh Y, Sekiguchi R, Shin-Ya K, Kusakabe H, Isono K (1988) A new antifungal antibiotic, cystargin: fermentation, isolation and characterization. J Antibiot 41:1763–1768

Vanittanakom N, Loeffler W, Koch U, Jung G (1986) Fengycin – a novel antifungal lipopeptide produced by *Bacillus subtills* F-29-3. J Antibiot 39:888–901

Waksman SA (1937) Associative and antagonistic effects of microorganisms. I. Historical review of antagonistic relations. Soil Sci 43:51–68

Waksman SA (1941) Antagonistic relations of microorganisms. Bacteriol Rev 5: 231–291

Waksman SA (1947) What is an antibiotic or an antibiotic substance? Mycologia 39:565–569

Waksman SA, Lechevalier HA (1962) The search for antibiotics: screening programs. In: The actinomycetes, vol III. Antibiotics of actinomycetes, Chapter 3. Williams and Wilkins, Baltimore, pp 20–30

Weltring KM, Turgeon BG, Yoder OC, VanEtten HD (1988) Isolation of a phytoalexin-detoxification gene from the plant pathogenic fungus *Nectria haematococca* by detecting its expression in *Aspergillus nidulans*. Gene 68:335–344

Wichmann CF, Liesch JM, Schwartz RE (1989) L-671, 329, a new antifungal agent. II. Structure determination. J Antibiot 42:168–173

Yamaguchi H, Hiratani T, Baba MN, Osumi M (1985) Effect of aculeacin A, a wall-active antibiotic, on synthesis of the yeast cell wall. Microbiol Immunol 29: 609–623

Zabriskie TM, Klocke JA, Ireland CM, Marcus AH, Molinski TF, Faulkner DJ, Xu C, Clardy JC (1986) Jaspamide, a modified peptide from a *Jaspis* sponge, with insecticidal and antifungal activity. J Am Chem Soc 108:3123–3124

CHAPTER 4

Screening and Evaluation In Vitro

ROBERT G. WILSON and JOHN F. RYLEY

A. Purpose of Screening

In any large-scale programme aimed at drug discovery, screening procedures will be necessary in order to identify compounds of potential interest. Candidate substances for screening may include chemical compounds selected at random or according to particular structural features from an existing chemical collection, compounds designed and synthesised specifically by project chemists and broths or extracts of natural product origin. The purpose of an antifungal screen is simply to provide a yes/no answer to the question, 'Is there sufficient interaction between this sample and fungi to warrant further investigation?' This further investigation of compounds of potential interest is termed evaluation.

The process of screening is used in order to deal with potentially very large numbers of samples, so that a manageable number can be selected and evaluated further to discover whether or not they are of any real interest. Screening is rather like fishing with a net. The fisherman decides what sort of fish he wants to catch and then uses a net of appropriate mesh. A net with large holes will retain only the biggest fish; a net with finer mesh will still catch these but will also retain smaller fish. In operating an in vitro screen the size of 'mesh', i.e. the criteria acceptable as 'sufficient interaction', may be modified in the light of the average weekly yield of the screen in terms of active compounds and the effort and facilities which are available for the further processes of evaluation. The essentials of an efficient screen include high sample throughout, simplicity and economy of operation, small sample requirements and unambiguity of interpretation. It matters little if the screen identifies compounds which are later found to be of no interest; it matters considerably if the screen fails to identify compounds of real potential interest, i.e. produces false negatives.

Our objective is to find new therapeutic agents for use in humans. Whether a compound which has shown interaction with a fungus in a simple system in vitro will be effective in vivo depends on many factors including absorption, appropriate distribution within the body, lack of premature metabolism to an inactive form and, of course, freedom from toxicity. Although there may be pharmacokinetic and metabolic differences between laboratory animals and humans, screening in vivo would be expected to be more relevant to the ultimate objective than screening in vitro. Screening in vivo may also identify compounds – by no means an unknown occurrence – which require metabolism before they show activity. Screening in vivo, however, is more expensive, requires the use of large numbers of laboratory animals, does not allow the use of a wide spectrum of organisms and, perhaps most important of all from the practical point of view, requires more compound than a simple in vitro test. Ideally, therefore, an initial screen should be done in vitro.

B. Methods of Screening

In an initial in vitro screen we wish to identify activity against as wide a range of fungi as possible and, in order to be able to decide whether it is worth proceeding further, to quantify that activity as far as is practicable. Three basic methods can be considered: agar dilution, agar diffusion and broth dilution. In an agar dilution system the test compound is incorporated in a molten agar-based medium, a plate is poured and subsequently inoculated. Using a multipoint inoculator a large number of different organisms can be tested on a single plate. Following incubation, plates are read visually, scoring for each organism normal growth, reduced growth or no growth. Where activity is found, the test can be repeated using plates containing serial dilutions of the compound in order to determine the minimum inhibitory concentration (MIC) against each organism.

In the agar diffusion assay each plate is seeded with a single organism, wells are cut in the agar, or stainless steel cylinders are placed on the agar, and each reservoir is charged with test substance. Following incubation the zones of inhibition of growth round the reservoirs are measured; the more active the compound, the larger the zone. Although only a single organism is incorporated in each plate, one plate can be used to test several compounds and their relative potencies determined from the respective zone sizes. With poorly soluble compounds which diffuse insufficiently in the agar, the zone of inhibition may not reflect the true antifungal potential of the compound; itraconazole is a good example of this problem.

In a broth dilution assay the compound is incorporated in a liquid medium which is then inoculated with the fungus and incubated. After a specified time, growth – or absence of growth – can be detected by visual observation and an MIC determined or the level of growth quantified by nephelometry or spectrophotometry. Although each compound and each organism require a separate tube, the broth dilution system is capable of miniaturization and automation.

Each system has its advantages and disadvantages, and because we desire to have an indication of the activity with a wide range of fungal organisms, we feel that the most practicable and adaptable system at the *screening* stage is the agar dilution assay.

C. Choice of Organisms and Conditions

The most prevalent fungal diseases are caused by various species of *Candida* or by dermatophytes, while the most serious infections may involve *Candida*, *Cryptococcus*, *Aspergillus*, or the 'American mycoses', *Coccidioides*, *Paracoccidioides*, *Histoplasma*, *Blastomyces*, etc. Because compounds of potential interest are not necessarily going to be wide spectrum in their activity, it is desirable to use as many organisms as possible in the primary screen, but due to potential hazards to the operator it is advisable to avoid some of the latter organisms at the initial screening stage. A number of different strains of the most important species may be used, including drug-resistant strains; thus, we have used an amphotericin-resistant strain of *Candida albicans* when screening natural product broths in order to identify polyenes which we did not wish to pursue.

With an agar dilution assay, in which a whole variety of different organisms are growing on the same plate, compromise over conditions will be necessary. The same medium is not necessarily ideal for each organism or type of compound. Thus, anti-metabolites such as 5-fluorocytosine (5-FC) will only inhibit yeasts in a simple defined medium, while most fungi require complex media for growth. As fungi differ markedly in their rates and optimal temperature for growth, the incubation conditions for any screen involving several different fungal genera must be a compromise. Under such circumstances some species will not achieve maximum growth, while others will be well into the stationary phase when the plates are read; nevertheless, it is possible to show activity against various species, even if they are not all growing under ideal conditions, and thus fulfil the purpose of the screen. Perhaps the most significant omission in such a simple screen, particularly in the azole era, is *C. albicans* growing in the mycelial phase. Mutants of *Candida* which will grow in the mycelial phase on solid media exist but are not generally available. To rectify this omission we have operated a concurrent screen using one strain of *C. albicans* growing in the mycelial phase in Eagle's minimum essential medium (MEM) with serum.

D. Choice of Media

Sabouraud's dextrose agar (SDA) has for long been the most widely used medium for growing pathogenic fungi. SHADOMY et al. (1982) in a comparison of bifonazole with clotrimazole used three different media and a large number of yeasts, dermatophytes and miscellaneous fungi. They observed that with yeasts in particular, lower MICs were found when Kimmig's agar was used rather than SDA or casein yeast extract glucose (CYEG). As a result of this paper we have used Kimmig's agar in place of SDA in our screen for some time with satisfactory results. In a recent unpublished study we investigated the antifungal activity of ketoconazole, itraconazole, fluconazole and the bistriazole ICI 195,739 against *C. albicans*, *Trichophyton quinckeanum* and *Aspergillus fumigatus* growing on 15 different media used in mycology, bacteriology or tissue culture by agar diffusion assay; further assays by agar dilution and broth dilution were carried out using 6 of the media. The overall conclusion was that no one medium was satisfactory for all compounds against all organisms using all three assay systems. Hardly surprising!

Thus, using an agar diffusion system, *C. albicans* was most sensitive to all four compounds when iso-sensitest agar (IST) was the assay medium, although much higher concentrations of fluconazole, which is the most soluble of the four compounds tested and possibly the most readily diffusable in agar, were required to produce zones of inhibition. Likewise, the greatest sensitivity was achieved when *T. quinckeanum* was grown on diagnostic sensitivity test agar (DST) and *A. fumigatus* on brain heart infusion agar (BHI), although with the latter organism we were unable to produce any zones of inhibition with fluconazole at 256 μg/ml using any of the 15 media tested.

Although *C. albicans* had shown much reduced sensitivity on casitone complex agar (CC) in agar diffusion assays, the lowest MICs by agar dilution of all four compounds were achieved in this medium. For example, ICI 195,739 had an MIC of $\leq$0.12 μg/ml compared with 16 μg/ml in yeast morphology agar (YMA) or IST. Indeed, CC was the only one of the 6 media tested in which MICs for fluconazole and itraconazole could be obtained by agar dilution. Although CC proved a satisfactory assay medium for *C. albicans*, it would not support sufficient growth of *T. quinckeanum* to allow MICs to be determined. For agar dilution assays using this organism, lowest MICs were achieved on IST, which also proved to be a very satisfactory medium for MIC determinations against *A. fumigatus*. Under these test conditions there was a general trend for MIC values to increase with prolonged periods of incubation.

C. albicans grew so well in all 6 liquid media that MICs could be determined at 24 h, at which time the lowest MICs were recorded for all four antifungals in tissue culture medium (TC); however, there was a marked increase of MIC with incubation time. TC was the only medium of the 6 tested in which an MIC could be obtained for fluconazole with *C. albicans* and then only if the assay was read at 24 h. By contrast, growth of *T. quinckeanum* in TC was so poor that MICs could not be determined.

This study highlights the difficulties encountered when trying to devise an assay system for more than one compound and more than one organism. Moreover, for azole antifungals in particular, widely different MICs can be obtained for a single combination of antifungal and fungus within a particular assay system simply by altering the type of medium. Likewise, maintaining the same medium but altering the method of MIC determination can grossly influence the result. Of particular note is that the antifungal activity of fluconazole, which has undoubted activity in vivo, was hardly detectable in most of the systems employed. It is possible to establish retrospectively assay systems to identify one particular attribute of a specific compound or indeed to rank a series of antifungals, but this is a very different situation from that of a generalised screen with which one is seeking to identify prospectively antifungal activity. A generalised screening procedure may be expected to have little more than a qualitative significance. Extrapolation of results to an in vivo situation will be difficult and often misleading. However, if compounds are in short supply or the number of compounds is very large, there may be no alternative to a preliminary in vitro screen.

E. A Workable In Vitro Screen

At one time our agar dilution screen utilized 8 yeasts grown on YMA and 11 dermatophytes grown on SDA in a two-compartment petri dish (RYLEY et al. 1981). We subsequently simplified the system by growing all organisms on Kimmig's agar in a single-compartment dish. Although Kimmig's agar was in no way outstanding in the agar diffusion studies mentioned in the last section, it seems to be a quite satisfactory medium for an agar dilution screen; MICs are equivalent to or lower than those found with YMA and SDA (RYLEY and RATHMELL 1984).

In our screen, compounds are dissolved in dimethyl sulphoxide (DMSO) at a concentration of 10 mg/ml and incorporated into molten agar at 50 μg/ml. By means of a Denley multipoint inoculator the surface of the agar is inoculated with calibrated suspensions of 9 yeasts and 11 fungi (Table 1). After 3 days incubation at 30°C, activity is determined by absence of growth of the fungus. Such a screen gives an early indication of the breadth of activity of the compounds being tested and their potential as broad-spectrum antifungal agents or yeast- or dermatophyte-specific agents. Compounds which show activity against several yeasts and/or dermatophytes at 50 μg/ml are retested at 100, 25, 6.2 and 1.6 μg/ml to determine relative potency. Table 1 contains data for a selection of antifungal agents tested under these conditions using doubling dilutions over a concentration range of 100–0.1 μg/ml. Conclusions which might be drawn from these data are that amphotericin B, ketoconazole, ICI 195,739, clotrimazole and miconazole are all potential broad-spectrum agents, whilst the activities of griseofulvin and terbinafine are restricted to dermatophytes. However, one could be misled into believing that itraconazole and fluconazole have no activity against yeasts and that 5-FC has no antifungal activity at all. Beware of the pitfalls of in vitro screens!

Because of the apparently poor activity of azoles against the blastospore form of *C. albicans* under the test conditions described above, all compounds submitted to our screen were also tested against the mycelial form of *C. albicans*. An overnight culture of *C. albicans* serotype A (NCPF 3153) in Eagle's MEM with 10% foetal calf serum (FCS) is adjusted to a standardized concentration in Eagle's MEM + 1% FCS as an inoculum; 2 ml volumes of this are dispensed into wells of multi-well plates, and aliquots of diluted

Table 1. Antifungal activities of various compounds in standard in vitro screen

Organism	Antifungal agent									
	Amphotericin B	Griseofulvin	Terbinafine	5-Fluorocytosine	Clotrimazole	Miconazole	Ketoconazole	Itraconazole	Fluconazole	ICI 195,739
Candida albicans NCPF 3153	<0.1	>100	>100	>100	25	12.5	25	>100	>100	6.2
C. albicans NCPF 3156	<0.1	>100	>100	>100	25	12.5	25	1.6	>100	12.5
C. albicans B2630	<0.1	>100	>100	>100	25	12.5	25	>100	>100	12.5
C. albicans 6406/8[a]	1.6	>100	12.5	>100	50	12.5	25	>100	>100	12.5
C. tropicalis	<0.1	>100	>100	>100	25	12.5	6.2	>100	>100	3.1
C. parapsilosis	<0.1	>100	0.8	>100	25	12.5	50	>100	>100	6.2
C. parapsilosis WL	<0.1	>100	3.1	>100	1.6	6.2	0.2	1.6	12.5	0.2
Torulopsis glabrata	<0.1	>100	<0.1	>100	100	0.8	6.2	>100	100	12.5
Cryptococcus neoformans	<0.1	>100	0.4	>100	3.1	<0.1	0.4	0.4	12.5	0.4
Trichophyton mentagrophytes	<0.1	3.1	<0.1	>100	6.2	1.6	3.1	0.4	100	1.6
T. quinckeanum	<0.1	0.8	<0.1	>100	3.1	<0.1	<0.1	0.2	6.2	0.8
T. interdigitale	<0.1	3.1	<0.1	>100	3.1	0.4	1.6	0.2	100	1.6
T. rubrum	<0.1	3.1	<0.1	>100	1.6	0.8	1.6	0.2	50	0.4
T. tonsurans	<0.1	3.1	<0.1	>100	6.2	0.8	1.6	0.4	100	1.6
Microsporum canis	<0.1	0.8	<0.1	>100	3.1	0.8	3.1	0.8	100	1.6
M. gypseum	<0.1	1.6	<0.1	>100	3.1	1.6	3.1	0.4	100	0.8
Epidermophyton floccosum	<0.1	0.4	<0.1	>100	3.1	<0.1	0.4	<0.1	1.6	<0.1
Prototheca zopfii	<0.1	>100	50	>100	>100	50	25	100	>100	>100
Scopulariopsis brevicaulis	0.4	>100	1.6	>100	25	50	6.2	>100	>100	>100
Hendersonula toruloidea	<0.1	3.1	<0.1	>100	12.5	0.4	0.8	0.4	25	1.6
Mycelial *C. albicans* NCPF 3153	0.1	>12	1	0.1	0.01	0.01	<0.01	<0.01	<0.01	<0.01

Figures represent the highest MIC (μg/ml) recorded from two tests using doubling dilutions of compounds.

[a] Amphotericin-resistant strain.

compound are added to give a final concentration of 12 μg/ml. The plates are incubated overnight at 37°C in an atmosphere of 5% CO_2:air after which the degree of mycelial development is observed using an inverted microscope. Compounds which are active at 12 μg/ml are retested at 12, 1, 0.1 and 0.01 μg/ml. The data in Table 1 confirm the potency of azoles in such a test system and highlight the differences in MIC values which can be achieved for this type of compound against the yeast or mycelial forms of *C. albicans*. It should be noted that amphotericin B is equiactive against both morphological forms, that the lack of anti-yeast activity of griseofulvin and terbinafine is confirmed and that of 5-FC is detectable in this test system.

F. Interpretation of Screen Results

Having screened a batch of compounds and obtained a series of MICs for each, the questions arise: does any require further investigation in vitro, and is any of sufficient interest for screening in vivo? In general we would not do any further work in vitro until we had established some sort of activity in vivo. The crucial question is what sort of activity in vitro is necessary to make screening in vivo worthwhile? Based on the performance of standard antifungals in our screen we use as criteria an MIC of 25 against *Candida* yeast, 0.1 against mycelial *Candida* or 6.2 against dermatophytes as end-points for follow-up in vivo. Other factors to take into account are the chemical structure or class of the compound, particular strategies which may be adopted in the exploration of a specific series of compounds, and such practical questions as the amount of compound available and the capacity of the in vivo screen in relation to the number of compounds coming through the in vitro screen. Only when the antifungal activity of a compound has been confirmed in vivo and is of such magnitude that it warrants interest should any consideration be given to further in vitro evaluation.

G. Relevance of Screen

Antifungal activity in vitro is no guarantee of activity in vivo, nor does it predict the extent of any such activity. Although this is particularly true of the azoles and *Candida*, it is by no means restricted to this class of compound or type of fungus. This situation can be difficult for anyone with a background in antibacterial chemotherapy to appreciate or understand. With antibacterial agents, MICs against a range of species are the major criteria by which a compound is judged before further investigations take place; in vivo studies concentrate on pharmacokinetics rather than behaviour in models of infection. Development of a compound to the stage of being a marketable drug is accompanied by the determination of more and more MICs against an ever increasing range of species and strains of bacteria, while clinical use is often controlled by sensitivity determinations on isolates from the particular patient. Not so with antifungals. MIC is almost a meaningless concept, depending as it does so much on the particular compound and on the type of medium and conditions under which the test is done. Therapeutic response – or lack of it – cannot be predicted by any consideration of MIC and plasma drug levels. The triazoles itraconazole and fluconazole and the imidazole ketoconazole have been shown to be efficacious at dose levels which could not generate concentrations in the body approaching the MICs recorded in Table 1. ODDS (1985) remarks that

> in the field of antifungal chemotherapy, the idea that an MIC is a clinically useful item of information has never been well proved, and it can occasionally become a positive handicap when the drug under consideration is one of the imidazole- or triazole-derivative family of antifungal agents... It should be possible to test any azole antifungal agent against any fungal isolate and manipulate test conditions in such a way as to achieve any desired MIC... So acute has the general problem become of noncorrelation of azole MICs with activity in vivo that at least three manufacturers with considerable experience in antifungal chemotherapy no longer rely on sensitivity tests in vitro to screen for novel antifungal compounds, since few of the most recently developed azoles show any significant inhibitory activity in vitro at all.

Is there therefore any point in testing compounds in vitro, and can anything be done to improve the situation? Under many circumstances, due either to shortage of compound or to sheer numbers of samples requiring screening, an initial in vitro approach is all that is possible. Efforts are being made to improve testing conditions so that they better reflect in vitro the undoubted potency of specific drugs in vivo, but the extent to which these retrospective studies will enable reliable *predictive* screens to be established for new classes of compound is open to question. VAN CUTSEM et al. (1986) reported an interesting retrospective study with miconazole, ketoconazole and itraconazole. Medium pH was unimportant for miconazole, but increased pH gave 'more valuable' results for ketoconazole and itraconazole. In media enriched with serum proteins, the activity of miconazole decreased, that of ketoconazole remained stable or increased, and that of itraconazole increased. The choice of correct solvent was important to show good activity for itraconazole, and they point out that due to poor solubility, agar diffusion tests will not adequately measure the real potency of the compound. A large number of strains of *C. albicans* and of dermatophytes were tested in BHI or Sabouraud's broth under standard conditions. A particularly disconcerting finding was that in animal infections the strains which needed higher growth-suppressing concentrations in vitro responded equally well to drug treatment as strains sensitive in vitro to lower concentrations. We have experienced an entirely similar situation. SHADOMY et al. (1984) examined 17 isolates of *C. albicans* by agar dilution and obtained MICs varying from 0.06 to 128 μg/ml with ketoconazole and 0.06 to 64 μg/ml with the azole ICI 153,066. We had the opportunity to assay these same isolates in vivo using a model of vaginal candidosis in the mouse and found minimum effective doses of 25–50 mg/kg × 5 for ketoconazole and 1–2.5 mg/kg for ICI 153,066 irrespective of the sensitivity of the strain in vitro.

During the course of our search for a new azole antifungal we have assayed many of the compounds against *C. albicans* in YNB by broth dilution, expressing the result as an IC_{50} (concentration required to give 50% inhibition of growth compared with untreated controls) and against vaginal candidosis in mice (Boyle et al. 1987). Plots of log IC_{50} against log minimum effective dose in mice showed good correlation in a group of 17 bistriazole and in one subset of a group of 43 monotriazole tertiary alcohols. Correlations, however, only hold within close chemical groups, and even here some compounds do not behave as expected, possibly due to factors such as metabolic instability. No correlation was possible across structurally divergent series, emphasising again the difficulties which prevail when trying to establish a test system for compounds of more than one chemical type.

Richardson et al. (1986) found ketoconazole active at 25 μg/ml against *C. albicans* in an agar dilution assay on diagnostic test agar, but fluconazole was inactive at 100 μg/ml. When they used a tissue culture agar (a defined medium similar to Synthetic Amino Acid Medium Fungal, SAAMF), they were able to obtain MICs of 0.01 and 0.8 μg/ml for ketoconazole and fluconazole, respectively. In a model of vaginal candidosis in mice, ketoconazole cured 50% of the animals at 60 mg/kg, while fluconazole showed similar effects at 4.4 mg/kg. Serum protein binding is 99% for ketoconazole, but only 11% for fluconazole. They then carried out pharmacokinetic studies in mice dosed with ketoconazole at 60 mg/kg or fluconazole at 4.4 mg/kg and plotted serum concentrations of unbound drug against time. They showed that levels of unbound drug exceeded MIC in tissue culture agar for around 9 h in each case, and suggested that the superiority of fluconazole in vivo is undoubtedly a consequence of its high, sustained blood levels and its low protein binding in spite of its poor performance in vitro. They fail, however, to explain why results obtained with tissue culture agar are more relevant to the in vivo situation than those obtained with other media or to substantiate the significance of serum protein binding to drug activity in the vagina.

One of the problems involved in the measurement of MICs with azoles or 5-FC is that the compounds cause partial inhibition of fungal growth over a wide range of concentrations, making end-points difficult to determine, subjective and potentially unreliable. In an attempt to overcome this problem, Odds and Abbott (1984) suggested calculating relative inhibition factors (RIF) on the premise that measurement of the area under the dose-response curve for an antifungal agent gave estimates of inhibitory activity which were more reproducible than MIC determinations. Moreover, these measurements take account of partial inhibitory effects. They evaluated 9 antifungal agents (azoles, polyenes and 5-FC) against 44 fungal isolates (yeasts, aspergilli and dermatophytes) at 7 different concentrations (0.01–10 μg/ml) in Eagle's MEM containing glutamine and 10% horse serum. Cultures were incubated under 5% CO_2 in air at 37°C for yeasts and aspergilli, and in air at 30°C for dermatophytes. Samples were taken while still in the exponential growth phase for the determination of viable fungal biomass as measured by ATP content using bioluminescence spectrophotometry and a luciferin/firefly lantern extract system. Growth was expressed as a percentage of that in drug-free controls. RIFs were then calculated by adding these values for the 7 different drug concentrations and dividing by 7. A RIF close to 0% indicates susceptibility to the drug while a value close to 100% indicates lack of response. Growth of control cultures of *C. albicans* was in the mycelial phase, whereas growth in the presence of low concentrations of azoles was as yeasts; measurement of fungal biomass by ATP determination does not differentiate between these. The choice of concentrations over which growth is measured is crucial and will differ from one type of agent to another. An inspection of RIF values obtained with the compounds and fungi tested indicates a tremendous variation from one combination to another, and it is not easy to see how significant comparisons can be made. Correlation between RIF and MIC as determined in YNB broth was limited in general; with individual azoles it was never good, and overall for all five imidazoles against yeasts there was no correlation between RIF and MIC. In a subsequent study ODDS et al. (1984) compared 9 more azoles and the morpholine amorolfine with the previous 9 compounds investigated. With RIFs against *Candida* spp. in the range of 44%–77% compared with 54%–69% in the previous series, it is difficult to see what significance can be attached to a particular value, especially from the point of view of predicting activity in the clinical situation. In fairness it should be pointed out that RIF values for all the azoles against the three ketoconazole-resistant isolates of *C. albicans* were outside these limits, though rarely approaching 100%. The value of this approach requires extensive verification with fungal isolates known to be refractory to therapy.

In an entirely different approach aimed at 'improving' MIC estimations with fluconazole, ODDS et al. (1986) showed that incorporating doxycycline (200 μg/ml) or other antibiotics which bind to 80*S* ribosomes, thereby blocking protein synthesis, resulted in MICs in DST agar of the same order as those found in tissue culture agar without antibiotic for both fluconazole and five other azoles; similar results for fluconazole were obtained in SDA and BHI liquid media containing antibiotics. Further studies with doxycycline in YNB broth with glucose and serum indicated that the effect was restricted to *Candida* species. Fluconazole was still the least active of the azoles tested. Reproducibility between tests conducted in microdilution plates was claimed to be good, but MICs did vary with the medium and conditions used. Although these findings are most interesting and could be relevant when screening for new azole antifungal agents, their value in a generalised screen requires investigation. The basic problem of devising a predictive in vitro screen remains.

H. Evaluation In Vitro

Once a compound with promising activity in vivo reaches the stage of development, in vitro data with large numbers of clinical isolates and an ever increasing range of species will be expected by potential trialists and regulatory authorities irrespective of the true value of such studies. In order to play the numbers game effectively, a rigorously standardised protocol is necessary. VAN CUTSEM et al. (1987) reported on just such a study with itraconazole which utilised 2813 strains belonging to 149 different species of fungi! Serial decimal dilutions of itraconazole dissolved in DMSO were made in BHI broth over the concentration range 100–0.001 μg/ml and inoculated with the fungi in question. Final evaluation was done after 14 days incubation at 37°C (an amazing length of time!); activity was defined as inhibition of growth by more than 90% at this time when compared with controls. The medium and conditions were selected "since the results obtained in this medium were more relevant to those obtained after oral or parenteral treatment in vivo." Although the results do suggest that itraconazole is a very active compound, with many strains responding to 0.1 μg/ml, it is not immediately obvious that the data mirror the useful clinical profile of the drug; in the absence of strictly comparable data it is not possible to decide whether itraconazole might be expected to produce a better response than an alternative therapy.

In a similar previous study (VAN CUTSEM et al. 1986) comparative data for ketoconazole and itraconazole were given. This could have been helpful were it not for the demonstration that some strains of dermatophytes and *C. albicans* which were least sensitive in vitro responded equally well in animal models of infection as strains which were most sensitive in vitro. Similar evaluations have recently been presented for terbinafine by CLAYTON (1987) and by PETRANYI et al. (1987), for amorolfine by POLAK and DIXON (1987) and for bifonazole by YAMAGUCHI et al. (1987). Because of the dependence of MICs on the conditions of the assay and the unpredictable inter-laboratory variations, such tables of activities can be little more than 'window dressing'.

SHADOMY and his group in Richmond, Virginia, have been notable among the independent generators of large scale in vitro data on development compounds and also as a service and reference laboratory performing in vitro tests with clinical isolates of pathogenic fungi and established or experimental antifungal agents. Although their methodology has changed over the years, and some of their published studies have concerned single compounds, other studies (e.g. SHADOMY et al. 1984) have generated potentially helpful comparative data. In a very honest and useful distillation of his vast experience, SHADOMY (1987) could do no more than underline the lack of predictability and reproducibility associated with in vitro testing. Among many examples he cites an exhaustive in vitro study with 181 isolates of *Cryptococcus neoformans* and 5-FC by both dilution and diffusion methods. On the basis of MICs, isolates were assigned to one of four susceptibility classes. 'Unfortunately, little or no correlation could be demonstrated between in vitro results and clinical responses observed in 160 patients from whom the isolates were obtained.'

Nevertheless, attempts to standardise antifungal susceptibility testing in vitro continue. GALGIANI (1986, 1987a,b) reviewed the problems and the attempts being made to solve them in the USA in studies sponsored by the National Committee for Clinical Laboratory Standards, while Drouhet (1988) examined similar endeavours being made in France and other parts of Europe. Guinet et al. (1988) reported recently on the first multicentre study of a commercially available micromethod for yeast susceptibility testing (Mycototal, Behring Diagnostic). The kit permits sensitivity testing of yeasts against 5-FC, amphotericin B and five imidazoles, based on the principle of determination of a category result (i.e. susceptible, intermediate or resistant) with two critical concentrations of each agent based on serum levels being tested for each isolate. The reproducibility between laboratories was 96.3% with an average repeatability within laboratories of 99.3%, and a concordance with reference MICs of 91.5%. Most of the discrepancies observed were for strains found resistant by mycototal but susceptible by MIC tests. To be of real value such a system must evolve to include the most recent triazoles fluconazole and itraconazole, and the belief of the authors that "Mycototal will be of considerable help in clarifying the confusing area of antifungal susceptibility testing" remains to be proved. Screening in vitro will continue, however unsatisfactory the predictive value may be, as long as it is necessary to test large numbers of samples available only in small quantities. Where research programmes are concentrated on specific chemical types, it may be possible to develop in vitro test systems with a more predictive value. Extensive in vitro evaluation of new compounds will continue because the data, however meaningless it may be, are expected by those in a position to progress or hinder the development of the new compound.

J. Features of Activity

Although the predictive value of MICs obtained in vitro may be suspect, useful data on the type of activity of a compound can be obtained by in vitro studies; such investigations may properly include investigations of fungicidal as opposed to fungistatic activity, synergy or antagonism with other compounds and studies on the development of resistance.

In an attempt to provide conditions which more accurately match the host environment, many investigators have chosen to use a medium supplemented with serum at a pH of 7.0–7.4. Certainly for azoles this has resulted in a considerable lowering of MIC values. In an evaluation programme, it could be of value to investigate the influence of pH on antifungal activity, e.g. Minagawa et al. (1983) showed that in buffered Sabouraud medium, MICs for ketoconazole varied from 40 μg/ml at pH 3 to 0.2 μg/ml at pH 7, more than a 1000-fold difference. Whilst the conditions specified above may reflect the average host environment, there are marked variations in pH, oxygen tension, etc. throughout the body such that it may be necessary to devise specific tests to address the influence of particular environmental conditions on the activity of the antifungal under investigation.

For conventional MIC determinations, the antifungal is added to a suspension of microorganisms at the start of the growth cycle. This is a very different situation to that which exists when therapy is commenced in an infected host. It is of value therefore to determine how the activity of an antifungal is influenced by the time of drug addition or the phase of growth of the fungus. This can be accomplished by sequential photometric monitoring of cultures or by viable count determinations.

Reference was made earlier to the apparent differences in sensitivity of the mycelial and blastospore forms of *C. albicans* to azole antifungals. ODDS et al. (1985) compared the effects of six azoles on the growth and morphology of *C. albicans* hyphae with those of amphotericin B and 5-FC. Morphology was affected by the latter two only at concentrations which inhibited growth, whereas all azole antifungals caused alteration to the morphology at concentrations lower than those which affected growth. For example 10 nanomoles of all azole compounds inhibited branch formation of hyphae whereas 10 micromoles were required to stop hyphal development when the fungus grew mainly in the form of budding yeast cells.

Similar studies on arthrospores and microconidia of *Trichophyton mentagrophytes* have been reported by SCOTT et al. (1984). Higher concentrations of imidazole antifungals were required to inhibit swelling and germination of the spores than to inhibit growth of the fungus. Concentrations which resulted in 90% inhibition of germ-tube formation were about four fold lower for microconidia than for arthrospores. Under these test conditions, ketoconazle was the least effective of the drugs, although it has been used successfully for the treatment of dermatophytoses. The same group of workers had previously shown MICs of imidazoles to be similar for the mycelial and spore forms of *T. mentagrophytes* (WRIGHT et al. 1983).

There have been numerous investigations of the fungicidal properties of antifungal drugs. Unfortunately, published reports, particularly for the imidazoles, have provided conflicting assessments of their fungicidal potencies. During the development of ICI 153,066 we investigated its fungicidal activity compared with six other imidazole antifungals against *C. albicans* using both viable count estimations and regrowth following subculture as parameters (WILSON 1985). ICI 153,066 and ketoconazole were only fungistatic in their activity whereas miconazole, tioconazole and zinoconazole caused 90%–100% kill at or near their respective MICs. When the pH of the medium was increased from 5.6 to 7.0–7.4, there was a marked reduction in the fungicidal activitics of clotrimazole, miconazole and zinoconazole. The addition of 10% serum to the medium reduced both the fungistatic and -cidal activities of all the compounds under investigation, including tioconazole, the most potent fungicide of those tested. Most in vitro tests have a fixed incubation period of 24 or 48 h for yeasts and up to 7 days for dermatophytes or other fungi. Some investigators have attempted to establish the relative importance of drug concentration compared with contact time. RUMLER et al. (1984) showed that for 5-FC, bifonazole and BAY N 7133 (vibunazole), as with clotrimazole and nystatin previously, only short contact times up to 1 h were required at the appropriate MIC to achieve maximum inhibitory effects against *C. albicans*. Prolongation of the contact time does not result in an increased inhibitory activity. From such in vitro experiments one can conclude that for successful therapy in vivo, it is the drug concentration at the site of infection which is of paramount importance. Such data could be of direct value in the evaluation of a topical antifungal but equally can relate to systemic antifungals when combined with serum levels achieved following administration.

The search for new antifungals in recent years has concentrated principally on the imidazole and triazole areas of chemistry. A common feature of the azole antifungals is their ability at low concentrations to block the demethylation of lanosterol to ergosterol, a vital component of the fungal membrane. However, certain azoles have the capacity for fungicidal activity at high concentrations by direct membrane damage (SUD and FEINGOLD 1981). A case could be argued that to achieve substantial improvement over present day antifungal chemotherapy, true fungicidal activity is a prerequisite. Therefore, a test system for detecting fungicial activity would be required in the screening cascade of any research project. The capacity for direct membrane damage is not universal amongst the azoles as demonstrated by a series of studies summarised in an editorial by BEGGS and HUGHES (1987). Miconazole, sulconazole and ketoconazole are capable of killing both proliferating *C. albicans* cells in the early logarithmic growth phase and starved cells of *C. parapsilosis* in pH 7 buffer. Their effect therefore appears to be independent of the growth phase whereas oxiconazole, which had an intermediate effect against resting *C. parapsilosis* cells, was devoid of any fungicidal activity against growing *C. albicans* cells. In both systems butoconazole showed an intermediate fungicidal effect, while ketoconazole was purely fungistatic irrespective of growth phase. None of the recent triazole antifungals, vibunazole, fluconazole or ICI 153,066, was capable of killing proliferating *C. albicans* cells.

In an attempt to improve suboptimal therapy or to reduce unwanted toxicity, various combinations of antifungal agents have been examined. Numerous in vitro studies have reported additive or synergistic effects against yeasts for amphotericin B combined with 5-FC, rifampicin or tetracycline. Reports for imidazole and amphotericin B combinations have been somewhat conflicting, with some interactions proving to be antagonistic (DUPONT and DROUHET 1979). The usual technique for studying such interactions is a 'checkerboard' serial dilution test. If inhibition of growth is observed in the combination containing $\frac{1}{4}$ MIC of each antifungal, then the combination is considered synergistic. The advent of microtitre plates and multichannel dispensers has made such experiments much easier to perform. If required, such studies can be done using agar dilution rather than broth dilution (DUPONT and DROUHET 1979). In the same publication these authors described a technique for studying interactions between antifungal agents which involves cutting in the agar four channels at right angles to one another in the form of a square but not connected, into which can be placed solutions of the antifungals under investigation. Following incubation, the shape of the inhibition area in the angle between adjacent channels is indicative of the type of interaction.

ODDS (1982) undertook a complex investigation of the interactions of amphotericin B, 5-FC, ketoconazole and miconazole in all combinations against three isolates of *C. albicans*, three other *Candida* species, two *Cryptococcus neoformans* strains and three isolates of *Aspergillus fumigatus*. The fungi were grown in a tissue culture medium and incubated in an atmosphere of 5% CO_2 in air. At a point during the logarithmic growth phase, the viable fungal biomass was assayed by bioluminescence spectrophotometry and expressed as a percentage of viable biomass in drug-free controls. Calculation of the area under the inhibition curves gave more consistent and reproducible data than MIC determinations. By both methods of assessment, the combination of amphotericin B and 5-FC usually showed an additive effect. The most antagonistic effects were seen using a combination of ketoconazole and miconazole as judged by MIC but not by the inhibition quotient derived from the area under the curves. Overall, the predominant interactions were additive or synergistic. In the evaluation of new antifungals one might feel it necessary to perform such experiments to determine the extent of interaction with other available antifungals, but the interpretation of such experiments is fraught with difficulties, and their relevance to in vivo therapy is questionable.

Drug resistance in fungi of medical importance is not as great a problem as in other branches of antimicrobial chemotherapy, with the singular exception of the natural and induced resistance of yeasts to 5-FC. Nevertheless, in the evaluation programme for a new antifungal agent it would be prudent to explore in vitro the potential for the development of resistance to the compound, and cross-resistance with existing agents. The most common technique employed is that of serial subculture of the organism in media containing increasing concentrations of the antifungal. This can be performed in liquid media but is probably best done on solid media as the 'resistant' colonies can readily be picked off for subculture. An alternative method is to use gradient plates consisting of a sloped layer of drug-free agar overlaid with antifungal-containing agar to produce a concentration gradient across the plate. Such a technique reduces the need to use a series of plates containing a range of concentrations. By such methods it is possible to produce mutants of yeasts and dermatophytes which are ergosterol deficient and therefore resistant to polyene antibiotics. However, when such mutants are cultured in drug-free media they invariably revert to their initial susceptible state. Fungi sensitive to griseofulvin can be made resistant in vitro by serial subculture, but unlike polyene-resistant mutants, susceptibility does not return if the fungus is cultured in drug-free media. Attempts to produce azole-resistant mutants by such in vitro techniques have been singularly unsuccessful. However, there have been at least four documented cases of resistant clinical isolates emerging during prolonged ketoconazole therapy. We were able to investigate two of these isolates in a series of in vitro and in vivo models (RYLEY et al. 1984). The sensitivities of the two relapse isolates AD and KB were similar to that of a reference strain of *C. albicans* and 36 other clinical isolates when MICs were determined by agar dilution. However, isolates AD and KB showed greatly reduced sensitivity when assayed by other methods comprising IC_{50} determination in liquid medium, MIC determination by two agar diffusion methods and estimations of concentrations required to inhibit mycelial formation. In all systems, the relapse isolates showed cross-resistance to the triazole antifungal ICI 153,066. Similar cross-resistance was seen to miconazole, clotrimazole and econazole. When evaluated in vivo in three models of infection, they were consistently less sensitive than other isolates to treatment with ketoconazole or ICI 153,066. Unfortunately, there has been an insufficient number of cases of resistance to azole antifungals to permit the determination of which in vitro test system might be most appropriate for sensitivity testing in conjunction with antifungal chemotherapy regimens. Before such sensitivity testing of clinical fungal isolates can become useful in the same context as antibacterial sensitivity testing, the meaning of the in vitro-derived MIC or other parameter for a given antifungal agent must be established. Data do exist for 5-FC and griseofulvin, and to a very limited degree for polyenes and imidazoles, which correlate lack of clinical response with reduced in vitro sensitivity, but we are not yet at the stage in which methods of sensitivity testing of antifungal agents are sufficiently standardised to be used in a predictive mode.

K. Conclusions

Methods are available for screening potential antifungal compounds in vitro; the agar dilution method is probably the most satisfactory for a high throughput screen utilising a wide variety of strains and species of fungi. Although general screens are easy to perform, difficulties arise when trying to assess the significance of the results obtained. MICs measured in vitro vary considerably with the conditions under which they are obtained and have little predictive value in terms of activity or the extent of any such activity in vivo. It is possible to modify and define conditions so that more predictive in vitro data can be obtained, but such modifications are only applicable to narrow chemical classes of compound; a generalised predictive screening format still eludes us. In vitro studies are probably more appropriate and reliable when investigating such features as fungicidal as opposed to fungistatic activity, synergy or antagonism between compounds and potential for developing drug resistance. Nevertheless, screening in vitro will continue in situations in which sample numbers are too great or inadequate amounts of compound are available for screening in vivo, and evaluation in vitro will continue in order to satisfy potential clinicians and regulatory authorities.

References

Beggs WH, Hughes CE (1987) Exploitation of the direct cell damaging action of antifungal azoles. Diag Microbiol Infect Dis 6:1–3
Boyle FT, Ryley JF, Wilson RG (1987) In vitro-in vivo correlations with azole antifungals. In: Fromtling RA (ed) Recent trends in the discovery, development and evaluation of antifungal agents. J R Prous, Barcelona, pp S1:31–S1:41
Clayton YM (1987) The in vitro activity of terbinafine against uncommon fungal pathogens. In: Fromtling RA (ed) Recent trends in the discovery, development and evaluation of antifungal agents. J R Prous, Barcelona, pp 433–439
Drouhet E (1988) Standardization of antifungal susceptibility testing. An introductory overview. Proc Xth ISHAM Congress, Barcelona, pp 203–209
Dupont B, Drouhet E (1979) In vitro synergy and antagonism of antifungal agents against yeast-like fungi. Postgrad Med J 55:683–686
Galgiani JN (1986) Antifungal susceptibility testing: recent findings and experience. Antimicrobic Newsletter 3:17–22
Galgiani JN (1987a) Antifungal susceptibility tests. Antimicrob Agents Chemother 31:1867–1870
Galgiani JN (1987b) The need for improved standardization in antifungal susceptibility testing. In: Fromtling RA (ed) Recent trends in the discovery, development and evaluation of antifungal agents. J R Prous, Barcelona, pp 15–24
Guinet R, Nerson D, De Closets F, Dupouy-Camet J, Kures L, Marjollet M, Poirot JL, Ross A, Texier-Maugein J, Volle PJ (1988) Collaborative evaluation in seven laboratories of a standardized micromethod for yeast susceptibility testing. J Clin Microbiol 26:2307–2312
Minagawa H, Kitaura K, Nakamizo N (1983) Effects of pH on the activity of ketoconazole against *Candida albicans*. Antimicrob Agents Chemother 23:105–107
Odds FC (1982) Interactions among amphotericin B, 5-fluorocytosine, ketoconazole, and miconazole against pathogenic fungi in vitro. Antimicrob Agents Chemother 22:763–770
Odds FC (1985) Laboratory tests for the activity of imidazole and triazole antifungal agents in vitro. Semin Dermatol 4:260–270
Odds FC, Abbott AB (1984) Relative inhibition factors – a novel approach to the assessment of antifungal antibiotics in vitro. J Antimicrob Chemother 13:31–43
Odds FC, Webster CE, Abbott AB (1984) Antifungal relative inhibition factors: BAY 1-9139, bifonazole, butoconazole, isoconazole, itraconazole (R 51211), oxiconazole, Ro-14-4767/002, sulconazole, terconazole and vibunazole (BAY n-7133) compared in vitro with nine established antifungal agents. J Antimicrob Chemother 14:105–114
Odds FC, Cockayne A, Hayward J, Abbott AB (1985) Effects of imidazole- and triazole-derivative antifungal compounds on the growth and morphological development of *Candida albicans* hyphae. J Gen Microbiol 131:2581–2589
Odds FC, Abbott AB, Pye G, Troke PF (1986) Improved method for estimation of azole antifungal inhibitory concentrations against *Candida* species, based on azole/antibiotic interactions. J Med Vet Mycol 24:305–311
Petranyi G, Meingassner JG, Mieth H (1987) Antifungal activity of the allylamine derivative terbinafine in vitro. Antimicrob Agents Chemother 31:1365–1368
Polak A, Dixon DM (1987) Antifungal activity of amorolfine (Ro 14-4767/002) in vitro and in vivo. In: Fromtling RA (ed) Recent trends in the discovery, development and evaluation of antifungal agents. J R Prous, Barcelona, pp 555–573
Richardson K, Andrews RJ, Marriott MS, Tarbit MH, Troke PF (1986) Correlation of in vitro and in vivo activity of azole antifungals. In: Iwata K, Vanden Bossche H (eds) In vitro and in vivo evaluation of antifungal agents. Elsevier, Amsterdam, pp 147–149
Rumler W, Heins S, Heins J (1984) Relations between the concentration and the contact-time in the antifungal activity of 5-fluorocytosine, bifonazole and BAY N 7133 to *Candida albicans*. Mykosen 27:436–442

Ryley JF, Rathmell WG (1984) Discovery of antifungal agents: in vitro and in vivo testing. In: Trinci APJ, Ryley JF (eds) Mode of action of antifungal agents. Cambridge University Press, Cambridge, pp 63–87 (Br Mycol Soc Symp No 9)

Ryley JF, Wilson RG, Gravestock MB, Poyser JP (1981) Experimental approaches to antifungal chemotherapy. Adv Pharmacol Chemother 18:49–176

Ryley JF, Wilson RG, Barrett-Bee KJ (1984) Azole resistance in *Candida albicans*. Sabouraudia: J Med Vet Mycol 22:53–63

Scott EM, Gorman SP, Wright LR (1984) The effect of imidazoles on germination of arthrospores and microconidia of *Trichophyton mentagrophytes*. J Antimicrob Chemother 13:101–110

Shadomy S (1987) Preclinical evaluation of antifungal agents: design of in vitro screens. In: Fromtling RA (ed) Recent trends in the discovery, development and evaluation of antifungal agents. J R Prous, Barcelona, pp S1:1–S1:10

Shadomy S, Dixon DM, May R (1982) A comparison of bifonazole (BAY H 4502) with clotrimazole in vitro. Sabouraudia 20:313–323

Shadomy S, Espinel-Ingroff A, Kerkering TM (1984) In-vitro studies with four new antifungal agents: BAY n 7133, bifonazole (BAY h 4502), ICI 153,066 and Ro 14-4767/002. Sabouraudia: J Med Vet Mycol 22:7–15

Sud IJ, Feingold DS (1981) Heterogeneity of action mechanisms among antimycotic imidazoles. Antimicrob Agents Chemother 20:71–74

Van Cutsem J, Van Gerven F, Janssen PAJ (1986) The in vitro evaluation of azoles. In: Iwata K, Vanden Bossche H (eds) In vitro and in vivo evaluation of antifungal agents. Elsevier, Amsterdam, pp 51–64

Van Cutsem J, Van Gerven F, Janssen PAJ (1987) The in vitro and in vivo antifungal activity of itraconazole. In: Fromtling RA (ed) Recent trends in the discovery, development and evaluation of antifungal agents. J R Prous, Barcelona, pp 177–192

Wilson RG (1985) Factors which affect the fungicidal activity of imidazoles and triazoles. IXth ISHAM Cong, Atlanta, Georgia, Abst R1–9

Wright LR, Scott EM, Gorman SP (1983) The sensitivity of mycelium, arthrospores and microconidia of *Trichophyton mentagrophytes* to imidazoles determined by in vitro tests. J Antimicrob Chemother 12:317–327

Yamaguchi H, Hiratani T, Uchida K (1987) The in vitro activity and evaluation of bifonazole. In: Fromtling RA (ed) Recent trends in the discovery, development and evaluation of antifungal agents. J R Prous, Barcelona, pp 335–352

CHAPTER 5

Screening and Evaluation In Vivo

JOHN F. RYLEY

A. Preliminary Considerations

If, as has been suggested, screening in vitro can be misleading and unreliable, it is even more important that in vivo screens should be relevant and that they should be able to cope with large numbers of compounds in restricted quantity. Although topical activity may be achievable in a new compound, a profusion of topical antifungals of differing chemical types is already available. As the current medical need is rather for safer and more effective drugs which can be given by mouth or by injection, the following discussion will be mostly concerned with systemic activity. The purpose of the screen is firstly to detect in vivo antifungal activity and then to indicate whether or not that activity is worth further investigation (as systemic activity in vivo is rare, it *will* be worth further investigation!). Because of varying fungal susceptibilities, compounded by the distribution patterns of compounds in the body and the different sites of fungal location, some indication of the *effective* spectrum of activity is desirable; e.g. although *Candida albicans* is basically susceptible to amphotericin B and systemic infections do show a response to treatment, vaginal ones do not. Other compounds will be basically narrow in their spectrum of activity, e.g. griseofulvin and terbinafine only have utility against dermatophytes, 5-fluorocytosine only against yeasts and cilofungin (LY 121019) only against two species of *Candida*. As there appears to be commercial viability in narrow spectrum antifungal agents as well as a medical need, the screen should be able to detect both types of activity. Extrapolation from mice to humans is never easy, and so comparison with already established antifungals will be important in assessing the possible significance of activity detected in the screen.

At the screening stage the amount of compound available for testing will be very limited. Although admirable models of infection in rats, hamsters or guinea pigs are available, it cannot be over-emphasised that models involving mice are greatly to be preferred becaused they will consume far smaller quantities of compound. In order to obtain the maximum amount of information from a limited amount of compound, I have used multiple infections; initially, I used mice carrying two infections and latterly modified this to a model involving four infections in the same mouse. *C. albicans* is an important cause of serious fungal disease; its widespread occurrence and the fact that it does not apparently produce disease in healthy individuals means that working with the organism presents little hazard. Not so with some of the causative agents of the 'American mycoses', e.g. *Coccidioides immitis*. Work with such organisms requires stringent precautions, and expensive facilities must be used; thus, it is not appropriate at the screening stage. In fact, work will only be undertaken when a very promising compound with an apparently wide spectrum activity is discovered and then sensibly only in a specialised laboratory. Working with aspergillus, cryptococcus or dermatophytes presents minimal hazard; accidental infections with the latter can be easily treated. Such considerations of safety therefore allow the use of quite a variety of different fungi which make it possible to detect wide spectrum as well as more restricted antifungal activity.

B. Types of Screen

There are basically two types of fungal infection: lethal ones, where response to treatment is measured by prevention of or delay in death, and non-lethal ones, where the severity of infection can be assessed visually, by culture from superficial sites or by viable fungal counts from internal organs. Fluconazole was discovered using an acute systemic infection with *C. albicans* in the mouse (RICHARDSON et al. 1985). Control mice inoculated i.v. with 10^7 blastospores were all dead within 48 h, the time when the screen was read. Treatment with fluconazole or other azoles given 1, 4 and 24 h following inoculation allowed survival at 48 h, and by using a range of doses, a 50% effective dose (ED_{50}) for each compound could be calculated. This dose has no absolute significance, since sterilisation was not achieved, and much higher doses had to be used if the test was prolonged beyond 48 h. The screen, however, is simple to perform, it does detect activity, and ED_{50}s have some comparative significance. With an ED_{50} of 0.08 mg/kg for fluconazole, compound requirements will be pleasingly small in such a screen. Like the version of the mouse protection test universally used in antibacterial research, ED_{50}s in this test bear little relation to the much larger doses of compound required to produce an effect in other models of infection. Assay of compounds for prevention of death in systemic fungal infections is appropriate in the development of a promising compound, but such procedures are ethically questionable if used at the *screening* stage. More acceptable are non-lethal infections in which activity is quantitated in another way. Because of the prevalence and economic importance of vaginal candidosis, a vaginal infection was used in mice as the basis of our screen. Compound requirements were greater, and reading the test – which involved plating out vaginal samples on BiGGY agar (Bismuth sulphite – Glucose-Glycine-Yeast; Difco) – was more time consuming. These limitations, however, were perfectly acceptable. Because of the prevalence and economic importance of dermatophytes, we also inoculated our mice with *Trichophyton quinckeanum* on the back. For the expenditure of effort involved in a simple inoculation and the visual scoring of ringworm lesions at the end of the experiment, further useful information was obtained without the expenditure of more compound or more animals. No interference between the infections was observed. With the increasing importance of systemic infections resulting from high technology medicine and the AIDS situation, I enlarged the screen to include in the same mice a non-lethal systemic infection with *C. albicans* and a lung infection with *Cryptococcus neoformans*. The response of these infections to treatment was determined by culturing aliquots of kidney and lung homogenates at the end of the test. Unfortunately, I have not been able to think of a way of incorporating the other pathogen of current importance, *Aspergillus fumigatus*, in the multi-infection model in such a way that it does not interfere with the other four infections! Although such a multi-infection model provides much more information without the expenditure of any more compound or animals or time and effort in dosing, much more effort is involved in setting up the test and taking it off. In any screening situation in which high throughput of compounds is essential, simplicity of operation and effort involved is important; in any particular screening campaign a compromise will have to be made between information required and the complexity of the screen within the constraints of effort available.

C. The Multi-Infection Screen

The multi-infection screen was described by RYLEY and MCGREGOR (1988). Briefly, female mice weighing 25–30 g are injected subcutaneously on a Friday (day −4) with 0.5 mg estradiol benzoate as a ball-milled suspension in 0.25 ml 0.5% Tween 80; this is sufficient to induce estrus for a period of 10 days. The following Tuesday (day 0) the fur on their backs is clipped, and the mice are then inoculated successively with 10^5 *C. albicans* in 0.2 ml saline given intravenously, 10^7 *C. neoformans* in 50 μl saline administered intranasally under light halothane anaesthesia, *C. albicans* introduced intravaginally with a blunt-ended Pasteur pipette until run-out using a suspension of 10^8/ml, and finally with a suspension of *T. quinckeanum* spores at 7×10^7/ml applied liberally to the back with a brush following light scarification of the clipped area with a piercing saw blade. Mice are caged in groups of five and dosed orally once daily on days 0–3; with a test involving 150 mice this means the first dose is administered within 4 h of the first intravenous inoculation. On day 6 (Monday) dermatophyte lesions are scored visually on an arbitrary scale of 0–4, and a specimen obtained from the vagina with a wire loop is plated out on BiGGY agar (Difco); after incubation at 37°C for 48 h, growth is scored visually on a scale of 0–4. Following vaginal sampling on day 6, the mice are killed, and the kidneys dissected out and placed in 5 ml saline in a plastic universal container; the lungs are similarly treated. The organs are then homogenised with a Ystral X 10/20 homogeniser, diluted 1/10–1/1000 with saline, and 50-μl samples spiral plated onto Sabouraud glucose agar containing penicillin G (500 units/ml) and streptomycin sulphate (100 mg/l) with a Spiral Plater model D. Following incubation of kidney plates at 37°C for 24 h and lung plates at 30°C for 48 h, growth is scored or actual colony counts done.

Nine antifungal agents were tested in this screen at a series of doses, and the effect of each compound on each infection graded as active, slightly active or not active. Table 1 indicates the minimum effective dose giving full activity in each case, with a figure in brackets giving the minimum dose which showed incomplete but nevertheless obvious activity, if this occurred. There was no discernible interference between the four infections or their responses to treatment. This was demonstrated by evaluating each compound against each infection on its own in further mice; the results in a single infection did not differ from those in the multi-infection screen by more than one dose increment either way for any of the compounds. The only unusual influence observed was that estradiol treatment, necessary to support the vaginal infection with *C. albicans*, also appeared to promote heavier dermal infections with *T. quinckeanum*. The screen was designed with weekly operation in view, and since the most labour-intensive operations are associated with setting it up and terminating it, its duration has been restricted to 6 days; with a 5-day week, this allows daily dosing for 4 days. Two technicians should be able to handle 30 groups of five mice in such a screen each week. Although the mice carried four different infections, there was no indication of distress to the animals during the period of the screen with the inocula of the various organisms chosen; had the mice been kept for a longer period, then some animals would have died from the kidney infection, and possibly clinical symptoms would have occurred as a result of the lung infection.

The screen can be modified and simplified by leaving out one, two or even three of the four infections; whether this is done will depend among other things on the chemical types of compound being tested, the number of compounds to be tested each week, and the technical effort available. It can be noted from Table 1 that the five azoles showed roughly equivalent activity against all four infections; what is different is the potency from compound to compound. In a screening campaign involving only azoles, in which the initial aim is to detect activity and give an indication as to whether that activity is worth further investigation, it would be sufficient to use only one of the infections in the screen. From the practical point of view vaginal *C. albicans* would probably be the simplest. If, however, the compounds for screening are not azoles, use of a single infection could result in missing narrow-spectrum but still very useful compounds such as griseofulvin, terbinafine or 5-fluorocytosine, or even compounds such as amphotericin, which have a wide spectrum of activity in vitro, but whose performance in vivo depends very much on the location of the fungus in the body. If a compound showing excellent activity at the screening stage is of real interest because of chemical structure and other properties, a fair idea may be gained of its potential by careful comparison with established antifungals in the full screen.

Table 1. Activities of nine antifungal agents in a multi-infection mouse screen

Compound	Minimum effective dose (mg/kg × 4)			
	T. quinckeanum	Vaginal *C. albicans*	Systemic *C. albicans*	*C. neoformans*
Amphotericin B	25 (5)[a]	NA 100[b]	2.5	50 (5)
5-Fluorocytosine	NA 500	NA 500	25	NA 500
Griseofulvin	250 (100)	NA 500	NA 500	NA 500
Ketoconazole	25	25	50	100
Itraconazole	10	25	25	25
SCH 39304 (SM 8668)	(100–1)	10 (5)	2.5 (1)	5 (2.5)
Fluconazole	5	2.5	5 (1)	5
ICI 195,739	1 (0.5)	0.5	1 (0.5)	2.5 (1)
Terbinafine	25	NA 250	NA 250	NA 250

[a] Figures are minimum effective doses for virtually complete control, while in brackets are minimum effective doses at which partial activity was seen.
[b] NA, not active.

D. Further Evaluation

Once interesting activity has been established for a particular compound in the screen, it may be necessary to confirm that activity using similar infections in different hosts or under different conditions, and to see whether activity extends to more exotic species of fungi.

I. Candidosis

1. Rat Vaginitis

Vaginal infections with *C. albicans* may be readily produced in ovariectomised, estrogen-treated rats (SCHOLER 1960). I have been unable, however, to establish vaginal infections in guinea pigs, rabbits, dogs or marmosets following a variety of surgical and chemical manipulations, although HARE and LOEBENBERG (1988) have recently described a model using hamsters which does not require the use of ovariectomy or hormone treatment. In this system hamsters are inoculated intravaginally on 3 consecutive days following gentle irritation of the vagina with a cotton swab. Infected animals are identified by culturing on day 5 and used for test. The progress of infection is followed by culturing samples taken with cotton swabs. Because of the lack of preconditioning requirements, this infection has potential for drug evaluation; for screening purposes the mouse is still to be preferred due to reduced compound requirements. For the more widely used rat model, female rats weighing 100–120 g are ovariectomised via a dorsal midline incision and treated every 2 weeks with 0.1 mg estradiol undecylate in sesame oil (Progynon: Schering) intramuscularly. Three days after the first treatment they are inoculated with a suspension of *C. albicans* at 10^8/ml in saline introduced into the vagina until run-out using a blunt-ended Pasteur pipette. The infection peaks at 2–3 weeks and then declines to give a low level chronic infection. The infection may be followed by sampling onto BiGGY agar with a wire loop (most convenient), by washing out the vagina with saline and culturing the washings, or by removing the vagina, homogenising, diluting, spiral plating and counting (RYLEY and MCGREGOR 1986). Using a similar schedule of treatment and sampling to that used in the mouse screen, compounds may appear more potent in rats than in mice; the most extreme example we have seen is itraconazole, active in the mouse at 25 mg/kg and in the rat at 1 mg/kg (RYLEY et al. 1988b). Both the mouse and rat models may be used to compare the ability of a compound to prevent infection (treatment started at the time of inoculation) with its ability to cure an established infection (treatment started say 3 days after inoculation). Likewise, it is useful to investigate the ability of the compound to eliminate infection using a single dose or at least a short course of treatment, since this must be the ultimate clinical aim. The models may also be used to investigate topical activity; treatment with a crude formulation in polyethylene glycols or a more refined pharmaceutical formulation may be given once or twice daily for a period and the effect on the infection studied (RYLEY et al. 1988b).

2. Intestinal Infections

C. albicans exists as a commensal in the gut of many people; this reservoir may act as a source of infection for the vagina and may under certain circumstances disseminate to internal organs and give systemic infection. It is therefore important to investigate the ability of novel compounds to eliminate this intestinal reservoir. Intestinal infections are difficult to produce in mature rodents but can readily be induced in mice inoculated at 6 days of age (HERRERA and GUENTZEL 1982). I have inoculated mice at this stage with 10^7 *C. albicans* in 0.1 ml delivered into the stomach with a fine metal catheter (day 0). Oral treatment was given in the same way over days 6–12, and mice were killed on day 17 for total homogenate counts on the stomach and intestinal tract. One litter was used for each treatment, and mice remained with their dam throughout the experiment (RYLEY et al. 1988b). Mice inoculated at 6 days of age will retain their infection for many weeks. Although dissemination from the intestinal tract may occur in humans in the presence of predisposing causes, dissemination in mice following treatment with antibiotics and cytotoxic agents is rarely sufficient to permit reliable evaluation of potential drugs; liver or kidney counts seldom exceed 10^3 cfu per mouse.

3. Systemic Infections

Systemic infections with *C. albicans* in mice, rats, guinea pigs and rabbits have been used in drug evaluation studies. For a few days following the intravenous inoculation of mice with *C. albicans*, fungi can be recovered from a variety of internal organs in ever decreasing numbers; only in the kidney is a progressive infection observed. High inocula produce early death with low kidney counts but with elevated blood urea and creatinine and a copious production of urine of low specific gravity. Moderate inocula produce infections which some mice survive; kidney fungal counts are higher for a time, and recovery may be faster in one kidney than the other. Low inocula produce transient kidney infections without mortality or changes in blood and urine chemistry (RYLEY et al. 1988a). Compounds can be evaluated in mice for prophylactic activity (if compound administration starts before or at the time of inoculation) or for therapeutic activity (if dosing is delayed for some time after inoculation). The infection can be followed by observations on mortality patterns after high inocula or by kidney fungal counts on groups of mice killed at intervals following smaller inocula. For experiments involving mortality, it is desirable to use inocula which will kill all untreated control mice within 5–7 days; this inoculum will vary with the strain of *C. albicans* used. Inocula greater than 10^7 per mouse should be avoided, since early deaths may be produced by obstructive rather than truly pathogenic mechanisms. Compounds appear more active the nearer to the time of inoculation that dosing is started and the earlier the experiment is terminated. Response to treatment may be illustrated graphically in terms of mortality patterns (e.g. POLAK 1987) or by calculation of mean survival times. Estimates of ED_{50} may be made, though at the evaluation stage one is more interested in a compound's potential for curing all patients treated rather than only half of them! With these severe infections, treatment usually causes a delay in mortality rather than permanent protection, although this may not be apparent if the experiment is terminated at 2–3 weeks, which has usually been the case in published studies. In an investigation with a new azole, ICI 195,739, I have recently compared treatments lasting 3, 10, 30 or 90 days, mortality being recorded for at least 70 days following cessation of treatment (RYLEY et al. 1988b). As may be seen from Fig. 1, the effect of the compound depended on the length of the treatment period, and delayed mortality would have been missed had the experiment been terminated at 2–3 weeks. Mice survived as long as dosing continued, but only with the 90-day treatment period was long-term survival achieved. Although this behaviour might be expected with a fungistatic azole, it may also be noted with other types of compound unless dosing is continued, e.g. POLAK (1987). The ability to cure rather than ameliorate infection is more obvious in experiments in which lower inocula are used and mice are sacrificed at intervals or at the end of the experiment for determination of kidney fungal counts (e.g. RYLEY et al. 1988b); such experiments indicate potential for elimination of infection rather than merely a reduction below a lethal threshold.

Similar evaluation experiments may be done using rats (e.g. GALGIANI and VAN WYCK 1984; RICHARDSON et al. 1985), although the procedure is more expensive in terms of compound and animals, with no apparent advantage in information generated. Guinea pigs likewise may be used, with the possibility of generating additional data if a dermatotropic strain of *C. albicans* is employed, and rabbits if there is an additional interest in eye infections (see later). In any of these situations, animals may be made neutropenic by injection with cyclophosphamide (200 mg/kg for mice) 4 days before inoculation to simulate the situation in immunocompromised patients. The result is an apparent increase in the virulence of the organism and an increase in the dose of compound required to produce any particular degree of response.

4. Skin Infections

Skin candidosis can be induced in large guinea pigs stressed by the injection of alloxan at 200 mg/kg 24 h before inoculation of clipped but intact skin (VAN CUTSEM and THIENPONT 1971). Treatment may be administered orally or topically and the infection followed by scoring the lesions at intervals (VAN CUTSEM and THIENPONT 1972). This group have produced skin lesions in guinea pigs reminiscent of those currently being observed in heroin addicts (VAN CUTSEM et al. 1985). Male guinea pigs are inoculated intravenously with a non-lethal dose of 8×10^3 cfu of *C. albicans* per g body wt. Pinpoint eruptions appear on the skin 4–5 days later, and these subsequently become

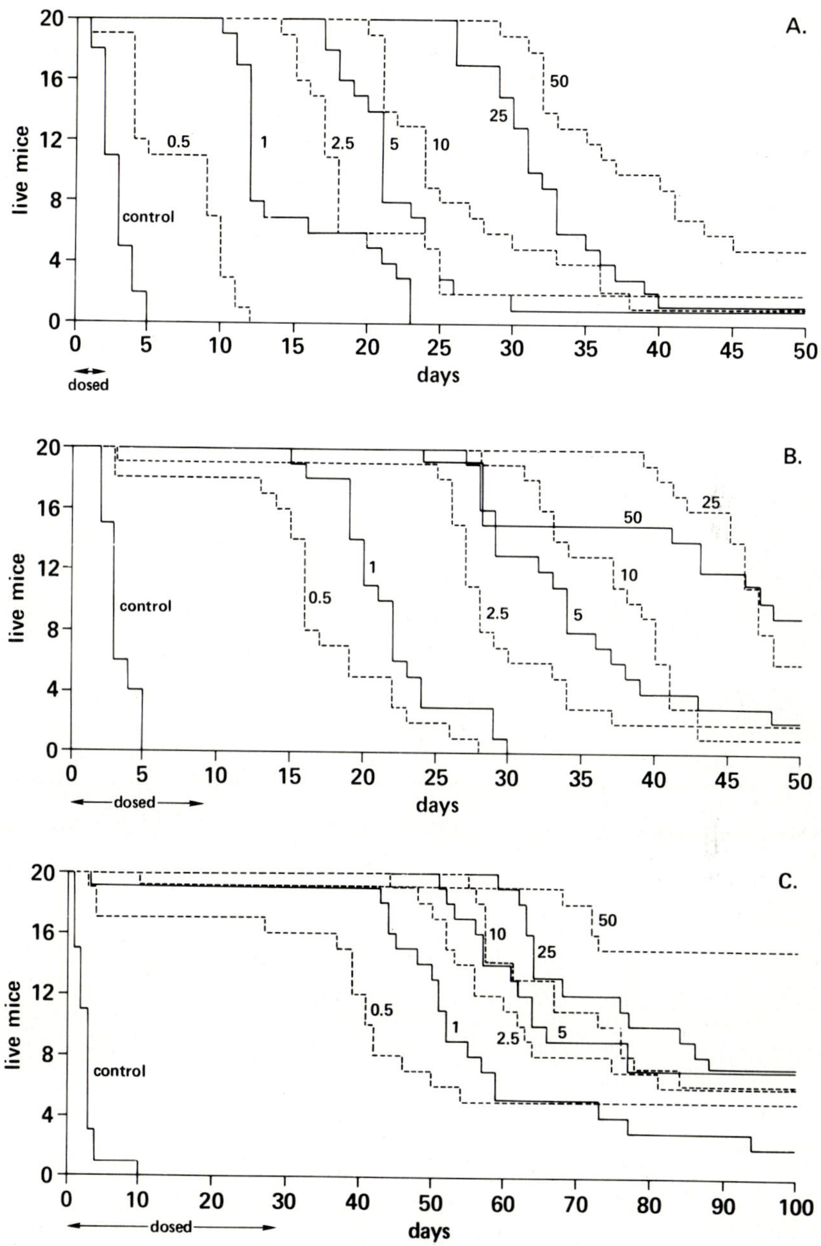

Fig. 1A–C. Mortality patterns in mice inoculated intravenously with *C. albicans* (4.5×10^6 cfu) and treated orally with ICI 195,739 over days 0–2 (**A**), 0–9 (**B**), or 0–29 (**C**) in doses (mg/kg per day) indicated on graphs inflammatory and erythematous; vesicles are formed containing exudate and blastospores, and yeasts invade the epithelial layers and undergo transformation to hyphae and pseudohyphae. The infection can be followed by visual scoring of the lesions, and of course at the end of an experiment involving systemic treatment, kidney fungal counts can be done to assess the effect on the systemic component of the infection. RAY (1985) may be consulted for a more comprehensive review of possible experimental models of skin candidosis.

5. Other Infections

Although infection of the intestine of rodents with *C. albicans* is difficult to induce, RUSSELL et al. (1976) have produced long-lasting colonisation of the mouth in rats given 0.1% tetracycline in the drinking water; the system could presumably be used in drug evaluation. Palatal candidosis is a frequent problem in denture wearers. SHAKIR et al. (1981) described an elegant model to simulate this condition in rats. Rats fitted with an acrylic plate inoculated with *C. albicans* and wired to the teeth of the upper jaw develop palatal lesions similar to those seen in humans. MARTIN (1989) has used this model with effect to demonstrate the potential of fluconazole in the treatment of this condition; an open trial in humans confirmed the predictive value of the model.

C. albicans administered intravenously to rabbits produces pyelonephritis; PERFECT et al. (1986) have used this model in a comparison of itraconazole with fluconazole. If a polyethylene catheter is inserted across the aortic valve prior to intravenous inoculation, mycotic endocarditis is also produced; PERFECT and DURACK (1985) used this system to evaluate the potential of a new derivative of amphotericin B. In addition to endocarditis and pyelonephritis, intravenous inoculation of rabbits with *C. albicans* also induces endophthalmitis; SAVANI et al. (1987) used this feature of the model in a study with ketoconazole, itraconazole and fluconazole. Fluconazole penetrated most readily into the eye, and all three compounds were able to reduce the number of fungi found in the eye when therapy was initiated within 24 h of inoculation; only ketoconazole gave a significant reduction in counts when therapy was delayed for 7 days.

An interesting model with potential chemotherapeutic application has been described by KRAUSE and SCHAFFNER (1988) in connection with some immunology studies. Mice were injected subcutaneously on the back with 2 ml air, and the sac induced was refilled every 3–4 days; no irritant such as croton oil was used. Seven days after the first injection of air, 10^5–10^7 *C. albicans* in 0.1 ml was introduced into the sac. If cyclosporin A dissolved in olive oil was given orally daily at the rate of 40 mg/kg starting 2 days before inoculation, thrush-like lesions were produced on the lining of the sac. POLAK and SCHAFFNER (1989) have subsequently described the use of this model in the evaluation of a number of antifungal agents; they found cyclophosphamide or cortisone to be more satisfactory immunosuppressive agents than cyclosporin A. A more artificial system for pharmacokinetic/activity studies had been described by HUGHES et al. (1986). Semipermeable visking chambers were implanted subcutaneously in rabbits and inoculated with *Candida* spp.; fungal growth and chamber drug concentrations were followed after the administration of ketoconazole ± 5-fluorocytosine.

II. Dermatophytosis

Since the classic demonstration by GENTLES (1958) of oral activity with griseofulvin, the guinea pig has been the favourite animal for work with dermatophytes; rabbits, dogs and monkeys may also be used, but these hosts offer no obvious advantage in terms of cost, convenience or information generated. Infections can readily be produced with suitable strains of *Trichophyton mentagrophytes* and *Microsporum canis*; most workers have been unable to produce experimental infections with *Trichophyton rubrum*, the most prevalent dermatophyte affecting humans, although TROKE (1987) was apparently more successful. In order for infection to develop it is necessary to scarify lightly (with sandpaper, scalpel blade, fine saw, wire brush, etc.) the skin of the guinea pig prior to inoculation, or to occlude the intact skin following inoculation (KERBS and ALLEN 1978). This latter procedure may be simply a device to raise the CO_2 tension at the skin surface which is believed to be necessary for fungal transformation and invasion (ALLEN and KING 1978). From the practical point of view, particularly when large numbers of animals are involved, inoculation with scarification is by far the simpler procedure and avoids the problem of maintaining occlusion on animals which object to being permanently bandaged or taped.

Fungal growth occurs in the surface layers of the skin during the first few days after inoculation followed by invasion of the hair follicles. During the 2nd week surface growth of the fungus is gradually eliminated, while penetration of the hair follicles increases, accompanied by spore production. The intensity of infection declines during the 3rd week, and fungal elements are usually eliminated by day 28. Macroscopically, infection first shows around the 5th day as an area of reddening, soon accompanied by the production of fine scale. The erythema increases over the next few days, and the scale gradually gives way to a crust or scab. The lesions are raised, and the skin thickens. Lesions appear to reach maximum severity 10–12 days after inoculation. As the animals recover, hair loss in heavy infections is pronounced; bald patches in such animals are transformed by hair regrowth within a couple of weeks. Because infections are self-limiting, drug evaluation studies are not concerned with a cure/no cure situation but rather a modification in the rate of spontaneous healing. In general the effectiveness of a compound in speeding up the rate of healing depends on how early in the course of infection treatment is started (Fig. 2B). With initial studies in guinea pigs, treatment is started 3 days after inoculation, at a time when hyphal growth in the keratin layers of the skin is well established and migration to the hair follicles is under way, but before macroscopic signs of infection are evident. Infection may be followed by culturing skin scrapings, by the 'hair root invasion test' of PETRANYI et al. (1982) or by simply assessing the lesions clinically and ascribing an arbitrary score based on scaling, erythema and thickening; I prefer this latter method (RYLEY et al. 1981; RYLEY and RATHMELL 1984). The model is equally applicable for oral or topical treatment. Figure 2 illustrates the response to treatment by a variety of oral or topical agents and also demonstrates the effect on response of the time when treatment is initiated.

Of possible slight relevance to immunocompromised hosts (NOVICK et al. 1987) is a model of experimental systemic dermatophytosis described by VAN CUTSEM and JANSSEN (1984). After a variety of animals had been inoculated intravenously with a large range of dermatophytes, *T. mentagrophytes* in guinea pigs was selected for further study. Unlike the situation following cutaneous inoculation, a generalised infection was produced, with fungi recoverable from the lung, liver and kidneys of many animals; granulomas or mycetomas developed in the lungs, often accompanied by bronchopneumonia. There was a generalised skin infection, and the soles of the feet and the nails were frequently involved. Inflammation was not as pronounced as that which follows cutaneous inoculation, and the skin infection persisted, probably due to continual reinfection from hyphal masses in the internal organs. This model has been used in the evaluation of itraconazole (VAN CUTSEM et al. 1987).

III. Cryptococcosis

Cryptococcosis starts as a pulmonary infection, which in some cases disseminates and spreads to the brain, causing meningitis; this type of infection is currently of particular importance in connection with AIDS. Experimental models of cryptococcosis have been described in mice, rats and rabbits. I have already described the screen which utilises intranasal inoculation of mice with *C. neoformans*. For evaluation studies such an infection can be used with the start of treatment delayed until a few days after inoculation. The progress of infection and response to treatment can be followed by observations on mortality and by fungal counts on lungs and brains of groups of mice killed at intervals. In the evaluation of ICI 195,739 (RYLEY et al. 1988b) I used such a model and also an infection produced by intravenous inoculation with *C. neoformans*, response to treatment being measured in terms of protection from mortality. GRAYBILL and AHRENS (1984) used infections in mice produced by intraperitoneal or intracranial inoculation in the evaluation of itraconazole and employed athymic as well as normal mice in a comparison of ketoconazole with two experimental drugs (GRAYBILL et al. 1983b); athymic mice are more susceptible to cryptococcosis than normal mice. GRAYBILL et al. (1983a) described an infection in rats induced by direct inoculation into the bronchi. The infection was self-limiting in normal rats but was progressive with dissemination in athymic rats. Although the work was described in

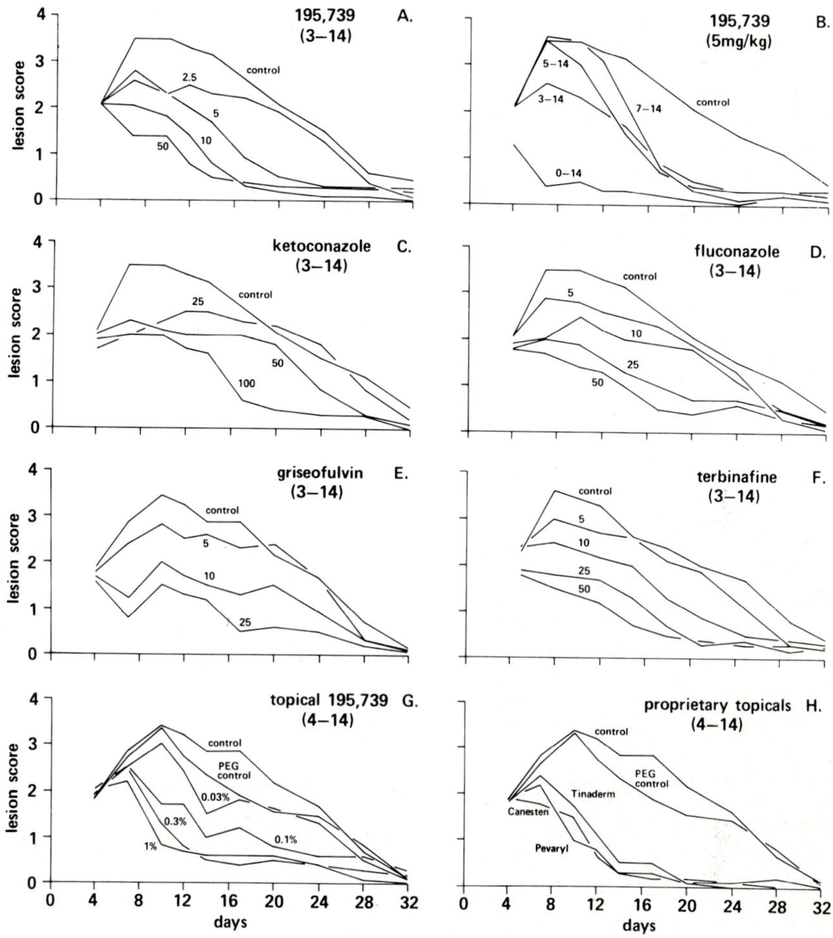

Fig. 2A–H. Response of *Trichophyton mentagrophytes* infection in guinea pigs to oral or topical treatment with antifungal agents. Doses of compound (mg/kg oral or % w/v topical) and period of treatment are indicated on the graphs. Tinaderm contains 1% tolnaftate, Canesten 1% clotrimazole and Pevaryl 1% econazole nitrate

connection with immunological studies, the model could have chemotherapeutic applications.

Because of the importance of the meningeal form of the disease, Perfect et al. (1980) developed a model of chronic meningeal infection in cortisone-treated rabbits. Following intracisternal inoculation, a progressive infection developed which was fatal in 2–12 weeks. The incidence and severity of infection were related to cortisone dose rather than inoculum size. Infection was followed by aspirating cerebrospinal fluid at intervals for culture and quantitation. In a chemotherapy trial with amphotericin B, 5-fluorocytosine and ketoconazole, alone and in combination, treatment reduced spinal fluid counts, but some untreated control rabbits appeared to show declining rather than progressive infection as well.

Certain strains of *C. neoformans* seem to be dermotropic; FROMTLING et al. (1988) described a rhinotropic strain which produced large granulomatous lesions of the nose as well as nodular lesions of the ears, feet and tail following intravenous inoculation of mice; the brains, lungs, liver, kidneys and spleen were also infected. POLAK and DIXON (1988) used a similar rhinotropic isolate for chemotherapy studies in mice. The best activity was seen with ICI 195,739, followed by fluconazole, itraconazole and ketoconazole; amphotericin B was only active in high doses, and 5-fluorocytosine when given early in the course of infection. VAN CUTSEM et al. (1986) managed to produce cryptococcomas scattered over the skin of guinea pigs following intravenous inoculation with a selected strain, a model which was subsequently used in the evaluation of itraconazole (VAN CUTSEM et al. 1987).

IV. Aspergillosis

Aspergillus is an important pathogen in immunocompromised individuals, and efficacy in this condition has been particularly sought in the ketoconazole-itraconazole-saperconazole development. Three basic models using mice have been developed for drug evaluation studies. GRAYBILL et al. (1983c) inoculated BALB/c mice intravenously or cortisone-treated mice intranasally and evaluated the response to treatment with ketoconazole or BAY n 7133 by observations on mortality, supplemented in some instances by fungal counts on lungs at the end of the experiment. Similar studies with itraconazole were described by GRAYBILL and AHRENS (1985) and with ICI 195,739 by RYLEY et al. (1988b), although when using the same strain of *A. fumigatus* as Graybill, I was unable to produce infection in mice by intranasal inoculation. ACKERBAUER et al. (1985) described a model for drug evaluation which involved direct inoculation of one kidney with spores of *A. fumigatus* followed by fungal counts on the kidney 3 days later.

V. Other Mycoses

As interest in a development compound increases, investigations of activity in some of the less common and often more refractory mycoses will be in order.

1. Coccidioidomycosis

C. immitis is one of the most dangerous fungal pathogens for experimentalists to use, and evaluations should only be carried out by competent individuals having all the necessary facilities for isolation and confinement. Levine has developed the most elaborate models for evaluating drugs in this condition, and his approach is well summarised in a comparison of BAY n 7133 and BAY 19139 with ketoconazole (LEVINE 1984). Mice were inoculated intranasally with graded doses of arthroconidia of *C. immitis*. In phase A studies treatment was started on day 4, at a time when infection was restricted almost entirely to the lungs, and continued 5 days a week to day 22. Response to treatment was assessed in terms of protection from mortality and recovery of fungi from lung, liver, spleen and kidney when the experiment was terminated on day 34. In phase B studies a lower inoculum was used, and treatment was not started until day 12, at which time the animals were moribund. Treatment was continued 5 days a week until day 84, and survivors were necropsied for culture of internal organs 15 days later. Again response to treatment was gauged in terms of mortality and organ culture. In phase C studies treatment was administered over days 36–120 following inoculation with a dose of arthroconidia which killed around 20% of the mice before treatment was started. The purpose of this latter phase was to see whether treatment would prevent death in animals with deep-seated illness and to investigate whether biocure was possible. With meningeal infections in view, GRAYBILL et al. (1986b) used mice inoculated intracerebrally with endospores of *C. immitis* in an evaluation of fluconazole.

2. Paracoccidioidomycosis

The most useful model for drug evaluation in this condition would seem to be that described by LEFLER et al. (1985a). Mice were inoculated intranasally; because of the acute nature of the model, treatment was started within 24 h of challenge. Treatment was continued for 4 weeks, and observations made on mortality and recovery of fungi from lung, spleen and liver at the end of the experiment. A more prolonged investigation was described by UEDA et al. (1987) which involved intravenous inoculation and immunological and histopathological studies in the assessment of response to treatment.

3. Histoplasmosis

In connection with the evaluation of fluconazole, GRAYBILL et al. (1986a) described a mouse model of histoplasmosis. Inoculation was intranasal, and both intact and athymic mice were employed. The course of infection and response to treatment were followed by observations on mortality, histoplasmin antigen concentrations in bronchoalveolar lavage fluid and fungal burdens in lungs from groups of mice killed at intervals. KOBAYASHI et al. (1986) in another evaluation of fluconazole using intravenous inoculation of mice, followed mortality over a period of 4 weeks and then determined terminal counts of fungi in the spleen. POLAK and DIXON (1986) in a similar study with fluconazole assessed the speed of response to treatment by doing counts on spleens taken from groups of animals killed at daily intervals over the first 6 days of a 3-week experiment.

4. Blastomycosis

LEFLER et al. (1985b) inoculated mice intranasally with yeast forms of *Blastomyces dermatitidis* in order to compare the efficacy of a number of developmental antifungals with ketoconazole and amphotericin B. A progressive focal pneumonia was followed by extrapulmonary dissemination in mice which survived long enough. Treatment was for 2 or 4 weeks, starting 3 days after inoculation. Response to treatment was assessed in terms of protection from mortality and the presence of fungi in lungs, spleen, liver and kidneys of animals which survived in experiments that ran for up to 9 weeks.

5. Sporotrichosis

Two somewhat artificial models have been described in attempts to predict the utility of compounds for this condition. SCHAUDE and MEINGASSNER (1986) implanted chambers fitted with 0.45 μm or 3.0 μm membranes subcutaneously in mice. Chambers were inoculated with 10^5 cfu of *Sporothrix schenckii* yeast before implantation. Mice were dosed 2 h before and 2, 4, 24, 48 and 72 h after implantation. Chambers were removed 24 h after the last dose and populations of surviving fungi determined by culture. In an evaluation of itraconazole, VAN CUTSEM et al. (1987) inoculated guinea pigs in the left testis, treated the animals daily for 4 weeks, and 1 week later killed the animals and cultured the liver and right testis to assess the extent of dissemination of the infection.

6. Miscellaneous Mycoses

POLAK (1984a,b) described models in mice relevant to the treatment of chromomycosis and phaeohyphomycosis. Selection of suitable strains of organisms was crucial. Mice were inoculated intravenously with 8×10^7 cfu of *Fonsecaea pedrosoi*; a few mice died early on, but the majority survived for up to 7 weeks. There was a gradual weight loss, reaching 35% after 7 weeks. After 3–4 weeks the legs became swollen, and black spots appeared on the tail; by 7 weeks the tail and legs had become dark in colour and full of nodules. The head also showed some deformations, and the animals died within the next few days. The lungs, brain and kidneys showed granulomatous lesions, but the liver and spleen were clear. Drug was administered daily for 29 days from the time of inoculation, and the effects of treatment assessed at 30 and 60 days in terms of mortality and lesions on the legs and tail.

Most mice inoculated intravenously with 6×10^6 cfu *Wangiella dermatitidis* died within a week, due mainly to heavy multiplication of the fungus in the brain. For chemotherapy experiments, three or six doses of compound were given, the first at the time of inoculation. Mortality was followed over a period of 20 days, or fungal counts in brain tissues were determined 4 days after inoculation.

VAN CUTSEM et al. (1988), recognising the importance of zygomycetes as agents of opportunistic infection, studied the pathogenicity and histopathology of two species of *Rhizopus* inoculated into mice and rats made diabetic with streptozotocin and in normal guinea pigs. With suitable inocula, fatal infections were produced in which most internal organs were invaded; the guinea pig was suggested as the best host for chemotherapeutic studies.

E. Extrapolation to Clinical Use

Having established antifungal activity for a new compound in a series of animal models of infection, the questions arise as to whether or not the compound will be effective in humans, and what sort of dose would be appropriate. Unlike the situation with antibiotics and bacteria, there is no way of predicting antifungal activity in humans, let alone the degree of such activity, on a basis of MIC determinations in vitro and pharmacokinetic considerations. Although the limited numbers of examples available do suggest that activity in animal models of infection indicates probable activity in humans, experience with fluconazole and itraconazole demonstrates that a straight transfer of doses in terms of mg/kg is not appropriate (RYLEY et al. 1988b). Likewise, it is unrealistic to try to define a plasma drug level associated with activity in an animal model and seek to achieve that same plasma level in the human situation. The most hopeful way of arriving at a possible human dose for a developmental compound seems to be to apply a 'potency ratio' argument. This means that if a developmental compound is 'n' times as potent as a compound in clinical use in an animal model of infection, then it is likely to be 'n' times as potent as that standard in humans also. Hence, at the screening stage and at all stages of evaluation it is important to have the models standardised with compounds already in clinical use.

References

Ackerbauer H, Meingassner JG, Mieth H (1985) Experimental renal infection with *Aspergillus fumigatus* in mice: a chemotherapeutic model of an organic mycosis. Mykosen 28:244–250

Allen AM, King RD (1978) Occlusion, carbon dioxide, and fungal skin infections. Lancet i:360–362

Fromtling RA, Abruzzo GK, Ruiz A (1988) *Cryptococcus neoformans*: a central nervous system isolate from an AIDS patient that is rhinotropic in a normal mouse model. Mycopathologia 102:79–86

Galgiani JN, Van Wyck DB (1984) Ornithyl amphotericin methyl ester treatment of experimental candidiasis in rats. Antimicrob Agents Chemother 26:108–109

Gentles JC (1958) Experimental ringworm in guinea pigs: oral treatment with griseofulvin. Nature 182:476–477

Graybill JR, Ahrens J (1984) R 51211 (itraconazole) therapy of murine cryptococcosis. Sabouraudia: J Med Vet Mycol 22:445–453

Graybill JR, Ahrens J (1985) Itraconazole treatment of murine aspergillosis. Sabouraudia: J Med Vet Mycol 23:219–223

Graybill JR, Ahrens J, Nealon T, Paque R (1983a) Pulmonary cryptococcosis in the rat. Am Rev Resp Dis 127:636–640

Graybill JR, Kaster SR, Drutz DJ (1983b) Comparative activities of Bay n 7133, ICI 153,066, and ketoconazole in murine cryptococcosis. Antimicrob Agents Chemother 24:829–834

Graybill JR, Kaster SR, Drutz DJ (1983c) Treatment of experimental murine aspergillosis with BAY n 7133. J Infect Dis 148:898–906

Graybill JR, Palou E, Ahrens J (1986a) Treatment of murine histoplasmosis with UK 49,858 (fluconazole). Am Rev Resp Dis 134:768–770

Graybill JR, Sun SH, Ahrens J (1986b) Treatment of murine coccidioidal meningitis with fluconazole (UK 49,858). J Med Vet Mycol 24:113–119

Hare RS, Loebenberg D (1988) Animal models in the search for antifungal agents. ASM News 54:235–239

Herrera C, Guentzel MN (1982) Mice with persistent gastrointestinal *Candida albicans* as a model for antifungal therapy. Antimicrob Agents Chemother 21:51–53

Hughes CE, Peterson LR, Beggs WH, Gerding DN (1986) Ketoconazole and flucytosine alone and in combination against *Candida* spp. in a neutropenic site in rabbits. J Antimicrob Chemother 18:65–72

Kerbs S, Allen AM (1978) Effect of occlusion on *Trichophyton mentagrophytes* infections in guinea pigs. J Invest Dermatol 71:301–304

Kobayashi GS, Travis S, Medoff G (1986) Comparison of the in vitro and in vivo activity of the bis-triazole derivative UK 49,858 with that of amphotericin B against *Histoplasma capsulatum*. Antimicrob Agents Chemother 29:660–662

Krause M, Schaffner A (1988) Comparison of immune mechanisms against *Candida albicans* in models of localized and systemic infection in mice. 28th Intersci Conf Antimicrob Agents Chemother, Los Angeles, Abstr 1287, p 341

Lefler E, Brummer E, McEwen JG, Hoyos GL, Restrepo A, Stevens DA (1985a) Study of current and new drugs in a murine model of acute paracoccidioidomycosis. Amer J Trop Med Hyg 34:134–140

Lefler E, Brummer E, Perlman AM, Stevens DA (1985b) Activities of the modified polyene *N*-D-ornithyl amphotericin methyl ester and the azoles ICI 153,066, Bay n 7133, and Bay 1 9139 compared with those of amphotericin B and ketoconazole in the therapy of experimental blastomycosis. Antimicrob Agents Chemother 27:363–366

Levine HB (1984) A direct comparison of oral treatment with BAY-n-7133, BAY-1-9139 and ketoconazole in experimental murine coccidioidomycosis. Sabouraudia: J Med Vet Mycol 22:37–46

Martin MV (1989) A comparison of fluconazole and ketoconazole in the treatment of rat palatal candidosis. J Med Vet Mycol 27:63–70

Novick LN, Tapia L, Bottone EJ (1987) Invasive *Trichophyton rubrum* infection in an immunocompromised host. Am J Med 82:321–325

Perfect JR, Durack DT (1985) Comparison of amphotericin B and *N*-D-ornithyl amphotericin B methyl ester in experimental cryptococcal meningitis and *Candida albicans* endocarditis with pyelonephritis. Antimicrob Agents Chemother 28: 751–755

Perfect JR, Lang SDR, Durack DT (1980) Chronic cryptococcal meningitis: a new experimental model in rabbits. Am J Pathol 101:117–194

Perfect JR, Savani DV, Durack DT (1986) Comparison of itraconazole and fluconazole in treatment of cryptococcal meningitis and candida pyelonephritis in rabbits. Antimicrob Agents Chemother 29:579–583

Petranyi G, Leitner I, Mieth H (1982) The 'hair root invasion test', a semi-quantitative method for experimental evaluation of antimycotics in guinea pigs. Sabouraudia 20:101–108

Polak A (1984a) Experimental infection of mice by *Fonsecaea pedrosoi* and *Wangiella dermatitidis*. Sabouraudia: J Med Vet Mycol 22:167–169

Polak A (1984b) Antimycotic therapy of experimental infections caused by dematiaceous fungi. Sabouraudia: J Med Vet Mycol 22:279–289

Polak A (1987) Combination therapy of experimental candidiasis, cryptococcosis, aspergillosis and wangiellosis in mice. Chemotherapy 33:381–395

Polak A, Dixon DM (1986) Fungistatic and fungicidal effects of amphotericin B, ketoconazole and fluconazole (UK 49,858) against *Histoplasma capsulatum* in vitro and in vivo. Mykosen 30:186–194

Polak A, Dixon DM (1988) Chemotherapeutic activity in a mouse model of cryptococcosis with cutaneous and nasal involvement. Mycoses 31:501–507

Polak A, Schaffner A (1989) A new experimental model of localized candidosis for the study of antifungal chemotherapy. Mycoses 32:398–404

Ray TL (1985) Animal models of experimental *Candida* infections of the skin. In: Maibach HI, Lowe NJ (eds) Models in dermatology, vol I. Karger, Basel, pp 41–50

Richardson K, Brammer KW, Marriott MS, Troke PF (1985) Activity of UK 49,858, a bis-triazole derivative, against experimental infections with *Candida albicans* and *Trichophyton mentagrophytes*. Antimicrob Agents Chemother 27:832–835

Russell C, Jones JH, Gibbs ACC (1976) The carriage of *Candida albicans* in the mouths of rats treated with tetracycline briefly or for a prolonged period. Mycopathologia 58:125–129

Ryley JF, McGregor S (1986) Quantification of vaginal *Candida albicans* infections in rodents. J Med Vet Mycol 24:455–460

Ryley JF, McGregor S (1988) A multi-infection model for antifungal screening in vivo. J Antimicrob Chemother 22:353–358

Ryley JF, Rathmell WG (1984) Discovery of antifungal agents: in vitro and in vivo testing. In: Trinci APJ, Ryley JF (eds) Mode of action of antifungal agents. Cambridge University Press, Cambridge, pp 63–87 (Br Mycol Soc Symp No 9)

Ryley JF, Wilson RG, Gravestock MB, Poyser JP (1981) Experimental approaches to antifungal chemotherapy. Adv Pharmacol Chemother 18:49–176

Ryley JF, McGregor S, Lister SC, Jackson KP (1988a) Kidney function in experimental systemic candidosis of mice. Mycoses 31:203–207

Ryley JF, McGregor S, Wilson RG (1988b) The activity of ICI 195,739, a novel orally active bis-triazole, in rodent models of fungal and protozoal infection. Ann N Y Acad Sci 544:310–328

Savani DV, Perfect JR, Cobo LM, Durack DT (1987) Penetration of new azole compounds into the eye and efficacy in experimental *Candida* endophthalmitis. Antimicrob Agents Chemother 31:6–10

Schaude M, Meingassner JG (1986) A diffusion chamber technique for testing of antifungal drugs against *Sporothrix schenckii* in vivo. J Med Vet Mycol 24:297–304

Scholer HJ (1960) Experimentelle Vaginal-Candidiasis der Ratte. Path Microbiol 23: 62–68

Shakir BS, Martin MV, Smith CJ (1981) Induced palatal candidosis in the Wistar rat. Arch Oral Biol 26:787–793

Troke PF (1987) Efficacy of fluconazole in animal models of superficial and opportunistic systemic fungal infection. In: Fromtling RA (ed) Recent trends in the discovery, development and evaluation of antifungal agents. J R Prous, Barcelona, pp 103–112

Ueda AK, Franco M, Fabio SA, Prestes FR (1987) Ketoconazole in the treatment of experimental murine paracoccidioidomycosis. Mycopathologia 98:27–34

Van Cutsem J, Janssen PAJ (1984) Experimental systemic dermatophytosis. J Invest Dermatol 83:26–31

Van Cutsem J, Thienpont D (1971) Experimental cutaneous *Candida albicans* infection in guinea pigs. Sabouraudia 9:17–20

Van Cutsem JM, Thienpont D (1972) Miconazole, a broad-spectrum antimycotic agent with antibacterial activity. Chemotherapy 17:392–404

Van Cutsem J, Fransen J, Van Gerven F, Janssen PAJ (1985) Oral treatment with ketoconazole in systemic candidosis of guinea-pigs: microbiology, hematology and histopathology. Sabouraudia: J Med Vet Mycol 23:189–198

Van Cutsem J, Fransen J, Van Gerven F, Janssen PAJ (1986) Experimental cryptococcosis: dissemination of *Cryptococcus neoformans* and dermotropism in guinea-pigs. Mykosen 29:561–575

Van Cutsem J, Van Gerven J, Janssen PAJ (1987) Activity of orally, topically, and parenterally administered itraconazole in the treatment of superficial and deep mycoses: animal models. Rev Infect Dis 9:S15–S32

Van Cutsem J, Fransen J, Janssen PAJ (1988) Experimental zygomycosis due to *Rhizopus* spp. infection by various routes in guinea-pigs, rats and mice. Mycoses 31:563–578

Section II. Drug Development

Introduction

John F. Ryley

Discovering a novel potential antifungal agent with activity in vivo is not easy or cheap. When I began my research career in the immediate post Second World War years, it was a relatively simple matter to get a compound active in an animal model of infection tested in humans. Toxicology was in its infancy and the disciplines of drug metabolism and pharmacokinetics embryonic. Some compounds became useful and established drugs, others just did not make the grade. As time progressed, preclinical investigations increased, but for example griseofulvin in the late 1950s was evaluated in humans by Harvey Blank in the USA within weeks of Gentle's letter to Nature describing its activity against ringworm in guinea pigs and has subsequently become a valuable drug which has stood the test of time. It was only after the thalidomide tragedy in the early 1960s that extensive preclinical evaluation and regulatory procedures burgeoned in the hope of avoiding a similar situation in the future. Sally Eardley, a colleague from ICI, has written a delightful chapter (11) chronicling regulatory developments over the past 3500 years. Although she has had no experience with antifungal drugs, I find her contribution fascinating to read, since it so graphically explains the situation in which we find ourselves at this time. It is important to realise that of the £100 million which may be spent today before a new drug can be marketed, at least two-thirds of this will be spent on the various aspects of development covered in this section, while only one-third will have been spent discovering the drug in the first place. Consideration of such figures emphasises the fact that drug development, if not drug discovery also, can only be handled by large multinational pharmaceutical companies with their vast resources. Consideration of such figures stresses too the hard fact of life that the management of such companies will not sanction research into therapeutic areas in which there is no hope of recouping the enormous costs of research and development from ultimate sales. As I have worked on various aspects of tropical medicine and medical mycology over the past 40 years, this has been personally one of the most difficult lessons to learn and situations with which to come to terms.

I owe much to Annemarie POLAK for the help she gave as I sought to transfer my affections from protozoology to medical mycology some 12 years ago, and she had been true to form in writing a most helpful chapter (6) on mode of action studies. This chapter is complementary to Chap. 2 and emphasises how knowledge of the mode of action of a drug can contribute to a better understanding of the limitations and practical considerations in its usage as well as providing yet more ideas for the synthetic chemist. An antifungal agent will only be of practical use if it reaches the site of infection and remains long enough in an active form to exert its therapeutic effects, hence the importance of pharmacokinetic studies as reviewed by Mike TARBIT (Chap. 7). In this chapter he advances pharmacokinetic reasons to explain the apparent lack of correlation between in vitro and in vivo activity with azoles, particularly fluconazole. While all these points are very appropriate, they do not explain all the problems raised in Chap. 4, and of course full pharmacokinetic investigations of compounds are not possible at the screening stage. I am particularly grateful to him for writing this chapter at very short notice. Routine toxicological investigations are required for regulatory purposes for any type of drug destined for human use, and their design depends more on the anticipated schedule of administration than the condition for which the drug will be used. Such routine studies with ketoconazole revealed teratogenicity in rats, fragility of leg bones in rats and lipofuscin deposition in certain tissues of dogs. These features have not shown up in clinical experience, but instead hepatotoxicity and disturbances consequent on the inhibition of testosterone and adrenal steroid synthesis – effects not anticipated by regulatory toxicology studies – have been seen. Rather than have a chapter on routine toxicology, I have chosen to highlight two areas of special toxicology particularly relevant to the current antifungal scene. The hepatotoxicity seen with ketoconazole is virtually impossible to predict by classic toxicological methods, and evidence for hormonal disturbances is only indirect. Experience has suggested that possibly a more practical approach is to study the effects of candidate drugs on the relevant enzymes of the host and fungus at cellular or subcellular levels, seeking to establsh sufficient differences in affinity or inhibitory activity. Mike TARBIT, who was involved in the development of fluconazole, and Andy ROBERTSON and Ann LAMBERT, who are experienced biochemical endocrinologists, have written of their experiences with azole derivatives in this area (Chap. 8). Although there has been no suggestion whatsoever of teratogenicity in clinical practice, many azoles can cause teratogenic malformations in rats and rabbits. Because our company has been particularly sensitive about this issue, teratological evaluation was an important early step in the screening cascade which led to ICI 195,739. Investigations in animals are expensive in terms of time, compound and effort, so that the in vitro approach developed by a former colleague Oliver FLINT was potentially a welcome and very practical contribution to our research programme. Oliver FLINT and my chemical colleague Tom BOYLE describe in Chap. 9 some of the issues and problems concerning structure-activity relationships arising out of this programme.

Practical experience over the years in the antifungal field has indicated just how much difference formulation can make to the biological availability of both topical and systemic drugs. In Chap. 10 a fairly recent recruit to the mycological field, Heinz HÄNEL, describes some of these developments, including particle size studies with griseofulvin, the exciting new potential inherent in the now ancient drug amphotericin B due to liposomal formulation, and experimental methods used to enhance penetration and develop more effective topical properties for the treatment of skin and nail infections. Eventually the moment of truth arrives! A compound showing promise in experimental models of infection has been demonstrated to be safe in experimental animals, and permission is granted to administer it to humans. We are still a long way from adding a new drug to the clinician's armamentarium, but at least the long process of clinical trial can begin. The manufacturer, the clinician and not least the regulatory authorities all need to be convinced that the compound is both efficaceous and safe in humans and represents a real therapeutic advance. Tom JONES has gained much recent experience in clinical trials with naftifine and terbinafine and has collaborated with a former colleague John STERN, now involved in treating AIDS patients, in writing a rather provocative chapter (12) on some of the issues germane to the planning and conduct of clinical trials.

CHAPTER 6

Mode of Action Studies

Annemarie Polak

A. Introduction

There are two approaches to the discovery of new antifungal drugs: the rational and the empirical. Up to now, none of the antifungal drugs available has been found on the basis of a truly rational approach. This may largely be explained by the unfortunate fact that fungi, like their human hosts, are eucaryotic organisms and hence the number of potential targets for specific drug action is limited. Furthermore, basic research on the biochemistry and physiology of the fungal cell was until recently rather neglected in contrast to the profound biochemical knowledge accumulated for bacterial cells. For a successful rational approach to designing antifungals it is important that detailed knowledge of the enzymatic steps used by fungal cells be available. Besides basic research on the biochemistry of fungi, mode of action studies with existing antimycotics may contribute to a deeper insight into the metabolism of fungal cells. Such mode of action studies are urgently needed and should not only be performed in industrial laboratories but also in an academic environment.

The deeper the knowledge of fungal metabolism and of individual enzymatic steps becomes, the greater will be the chance of designing a drug which is not only active at the level of the target enzyme but also inhibits the fungal cell in the organs of the host. Up to now, no such direct rational approach has succeeded. It has been possible, however, based on the knowledge of the mode of action, to improve the specificity of antifungal activity of an empirically discovered drug. An excellent example of this approach is found in the imidazole and triazole derivatives. Biochemical studies have established that the azole group binds to a cytochrome P-450 of fungal and human cells. The structure of the molecule plays a role in specificity, and structural modifications were made which led to improved specificity. The newer azoles have a significantly higher affinity for the cytochrome P-450 of fungal cells and bind only weakly to that of human cells. As a consequence these new drugs have shown significantly fewer toxic side effects in clinical evaluation and represent an important improvement.

Biochemical studies have identified a number of potential targets for antifungal chemotherapy, including cell wall synthesis, membrane sterol biosynthesis, nucleic acid synthesis, nuclear division, metal chelation,

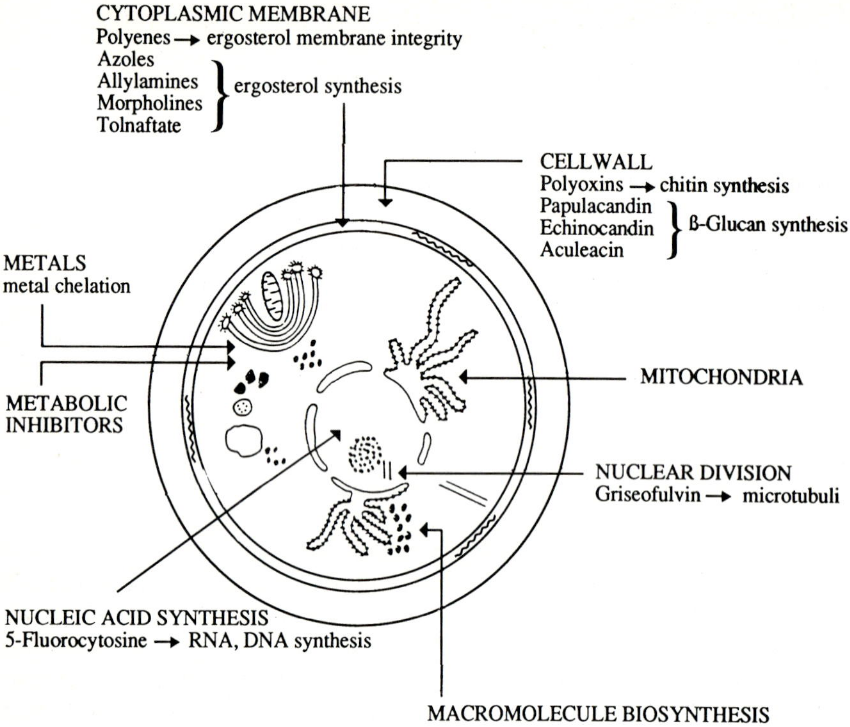

Fig. 1. Potential targets for antifungal activity

metabolic inhibition and macromolecular biosyntheses (Fig. 1). The inhibition of cell wall synthesis would be in theory highly specific, since only fungal cells build their cell wall with chitin and glucan. Despite this desired specificity, none of the clinically available drugs act there. On the contrary, most of the antifungals in clinical use interfere with enzymatic steps involved in the complicated synthesis of ergosterol, which are mostly not fungi-specific, the enzymes also being present in the host cells. The specificity required for a non-toxic antifungal drug has to be based on a difference in the affinity of the drug for the fungal and host enzymes or on different substrate requirements. A few enzymes situated late in the biosynthetic pathway are fungi-specific, but up to now no antifungal has been found to interfere with these enzymatic steps.

Basic biochemical research and mode of action studies are required to extend the present knowledge of fungal metabolism, not only to broaden the range of rational approaches to the development of an effective, non-toxic, antifungal drug but also to gain insight into the poorly understood areas of virulence and pathogenicity. In this chapter the mode of action of the various clinically available antifungals will be presented.

B. Target: Nucleic Acid Synthesis and Cell Division

I. 5-Fluorocytosine

The antifungal spectrum of fluorocytosine (5-FC; Fig. 2) relevant to human chemotherapy is limited to species of *Candida*, *Cryptococcus*, *Aspergillus* and dematiaceae. *Candida* and *Cryptococcus* are highly sensitive, with MICs ranging from 0.1 to 2 μg/ml, whereas aspergilli and dematiaceae are moderately sensitive, with MICs of 1–25 μg/ml. In yeast and dematiaceous fungi the drug becomes fungicidal after prolonged contact (SCHOLER 1980; SCHOLER and POLAK 1984).

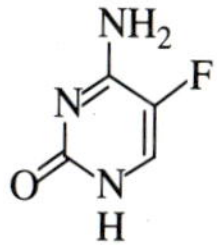

Fig. 2. 5-Fluorocytosine

5-FC is taken up by a cytosine permease normally responsible for the uptake of adenine, guanine, hypoxanthine and cytosine (POLAK and SCHOLER 1980; Fig. 3). The uptake of 5-FC can therefore be competitively inhibited by the pyrimidine cytosine and also by various purines. Inside the fungal cells 5-FC is rapidly deaminated to 5-fluorouracil, a molecule with well-known cytotoxic properties, by a cytosine deaminase. This is the critical enzyme which determines the antimicrobial spectrum of 5-FC: only fungi with an effective enzyme are sensitive. The low toxicity of the drug in the human host can be correlated with the absence or low activity of this enzyme in mammalian tissue. From 5-fluorouracil two different pathways have to be considered. In one, 5-fluorouracil is converted by uridine monophosphate pyrophosphorylase into 5-fluorouridylic acid which is further phosphorylated and incorporated into RNA; this incorporation is strongly antagonised by uridine. In the other, 5-fluorouracil is converted to 5-fluorodeoxyuridine monophosphate, a potent inhibitor of DNA synthesis at the level of thymidylate synthetase. 5-Fluorouracil itself cannot be given as an antimycotic drug since its uptake by the fungal cell is poor, and its toxicity to mammalian cells precludes systemic use in quantities necessary for chemotherapy, although sensitive fungi produce the cytotoxic drug after uptake of 5-FC.

In hydrolysates of purified ribosomal RNA and particularly of transfer RNA from fungi exposed to 5-FC enormous quantities of 5-fluorouracil have been found, replacing up to 70% of normal uracil. No unchanged 5-FC is found in the RNA nor is any fluorinated pyrimidine observed in the DNA of the fungi (POLAK and SCHOLER 1980).

RNA modified by incorporation of 5-fluorouracil behaves differently to normal RNA. Transfer RNA isolated from *Saccharomyces cerevisiae* was found to be still capable of amino acid acylation in vitro, but some amino

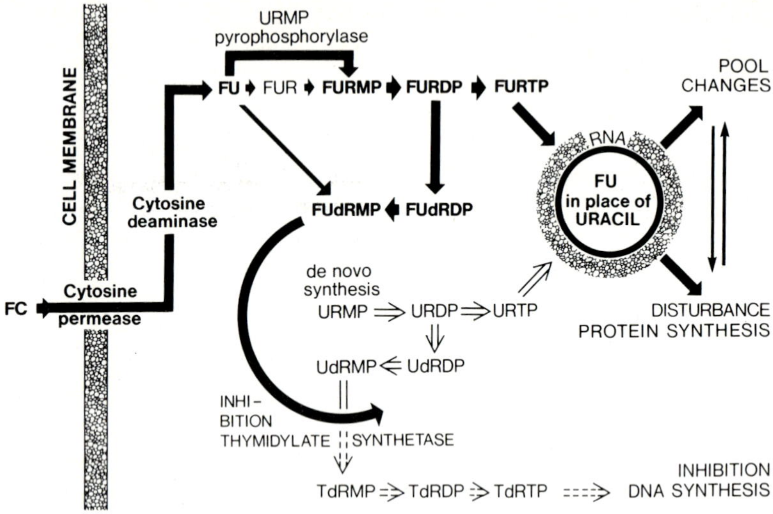

Fig. 3. Intrafungal pathway and mode of action of 5-fluorocytosine. *URMP*, uridine monophosphate; *URDP*, uridine diphosphate; *URTP*, uridine triphosphate; *UdRMP*, deoxyuridine monophosphate; *UdRDP*, deoxyuridine diphosphate; *TdRMP*, thymidine monophosphate; *TdRDP*, thymidine diphosphate; *TdRTP*, thymidine triphosphate; *FC*, flucytosine (5-fluorocytosine); *FU*, 5-fluorouracil; *FUR*, 5-fluorouridine; *FURMP*, 5-fluorouridine monophosphate; *FURDP*, 5-fluorouridine diphosphate; *FURTP*, 5-fluorouridine triphosphate; *FUdRMP*, 5-fluorodeoxyuridine monophosphate; *FUdRDP*, 5-fluorodeoxyuridine diphosphate

acids were found in excess and others in reduced proportions (GIEGE and WEIL 1970). 5-Fluorouracil-containing ribosomal RNA is still capable of forming 80*S* ribosomes but to a significantly lower extent, and it is not certain whether these 5-fluorouracil-containing ribosomes still produce normal or modified proteins (WAIN and POLAK 1981).

5-Fluorodeoxyuridine monophosphate can be detected in homogenates of 5-FC-treated *Candida albicans* cells, and a concomitant decrease in thymidylate synthetase activity is observed (WALDORF and POLAK 1983). The inhibition is most probably effected, as in bacterial and mammalian cells, by the formation of a stable ternary complex between the inhibitor, 5,10-methylenetetrahydrofolate and thymidylate synthetase. The 6-position of the analogue is bound covalently to the catalytic nucleophile of the enzyme via a thioether bond, and the 5-position is linked to carbon 1 of the 5,10-methylenetetrahydrofolate.

In vivo it is found that addition of 5-FC to logarithmically multiplying *C. albicans* yeasts or hyphae results in an immediate inhibition of DNA and RNA synthesis without influencing cell multiplication or hyphal elongation in the first hours of contact; the content of DNA and RNA per cell is therefore significantly reduced. This phenomenon of reduced DNA content can be demonstrated by counting the nuclei in 5-FC-treated *C. albicans* hyphae.

After 5 h of 5-FC exposure the mean number of nuclei per hypha is significantly smaller (1.56 nucleus/hypha) in comparison with the controls (2.97 nucleus/hypha). During the same period no reduction in hyphal length was observed. Furthermore, 5-FC does not influence the germination of *C. albicans* cells in serum. In an electron microscope study a significant enlargement of the nucleus of 5-FC-treated *C. albicans* was observed, and later the nucleus became translucent with filamentous components appearing within the cell wall, which became progressively thinner, probably as a result of an increase in cell volume without a concomitant increase in cell wall constituents (ARAI et al. 1977). These morphological changes are exactly analogous to those observed by COHEN and BARNER 1954 and COHEN et al. 1958 in bacterial and mammalian cells under the influence of DNA inhibitors and thus provide further evidence that a primary target of 5-FC is thymidylate synthetase inhibition.

In aspergilli addition of 5-FC immediately inhibits germination of the conidia and simultaneously inhibits hyphal growth and DNA or RNA synthesis. This is in contrast to the effect on *Candida* cells, in which no influence on hyphal growth but only on nucleic acid synthesis is seen at the first contact. Due to the fact that hyphal growth and DNA and RNA synthesis are inhibited to the same degree, no reduction in content of nucleic acids per cell can be observed in aspergilli (POLAK 1988a).

Protein synthesis in *C. albicans* is increased after an initial decrease for the first 6 h, the content of protein per cell reaching up to 200% of that of normal cells. The protein produced by cells exposed to 5-FC is most probably abnormal, but this has not yet been proven. However, abnormality in the function of enzymes has been observed in bacteria exposed to 5-fluorouracil, and also in some enzymes in 5-FC-treated *C. albicans* cells.

A marked increase in carbohydrate synthesis takes place from the first contact with 5-FC in all species of *Candida*, dematiaceous fungi and aspergilli. In yeasts the content of carbohydrate in treated cells reaches up to 380% of that in normal cells. Increased synthesis of both carbohydrate and protein accounts for the increase in size and dry weight of 5-FC-treated fungal cells. The increase is mainly in the storage polysaccharides glycogen and glucan and is virtually absent in mannan, which is the main cell wall constituent in *C. albicans*. This is consistent with the electron microscope study which showed a thinner cell wall in 5-FC-treated cells.

The pool of all small metabolites in *C. albicans* yeast cells incubated with 5-FC definitely increases. This has been specifically documented for the total amino acid pool and the total carbohydrate pool. There were profound changes in the concentrations of individual amino acids, which were sometimes increased, sometimes unchanged and sometimes even decreased. Similar changes in the total pool and the amino acid pool have also been observed in bacteria and *Candida utilis* exposed to 5-fluorouracil. All these events take place at an early phase of the contact with 5-FC and therefore represent its primary action (WALDORF and POLAK 1983). It cannot be stated which pathway of the two is more important. In resistant *C. albicans* cells the incorporation of 5-fluorouracil into RNA could be correlated with sensitivity (POLAK and SCHOLER 1975), i.e. the lower the incorporation, the more resistant is the fungus. However, it is still possible that inhibition of DNA synthesis plays a more important role than incorporation of 5-fluorouracil into RNA.

In yeast cells of *Candida* and *Cryptococcus* inhibition of DNA synthesis is not paralleled by an inhibition of protein and carbohydrate synthesis. Both proteins and carbohydrates are produced in excess, a phenomenon already observed in mammalian cells or bacteria treated with 5-fluorouracil or with other DNA inhibitors. This phenomenon, called unbalanced growth, occurs as a consequence of inhibited DNA synthesis. In bacteria it could be shown that DNA inhibition followed by unbalanced growth is bactericidal (COHEN and BARNER 1954; COHEN et al. 1958). This is also true for 5-FC in *C. albicans*. *Cryptococcus* and dematiaceous fungi, in which 5-FC exerts a fungicidal activity as well as a fungistatic effect. In 5-fluorouracil-treated bacteria, which were simultaneously exposed to thymidine, it could be shown that incorporation of 5-fluorouracil into RNA resulted in bacteriostatic but not in bactericidal activity. It may be thus concluded that the same differences are also true for 5-FC after deamination to 5-fluorouracil, i.e. 5-fluorouracil incorporation into RNA leads to a cytostatic effect, whereas inhibition of DNA synthesis leads to a fungicidal effect.

In aspergilli, in which the inhibition of cells runs parallel with the inhibition of DNA and RNA synthesis, the phenomenon of unbalanced growth is not observed; 5-FC is only fungistatic. The conclusion is that the phenomenon of unbalanced growth leads to a fungicidal effect, whereas a simultaneous inhibition of multiplication and nucleic acid synthesis leads only to a cytostatic effect.

The study of 5-FC-resistant mutants has been an important key to the above mentioned biochemical pathways and has to some extent also contributed to the identification of the antifungal's intracellular metabolites. Resistance to 5-FC may be produced by lack or deficiency of an enzyme at any step of the pathway (see Fig. 3) or by a surplus of de novo synthesis of normal pyrimidines competing with the fluorinated metabolites. Five types of resistant mutants in *S. cerevisiae* have been distinguished, having variously a deficiency in cytosine permease, a deficiency in cytosine deaminase, a deficiency in URMP-pyrophosphorylase, a loss of feedback regulation leading to increased de novo synthesis or an increased de novo synthesis of pyrimidines caused by stimulation of orotidylic acid pyrophosphorylase (JUND and LACROUTE 1974). Newer studies using 5-FC as a genetic marker have revealed that *C. albicans* is diploid and heterozygous at the gene that determines the activity of uridine monophosphate pyrophosphorylase. In future, 5-FC may lead to further insight into the genetics of *C. albicans* (WHELAN et al. 1986).

Recently, a modified bacterial DNA has been synthesised containing 5-FC as a part of the GCGC recognition sequence of *Hha*I-methylase, a bacterial DNA-cytosine methyltransferase which methylates the internal cytosine residue of GCGC sequences in DNA (OSTERMAN et al. 1988). This modified synthetic DNA induced an inhibition of DNA cytosine methyltransferase which was shown to be due to an irreversible covalent inactivation. This study shows that under some circumstances 5-FC itself can be of lethal importance. However, in fungal cells no 5-FC has been seen in RNA or in DNA; 5-fluorouracil is the only active principle (POLAK and SCHOLER 1980).

In conclusion the biochemical pathway of 5-FC in sensitive fungi leads to the formation of 5-fluorouridine and to the incorporation of 5-fluorouracil into RNA which seems to inhibit fungal growth. Simultaneously, 5-fluorodeoxyuridine monophosphate is formed which inhibits thymidylate synthetase and as a consequence DNA synthesis and nuclear division are inhibited, leading to death of the fungal cells (reviewed by KERRIDGE 1986; POLAK and SCHOLER 1980).

II. Griseofulvin

Griseofulvin (Fig. 4) is an antibiotic produced by certain species of *Penicillium*, particularly *P. griseofulvum*. A variety of non-pathogenic fungal species are sensitive to griseofulvin, but of the fungi pathogenic to humans only the dermatophytes are sensitive, showing a minimal inhibitory concentration of 0.1–5 μg/ml (SCHOLER and POLAK 1984).

The most evident effect of griseofulvin on sensitive fungi is a "curling" phenomenon, which has been attributed to a change in the cell wall, making it abnormally soft or abnormally rigid at regular intervals. The pronounced distortion of the hyphae is associated with the fungistatic effect of the drug, whereas its fungicidal action is due to rupture of the cell wall. These phenomena were first hypothetically explained by an inhibition of cell wall synthesis, especially chitin synthesis. However, no inhibition of the synthesis of any cell wall constituent was ever demonstrated in the laboratory. The second effect of griseofulvin is an impairment of nuclear division due to an arrest of mitosis in metaphase. These observations, made as early as 1958 in both *Vicia faba* and the rat, stimulated various studies on the effect of the drug on macromolecular synthesis and nuclear metabolism.

Studies on *Basidiobolus ranarum* (GULL and TRINCI 1973), a fungus with a large nucleus (25 μm long) in each hyphal compartment, revealed that the radial growth of the fungus was decreased, and more than one nucleus

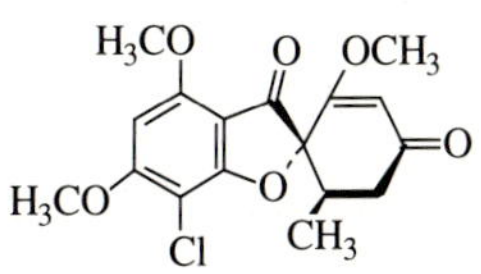

Fig. 4 Griseofulvin

appeared in each hyphal compartment. Mitosis was arrested in metaphase as a result of dissociation of the mitotic spindle; multipolar mitosis also occurred. No direct effect of griseofulvin on the synthesis of proteins or nucleic acids has been observed, and it seems to act specifically on the mitotic cycle by affecting microtubular structure or function. The interaction is different from that observed with colchicine, a known microtubular inhibitor. In the frog melanine model griseofulvin also acts on the function of the cytoplasmic microtubule (Malawista 1973).

Intensive studies with newer methods, e.g. light scattering, have revealed that griseofulvin inhibits microtubular formation in a concentration-dependent fashion. This inhibition may be caused by one of two interactions, either binding to microtubule-associated proteins or to tubulin dimers. To date more studies favour the latter hypothesis, but there is still a need for further studies to elucidate exactly the mechanism of griseofulvin-induced inhibition of microtubule assembly (Grisham et al. 1973).

The fact that griseofulvin also affects the cytoplasmic microtubules which are known to be involved in the intracellular transport of endogenous compounds may explain a variety of seemingly unrelated abnormalities in treated cells. Most probably the transport of newly synthesised cell wall constituents is disturbed, and this may lead to the characteristic "curling" effect of the hyphae. So it would seem that the microtubules are the primary target responsible for its antimycotic effect. Griseofulvin interacts with tubules from a variety of sources including rat brain, mammalian cells, various fungal cells and frogs. This raises the question of specificity. Thorough studies with *C. albicans* and *Escherichia coli*, two resistant species, and sensitive and resistant dermatophyte strains revealed that griseofulvin has to be taken up actively. In sensitive species a prolonged energy-dependent uptake over 48 h takes place. However, in resistant strains this prolonged uptake is replaced by a short energy-independent uptake which does not transport enough compound into the cell to be active on the tubules (El-Nakeeb and Lampen 1965). So one may conclude that only organisms possessing a transport system for griseofulvin are sensitive to the drug (reviewed by Kerridge 1986).

C. Target: Cell Membrane

Cell membranes of fungi contain a large amount of ergosterol which seems to have at least two important roles for fungal growth. It interacts with the phospholipid in the membrane, controlling the degree of membrane fluidity which is vital for the barrier function of the membrane as well as for the proper functioning of all membrane-bound enzymes. In addition to its function as a bulk sterol, micro amounts of ergosterol play a highly specific regulatory function – the so-called sparking effect (Rodriguez and Parks 1983).

It has been demonstrated in artificial and natural membranes that the more or less planar sterols like cholesterol and ergosterol are necessary to stabilise the physical properties of the phospholipid phases. When non-planar sterols are incorporated into the membranes the interaction of the sterol α phase with phospholipid acyl side chains is disturbed (by removing C12 contacts and weakening the interactions of C5 and C7). This disturbance induces changes in the lipid structure and phase transition resulting in growth inhibition (NES et al. 1978). Mutants with non-planar sterols in the membrane are not viable and can only grow in the presence of added sterols. They are also significantly more sensitive to host defense cells (PLEMPEL and BERG 1984).

The sterol content and conformation of the sterols is of vital importance for membrane stability, and as a consequence ergosterol is one of the most important components of fungal cells. Interaction with ergosterol biosynthesis will have a drastic effect on fungal cell metabolism and leads to cell growth inhibition or even cell death. Most likely for this reason antimycotics that have been discovered empirically (polyenes, azole derivatives, morpholines, allylamines and tolnaftate) have their primary effect on the plasma membranes. Polyene macrolide binding to ergosterol located in the fungal membrane destroys directly the integrity of the membrane whereas all other antimycotics inhibit the synthesis of ergosterol and affect the integrity of the membrane indirectly.

I. Polyene Macrolides

Polyene antibiotics are all produced by species of *Streptomyces* and consist of a macrolide ring closed by a lactone. On one side of the ring there are several conjugated carbon-carbon double bonds, and on the opposite side there is a similar number of free hydroxyl groups which accounts for the amphipathic properties of these compounds.

The spectrum of antifungal activity of amphotericin B (Amph B; Fig. 5) is very broad. Most fungal species pathogenic to humans including *Candida* spp., *Cryptococcus neoformans*, *Aspergillus fumigatus*, *Histoplasma capsulatum, Paracoccidioides brasiliensis. Coccidioides immitis* and *Mucoraceae* are inhibited at least fungistatically at concentrations around 1 μg/ml. Dermatophytes, the dematiaceous fungi and species of *Madurella* are considered

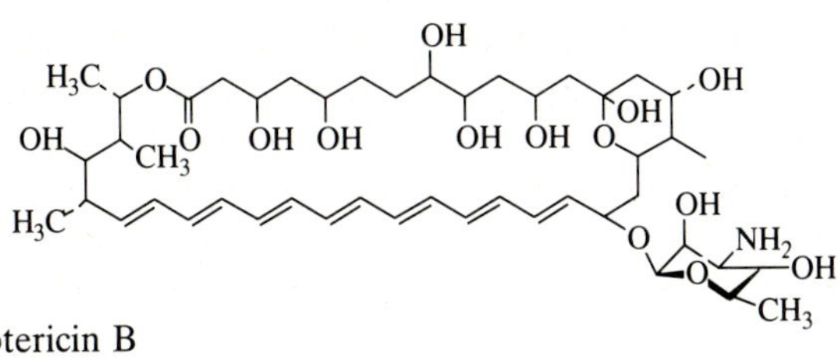

Fig. 5. Amphotericin B

resistant, with MIC values > 10 μg/ml. *Mucoraceae* and *Aspergillus flavus* are only moderately sensitive (SCHOLER and POLAK 1984).

The inhibitory effect of polyene antibiotics is specific for eucaryotic cells, i.e. all cells containing sterols in the cytoplasmic membrane. Their mode of action is based on a complex binding to the sterols in the membrane, but they also show affinity for lipids other than sterols, depending on their structure (ZYGMUNG and TAVORMINA 1966). The fact that Amph B has a rather strong specificity for ergosterol over cholesterol, the main sterol of mammalian membranes, is the key to the relatively low toxicity of this compound to human hosts. Other macrolides, for example filipin, possess the same affinity for cholesterol and ergosterol and are therefore unsuitable for use in humans (KOTLER-BRAJTBURG et al. 1974). The toxicity of Amph B observed during chemotherapy is due to the fact that it does also bind to mammalian membranes to some extent, and this is sufficient to interfere with their integrity.

The first result of the interaction of Amph B with sensitive cells is a leakage of potassium ions. This led to the suggestion that the primary effect of Amph B was to render the plasma membrane specifically permeable for K^+ ions, cell death being explained by the associated uptake of protons leading to acidification of the cell (MARINI et al. 1961). However, PALACIOS and SERRANO (1978) showed that in *S. cerevisiae* maltose fermentation was significantly more susceptible to Amph B than glucose fermentation. Maltose transport in *S. cerevisiae* is known to be an active process which derives energy from a proton gradient. Further inhibition was not antagonised by the addition of potassium ions. Based on these observations PALACIOS and SERRANO postulated that the primary effect of Amph B is to render the membrane permeable to protons. The proton gradient – catalysed by an ATPase located in the plasma membrane – has a central role in the functioning of the plasma membrane. It energises the uptake of amino acids and other nutrients and maintains the internal pool of potassium ions intact; furthermore, it has an important role in the regulation of growth of fungal cells.

The release of potassium ions observed at fungistatic concentrations of the drug is nowadays considered a secondary event due to drug-induced proton permeability. Various studies have shown that the fungicidal effect of Amph B may not be due to the efflux of potassium ions but more to an irreversible inhibition of the action of ATPase located in the membrane (CHEN et al. 1978).

The interaction of Amph B with lipid bilayers has been studied both in sensitive cells and in liposomal vesicles and black films (LAMPEN et al. 1962; LAMPEN 1966; YAMAGUCHI and IWATA 1979; reviewed by KERRIDGE 1986; MEDOFF and KOBAYASHI 1980). Based on these studies, various molecular models have been proposed to explain how the complex of Amph B and lipids in the membrane is constructed and how it renders the membrane permeable to various compounds. The hydrophobic part of Amph B would seem to interact with a sterol molecule or with the acyl side chain of a phospholipid present in the membrane. Some models suggest that 8 polyene molecules aggregate to form a hollow cylinder in which their hydrophilic surfaces are directed inwards to produce an aqueous pore (De Kruijff et al. 1974; Kerridge 1986; Thomas 1986). Such a pore structure has never been observed by electron microscopy, but the diameter of the cylinder (0.8 Å) would be too small to be seen by this method. Studies using various physical methods including electrical conduction measurements on black films have provided some evidence for the formation of an antibiotic-induced aqueous pore, but conclusive evidence has as yet proved elusive.

According to such a model, polyene molecules present on one side of the artificial membrane form an aqueous pore of a length corresponding to half of the membrane depth, and this pore shows cationic specificity. A proper channel through the total membrane would only be possible when two cylinders came together. This event has been shown to happen specifically when the polyene molecules were present on both sides of an artificial membrane, and this channel was anion specific. In fungal cells most probably only half an annulus can be built since Amph B has never been found in the intracellular membrane, most probably due to lack of transport of the drug through the plasma membrane. The formation of such an aqueous pore in the membrane would in any case not be able to explain why Amph B induces an enhanced penetration for compounds such as rifampicin, tetracycline, 5-FC and DNA at concentrations far below its MIC.

In fact an explanation of the effect of Amph B on the permeability of the fungal membrane does not require the formation of a non-static aqueous pore. A disturbance of ergosterol function in the membrane by complexing with Amph B is sufficient. Sterols in the membrane play a major role in controlling the fluidity of the lipid bilayer, involving interaction with the acyl chain of the phospholipid present in the membrane. When Amph B binds to ergosterol, it disturbs this important interaction and induces local changes in the physical state of the lipid bilayer, and as a consequence the membrane is rendered permeable for various compounds. At high concentrations of Amph B, there is a gross and visible disorganisation of the membrane structure associated with a loss of both low and high molecular weight cellular constituents.

The appearance of mutants resistant to Amph B is not a clinical problem. The appearance of secondary resistance to the drug has remained an extremely rare occurrence despite its extensive use in chemotherapy for many years, although polyene-resistant mutants are easily obtained in the laboratory. They are generally distinguished from parent strains by an altered cell membrane lipid composition. Such mutants have proved useful for studying sterol biosynthesis in yeasts.

Phenotypic changes in Amph B sensitivity also occur during growth of *C. albicans*. Stationary yeast cells show high Amph B resistance (Gale 1986). Gale demonstrated that in the stationary phase a permeability barrier to polyene macrolides is built up in the fungal cell wall, and he identified an increase in glucan content as the cell wall factor responsible for this effect. All compounds decreasing the activity of endogenous β-glucanase increase resistance, whereas all compounds increasing the activity of this enzyme render the cells sensitive to the drug (polyene macrolide, reviewed by KERRIDGE 1986; MEDOFF and KOBAYASHI 1980; THOMAS 1986).

II. Ergosterol Biosynthesis Inhibitors

1. Imidazole and Triazole Derivatives

Imidazole derivatives (Fig. 6) are commonly considered broad spectrum antimycotics which also show activity against gram-positive bacteria. However, the fungistatic concentrations for the most and the least sensitive pathogenic fungal species differ by factors of up to 1000. For example, the average MIC of ketoconazole against *H. capsulatum* is reported to be 0.01 μg/ml but is 10 μg/ml against *C. albicans*. In general the imidazoles are fungistatic, although some (for instance miconazole) are fungicidal at higher concentrations. Chemotherapeutic activity in vitro is markedly dependent on methodology and affected by environmental conditions. This may be the reason for the reported differences in the sensitivity of fungi to these compounds and the difficulties in reproducibly determining the minimal growth inhibitory concentration (SCHOLER and POLAK 1984). Of the newer triazoles, fluconazole does not show high in vitro activity in comparison with other imidazole derivatives but exerts a significantly better action in animal experiments than expected from the in vitro data. Itraconazole has a broader spectrum, being highly fungistatic and fungicidal against *Aspergillus* species.

Electron microscopic and biochemical studies have revealed that all azole derivatives interfere with the cell membrane of the fungus (BORGERS 1985; BORGERS and VAN DE VEN 1987; VAN DEN BOSSCHE et al. 1984b; YAMAGUCHI and IWATA 1979). Both imidazole and triazole derivatives disturb the cytochrome P-450-dependent lanosterol C_{14}-demethylase system at concentrations as low as 10^{-11} M. This results in a depletion of ergosterol and accumulation of C_{14}-methyl sterols in the fungal cytoplasmic membrane. Interactions with other biochemical targets causing inhibition of fatty acid desaturase, direct interaction with the barrier function of the membrane, accumulation of toxic peroxides resulting from the effect on oxidation enzymes and inhibition of respiration have been also observed. The latter has even been considered as the primary target for ketoconazole.

It is generally agreed that fungistatic activity is related to an interaction with the cytochrome P-450-dependent C_{14}-demethylase system whereas fungicidal activity is associated with the leakage of cytoplasmic constituents and/or gross alteration of the cell membrane. Inhibition of the biosynthesis of ergosterol has been observed not only in vitro but also in fungal cells multiplying in host organs and in cell-free systems. These observations indicate that this is the primary target of azole or triazole derivatives.

On a molecular basis the C_{14}-demethylation of lanosterol is catalysed by

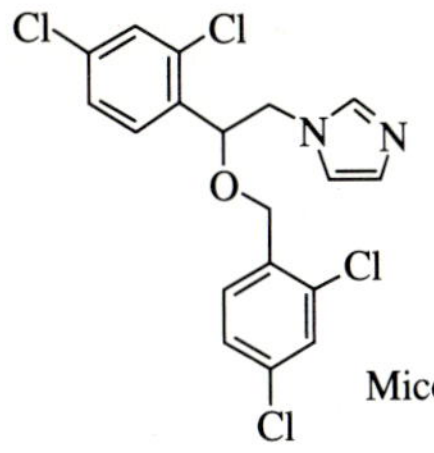

Miconazole

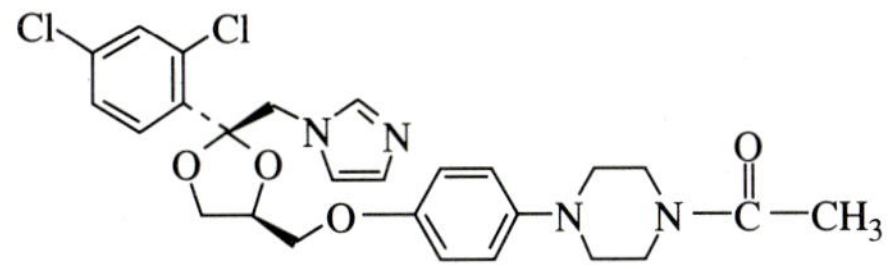

Ketoconazole

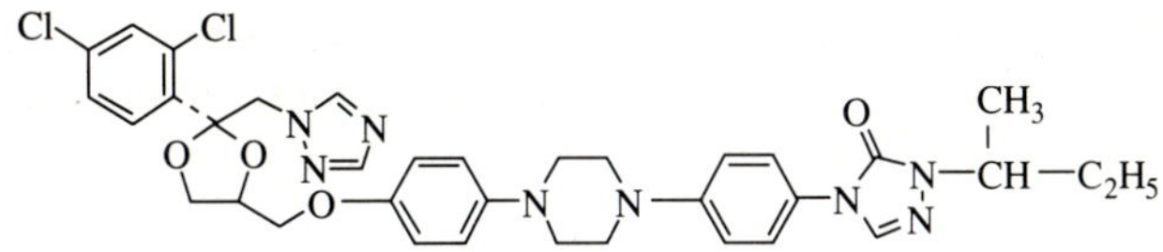

Itraconazole

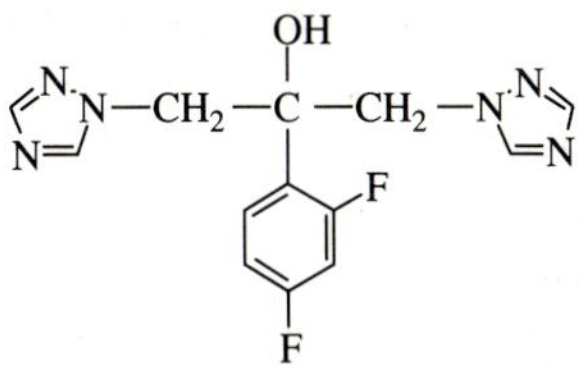

Fluconazole

Fig. 6. Azole antifungals

the cytochrome P-450-NADPH cytochrome P-450-reductase system. There are three oxygenation steps necessary to remove the methyl carbon group as formic acid, resulting in the production of a sterol with a double bond at C14. The fact that in the presence of azole derivatives C_{14}-methyl sterols and not the alcohol or aldehyde derivatives accumulate suggests that the first oxidation step is inhibited.

Various studies with all kinds of azole or triazole derivatives clearly show that these inhibitors interact with cytochrome P-450 in fungal microsomes yielding type II binding spectra, with an absorption maximum at 430 nm and a minimum at 393 nm. From a type II spectral change it can be concluded that they bind with the unhindered nitrogen (N_3 in the imidazole, N_4 in the triazole ring) to the 6 coordination position of the heme iron atom, which in the resting form of ferric cytochrome P-450 is occupied by water. Upon reduction of the iron, this 6th ligand normally becomes the site of dioxygen (O_2) binding, a step required to initiate oxidation of the C_{14}-methyl group of lanosterol. In the presence of inhibitors the formation of the superoxide Fe^{3+} complex ($Fe^{3+}O_2^-$) needed for the hydroxylation of methyl sterols no longer takes place, and a decreased synthesis of ergosterol and concomitant accumulation of C_{14}-methylated sterols result.

In all studies a clear correlation between the intensity of the difference spectra ($OD_{max}-OD_{min}$) and the inhibitor concentration was observed. However, the values at the saturation concentration differ from inhibitor to inhibitor. Additionally, the interaction of the various azoles with the heme iron was differently sensitive to carbon monoxide. Carbon monoxide removed miconazole from the 6th position whereas itraconazole was not displaced. These observed differences in behaviour have been explained not by a difference in the binding capacity of the nitrogen heterocycle with a heme iron but by different degrees of interaction with the apoprotein (VANDEN BOSSCHE et al. 1986), which is responsible for the affinity of the inhibitor to cytochrome P-450 isoenzymes.

VANDEN BOSSCHE et al. (1986) conclude in their review that for a prediction of the inhibitory effect on a P-450-dependent reaction the degree and velocity of the conversion of the reduced cytochrome P-450-drug complex into the cytochrome P-450-carbon monoxide complex may be the best indication. Since the cytochrome P-450-dependent enzyme systems are present not only in fungal but also in human cells, the usefulness of imidazole or triazole derivatives as antifungals is strongly dependent on the specificity of their binding. Various side effects observed during chemotherapy may be explained by interaction with other P-450 systems. For instance, azoles may interfere with cholesterol biosynthesis, with hormonal synthesis such as androgen or testosterone and also with several liver enzymes needed for inactivation of toxic and carcinogenic agents. Clotrimazole, for instance, most effectively inhibits hepatic hydrocarbon hydrolase. The therapeutic margin of azoles has usually been ascribed to marked differences in binding to fungal and to host cytochromes P-450. Recent studies with the silicon analogue flusilazole show similar affinities with purified yeast and rat liver enzymes and suggest that selectivity may not be due to inherent sensitivity differences between fungal and mammalian 14α-demethylase but rather to a protective effect afforded by other susceptible isozymes present in mammalian systems (TRZASKOS and HENRY 1989).

Other targets for the interaction of azole derivatives besides the inhibition of sterol biosynthesis have been found. The inhibition of respiration due to an interaction with cytochrome c oxidase in mitochondria of *C. albicans* was even considered as a primary action of ketoconazole from which the inhibition of ergosterol biosynthesis – a strictly aerobic synthesis – would naturally follow (SHIGEMATSU et al. 1982; UNO et al. 1982). A general role for the effect on respiration may also be indicated by the finding that under anaerobic conditions the fungistatic potency of azole derivatives is significantly lower than under aerobic conditions.

Further studies indicate an influence of azole and triazole derivatives on various mitochondrial enzymes, the activity of mitochondrial ATPase, succinate dehydrogenase and peroxidase being significantly decreased and that of catalase increased. At high concentrations of miconazole both peroxidase and catalase activities were totally abolished, inducing an increased internal concentration of H_2O_2. This accumulation of toxic peroxides may be one reason for the fungicidal effect of miconazole. In the presence of azole derivatives, fatty acid desaturation and fatty acid elongation, both aerobic events, are impaired. Whether all these observed interactions are primary targets of azole derivatives or whether they are only a consequence of the interaction with sterol biosynthesis is not yet clear (VANDEN BOSSCHE et al. 1982).

Apart from the interference with enzymes at a molecular level, a direct interaction with the bilayer function of the cytoplasmic membrane can be observed at high concentrations of some azole derivatives. This direct influence is antagonized by unsaturated or unesterified fatty acids and not by sterols. Computer modelling and differential scanning calorimetry studies have clearly shown a different drug orientation in the bilayer for miconazole and ketoconazole. The 2-dichlorophenyl group of miconazole is inserted in the hydrophobic phase of the bilayer whereas with ketoconazole the piperazine moiety is inserted into the hydrophobic region and the dichlorophenyl group into the hydrophilic phase. The orientation of ketoconazole in the bilayer does not induce a disruption of membrane function, but the miconazole orientation has this effect (BRASSEUR et al. 1983). This differential influence on the cell membrane bilayer may be the reason for the fungicidal effect of miconazole which is not observed with ketoconazole. It has to be mentioned that the fungicidal effect is only seen at high concentrations but may nonetheless be the reason for the topical antibacterial and fungicidal properties of miconazole. Itraconazole, a triazole derivative, also exerts a fungicidal effect on aspergilli, and from all data available it is clear that this is not due to inhibition of sterol biosynthesis. However, there are as yet no results indicating that the orientation of itraconazole in the lipid bilayer is the cause of this fungicidal activity.

As the azoles interfere with both barrier function and fluidity of the membrane, they induce as a consequence an alteration in the activity of cell membrane-bound enzymes such as chitin synthase and ATPase. In normal growing cells chitin synthase is in a latent state in the plasma membrane and is activated only locally for hyphal growth or building up of septa. In azole-treated cells, however, the enzyme seems to be uniformly activated and causes irregular accumulation of chitin in the membrane. Chitin synthesis is more important in mycelial growing *Candida* cells than in yeast forms, and the higher in vitro activity of azole derivatives in the mycelial form than yeast forms is a further indication that a secondary target of the azole derivatives is the inhibition of the chitin synthesis.

The primary target of azole and triazole derivatives is clearly the C_{14}-demethylase. Whether growth inhibition and especially the fungicidal effect are a consequence of the ergosterol depletion, accumulation of an unnatural sterol or a direct action on the membrane function has yet to be definitely elucidated (reviewed by KERRIDGE 1986; THOMAS 1986; VANDEN BOSSCHE et al. 1984a, b, 1986).

2. Morpholine Derivatives

Amorolfine (Fig. 7), the only morpholine derivative in clinical use, exhibits activity against fungi pathogenic to plants and humans. The highest fungistatic and fungicidal activity is observed against dermatophytes (MIC 0.06 μg/ml) followed by dimorphic fungi (MIC 0.1 μg/ml), dematiaceous fungi (0.07 μg/ml) and yeasts (0.5 μg/ml); moulds are inconsistent in their sensitivity, aspergilli being resistant (MIC > 100 μg/ml), *Alternaria* and *Scopulariopsis* being highly sensitive (0.3 μg/ml). (For more detailed biological data see Chap. 21.)

Cell growth changes drastically under amorolfine treatment. Dermatophytes show enlarged hyphal diameters, cell size in *C. albicans* is significantly increased, and germ tube formation is reduced. Under TEM study of both *C. albicans* and *Trichophyton mentagrophytes* the appearance of electron-transparent areas and vacuoles in the cytoplasm can be observed together with destruction of the cytoplasmic membrane and the formation of numerous vesicles and deposits in the cell wall, which is significantly thickened. All these changes strongly resemble the damage caused by azole derivatives (MÜLLER et al. 1987).

On the molecular level amorolfine exerts no effect on respiration, RNA, DNA, carbohydrate or protein synthesis before cessation of growth. However, incorporation of radiolabelled acetate reveals a stimulated synthesis of lipids in *C. albicans* and plant pathogenic fungi at concentrations not affecting growth (KERKENAAR 1987; POLAK-WYSS et al. 1985; POLAK 1988b). Analyses of the fatty acids in *C. albicans* show a shift to higher amounts of $C_{16\text{-}0}$ fatty acids whereas the $C_{18\text{-}1}$ fatty acids diminish. More important changes, however, are observed in the sterol patterns of all sensitive fungi treated with amorolfine. In all species tested the bulk sterol (ergosterol in *C. albicans* or

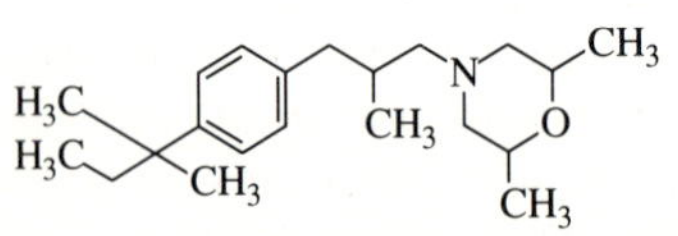

Fig. 7. Amorolfine

ergosta-5, 22-dienol in *H. capsulatum*) disappears, the degree of the effect on the whole cells being both time- and concentration-dependent, indicating a definite correlation between the observed changes in the sterol pattern and growth inhibition (POLAK-WYSS et al. 1985; POLAK 1988b).

In *C. albicans* ignosterol, a sterol containing a Δ_{14} double bond, accumulates. This accumulation takes place soon after contact with the drug, i.e. after one generation 10% of the sterol is already ignosterol, and this reaches 99% after 24-h incubation. The appearance of a Δ_{14}-sterol in treated cells indicates an inhibition of Δ_{14}-reductase, a step in the biosynthesis of ergosterol following C_{14}-demethylation. Upon inhibition of the Δ_{14}-reductase by amorolfine, further conversion of the sterol molecules proceeds to the fecosterol level. However, the Δ_7-Δ_8-isomerization no longer occurs. From these observations it was postulated that amorolfine, like other morpholine derivatives, in fact inhibits two steps in the pathway of ergosterol biosynthesis, namely the Δ_{14}-reductase and the Δ_7-Δ_8-isomerase.

In studies with a cell-free system of *S. cerevisiae*, amorolfine exhibited a high inhibitory activity on both enzymes with an IC_{50} of 2.93 μM for the Δ_{14}-reductase and an IC_{50} of 0.0018 μM for Δ_7-Δ_8-isomerase. Clearly, the affinity of amorolfine for the isomerase enzyme is significantly higher than that for the reductase. The same findings were also observed with fenpropidine and other morpholines. However, since the reductase step comes earlier in the pathway, this first inhibition is more important than the second for growth inhibition in whole cells (BALOCH and MERCER 1987).

This double inhibition has also been observed in aspergilli, *Histoplasma* and dermatophytes. In all these species ignosterol or ergosta-8,14,24(28)-trienol accumulate. However, in *Trichophyton* species this accumulation is only seen at low concentrations of the drug. At high concentrations (>10 μg/ml) sterol biosynthesis is already inhibited at the level of squalene, as shown by the enormous amounts of squalene which accumulate in amorolfine-treated cells. Whether this accumulation is due to a direct inhibition of squalene epoxidase or is induced by a regulatory mechanism is not yet clear, since up to now it has not been possible to study the direct effect of amorolfine on squalene epoxidase in cell-free systems of *T. mentagrophytes* (POLAK 1988b).

As the Δ_7-Δ_8-isomerase and the Δ_{14}-reductase show some similarities at the molecular level, it has been suggested that the Δ_7-Δ_8-isomerization reaction starts with an 8-hydrogenation, which is assumed to be an NADPH/H^+-dependent reduction of the 8-double bond similar to the NADPH/H^+-dependent reduction of the 14-double bond. The formation of a carbonium-ion, high-energy intermediate at C14 in the reductase and at C8 for the isomerase has been postulated. An alkyl morpholine, which at pH 7.4 forms morpholinium ions, shows electronic and structural similarities with these carbonium-ion, high-energy intermediates and may therefore have high affinity for the two enzymes and thus inhibit their action. It is interesting that the degree of inhibitory effect of morpholines on Δ_{14}-reductase and Δ_7-Δ_8-

isomerase varies depending on the configuration (*cis* or *trans*) and on the enantiomer (R or S) of the derivatives (Baloch and Mercer 1987).

Although it is clear that morpholine derivatives strongly inhibit sterol biosynthesis at two different enzymatic steps at least, it is still questionable whether this inhibition is the sole basis of toxicity to the fungal cell. It may be that not only the effect on the sterol pattern in the membrane, which is clearly the primary target of amorolfine and related morpholine derivatives, but also secondary effects (e.g. succinate cytochrome c-reductase) are together responsible for their fungicidal activity. Furthermore, accumulation of C_{14}-methyl sterols or Δ_8, Δ_{14}-sterols appears to be correlated with the deposition of chitin in the membrane and with the inhibition of membrane-bound chitin synthase (Kerkenaar 1987; Vanden Bossche et al. 1984b). Chitin is important in the growth processes of most fungi, and this secondary event may play an important role in the fungicidal effect of drug. Ignosterol, as C_{14}-methyl-sterols, does not fulfill the steric demands at C14 for a planar sterol α-phase which is needed for the proper functioning of the membrane and so, like the C_{14}-methyl-sterols accumulated during azole treatment, interferes with the membrane functions in fungal cells.

In conclusion amorolfine certainly inhibits sterol biosynthesis in fungi, which causes hyperfluidity of the membrane, which in turn leads not only to changes in membrane permeability that adversely affect the fungal metabolic processes but additionally induces abnormal chitin deposition leading to growth abnormalities.

3. Allylamines

Naftifine and terbinafine (Fig. 8) show in vitro antimycotic activity against a wide range of pathogenic fungi. The effect is exceptionally high against dermatophytes (MIC 0.003–0.2 μg/ml), good against filamentous and dimorphic fungi (MIC 0.1–1 μg/ml) but rather weak against yeasts, especially against *C. albicans* (MIC 6–100 μg/ml). Besides fungistatic activity a strong fungicidal effect is seen, especially in dermatophytes, and allylamines are highly effective in the treatment of dermatophytic infections. Whereas naftifine is applied topically, terbinafine can also be given systemically.

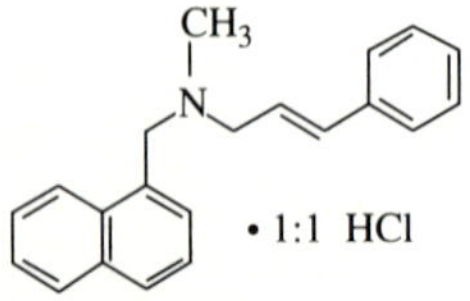

Naftitine • HCl

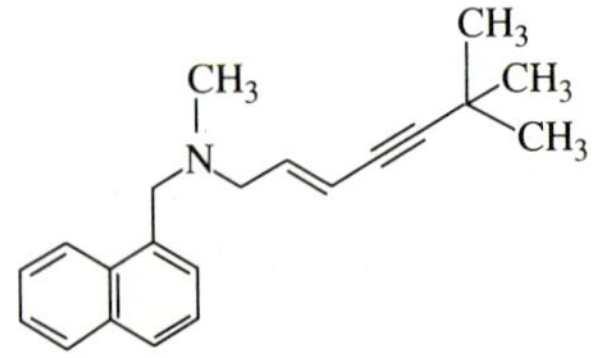

Terbinafine
(Sandoz, SF 86-327)

Fig. 8. Allylamines

Morphological changes observed in dermatophytes and in yeasts under the influence of allylamines include accumulation of lipid particles within the cytoplasm, alteration in the cytoplasmic membrane and a thickening of the cell wall. All these findings are consistent with an inhibition of membrane sterol synthesis (MEINGASSNER and SLEYTR 1982; MEINGASSNER et al. 1981).

Biochemical studies have revealed that in allylamine-treated fungal cells an accumulation of squalene and a concomitant decrease of ergosterol level takes place, again indicating the inhibition of sterol biosynthesis. This is observed in whole cells as well as in crude extracts of *C. albicans*. There is a clear correlation between the inhibition of growth and the degree of inhibition of sterol biosynthesis (RYDER 1984, 1985a; RYDER and DUPONT 1985), indicating that the primary action of allylamines is at the level of squalene epoxidation.

Differences in the sensitivity of sterol biosynthesis between species influence their susceptibility to these drugs, but some variations in the degree of growth inhibition are not so easy to explain. Penetration problems with allylamines do not seem to be a factor in lack of inhibition for this class of compound, since activity against squalene epoxidase in whole cells and crude extracts of *Candida* cells is always similar. It has been postulated that fungal species differ not only in their inherent susceptibility of ergosterol synthesis but also in their reaction to the intracellular accumulation of squalene. Dermatophytes and dimorphic fungi seem to be extremely susceptible to ergosterol depletion and/or accumulation of unnatural sterols or squalene. However, *Candida* spp. can grow anaerobically and in this condition produce low levels of ergosterol in the cytoplasmic membrane with high levels of squalene; thus, they can apparently better tolerate an alteration in sterol biosynthesis than filamentous and dimorphic fungi. Sterol biosynthesis in *C. albicans* cells treated with an allylamine continues to a reduced degree and may enable the fungal cells to grow at a very low rate, but in *T. mentagrophytes* sterol biosynthesis is completely inhibited at the level of epoxidation, and no ergosterol at all is produced in the presence of terbinafine (RYDER 1985b). This fact may be the reason for the rapid and complete inhibition of growth in these species. It is interesting that allylamines are fungistatic for species in which the MIC value is higher than the concentration required for 95% inhibition of the enzyme, but fungicidal for those in which the MIC is significantly smaller than the IC_{95} for the enzyme. This suggests that the fungicidal effect may not be the result of a depletion of ergosterol, of which the IC_{95} is a measure. RYDER (1984, 1985a) and RYDER and DUPONT (1985) have postulated that fungicidal activity is due to the high intracellular accumulation of squalene and not to the depletion of ergosterol, which is only fungistatic.

Another proposed explanation for the difference in the fungistatic and fungicidal effects of allylamines may prove to be relevant. Ergosterol depletion leads to a deregulation of chitin synthesis which is followed by chitin deposition in the cell membrane and to cell wall abnormalities. Fungi growing in the mycelial form, whose cell wall structure is based mainly on chitin, may respond to this secondary alteration much more strongly than yeasts, which have mainly glucan in their cell wall skeleton.

On a molecular basis the mechanism of action is not well understood. Allylamines are clearly not substrate analogues for the squalene epoxidase enzyme, and there is no indication that the inhibition by allylamines is mechanism-based. Squalene epoxidase is not a cytochrome P-450-dependent enzyme, and therefore the specificity and toxicological problems associated with the azole derivatives are avoided (RYDER AND DUPONT 1985). Despite the fact that it is an early and not a fungi-specific step in the pathway of sterol biosynthesis, the specificity of the allylamines for the enzyme is relatively good. The K_m value of terbinafine, for example, is 3×10^{-8} M for the *C. albicans* enzyme compared with 1×10^{-4} M for the rat liver enzyme. In a *C. albicans* crude extract a K_i value of 0.03 μM was measured, whereas for the rat liver enzyme it was 77 μM. Kinetic analyses performed to date suggest that allylamines inhibit the yeast enzyme non-competitively in microsomes and independently of the presence of an S200 supernatant. Inhibition of the rat liver enzyme, on the other hand, appears to be competitive and is affected by S200 addition. However, these results must be open to question, as the interpretation of kinetic experiments performed on crude preparations of membrane-bound enzymes using insoluble substrates are anything but reliable. Neither the fungal nor the mammalian enzyme has been purified, and there appear to be important differences between microsomal preparations from the two sources.

Thus, although the primary target of allylamines is clearly squalene epoxidation, whether the growth inhibition and especially the fungicidal effect are a consequence of ergosterol depletion or of squalene accumulation remains an open question. It may well be that the lethal effect on the cell is the result of a secondary event such as the disturbance of chitin synthesis or other important cell membrane-bound enzyme functions which have not yet been identified.

4. Thiocarbamate Antifungals

The thiocarbamate antifungals, tolnaftate and tolciclate (Fig. 9), exhibit strong antifungal activity only against dermatophytes (MIC 0.1–1 μg/ml); yeast cells are resistant (MIC > 100 μg/ml; SCHOLER and POLAK 1984). The mode of action of these two antifungals is based on an inhibition of ergosterol biosynthesis, leading to an accumulation of squalene. In *T. mentagrophytes* cells the inhibition of ergosterol biosynthesis correlates with the in vitro efficacy. A microsomal enzyme preparation from *C. albicans* has also been shown to be inhibited by tolnaftate and tolciclate, but in whole cells the compounds were clearly less effective inhibitors, suggesting that they do not penetrate the *Candida* cell wall. From the biochemical studies available (BARRETT-BEE et al. 1986; RYDER et al. 1986) it is apparent that a primary target of tolnaftate and tolciclate is squalene epoxidase, as for the allylamine

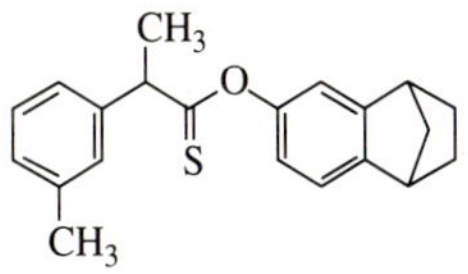

Tolciclate

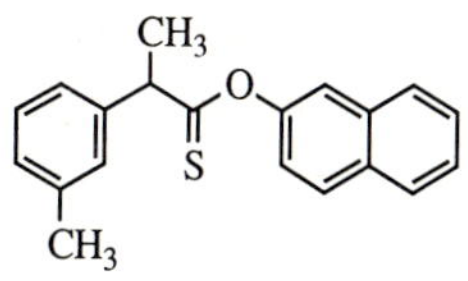

Tolnaftate

Fig. 9. Thiocarbamates

antifungals, but other mechanisms, secondary or primary, cannot be ruled out. The fact that both thiocarbamate and allylamines have a naphthalene moiety may indicate that this is involved in binding to the squalene epoxidase system and is the reason for the same primary target being responsible for antifungal activity of the two chemical classes.

5. Conclusions

The various inhibitors of ergosterol biosynthesis exert their effects through different enzymes in the biosynthetic pathway (Fig. 10) and induce different sterol patterns in treated cells, but they all inhibit growth and induce modification of cell morphology. Electron microscopy of fungal cells treated with such an inhibitor reveals destruction of the cell membrane, irregular deposition of chitin and significant thickening of the cell wall. This is observed in a variety of fungal species, and the same picture is evident regardless of the nature of the 'false' sterol (i.e. non-ergosterol sterol, or squalene in the case of the allylamines) that is accumulated. Added to the fact that these phenomena first become apparent considerably after the accumulation has reached a significant level, this suggests that it is the depletion of ergosterol rather than the structure or amount of unusual membrane components which adversely affects the cells.

It appears that all sterol biosynthesis inhibitors act essentially by disturbing the fluidity of the cell membrane, which not only alters its mechanical properties but also disturbs the regulation and function of the membrane-bound enzymes. The fungal membrane derives its properties from a specific interaction between ergosterol and phospholipids, and present evidence suggests that it is the inability of the accumulated precursors to mimic this specificity rather than their active disturbance of such interactions that leads to growth inhibition.

D. Target: Cell Wall Synthesis

Cell wall synthesis should be one of the most selective targets for antifungal drugs since the two major structural polysaccharides, chitin and β-glucan, are absent in human cells. Although a number of antifungal antibiotics which

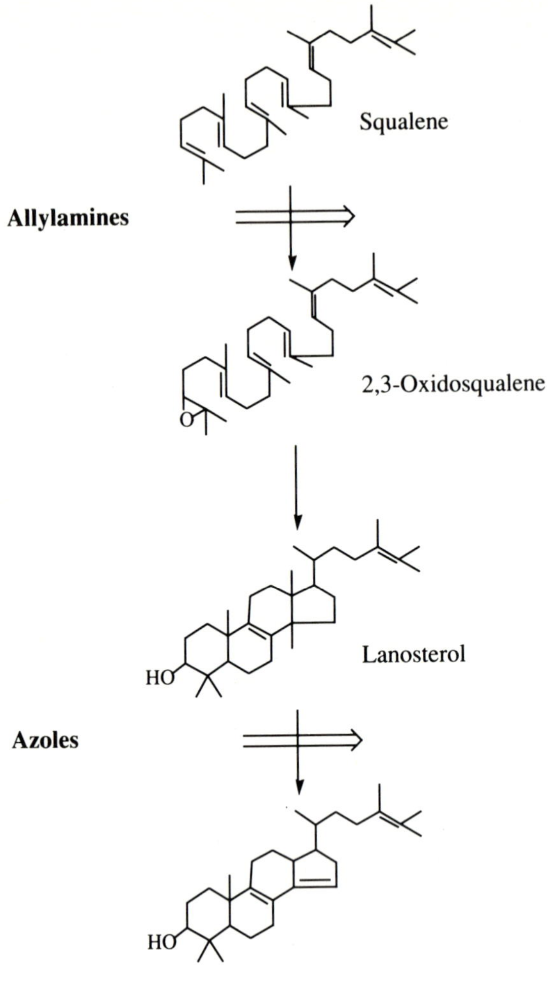

Fig. 10. Sterol biosynthesis in fungi

inhibit the synthesis of these polysaccharides and mannoproteins exist, only one, the semisynthetic echinocandin derivative LY121019 (cilofungin), has reached the stage of clinical evaluation.

I. Chitin Synthase Inhibition

Polyoxins and nikkomycins, both produced by *Streptomyces*, strongly inhibit the chitin synthase of *C. albicans* in vitro with K_i values lower than the K_m value for the normal substrate UDP GlcNAC. However, enormous discrepancies exist between the high inhibition at the level of the enzyme and the low inhibition of *Candida* cell growth. The compounds are taken up in

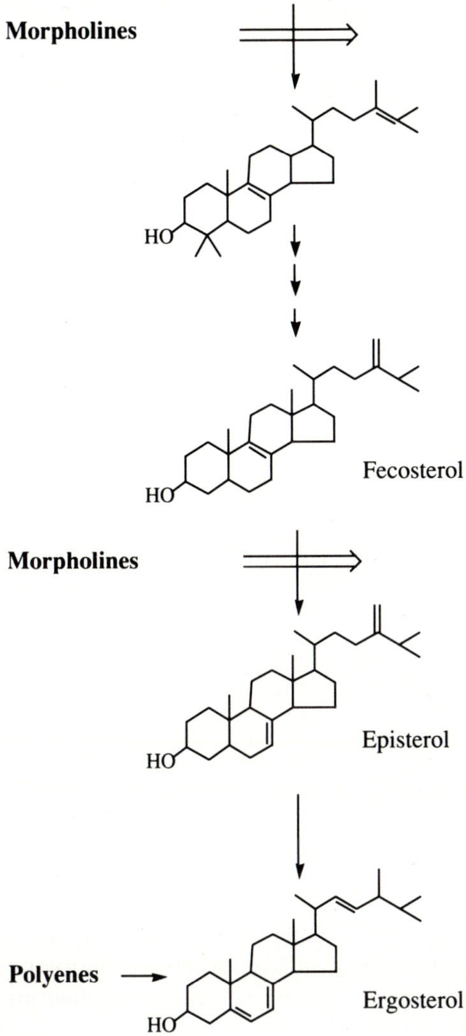

Fig. 10. (continued)

filamentous fungi and in yeasts by the peptide transport system which seems to be less efficient for these compounds in yeasts. Thus, the inhibitor does not reach the target enzyme in yeast, and any use as a clinical antifungal is precluded, although polyoxin is widely used in Japan as an agricultural fungicide.

II. Glucan Synthesis

Glucan synthesis is specifically inhibited by various antibiotics (Fig. 11): echinocandin produced by *Aspergillus nidulans* var. *echinulatus*, aculeacin produced by *Aspergillus aculeatus*, papulacandin produced by *Patularia*

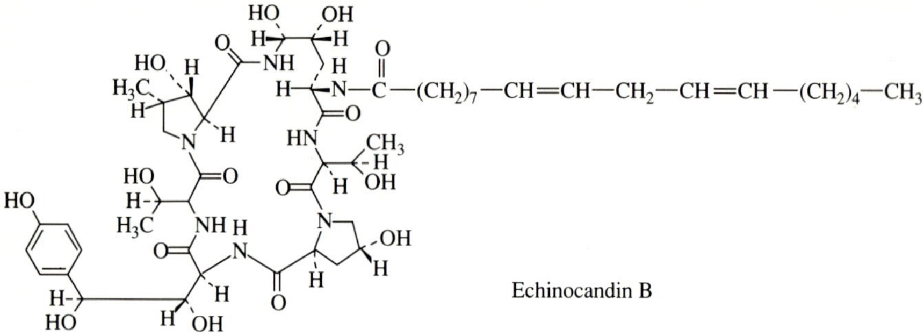

Echinocandin B

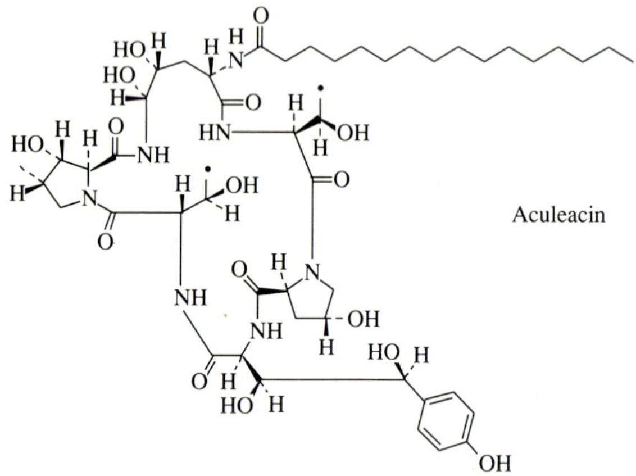

Aculeacin

Fig. 11. Inhibitors of glucan synthesis

spherosperma and a semisynthetic derivative of echinocandin, LY121019, now being evaluated for clinical use. All these antibiotics show a relative narrow antifungal spectrum, having no activity against moulds or dermatophytes, only against *Candida* species. The most susceptible species are *C. albicans* (MIC values below 0.2 μg/ml) and *C. tropicalis* (MIC values below 0.5). The other species *C. krusei*, *C. parapsilosis* and *Torulopsis glabrata* show MIC values between 0.2 and 10 μg/ml (GORDEE et al. 1984).

All the above mentioned antibiotics inhibit β-glucan synthesis both in vitro (at the enzyme level) and in vivo (on the whole cell) (BAGULEY et al. 1979; IWATA et al. 1982; SAWISTOWSKA-SCHRÖDER et al. 1984; VARONA et al. 1983; YAMAGUCHI et al. 1982). The antifungal effect on the cell is only seen in growing cells, not in resting ones. Incubation of sensitive growing cells with these antibiotics leads to a rapid aggregation of the cells, and the release of some cellular components which function outside the cells as a sort of cement to aggregate the rest of the cells. Furthermore, large distorted forms are induced which disrupt at low concentrations of the antibiotic (Fig. 12). This

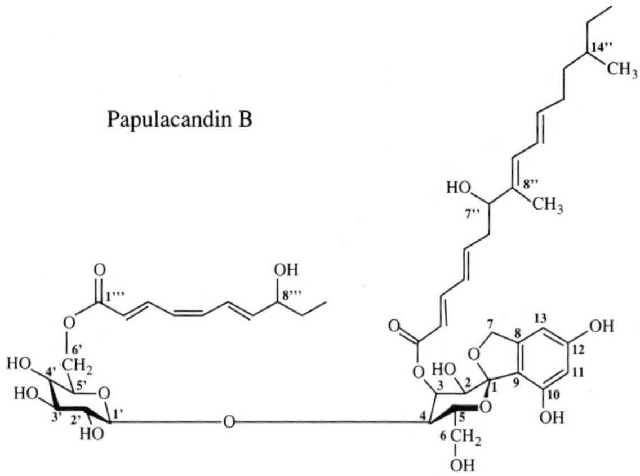

Papulacandin B

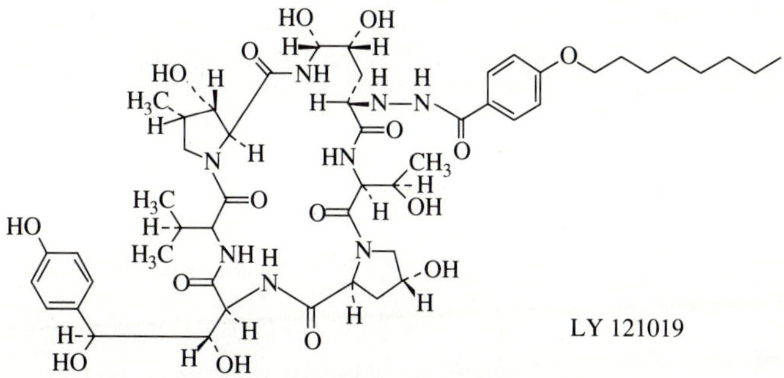

LY 121019

Fig. 11. (continued)

cell lysis can be prevented by osmotic stabilisers. All such antibiotics display an unexpected phenomenon at higher concentrations. The fungicidal effect is progressively reduced until at high concentrations the drug is not even fungistatic, but the yeasts grow in a special, bizarre form. An explanation for this phenomenon may be the amphiphilic nature of the antibiotics; at high concentrations in an aqueous medium they form micelles which no longer have access to the target site.

Glucan synthesis is also inhibited in *Geotrichum* by the above drugs, but in contrast to yeasts, its growth is not prevented (PEREZ et al. 1981). This is probably explained by the fact that in *Geotrichum* the cell wall skeleton is composed to a greater extent of chitin, which may replace the glucan skeleton inhibited by the antibiotics. In *C. albicans* and *S. cerevisiae*, however, the main skeleton is the glucan moiety and therefore an inhibition of its synthesis leads to a fungicidal effect. At the enzyme level a total inhibition of glucan synthase is never achieved. For instance, only 70% of the activity of the β-1,3-glucan synthase is inhibited by 0.8 μg/ml aculeacin. Higher concentrations

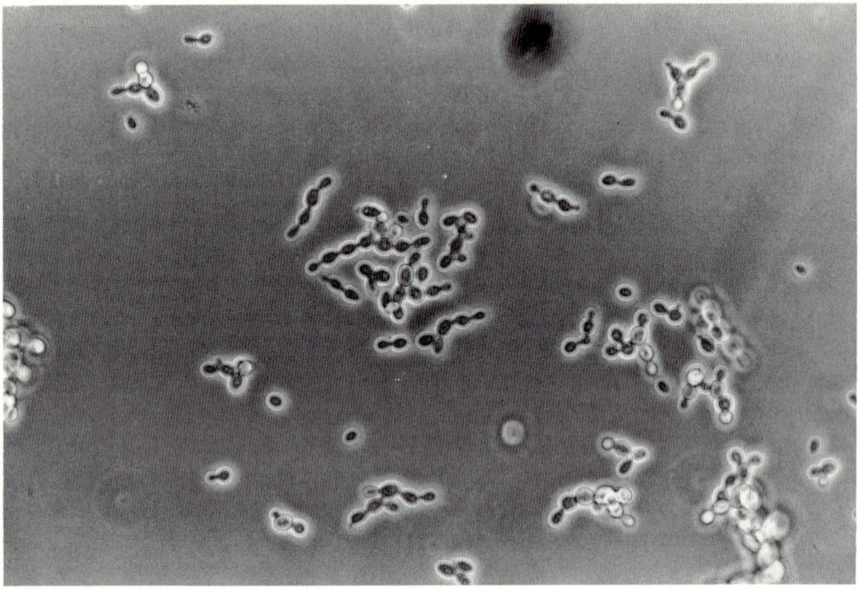

Fig. 12a

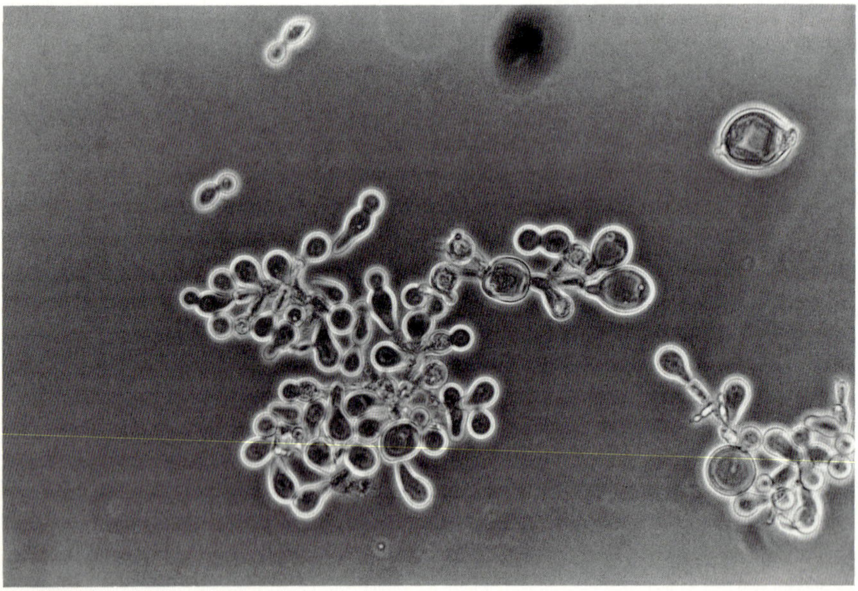

Fig. 12b

Fig. 12a–c. Influence of aculeacin on *Candida albicans* blastospores. **a** Control cells; **b** cells treated with 1 μg/ml for 24 h at 37°C; **c** cells treated with 1 μg/ml for 48 h at 37°C

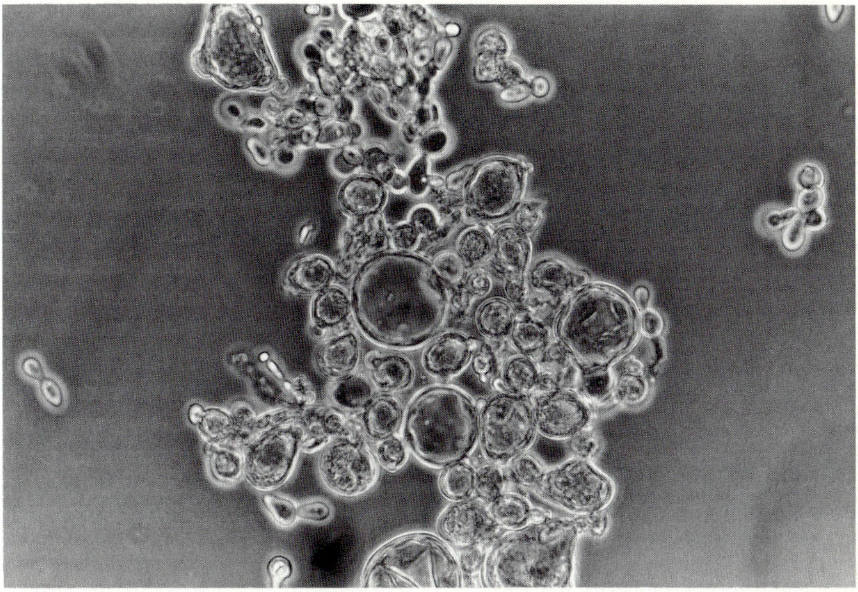

Fig. 12c

are less efficient, as is the case for the effect on the whole cell. The inhibition is characterised as non-competitive and mixed, in which the affinity of the substrate is increased by the addition of the inhibitor. The interpretation of kinetic data is difficult since the enzyme is present in a mixed membrane fraction, and up to now no studies on the purified enzyme have been possible. Variation of the structure of papulacandin has shown that the inhibitory effect at the enzyme level is dependent on the long fatty acid chain and on the phenol residue. Hydrogenation of the fatty acid leads to a reduction of enzyme activity, but penetration to the target seems better (Römmele et al. 1983).

All the above antibiotics specifically inhibit β-1,3-glucan synthase and have no effect on chitin synthase, mannan synthase or glucanase, but as yet none has proved its worth as a chemotherapeutic agent.

Acknowledgements. I wish to express grateful appreciation to M. Jenni for typing the text and to Dr. P. Hartman for stimulating discussions and critical appraisal of the manuscript.

References

Arai T, Mikami T, Yokoyama K, Kawata T (1977) Morphological changes in yeasts as a result of the action of 5-fluorocytosine. Antimicrob Agents Chemother 12: 255–260

Baguley BC, Römmele G, Gruner J, Wehrli W (1979) Papulacandin B: an inhibitor of glucan synthesis in yeast spheroplasts. Eur J Biochem 97:345–351

Baloch RI, Mercer EI (1987) Inhibition of sterol Δ^8-Δ^7-isomerase and Δ^{14}-reductase by fenpropimorph, tridemorph and fenpropidin in cell-free enzyme systems from *Saccharomyces cerevisiae*. Phytochem 26:663–668
Barrett-Bee KJ, Lane AC, Turner RW (1986) The mode of antifungal action of tolnaftate. J Med Vet Mycol 24:155–160
Borgers M (1985) Antifungal azole derivatives. In: Greenwood D, O'Grady F (eds) The scientific basis of antimicrobial chemotherapy. Cambridge University Press, Cambridge, pp 133–153 (Thirty-eighth symposium of the Society for General Microbiology)
Borgers M, Van de Ven MA (1987) Degenerative changes in fungi after itraconazole treatment. Rev Inf Dis 9:S33–S42
Brasseur R, Vandenbosch C, Vanden Bossche H, Ruysschaert JM (1983) Mode of insertion of miconazole, ketoconazole and deacylated ketoconazole in lipid layers. Biochem Pharmacol 32:2175–2180
Chen WC, Chou DL, Feingold DS (1978) Dissociation between ion permeability and the lethal action of polyene antibiotics on *Candida albicans*. Antimicrob Agents Chemother 13:914–917
Cohen SS, Barner HD (1954) Studies on unbalanced growth in *Escherichia coli*. Proc Natl Acad Sci USA 40:885–893
Cohen SS, Flaks JG, Barner HD, Loeb MR, Lichtenstein J (1958) The mode of action of 5-fluorouracil and its derivatives. Proc Natl Acad Sci USA 44:1004–1012
De Kruijff B, Gerritsen WJ, Oerlemans A, van Dijck PWM, Demel RA, Deenen LLM (1974) Polyene antibiotic-sterol interactions in membranes of *Acholeplasma laidlawii* cells and lecithin liposomes. II. Temperature dependence of the polyene antibiotic-sterol complex formation. Biochim Biophys Acta 339:44–56
El-Nakeeb MY, Lampen JO (1965) Uptake of ^{3}H-griseofulvin by micro-organisms and its correlation with sensitivity to griseofulvin. J Gen Microbiol 39:285–293
Gale E (1986) Nature and development of phenotypic resistance to amphotericin B in *Candida albicans*. Adv Microb Physiol 27:278–320
Giege R, Weil J-H (1970) Etude des tRNA de levure ayant incorporé du 5-fluorouracile provenant de la désamination in vivo de la 5-fluorocytosine. Bull Soc Chim Biol 52:135–144
Gordee RS, Zeckner DJ, Ellis LF (1984) In vitro and in vivo anti-*Candida* activity and toxicology of LY 121019. J Antibiot 37:1054–1065
Grisham LM, Wilson L, Bensch KG (1973) Antimitotic action of griseofulvin does not involve disruption of microtubules. Nature 244:294–296
Gull K, Trinci APJ (1973) Griseofulvin inhibits fungal mitosis. Nature 244:292–294
Iwata K, Yamamoto Y, Yamaguchi H, Hiratani T (1982) In vitro studies of aculeacin A, a new antifungal antibiotic. J Antibiot 35:203–209
Jund R, Lacroute F (1974) Génétique et physiologie de la résistance aux 5-fluoropyrimidines chez *Saccharomyces cerevisiae*. Bull Soc Franc Mycol Médicale III:5–8
Kerkenaar A (1987) The mode of action of dimethylmorpholines. In: Fromtling RA (ed) Recent trends in the discovery, development and evaluation of antifungal agents. JR Prous, Barcelona, pp 523–542
Kerridge D (1986) Mode of action of clinically important antifungal drugs. Adv Microb Physiol 27:1–72.
Kotler-Brajtburg J, Price HD, Medoff G, Schlessinger D, Kobayashi GS (1974) Molecular basis for the selective toxicity of amphotericin B for yeast and filipin for animal cells. Antimicrob Agents Chemother 5:377–382
Lampen JO (1966) Interference by polyene antibiotics (especially nystatin and filipin) with specific membrane functions. In: Newton BA, Reynolds PE (eds) Biochemical studies of antimicrobial drugs. Cambridge University Press, Cambridge, pp 111–130 (Sixteenth symposium of the Society for General Microbiology)
Lampen JO, Arnow PM, Borowska Z, Laskin AI (1962) Location and role of sterol at nystatin-binding sites. J Bacteriol 84:1152–1160
Malawista SE (1973) Microtubules and the movement of melanin granules in frog dermal melanocytes. Ann NY Acad Sci 253:702–710

Marini F, Arnow P, Lampen PO (1961) The effect of monovalent cations on the inhibition of yeast metabolism by nystatin. J Gen Microbiol 24:51–62

Medoff G, Kobayashi GA (1980) Antifungal agents – the polyenes. In: Speller DCE (ed) Antifungal chemotherapy. Wiley & Sons, Chichester, pp 3–33

Meingassner JG, Sleytr UB (1982) The effects of naftifine on the ultrastructure of *Candida parapsilosis*: a freeze fracture study. Sabouraudia 20:199–207

Meingassner JG, Sleytr UB, Petranyi G (1981) Morphological changes induced by naftifine, a new antifungal agent, in *Trichophyton mentagrophytes*. J Invest Dermatol 77:444–451

Müller J, Polak A, Jaeger R (1987) The effect of the morpholine derivate amorolfin (Roche 14-4767/002) on the ultrastructure of *Candida albicans*. Mykosen 30: 528–540

Nes WR, Sekula BC, Nes D, Adler JH (1978) The functional importance of structural features of ergosterol in yeast. J Biol Chem 253:6218–6225

Osterman DG, DePhillis GD, Wu JC, Matsuda A, Santi DV (1988) 5-Fluorocytosine in DNA is a mechanism-based inhibitor of *Hha*I methylase. Biochemistry 27:5204–5210

Palacios J, Serrano R (1978) Proton permeability induced by polyene antibiotics. A plausible mechanism for their inhibition of maltose fermentation in yeast. FEBS Lett 91:198–201

Perez P, Varona R, Garcia-Acha I, Duran A (1981) Effect of papulacandin B and aculeacin A on β-(1,3)-glucan-synthase from *Geotrichum lactis*. FEBS Lett 129:249–252

Plempel M, Berg D (1984) Reduction of the in vitro virulence of *Candida albicans* by pretreatment with subinhibitory azole concentrations in vitro. Dermatologica 169 [Suppl.1]:11–18

Polak A (1988a) Mode of action of 5-fluorocytosine in *Aspergillus fumigatus*. In: Vanden Bossche H, Mackenzie DWR, Cauwenbergh G (eds) *Aspergillus* and aspergillosis. Plenum, New York, p 165

Polak A (1988b) Mode of action of morpholine derivatives. Ann N Y Acad Sci 544:221–228

Polak A, Scholer HJ (1975) Mode of action of 5-fluorocytosine and mechanisms of resistance. Chemotherapy 21:113–130

Polak A, Scholer HJ (1980) Mode of action of 5-fluorocytosine. Rev Inst Past Lyon 13:233–244

Polak-Wyss A, Lengseld H, Oesterhelt G (1985) Effect of oxiconazole and Ro 14-4767/002 on sterol pattern in *Candida albicans*. Sabouraudia: J Med Vet Mycol 23:433–442

Rodriguez RJ, Parks LW (1983) Structural and physiological features of sterols necessary to satisfy bulk membrane and sparking requirements in yeast sterol auxotrophs. Arch Biochem Biophys 225:861–871

Römmele G, Traxler P, Wehrli W (1983) Papulacandins – the relationship between chemical structure and effect on glucan synthesis in yeast. J Antibiotics 36: 1539–1542

Ryder N (1984) Selective inhibition of squalene epoxidation by allylamine antimycotic agents. In: Nombela C (ed) Microbial cell wall synthesis and autolysis. Elsevier, Amsterdam, p 313

Ryder N (1985a) Specific inhibition of fungal sterol biosynthesis by SF 86-327, a new allylamine antimycotic agent. Antimicrob Agents Chemother 27:252–256

Ryder N (1985b) Effect of allylamine antimycotic agents on fungal sterol biosynthesis measured by sterol side-chain methylation. J Gen Microbiol 131:1595–1602

Ryder NS, Dupont MC (1985) Inhibition of squalene epoxidase by allylamine antimycotic compounds. A comparative study of the fungal and mammalian enzymes. Biochem J 230:765–770

Ryder NS, Frank I, Dupont MC (1986) Ergosterol biosynthesis inhibition by the thiocarbamate antifungal agents tolnaftate and tolciclate. Antimicrob Agents Chemother 29:858–860

Sawistowska-Schröder ET, Kerridge D, Perry H (1984) Echinocandin inhibition of 1,3-β-D-glucan synthase from *Candida albicans*. FEBS Letts 173:134–138

Scholer H (1980) Flucytosine. In: Speller DCE (ed) Antifungal chemotherapy. Wiley & Sons, Chichester, pp 35–106

Scholer HJ, Polak A (1984) Resistance to systemic antifungal agents. In: Bryan LE (ed) Antimicrobial drug resistance. Academic, Orlando, pp 393–460

Shigematsu ML, Uno J, Arai T (1982) Effect of ketoconazole on isolated mitochondria from *Candida albicans*. Antimicrob Agents Chemother 21:919–924

Thomas AH (1986) Suggested mechanisms for the antimycotic activity of the polyene antibiotics and the N-substituted imidazoles. J Antimicrob Chemother 17:269–279

Trzaskos JM, Henry MJ (1989) Comparative effects of the azole-based fungicide flusilazole on yeast and mammalian lanosterol 14α-methyl demethylase. Antimicrob Agents Chemother 33:1228–1231

Uno J, Shigematsu ML, Arai T (1982) Primary site of action of ketoconazole on *Candida albicans*. Antimicrob Agents Chemother 21:912–918

Vanden Bossche H, Ruysschaert JM, Defrise-Quertain F, Willemsens G, Cornelissen F, Maricahl P, Cools W, van Cutsem J (1982) The interaction of miconazole and ketoconazole with lipids. Biochem Pharmacol 31:2509–2517

Vanden Bossche H, Lauwers W, Willemsens G, Marichal P, Cornelisson F, Cools W (1984a) Molecular basis for the antimycotic and antibacterial activity of N-substituted imidazoles and triazoles: the inhibition of isoprenoid biosynthesis. Pesticide Sci 15:188–198

Vanden Bossche H, Willemsens G, Marichal P, Cools W, Lauwers W (1984b) The molecular basis for the antifungal activities of N-substituted azole derivatives. Focus on R 51 211. In: Trinci APJ, Ryley JF (eds) Mode of action of antifungal agents. Cambridge University Press, Cambridge, pp 321–341 (Symposium no 9 of the British Mycological Society)

Vanden Bossche H, Bellens D, Cools W, Gorrens J, Marichal P, Verhoeven H, Willemsens G, De Coster R, Beerens D, Haeltermann C, Coene MC, Lauwers W, Le Jeune L (1986) Cytochrome P-450: target for itraconazole. Drug Dev Res 8:287–298

Varona R, Pérez P, Durán A (1983) Effect of papulacandin B on β-glucan synthesis in *Schizosaccharomyces pombe*. FEMS Microbiol Lett 20:243–247

Wain WH, Polak A (1981) The effect of 5-fluorocytosine on the synthesis of 80S ribosomes by pathogenic fungi. Sabouraudia 19:187–197

Waldorf AR, Polak A (1983) Mechanisms of action of 5-fluorocytosine. Antimicrob Agents Chemother 23:79–85

Whelan WL, Markie D, Kwong-Chung KJ (1986) Complementation analysis of resistance to 5-fluorocytosine in *Candida albicans*. Antimicrob Agents Chemother 29:726–729

Yamaguchi H, Iwata K (1979) Effect of fatty acyl group and sterol composition on sensitivity of lecithin liposomes to imidazole antimycotics. Antimicrob Agents Chemother 15:706–711

Yamaguchi H, Hiratani T, Iwata K, Yamamoto Y (1982) Studies on the mechanism of antifungal action of aculeacin A. J Antibiot 35:210–219

Zygmung WA, Tavormina PA (1966) Steroid interference with antifungal activity of polyene antibiotics. Applied Microb 14:865–869

CHAPTER 7

Pharmacokinetic Aspects of Antifungal Therapy

MICHAEL H. TARBIT

A. Introduction

The pharmacokinetic study of drugs, analysis of the time course of a drug substance in the body, is no longer novel in clinical therapeutics. The application of the concepts of pharmacokinetics to the discovery and development of better therapeutic agents, particularly within the pharmaceutical industry, is growing rapidly. There are several aspects of this process which are particularly important in the development of antimicrobial agents. Thus, for example, drug discovery projects are now focussing on the need to achieve high systemic availability following oral administration; the potential benefit in targeting drugs to particular tissues such as the CNS or via specific routes of elimination such as in urine or body secretions to treat topical infections; and the need to obtain drugs with a sufficiently long duration of action to achieve once daily dosing. In addition, the relationship between the in vitro potency of drugs in primary screens and their efficacy in vivo is often poorly understood, and discovery project scientists often cannot rationalise the efficacy of their novel compounds in vivo without an awareness of their pharmacokinetics. Consequently, both the practising clinician and the project scientist need to have an understanding of what impact the pharmacokinetic profile of the drugs they propose for antifungal therapy will have on their efficacy.

The objective of this chapter is to discuss some of the fundamental pharmacokinetic concepts which relate to the therapeutic use of antifungal drugs and to present a critical review of the pharmacokinetics of some of the agents which are currently available in the clinic.

B. Pharmacokinetic and Metabolic Concepts

A thorough exposition of the fundamentals of pharmacokinetic concepts requires more than a single chapter, and the reader is directed to the excellent publications of ROWLAND and TOZER (1988) and GIBALDI and PERRIER (1982) for further information. However, the concepts which aid an understanding of the kinetics of antifungal drugs are outlined briefly in this section.

I. In Vitro Potency Versus In Vivo Efficacy

Whether it be the initial screening of potential antifungal agents emerging from a drug discovery programme or the sensitivity testing of a particular agent against a number of different fungal species, the primary testing of a novel agent usually occurs in vitro. The conditions of in vitro tests are such that the compound remains in contact with the organism at the same concentration throughout the period of exposure; generally there is no metabolism of the compound, and consequently metabolites are absent; there is little or no protein present to bind the drug, thus reducing the availability of "active" drug; the fungal organism may be present in a specific morphological form, e.g. yeast; and there is no involvement of any immune component.

These conditions can be described as a "static" test of the antifungal compound. When the same compound is administered in vivo, conditions are usually entirely different. Thus, following an oral dose the compound may not be completely absorbed from the gastrointestinal tract due to, for instance, low aqueous solubility or high molecular weight; following absorption, the drug has to pass first through the liver, the body's main organ of metabolism, where exposure to metabolism may remove part or all of the fraction of the dose absorbed. Once present in the systemic circulation, the drug may bind to proteins in both plasma and tissues, thus reducing the availability of effective drug. In addition, depending on its relative lipophilicity, the drug may be taken up extensively into lipid membranes in tissues which may or may not be the site of infection; this may markedly alter the circulating concentrations of the drug. Finally, the body will attempt to clear the drug from the system by metabolism and/or renal excretion; thus its concentration may change markedly with time. Under these conditions, the relative potency of an antimicrobial agent in vitro can be completely negated by its pharmacokinetic profile in vivo. One corollary to this effect of pharmacokinetics is that in vitro tests of antifungal agents should never be used as the sole selective index for candidate drugs. Indeed, the utility of in vitro tests for predicting the relative activity of antifungal drugs per se has often been called into question (ODDS 1980, 1986; see also Chap. 4). Recent attempts to correlate in vivo efficacy with in vitro potency of antimicrobial agents, however, have encouraged a view that some rationalisation is possible when the full pharmacokinetic profile of an agent is known (RICHARDSON et al. 1986; ROLINSON 1980; TROKE et al. 1988; WISE 1986).

II. Analysis of Samples

The minimal requirement for pharmacokinetic analysis is a set of data on blood or plasma concentrations of a drug related to time after the dose. To determine the concentrations of a drug, a precise, specific and accurate assay with the required degree of sensitivity is required. Bioassay is frequently used with antimicrobial agents, since this is usually rapid, often very sensitive and usually requires only small volumes of blood or plasma. However, caution should be practised in the use of such assays, since the impact of any bioactive metabolites of a drug circulating at concentrations which may be significantly higher than that of the parent drug may produce large errors in determining concentrations. The use of specific chemical assays, using liquid or gas chromatographs, is increasing in frequency due to the fact that modern detectors have improved sensitivity to the level achievable by bioassay, and these are now the methods of choice for accurate kinetic analysis.

III. Assessment of Absorption and Systemic Availability

Most drugs used clinically are administered orally; this is particularly so when treatment is given to outpatients. Consequently, determination of the extent of absorption of a drug into the systemic circulation following oral administration is fundamental to an assessment of the likely clinical utility of an antifungal drug. The systemic exposure to a drug is described by measurement of the area under the plasma, serum or blood concentration versus time curve (AUC). It obviously follows that the lower the AUC, the lower the systemic exposure. In principle the classic method used to determine the extent of systemic exposure to a drug following oral administration, its oral bioavailability, is to compare the AUC value following intravenous administration – when all of the dose is delivered to the systemic circulation – with the corresponding AUC value following oral administration. If these are similar when corrected for dose, then it is reasonable to conclude that all of the oral dose was absorbed into the systemic circulation. If the AUC value following oral administration is significantly lower than the corresponding intravenous value, it follows that absorption into the systemic circulation following oral administration is incomplete. The simple ratio of the AUC values (Fig. 1) will determine the fraction of the oral dose (often abbreviated as F) which is systemically available. Log transformation of the data is often used, as the elimination of drugs is a first-order rate process (see below): consequently for accurate comparison, the AUC values need to be corrected to infinity.

As outlined above, the accurate assessment of systemic availability requires intravenous administration of a drug. This is not always possible, particularly in human studies, if the drug is poorly soluble or cannot be formulated. Under these circumstances a minimum estimate of the extent of absorption of a drug may be made using radiolabelled drug and determining the fraction of radiolabel excreted in the urine. This method assumes that the drug was absorbed intact and was not broken down prior to absorption. The calculated figure represents a minimum value, because drug-related material may also be excreted via the bile into the faeces.

It is common practice in drug discovery programmes to use subcutaneous or intraperitoneal dosing as a parenteral route to obviate the need for intravenous formulation. Both of these dose routes involve an absorption phase which may or may not be complete. Consequently, in pharmacokinetic terms,

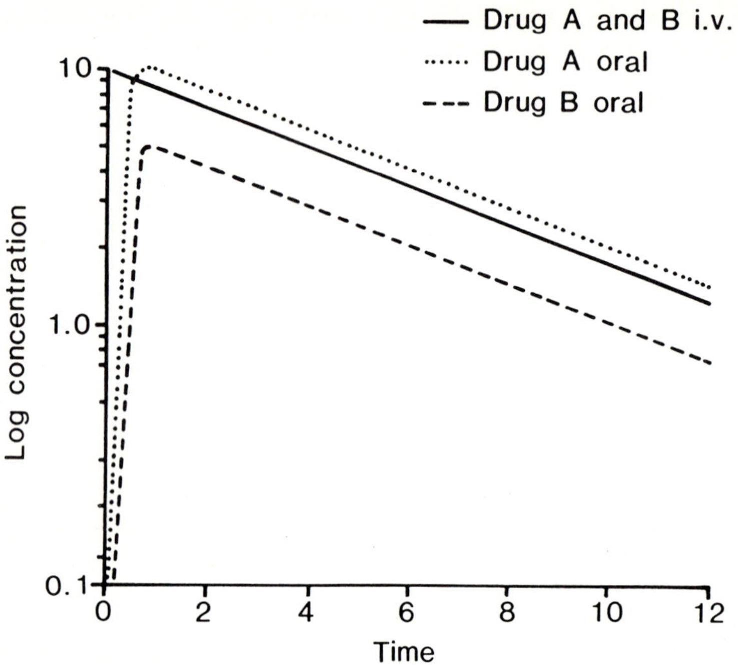

Fig. 1. Comparison of systemic exposure (area under curve) to two hypothetical drugs following intravenous and oral administration at the same dose level. Drug A exhibits complete oral bioavailability: $AUC_{po}/AUC_{iv} = 1$. Drug B exhibits oral bioavailability of 50%: $AUC_{po}/AUC_{iv} = 0.5$

they are less than ideal substitutes for the intravenous dose route, where all of the administered dose is presumed to be systemically available.

There are two major reasons why all of an orally administered drug may not reach the systemic circulation. The first is that the drug may not be absorbed from the gastrointestinal tract. This is frequently the case if the drug is highly lipophilic and exhibits poor aqueous solubility at the pH of the small intestine, the major site of absorption, since a drug needs to be in solution to be absorbed. Conversely, the drug may be a large, highly polar molecule, which is soluble at intestinal pH but is too polar to cross the lipophilic membranes of the intestinal wall. Both conditions apply to antifungal drugs currently used in therapy (see below).

The second reason for poor systemic availability of orally administered drugs relates to the fact that, following absorption, all materials pass through the liver en route to the heart and systemic circulation. The liver is the major organ of metabolism in the body and has a high capacity for metabolism of orally absorbed xenobiotics. Consequently, any drug which is metabolically labile may be metabolised extensively, or even completely, before it reaches the systemic circulation. Under these conditions a drug may be completely absorbed from the intestine but still exhibit very low or negligible blood levels. As described below, the first generation of imidazole antifungal agents were not therapeutically useful as oral drugs for this reason.

Thus, the systemic availability of an antifungal agent following oral administration depends upon a combination of its extent of absorption from the gastrointestinal tract and the extent to which it escapes metabolism by the liver on its first pass through the portal system. The importance of developing drugs with high oral bioavailability lies in the variation in absorption and metabolism usually observed within the patient population. Given a drug which exhibits low bioavailability, e.g. 5%, normal variation within the population may lead to a range of bioavailabilities from 1% to 10%, i.e. a tenfold range in systemic exposure. This may result in lack of efficacy at one end of the range and, with drugs with a narrow therapeutic index, toxicity at the other. Frequently, blood levels of such drugs show wide variations within the patient population and often require therapeutic monitoring in clinical use. Conversely, a drug which exhibits high bioavailability e.g. 90%, may show variation in bioavailability over the range 80%–100%; however, this represents a range of increase of only 20% and is less likely to cause significant problems.

IV. Distribution Parameters

Following the administration of an intravenous dose of an antifungal, the drug will distribute from the bloodstream into the tissues of the body. The extent to which this happens will depend upon the physico-chemical characteristics of the compound. Thus, highly lipophilic drugs which are not ionised at blood pH will pass out of the blood into the tissues rapidly. Drugs which are more polar, or which are partially ionised at blood pH, will distribute more slowly and/or less extensively. The parameter used to measure the extent of tissue distribution of a drug is the volume of distribution (often abbreviated as V). In simple definition, the volume of distribution term is the apparent volume of plasma (or serum) which the administered dose would have to occupy to result in the observed initial concentration in the plasma. If a dose of 1 mg was administered, and the initial concentration in plasma was 1 μg/ml, then the apparent volume of plasma required to account for the dose would be 1 l, i.e. V = 1 l. The importance of the volume term to the assessment of the utility of antifungal drugs is that it reflects how much of the dose is in the tissues and how much is circulating in the blood. A drug which exhibits a very low volume of distribution, for example, 10% of body volume, is likely to be located predominantly in the blood; this may not be appropriate for the treatment of soft tissue infections. Conversely, a high volume of distribution for a drug reflects, by definition, a significant uptake into tissues. This may lead to low circulating concentrations in well-perfused organs, such as the heart, kidneys and lungs, or low concentrations in the interstitial fluids. It is important to realise, however, that because the volume parameter relates the plasma concentration to an *apparent* plasma or blood volume, it rarely has any physiological relevance. Thus, very large volumes of distribution (e.g. 250 l), which apparently exceed the body volume (about 60 l), are possible; they merely indicate that concentrations in the tissues are much higher than those in the blood. Volume of distribution varies markedly with different antifungal agents, reflecting their spectrum of physicochemical characteristics, and has a significant bearing on their relative efficacy.

Volume of distribution is also an important factor in controlling the persistence of a compound in the body, since it determines the concentration of drug in the blood which flows through the organs of elimination. If the volume of distribution of a drug is high and concentrations in the blood are low, it will take longer for all of the dose resident in the body to pass through the metabolising or eliminating organs than if the volume is low and the drug is confined to the vasculature. As explained below, this has a significant impact on the half-life of a drug.

Another major distribution parameter which has a fundamental impact on the efficacy of antifungal drugs is the extent to which the drug is bound to plasma and tissue proteins. The determinants of the extent of drug binding to plasma proteins have not been fully elucidated, although lipophilicity and relative basicity or acidity appear to be involved. Drug bound to protein exists in an equilibrium with unbound drug in both plasma and tissues. The extent of binding to plasma proteins may differ from that for tissue proteins, and total concentrations in plasma and various tissues may, therefore, differ markedly. However, the equilibrium of drug distribution between plasma and tissues, including any infecting fungal organism, relates only to the unbound drug. Consequently, even though total drug concentrations may differ in plasma and in different tissues, the unbound drug concentrations will be the same. It is now well-recognised that it is the unbound fraction of a drug which represents the active antimicrobial form (WISE 1986). Consequently, it can be seen that a major determinant of the effective concentration of an antifungal compound in vivo will be the extent to which it binds to both tissue and plasma proteins, i.e. drugs exhibiting high potency in vitro but which are highly protein bound in vivo may require higher circulating concentrations to achieve comparable in vivo efficacy to compounds with lower potency but with low protein binding (Table 1).

Table 1. Comparison of effect of extent of protein binding on drug efficacy

	Drug A	Drug B
Antifungal potency in vitro	0.1 μg/ml	1.0 μg/ml
Protein binding	99%	10%
Effective concentration in vivo	0.1 μg/ml	1.0 μg/ml
Actual concentration required	10 μg/ml	1.11 μg/ml

It is important to realise therefore that because of differences in protein binding, compounds may exhibit efficacy dose levels which totally belie their relative potencies against the fungal organisms in in vitro tests.

V. Assessment of Duration of Action

The pharmacokinetic parameter most commonly used to describe the duration of exposure to or action of a drug is the plasma elimination half-life, the time for the concentration of the drug in plasma to decrease by half. As mentioned above,the elimination of a drug from the body, whether by metabolism or by renal excretion, is a first-order rate process, i.e. a process whose rate is determined by the concentration of the substance and a rate constant. The half-life of a drug (usually abbreviated to $t_{1/2}$) is a reflection of the rate constant for the eliminating process; indeed, the half-life can be calculated from the term:

$$t_{1/2} = \frac{0.693}{k}$$

where k is the rate constant for the eliminating process and 0.693 is the natural logarithm of 2.

However, the rate constant and its derivative the half-life do not indicate fully the intrinsic ability of the body to clear the drug since, as mentioned above, the concentration presented to the metabolising organ is determined by the volume of distribution. Thus, the elimination half-life of a drug is a hybrid parameter reflecting both the potential rate of metabolism of a compound and the volume into which the drug is distributed.

The parameter which describes the intrinsic ability of the body to clear a drug is the plasma clearance (usually abbreviated to Cl_p). The systemic exposure to two hypothetical drugs, following intravenous administration (when all of the dose is known to be systemically available), is shown in Fig. 2.

It is evident that, since the AUC for drug C is smaller than that for drug A, the body can 'clear' C more effectively than A, whether it be because C is more readily metabolised than A or more readily cleared by the kidneys. The simple measurement of these two AUC values could, therefore, define the relative 'clearances' for the two drugs. However, AUC will also vary with the size of the dose administered. Consequently, comparison of AUC values needs to be corrected for dose. Thus, clearance is defined as:

$$Cl = \frac{\text{Dose (mg)}}{\text{AUC } (\mu\text{g.h/ml})}$$

Weight terms cancel out in the equation, leaving a clearance value expressed in volume per unit time.

Clearance defines the volume of plasma which can be cleared of drug by the metabolising organ or the kidney per unit time. The higher the clearance

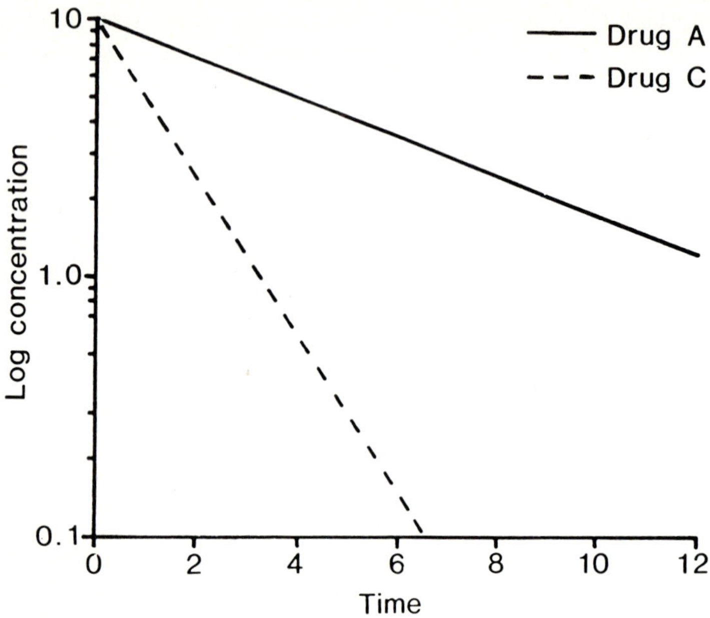

Fig. 2. Comparison of systemic exposure (area under curve) to two hypothetical drugs following intravenous administration at the same dose level. Drug A exhibits lower clearance than drug C

value, the higher the capacity of the clearing organ to eliminate the compound. This could indicate either high renal clearance for a metabolically stable compound, or significant metabolic vunerability for a compound that is not renally cleared. However, as mentioned above, the actual concentration of drug in the plasma cleared by the eliminating organ is determined by the volume of distribution. Consequently, the descriptor of elimination of a compound, the half-life, will depend upon both its volume of distribution and its clearance. As illustrated in Fig. 3, a drug with a high clearance and a small volume of distribution will have a short half-life as the clearing organ will effectively eliminate high concentrations of drug in the plasma. A drug with the same clearance (i.e. same AUC) but a larger volume of distribution (i.e. lower initial concentration) will have a longer half-life as the clearing organ will be exposed to only low concentrations of the drug at any one time.

The significance of these parameters in the development of successful antifungal agents is that a long duration of action for a systemic agent may be obtained either by producing molecules which are metabolically stable, i.e. exhibit low clearance, and which persist because the body cannot clear them effectively, or by producing lipophilic molecules which exhibit large volumes of distribution, which, even if they are metabolically vulnerable, will persist because the fraction of the dose present in the blood stream and exposed to the clearing organ will be low. As described below, both of these approaches

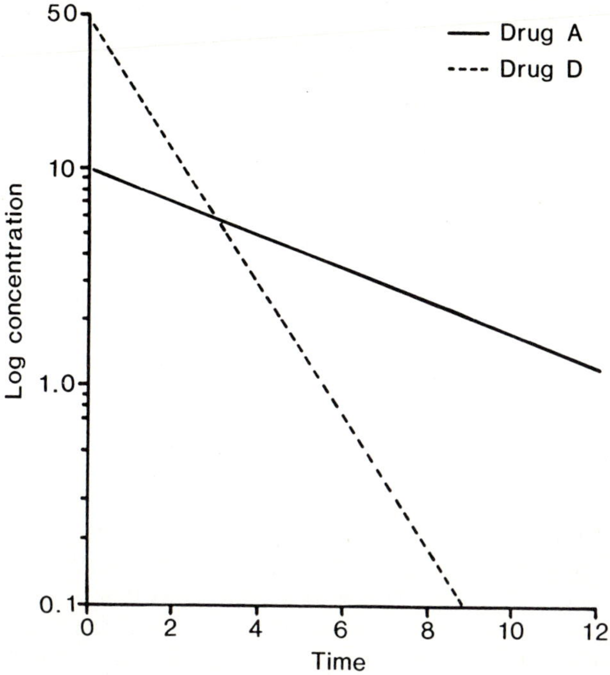

Fig. 3. Relationship between clearance, volume of distribution and half-life for two hypothetical drugs following intravenous administration at the same dose level. AUC values are equal, thus $Cl_A = Cl_D$: $V_A > V_D$. Thus $t_{1\;2}A > t_{1/2}D$

have been followed in the discovery of novel, long-acting, azole antifungal agents.

VI. Summary

Any project which sets out to discover novel, effective agents for the systemic treatment of fungal diseases should evaluate the parameters outlined above both in the animal models used to assess efficacy of their compounds and in human subjects. This is essential if an understanding is to be gained of the relatively complex relationship between in vitro and in vivo models, and if the project wishes to identify the most appropriate compounds for development or to eliminate those which are inappropriate, prior to incurring significant development costs.

C. Pharmacokinetics of Clinically Used Antifungal Agents

There are several comprehensive reviews on the pharmacokinetics of clinically used antifungal agents, including those by DANESHMEND and

WARNOCK (1983), GRAYBILL and CRAVEN (1983) and POLAK (1979). In addition several publications outline the pharmacokinetic profiles of individual agents. Thus the pharmacokinetic profiles of miconazole (BRUGMANS et al. 1972; HEEL et al. 1980), econazole (HEEL et al. 1978), clotrimazole (DUHM et al. 1974; SAWYER et al. 1975), ketoconazole (BRASS et al. 1982; DANESHMEND et al. 1981; GASCOIGNE et al. 1981; HEEL et al. 1982; HUANG et al. 1986; SYMOENS and CAUWENBERGH 1983) and fluconazole (BRAMMER and TARBIT 1987; HUMPHREY et al. 1985) in both laboratory animals and human subjects have been determined following their clinical introduction. This section will highlight aspects of the pharmacokinetic profiles of these agents which have a significant impact on their utility as antifungal agents.

I. Non-Azoles

1. Amphotericin B

Amphotericin B has been used to treat systemic fungal disease via the intravenous route for a number of years due to its relative efficacy, broad spectrum of activity and absence of suitable alternative therapy for intravenous administration. The drug is a polyene macrolide antibiotic of high molecular weight and poor solubility; consequently, it is very poorly absorbed following oral administration (CRAVEN et al. 1979). As such, therefore, its systemic use is confined to the hospitalised patient with serious systemic fungal disease. This is fortuitous, since the drug has a significant toxicity potential which, coupled with its poor and variable absorption, leads to a requirement for monitoring during use (BENNETT et al. 1979).

Protein binding of the drug is high, exceeding 90% in serum (BLOCK et al. 1974; BINDSCHADLER and BENNETT 1969), and this has a significant impact on its clinical utility. Diffusion of the drug into tissues is slow; the initial volume of distribution of the drug is low, and the drug is confined predominantly to the blood. Eventually, the drug occupies a volume of distribution of about 2 l/kg (ATKINSON and BENNETT 1978), indicating penetration into the tissues. Amphotericin B does not penetrate into the CNS effectively, probably due to a combination of its high protein binding and high molecular weight. Passage into bronchial secretions (PENNINGTON et al. 1974) and peritoneal, pleural and synovial fluids (POLAK 1979) is also very poor. The high protein binding of the drug also mitigates against renal filtration; consequently, concentrations of the drug in urine are low (ATKINSON and BENNETT 1978). Thus, the distribution parameters of amphotericin B are not favourable for the rapid treatment of soft tissue infections but do favour the treatment of infections in well-perfused organs such as the heart and lungs.

Amphotericin B has one advantageous pharmacokinetic feature relative to therapeutic effect in that it exhibits very low systemic clearance, reflecting a high degree of metabolic stability; the drug persists in the body for several days. Its initial half-life of elimination in humans is long, ranging between 24 and 48 h (ATKINSON and BENNETT 1978); however, there is evidence of a residual elimination phase which exhibits a half-life of about 15 days (ATKINSON and BENNETT 1978).

For the reasons outlined above, the pharmacokinetic profile of amphotericin B could be considered wholly inappropriate for a modern antifungal agent targeted at the systemic treatment of systemic and topical infections. Its continued use reflects the lack of alternative intravenous therapy emerging with the discovery of the first generation imidazole agents and may thus be affected by novel compounds in the current generation of triazole compounds, such as fluconazole, which exhibit high oral bioavailability and which can also be given intravenously (RICHARDSON et al. 1985).

2. 5-Fluorocytosine

5-Fluorocytosine (5-FC) is a relatively polar fluorinated pyrimidine which is used for the oral treatment of systemic infections by specific fungal species, reflecting its narrow spectrum of activity. The drug is well absorbed from the intestine and exhibits high oral bioavailability in normal human subjects (80%; SCHÖNEBECK et al. 1973). In addition, the binding of the drug to plasma proteins is very low, being about 4% over a concentration range of 2–55 μg/ml (BLOCK et al. 1974). In keeping with its polarity, the volume of distribution of the drug is moderate, 0.6–0.9 l/kg (WADE and SUDLOW 1972; DAWBORN et al. 1973; SCHÖNEBECK et al. 1973), approximating to the volume occupied by total body water. This volume suggests that the drug is evenly distributed throughout the tissues of the body.

The combination of low protein binding and polarity results in 5-FC penetrating effectively into the CNS and reaching high concentrations in body tissues and secretions. The relative polarity of the molecule renders it metabolically stable, since the metabolising enzymes are contained in lipophilic membranes; combined with the lack of protein binding of the molecule, this promotes its elimination by renal excretion. As a consequence, the drug is almost wholly cleared by renal excretion and has a plasma half-life of about 5 h (DAWBORN et al. 1973). In addition to its use for disseminated systemic mycoses, 5-FC represents a suitable agent to treat urinary tract infections.

In most respects the pharmacokinetic profile of 5-FC is ideal for an antimicrobial agent. The combination of good oral bioavailability, low protein binding, widespread distribution and metabolic stability is highly appropriate for the successful treatment of both topical and systemic infections. Unfortunately, it also exhibits a narrow spectrum of antifungal activity, is associated with a significant incidence of side effects and induces resistance in susceptible organisms. Its use has to be carefully monitored, and it is often confined to administration in combination with other agents in hospitalised patients.

II. First Generation Imidazole Drugs

The clinical problems associated with the use of both amphotericin B and 5-FC led to several significant efforts to identify agents which exhibit a broad spectrum antifungal activity but lower toxicity. The initial products of this research were the imidazole agents, clotrimazole (Büchel et al. 1972) and miconazole (Van Cutsem and Thienpont 1972), which were introduced in the early 1970s for the oral treatment of systemic mycoses. Two further close analogues of miconazole, tioconazole (Jevons et al. 1979) and econazole (Thienpont et al. 1975), were also initially in development for systemic treatment but were eventually confined to the topical treatment of superficial infections.

These imidazole agents failed to achieve wide usage in systemic treatment of fungal disease for several reasons, including auto-induction of metabolism and inappropriate side-effect profiles. However, in all cases the problems were complicated by pharmacokinetic properties which were not conducive to good antimicrobial therapy. Thus, the oral systemic bioavailability of clotrimazole (Menz et al. 1973; Ritter et al. 1982; Ritter 1985), miconazole (Brugmans et al. 1972; Boelaert et al. 1976), econazole (Midgley et al. 1981) and tioconazole (Marriott et al. 1983; Tarbit, unpublished data) is low and variable in both the laboratory animals used in efficacy and safety testing and in humans. This low bioavailability is probably predominantly due to extensive first-pass metabolism, since all of the compounds are lipophilic and exhibit high metabolic clearance. There is evidence from studies using radio-labelled drug to support the existence of a significant degree of first-pass metabolism in humans for econazole (Midgley et al. 1981), clotrimazole (Ritter 1985), miconazole (Brugmans et al. 1972) and tioconazole (Marriott et al. 1983; Tarbit, unpublished data). Incomplete absorption may also be important with miconazole (Brugmans et al. 1972) and clotrimazole (Seo et al. 1977) since significant amounts of unchanged drug are excreted in the faeces following oral administration, although these findings should be interpreted with caution, since there is evidence with tioconazole (McCrae et al., in prep.; Marriott et al. 1983), croconazole (Nakano et al. 1989) and econazole (Midgley et al. 1981) that labile conjugates of the parent drugs are formed in vivo and may be excreted in the bile. Breakdown of these conjugates in the gastrointestinal tract would produce unchanged drug in the faeces. In keeping with many drugs exhibiting significant first-pass metabolism (George and Shand 1982; Wilkinson and Shand 1975), clotrimazole (Seo et al 1977) and miconazole (Boelaert et al. 1976) have been shown to exhibit non-linear increases in exposure with increased dose levels.

The low systemic availability of the agents is compounded by large volumes of distribution, typified by that of 20 l/kg for miconazole (Heel et al. 1980), indicating that most of the dose is bound in the tissues, thus resulting in very low circulating concentrations in the plasma. Plasma protein binding is also uniformly high with these imidazoles, exceeding, for instance, 90% for miconazole (Stevens et al. 1976), 97% for econazole (Midgley et al. 1981) and 99% for tioconazole (Tarbit, unpublished data); circulating concentrations of the unbound, pharmacologically active form, are exceedingly low. This results in very low concentrations in plasma-derived fluids such as urine and secretions such as saliva, sweat, vaginal and intestinal secretions, which are often important in treating topical infections by systemic administration. In addition, since CSF levels are often in equilibrium with unbound drug concentrations in the plasma, penetration across the blood-brain barrier can be low.

A further complication associated with the use of these imidazoles is their propensity to induce metabolising enzymes, thus resulting in increased clearance and decreased systemic exposure with chronic use. Recent studies (HOSTETLER et al. 1989; RITTER and FRANKLIN 1987; RODGRIGUES et al. 1988) have shown that all of the first generation imidazole drugs are potent enzyme inducers in laboratory animals (see Chap. 8).

The only imidazole which has survived for systemic treatment of fungal infections is miconazole. This is due to the availability of an intravenous formulation, although the vehicle itself (cremophor EL) has an associated toxicity which limits its use to life-threatening mycoses.

III. Ketoconazole

The residual utility of first generation imidazole compounds for oral treatment of systemic infections was effectively removed by the introduction of ketoconazole as an oral drug in the treatment of systemic and superficial mycoses in the late 1970s. Ketoconazole exhibited a similar broad spectrum of activity against fungal organisms to that of miconazole and clotrimazole but appeared to be less potent in vitro (ODDS 1980). This apparent disadvantage, however, was overturned in vivo, where much higher blood levels of ketoconazole were evident following oral administration than for the first generation imidazoles.

The absorption of ketoconazole, although described as 'good' in several reviews (HEEL et al. 1982; DANESHMEND and WARNOCK 1988; SYMOENS and CAUWENBERGH 1983), appears to be variable in both animals and humans. Studies examining the disposition of radiolabelled ketoconazole in the rat (REMMEL et al. 1987) indicate that the compound is essentially completely absorbed from the gastrointestinal tract in this species. However, studies in the dog by BAXTER et al. (1986) and GASCOIGNE et al. (1981) show variations in the extent of excretion of what is presumably unabsorbed ketoconazole in the faeces. Absorption of the compound also appears variable in humans, with faecal levels of unabsorbed drug ranging from 25% to 65% of the dose in three fasted volunteers (GASCOIGNE et al. 1981).

The extent of absorption of a drug is affected by its solubility in the gastrointestinal tract, and since ketoconazole is a weak base (pKa 6.5; GASCOIGNE et al. 1981) which is only slightly soluble at intestinal pH, variations in gastric acidity are likely to have a marked impact on its solubility and hence its absorption. There is clear evidence that this is so in humans from the studies reported by VAN DER MEER et al. (1980).

The absolute bioavailability of ketoconazole in humans has not been reported since in the absence of a suitable formulation a reference intravenous dose cannot be administered. However, studies in the rat (REMMEL et al. 1987) and the dog (BAXTER et al. 1986) indicate that the absolute bioavailability in these species ranges between 30% and 50% at dose levels of 5 mg/kg and 22 mg/kg, respectively. Studies carried out in the dog at higher dose levels (TARBIT, unpublished data) indicate that bioavailability is non-linear in this species and ranges up to an apparent value of 100% with increasing dose. Studies carried out in the mouse with a range of oral dose levels (BORELLI et al. 1979) support this dose dependency, showing marked non-linearity in serum levels with increasing dose level. These findings reflect evidence emerging from several studies, including those of GASCOIGNE et al. (1981) and REMMEL et al. (1987) which indicate that ketoconazole undergoes first-pass metabolism in some animal species. The variations in bioavailability are thus likely to be due to significant dose-dependent saturation of metabolism. There is also some evidence in animal studies (REMMEL et al. 1987; TARBIT, unpublished data) that systemic clearance of the compound may be markedly altered after oral administration relative to that after IV administration, leading to apparent changes in bioavailability. This phenomenon is consistent with the well-defined inhibitory effects of these azole compounds on the hepatic cytochromes P-450 which are responsible for first-pass metabolism of the compound and which have been observed to lead to anomalous bioavailability calculations, often apparently exceeding 100%, for a number of experimental imidazole and triazole compounds, including ketoconazole (TARBIT, unpublished observations).

Recently, evidence has emerged to indicate that the non-linearities observed in animals at higher dose levels of ketoconzole are also evident in humans at therapeutic levels. Non-linear increases in systemic exposure with doses ranging between 100 and 800 mg have been reported by DANESHMEND et al. (1981, 1984), GASCOIGNE et al. (1981) and HUANG et al. (1986). In addition, the observed half-life of ketoconazole appears to increase with increasing dose (DANESHMEND et al. 1984), suggesting altered clearance of the drug at higher dose levels.

Notwithstanding the variations and non-linearities in absorption and systemic bioavailability, ketoconazole exhibits markedly higher plasma levels on a dose-normalised basis than either miconazole or clotrimazole. This is predominantly due to the relatively low volume of distribution of the drug, which is reported to be about 0.7 l/kg in both the rat (REMMEL et al. 1987) and the dog (BAXTER et al. 1986). A relatively modest dose of 200 mg of ketoconazole in humans results in peak circulating concentrations of about 2–3 μg/ml (DANESHMEND and WARNOCK 1988) compared with peak concentrations of about 1 μg/ml following 1 g doses of miconazole. The impact that relative bioavailability and volume of distribution have on the therapeutic use of such agents is evident in these comparative data.

In common with the other imidazole drugs, the protein binding of ketoconazole is high, exceeding 99% with human proteins (SYMOENS and CAUWENBERGH 1983); consequently, the drug also exhibits some of the problems associated with other imidazoles in treating topical infections. Although penetration into vaginal and skin secretions is satisfactory enough to achieve successful treatment of topical infections at these sites, possibly due to ionic trapping of the basic compound in the relatively acidic environments, the drug does not effectively cross the blood-brain barrier (BRASS et al. 1982; GASCOIGNE et al. 1981), and treatment of CNS infections is not very successful (CRAVEN et al. 1983). In addition, concentrations of the drug in saliva and milk are low and in keeping with the unbound concentrations in plasma (HEEL et al. 1982).

Again, in common with first generation imidazoles, the systemic clearance of ketoconazole is almost wholly metabolic. Excretion of unchanged drug in the urine accounts for less than 5% of the dose (HEEL et al. 1982). Systemic clearance of ketoconazole is low in the dog, being equivalent to about one-tenth of liver blood flow (BAXTER et al. 1986; HEYKANTS et al. 1987), and moderate in the rat, about one-quarter of liver blood flow (REMMEL et al. 1987), indicating that it is reasonably metabolically stable in these species. In the absence of an intravenous formulation, systemic clearance in humans cannot be determined. However, given that routes of metabolism appear similar in animals and humans (GASCOIGNE et al. 1981), it is reasonable to assume that the compound is relatively metabolically stable in humans. In this respect, ketoconazole represents an improvement over the first generation imidazoles which, typified by miconazole, exhibit systemic clearance greater than 50% of liver blood flow (calculated from LEWI et al. 1976).

Unlike the first generation imidazoles, the pharmacokinetic profile of ketoconazole has not presented major difficulties to its therapeutic use, although it is evident from the preceding paragraphs that the pharmacokinetic characteristics are not wholly ideal for an antimicrobial agent.

IV. Novel Triazole Agents

Two major new triazole antifungal drugs, fluconazole (RICHARDSON et al. 1985) and itraconazole (VAN CUTSEM et al. 1987a), were introduced for the systemic treatment of superficial and systemic fungal disease in the early 1980s. It is evident that the development of both drugs included an awareness of the need to achieve appropriate pharmacokinetic profiles (HEYKANTS et al. 1987; RICHARDSON et al. 1988). However, the end result of this research is drugs which differ markedly in particular aspects of their kinetic profile. Thus, fluconazole, a weakly basic bistriazole with comparatively high water solubility for this class of drug, can be administered both intravenously and orally to patients. In contrast, itraconazole, a triazole derivative of ketoconazole, is more lipophilic and less water soluble than ketoconazole and is not ideal for intravenous formulation. It is the marked difference in polarity of these two agents which has such a significant impact on their respective pharmacokinetic profiles.

The absorption of itraconazole appears to be variable and dependent upon formulation and fasted state in both animals and humans (HEYKANTS et al. 1987). Absolute bioavailability of itraconazole in the dog is 50% from an oral solution and 20% from capsules containing polyethylene glycol. The intake of food in human volunteers increases the absorption of the drug, presumably due to enhanced dissolution in the acidic stomach.

Following absorption, there is no clear evidence that itraconazole undergoes significant first-pass metabolism. Consideration of systemic clearance data after intravenous administration to the dog indicates that the drug is relatively metabolically stable. Consequently, significant first-pass metabolism would not be expected following an oral dose. Neverthelsss, the drug exhibits significant non-linearity in systemic exposure in relation to dose in human volunteers (HEYKANTS et al. 1987), indicating that the characteristic of these inhibitory agents (see above) to saturate the metabolising enzymes may be present.

In contrast to itraconazole, the absorption and systemic bioavailability of fluconazole appears essentially complete in animals and humans (HUMPHERY et al. 1985) and is unaffected by food intake or whether given as solution or capsule (BRAMMER and TARBIT 1987). In addition, the relationship between dose and systemic exposure to fluconazole is remarkably linear over a tenfold range in dose level (BRAMMER and TARBIT 1987). This linearity undoubtedly reflects the polarity of fluconazole and its relative lack of interaction with the metabolising enzymes which are essentially located in lipophilic membranes.

The distribution of the two triazole drugs is also markedly different. Itraconzole exhibits very high protein binding (99.8%) in human plasma (HEYKANTS et al. 1987). Consequently, its concentrations in body fluids which are in equilibrium with the unbound drug in plasma are very low. Total concentrations of bound and unbound drug in tissues are significantly higher than plasma concentrations, reflecting the strong binding of the drug to tissue proteins. It is possible that these tissue levels can act as a reservoir for the unbound, active form of the drug. Itraconazole, in common with the highly protein-bound imidazoles, does not effectively cross the blood-brain barrier into the CNS and appears in low concentrations in body fluids, including saliva and urine. This distribution pattern is reflected in a very large calculated volume of distribution (17 l/kg in the dog, HEYKANTS et al. 1987) compared with that for ketoconazole. The large volume has the advantage of contributing to a long plasma half-life for the drug, since it keeps the drug out of the blood circulating through the metabolising organs.

Fluconazole exhibits very low protein binding, about 11% in human plasma (HUMPHREY et al. 1985). This has a fundamental impact on its potential efficacy in several systemic and superficial infections. The drug penetrates freely across the blood-brain barrier, and concentrations in the cerebrospinal fluid are up to 64% of the corresponding plasma concentrations in healthy subjects and up to 94% in patients with meningeal disease

(BRAMMER and TARBIT 1987). Fluconazole is also freely secreted in saliva and alimentary fluids and has been shown to eradicate gut *Candida* following intravenous administration (TROKE, unpublished data). In addition, the drug is extensively filtered in the kidney and very high concentrations are found in urine, indicating a potential utility in urinary tract infections. Indeed, the drug has been introduced for the single-dose systemic treatment of vaginal candidosis (HENDERSON 1987).

In keeping with the polarity of fluconazole and its low protein binding, the drug occupies a volume of distribution equating to total body water. In some respects this is an ideal distribution for an antimicrobial agent, since it indicates an even distribution of active, unbound drug throughout the body.

The systemic clearance of both fluconazole and itraconazole is significantly lower in both animals and humans than that for ketoconazole. In this respect they represent a major advance in therapy, since both have plasma half-lives which exceed 24 h. Both can be considered as once daily therapy for the chronic treatment of fungal disease. One potentially adverse result of their long half-lives is that the time to achieve steady-state concentrations during chronic therapy will be prolonged. With a half-life of about 20 h for itraconazole (HEYKANT et al. 1987) and about 30 h for fluconazole (BRAMMER and TARBIT 1987), they will take up to a week to achieve a steady state level.

Both fluconazole and itraconazole appear to be effective treatments for a variety of fungal diseases (CAUWENBERGH and DE DONCKER 1987; HENDERSON 1987), and it is interesting to speculate that this may be for different reasons in relation to their kinetic profiles. Itraconazole appears to be a more potent antifungal agent than either fluconazole or ketoconazolein in vitro tests (MARRIOTT and RICHARDSON 1987; VAN CUTSEM et al. 1987b) and works in vivo predominantly because of this potency advantage and despite inappropriate pharmacokinetic characteristics of very high protein binding, low concentration in plasma and body fluids and relatively low systemic availability. In contrast, the apparent low potency of fluconazole in vitro is overturned in vivo by complete bioavailability, high plasma concentrations, low protein binding and even distribution throughout body fluids. As mentioned above, a comparison of the relative in vitro potencies of itraconazole and fluconazole and their repective in vivo efficacies, without an awareness of the impact of pharmacokinetics, would have offered little basis for understanding their antifungal activities. Recently, attempts to rationalise the systemic exposure to unbound drug concentrations for a number of agents, including fluconazole (TROKE et al. 1988), in animal models indicate that in vitro tests of antifungal agents, often discounted for the azole drugs (POLAK and DIXON 1987; Chap. 4), may be meaningful indicators of in vivo efficacy when due account is taken of the impact of their pharmacokinetic characteristics in vivo.

D. Conclusions

The preceding sections give ample illustration of the impact that the pharmacokinetics of an antifungal drug can have on its therapeutic use. What then would constitute the ideal pharmacokinetic profile for a novel agent? Undoubtedly one major target should be high oral bioavailability, if for no other reason than to avoid the necessity of having to manufacture and administer a large dose of a drug to ensure that a small proportion is absorbed into the system. More importantly, variability in blood levels is significantly decreased in drugs which are highly bioavailable, leading to a decreased requirement for therapeutic monitoring. Drugs which exhibit long half-lives, whether by enhanced metabolic stability or by large volumes of distribution, may also present a therapeutic advantage, since single-dose systemic therapy for both systemic and topical infections becomes a real possibility. In addition, once daily administration can also aid compliance in outpatient therapy. The ideal distribution parameters for an agent are more difficult to define since, as outlined above, these can represent a titration between relative potency and degree of tissue or protein binding. In addition, the ideal distribution of a drug will also reflect the particular sites of infection to be treated. In many respects a drug which is distributed into total body water (about 0.65 l/kg) can be considered as ideal as it indicates an even distribution throughout the body. Low protein binding is also undoubtedly advantageous for any agent required to treat both systemic infections and infections in topical sites bathed in secretions derived from plasma, since most of the drug in the body will be in the unbound or active form.

However, the ideal pharmacokinetic properties for an antifungal agent must also reflect an appropriate balance between the physicochemical characteristics required for efficacy – such as increased lipophilicity, since many antifungal target sites are in membranes – and those required to enhance metabolic stability and low protein binding, etc. – usually increased polarity. The modern means of bringing these two opposites into balance is to conduct pharmacokinetic studies in parallel with efficacy tests, so that the structure-activity relationships appropriate to the correct balance can be derived. As RICHARDSON et al. (1988) demonstrated, this can lead to a novel and exciting drug in a relatively short space of time.

References

Atkinson AJ, Bennett JE (1978) Amphotericin B pharmacokinetics in humans. Antimicrob Agents Chemother 13:271–276

Baxter JG, Brass C, Schentag JJ, Slaughter RL (1986) Pharmacokinetics of ketoconazole administered intravenously to dogs and orally as tablets and solution to humans and dogs. J Pharm Sci 75:443–447

Bennett JE, Dismukes WE, Duma RJ, Medoff G, Sande MA, Gallis H, Leonard J, Fields BT, Bradshaw M, Haywood H, McGee ZA, Cate TR, Cobbs CG, Warner JF, Alling DW (1979) A comparison of amphotericin B alone and combined

with flucytosine in the treatment of cryptococcal meningitis. N Engl J Med 301: 126–131
Bindschadler DD, Bennett JE (1969) A pharmacologic guide to the clinical use of amphotericin B. J Infect Dis 120:427–436
Block ER, Bennett JE, Livoti LG, Klein WJ, MacGregor RR, Henderson L (1974) Flucytosine and amphotericin B: haemodialysis effects on the plasma concentration and clearance. Ann Int Med 80:613–617
Boelaert J, Daneels R, Van Lunduyt H, Symoens J (1976) Miconazole plasma levels in healthy subjects and in patients with impaired renal function. In: Williams JD, Geddes AM (eds) Chemotherapy, Proc 9th Int Cong Chemother, London, vol 6. Plenum, New York, pp 165–169
Borelli D, Bran JL, Fuentes J, Legendre R, Leiderman E, Levine HB, Restrepo MA, Stevens DA (1979) Ketoconazole, an oral antifungal: laboratory and clinical assessment of imidazole drugs. Postgrad Med J 55:657–661
Brammer KW, Tarbit MH (1987) A review of the pharmacokinetics of fluconazole (UK-49,858) in laboratory animals and man. In: Fromtling RA (ed) Recent trends in the discovery, development and evaluation of antifungal agents. JR Prous, Barcelona, pp 141–149
Brass C, Galgiani JN, Blaschke TF, Defelice R, O'Reilly RA, Stevens DA (1982) Disposition of ketoconazole, an oral antifungal, in humans. Antimicrob Agents Chemother 21:151–158
Brugmans J, Van Cutsem J, Heykants J, Schuermans V, Thienpont D (1972) Systemic antifungal potential, safety, biotransport and transformation of miconazole nitrate. Eur J Clin Pharmacol 5:93–99
Büchel KH, Draber W, Regel E, Plempel M (1972) Synthesen und Eigenschaften von Clotrimazol und weiteren antimykotischen 1-Triphenylmethylimidazolen. Arzneimittelforsch 22:1260–1272
Cauwenbergh G, De Doncker P (1987) The clinical use of itraconazole in superficial and deep mycoses. In: Fromtling RA (ed) Recent trends in the discovery, development and evaluation of antifungal agents. JR Prous, Barcelona, pp 273–284
Craven PC, Ludden TM, Drutz DJ, Rogers W, Haegele KA, Skrdlant HB (1979) Excretion pathways of amphotericin B. J Infect Dis 140:329–341
Craven PC, Graybill JR, Jorgensen JH, Dismukes WE, Levine BE (1983) High-dose ketoconazole for treatment of fungal infections of the central nervous system. Ann Int Med 98:160–167
Daneshmend TK, Warnock DW (1983) Clinical pharmacokinetics of systemic antifungal drugs. Clin Pharmacokinet 8:17–42
Daneshmend TK, Warnock DW (1988) Clinical pharmacokinetics of ketoconazole. Clin Pharmacokinet 14:13–34
Daneshmend TK, Warnock DW, Turner A, Roberts CJC (1981) Pharmacokinetics of ketoconazole in normal subjects. J Antimicrob Chemother 8:299–304
Daneshmend TK, Warnock DW, Ene MD, Johnson EM, Potten MR, Richardson MD, Williamson PJ (1984) Influence of food on the pharmacokinetics of ketoconazole. Antimicrob Agents Chemother 25:1–3
Dawborn JK, Page MD, Schiavone DJ (1973) Use of 5-fluorocytosine in patients with impaired renal function. Br Med J 4:382–384
Duhm B, Maul W, Medenwald H, Patzschke K, Puetter J, Wegner LA (1974) The pharmacokinetics of clotrimazole ^{14}C. Postgrad Med J (July Suppl):13–16
Gascoigne EW, Barton GJ, Michaels M, Meuldermans W, Heykants J (1981) The kinetics of ketoconazole in animals and man. Clin Res Rev 1:177–187
George CF, Shand DG (1982) Presystemic drug metabolism in the liver. In: George CF, Shand DG, Renwick AG (eds) Clinical pharmacology and therapeutics. 1. Presystemic drug elimination. Butterworth, London, pp 69–77
Gibaldi M, Perrier D (1982) Pharmacokinetics, 2nd edn. Marcel Dekker, New York
Graybill JR, Craven PC (1983) Antifungal agents used in systemic mycoses: activity and therapeutic use. Drugs 25:41–62

Heel RC, Brogden RN, Speight TM, Avery GS (1978) Econazole: a review of its antifungal activity and therapeutic efficacy. Drugs 16:177–201
Heel RC, Brogden RN, Pakes GN, Speight TM, Avery GS (1980) Miconazole: a preliminary review of its therapeutic efficacy in systemic fungal infections. Drugs 19:7–30
Heel RC, Brogden RN, Carmine A, Morley PA, Speight TM, Avery GS (1982) Ketoconazole: a review of its therapeutic efficacy in superficial and systemic fungal infections. Drugs 23:1–36
Henderson JT (1987) Fluconazole – a significant advance in the management of human fungal disease. In: Fromtling RA (ed) Recent trends in the discovery, development and evaluation of antifungal agents. JR Prous, Barcelona, pp 77–79
Heykants J, Michiels M, Meuldermans W, Monbaliu J, Lavrijsen K, Van Peer A, Levron JC, Woestenborghs R, Cauwenbergh G (1987) The pharmacokinetics of itraconazole in animals and man: an overview. In: Fromtling RA (ed) Recent trends in the discovery, development and evaluation of antifungal agents. JR Prous, Barcelona, pp 223–249
Hostetler KA, Wrighton SA, Molowa DT, Thomas PE, Levin W, Guzelian PS (1989) Coinduction of multiple hepatic cytochrome P-450 proteins and their mRNAs in rats treated with imidazole antimycotic agents. Mol Pharmacol 35:279–285
Huang Y-C, Colaizzi JL, Bierman RH, Woestenborghs R, Heykants J (1986) Pharmacokinetics and dose proportionality of ketoconazole in normal volunteers. Antimicrob Agents Chemother 30:206–210
Humphrey MJ, Jevons S, Tarbit MH (1985) Pharmacokinetic evaluation of UK-49,858, a metabolically stable triazole antigungal drug, in animals and humans. Antimicrob Agents Chemother 28:648–653
Jevons S, Gymer GE, Brammer KW, Cox DA, Leeming MRG (1979) Antifungal activity of tioconazole (UK-20,349), a new imidazole derivative. Antimicrob Agents Chemother 15:597–602
Lewi PJ, Boelaert J, Daneels R, De Meyere R, Van Landuyt H, Heykants JJP, Symoens J, Wynants J (1976) Pharmacokinetic profile of intravenous miconazole in man: comparison of normal subjects and patients with renal insufficiency. Eur J Clin Pharmacol 10:49–54
Marriott MS, Richardson K (1987) The discovery and mode of action of fluconazole. In: Fromtling RA (ed) Recent trends in the discovery, development and evaluation of antifungal agents. JR Prous, Barcelona, pp 81–92
Marriott MS, Baird JRC, Brammer KW, Faccini J, Faulkner JK, Halliwell G, Jevons S, Monro AM, Nachbaur J, Perraud J, Tarbit MH (1983) Tioconazole, a new broad-spectrum antifungal agent: preclinical studies related to vaginal candidiasis. Gynak Rdsch 23 [Suppl 1]:1–11
Menz HP, Teltscher U, Bayer C, Oldershausen HF (1973) Zur Pharmakokinetik des oralen Antimykotikums Clotrimazole beim Menschen. Dtsch Med Wochenschr 98:1606–1609
Midgley I, Biggs SR, Hawkins DR, Chasseaud LF, Darragh A, Brodie RR, Walmsley LM (1981) The metabolic fate of [^{3}H]econazole in man. Xenobiotica 11:595–608
Nakano M, Nakajima Y, Iwatani K, Ikenishi Y, Nakagawa Y, Sugeno K (1989) Metabolism of the antimycotic agent, croconazole, in rabbits. Drug Metab Dispos 17:323–329
Odds FC (1980) Laboratory evaluation of antifungal agents: a comparative study of five imidazole derivatives of clinical importance. J Antimicrob Chemother 6:749–761
Odds FC (1986) A survey of old and new antifungal tests in vitro. In: Iwata K, Vanden Bossche H (eds) In vitro and in vivo evaluation of antifungal agents. Elsevier, Amsterdam, pp 13–19
Pennington JE, Block ER, Reynolds HY (1974) 5-Fluorocytosine and amphotericin B in bronchial secretions. Antimicrob Agents Chemother 6:324–326
Polak A (1979) Pharmacokinetics of amphotericin B and flucytosine. Postgrad Med J 55:667–670

Polak A, Dixon DM (1987) In vitro/in vivo correlation of antifungal susceptibility testing using 5-fluorocytosine and ketoconazole as examples of two extremes. In: Fromtling RA (ed) Recent trends in the discovery, development and evaluation of antifungal agents. JR Prous, Barcelona, pp 45–59

Remmel RP, Amoh K, Abdel-Monem MM (1987) The disposition and pharmacokinetics of ketoconazole in the rat. Drug Metab Dispos 15:735–739

Richardson K, Brammer KW, Marriott MS, Troke PF (1985) Activity of UK-49,858, a bis-triazole derivative, against experimental infections with *Candida albicans* and *Trichophyton mentagrophytes*. Antimicrob Agents Chemother 27:832–835

Richardson K, Andrews RJ, Marriott MS, Tarbit MH, Troke PF (1986) Correlation of in vitro and in vivo activity of azole antifungals. In: Iwata K, Vanden Bossche H (eds) In vitro and in vivo evaluation of antifungal agents. Elsevier, Amsterdam, pp 147–149

Richardson K, Cooper K, Marriott MS, Tarbit MH, Troke PF, Whittle PJ (1988) Design and evaluation of a systemically active agent, fluconazole. Ann NY Acad Sci 544:4–11

Ritter W (1985) Pharmacokinetic fundamentals of vaginal treatment with clotrimazole. Am J Obstet Gynecol 152:945–947

Ritter JK, Franklin MR (1987) Induction and inhibition of rat hepatic drug metabolism by N-substituted imidazole drugs. Drug Metab Dispos 15:335–343

Ritter W, Patzschke K, Krause U, Stettendorf S (1982) Pharmacokinetic fundamentals of vaginal treatment with clotrimazole. Chemotherapy 28 [Suppl]:37–42

Rodrigues AD, Wadell PR, Ah-Sing E, Morris BA, Wolf CR, Ioannides C (1988) Induction of the rat hepatic microsomal mixed-function oxidases by 3 imidazole-containing antifungal agents: selectivity for the cytochrome P-450IIB and P-450III families of cytochromes P-450. Toxicology 50:283–301

Rolinson GN (1980) The significance of protein binding of antibiotics in antibacterial chemotherapy. J Antimicrob Chemother 6:311–317

Rowland M, Tozer TN (1988) Clinical pharmacokinetics: concepts and applications. Lea and Febiger, Philadelphia

Sawyer PR, Brogden RN, Pinder RM, Speight TM, Avery GS (1975) Clotrimazole: a review of its antifungal activity and therapeutic efficacy. Drugs 9:424–447

Schönebeck J, Polak A, Fernex M, Scholer HJ (1973) Pharmacokinetic studies on the oral antimycotic agent 5-flurocytosine in individuals with normal and impaired kidney function. Chemotherapy 18:321–336

Seo, M, Iida H, Miura Y (1977) Basic experiments with clotrimazole administered orally. Curr Med Res Opinion 5:169–178

Stevens DA, Levine HB, Deresinski SC (1976) Miconazole in coccidioidomycosis. II. Therapeutic and pharmacologic studies in man. Am J Med 60:191–202

Symoens J, Cauwenbergh G (1983) Ketoconzole, a new step in the management of fungal disease. Prog Drug Res 27:63–84

Thienpont D, Van Cutsem J, Van Nueten JM, Niemegeers CJE, Marsboom R (1975) Biological and toxicological properties of econazole, a broad-spetrum antimycotic. Arzneimittelforsch 25:224–230

Troke PF (1987) Efficacy of fluconazole in animal models of superficial and opportunistic systemic fungal infection. In: Fromtling RA (ed) Recent trends in the discovery, development and evaluation of antifungal agents. JR Prous, Barcelona, pp 103–112

Troke PF, Marriott MS, Richardson K, Tarbit MH (1988) In vitro potency and in vivo activity of azoles. Ann NY Acad Sci 544:284–293

Van Cutsem JM, Thienpont D (1972) Miconazole, a broad-spectrum antimycotic agent with antibacterial activity. Chemotherapy 17:392–404

Van Cutsem J, Van Gerven F, Janssen PAJ (1987a) Activity of orally, topically, and parenterally administered itraconazole in the treatment of superficial and deep mycoses: animal models. Rev Infect Dis 9:S15–S32

Van Cutsem J, Van Gerven F, Janssen PAJ (1987b) The in vitro and in vivo antifungal activity of itraconazole. In: Fromtling RA (ed) Recent trends in the discovery, development and evaluation of antifungal agents. JR Prous, Barcelona, pp 177–192

Van Der Meer JWM, Keuning JJ, Scheijgrond HW, Heykants J, Van Cutsem J, Brugmans J (1980) The influence of gastric acidity on the bio-availability of ketoconazole. J Antimicrob Chemother 6:552–554

Wade DN, Sudlow G (1972) The kinetics of 5-fluorocytosine elimination in man. Aust NZ J Med 2:153–158

Wilkinson GR, Shand DG (1975) Commentary: a physiological approach to hepatic drug clearance. Clin Pharmacol Ther 18:377–390

Wise R (1986) The clinical relevance of protein binding and tissue concentrations in antimicrobial therapy. Clin Pharmacokinet 11:470–482

CHAPTER 8

Hepatic and Endocrine Effects of Azole Antifungal Agents

MICHAEL H. TARBIT, WILLIAM R. ROBERTSON, and ANN LAMBERT

A. Introduction

The group of drugs known collectively as the azoles, comprising a number of 1-substituted imidazole and triazole compounds, undoubtedly represents the modern approach to both topical and systemic treatment of fungal disease. The first generation of azole antifungals, lipophilic imidazole compounds such as clotrimazole, econazole and miconazole, exhibited poor systemic availability following oral administration, due to both poor absorption and extensive first-pass metabolism. Their use has consequently been essentially limited to topical treatment of superficial fungal infections. Ketoconazole, a more polar imidazole introduced into therapy in the late 1970s (THIENPONT et al. 1979), represented a breakthrough in the treatment of antifungal disease since it was the first imidazole agent with good oral bioavailability in humans (HEEL et al. 1982). Consequently, it was introduced for the treatment of both superficial and systemic fungal infections by oral administration. The subsequent extensive systemic use of ketoconazole resulted in the appearance of two major classes of side effect: drug-related idiosyncratic hepatitis and decreased plasma concentrations of steroid hormones. In addition, and somewhat less serious in impact, the drug has also been shown to interfere with the metabolism of a number of co-administered drugs.

The idiosyncratic symptomatic hepatitis caused by ketoconazole (for reviews, see LAKE-BAKAAR et al. 1987; LEWIS et al. 1984) appears to have an unknown aetiology, although the effect appears to be specific to this drug rather than the azole group of compounds, since despite findings of raised serum levels of hepatic enzymes following clotrimazole treatment (WENTA 1974), there are no reports of this type of hepatitis being associated with the use of other imidazole drugs. There has been a suggestion (HEIBERG and SVEJGAARD 1981) that the hepatic reaction to ketoconazole is immunological in nature since the toxicity often develops following the completion of dosing or re-appears upon re-challenge with ketoconazole. However, there is no firm evidence to support this finding, and current evidence suggests a drug-induced biochemical lesion. The hepatitis associated with ketoconazole has had a marked impact on its use as a systemic agent, particularly when considered for the treatment of relatively trivial superficial infections, and consequently its current use is confined to the treatment of serious systemic fungal disease.

The idiosyncratic side effects of ketoconazole illustrate a major potential problem in the development of a new drug. The clinical incidence of hepatitis associated with the use of ketoconazole has been quoted to be as low as 1 in 15000 patients (LEWIS et al. 1984). Under these circumstances and the uncertain aetiology of the hepatitis, it seems unlikely that a suitable model could be devised to screen other azole antifungals for similar effects. However, there are as yet no reports of similar idiosyncratic reactions with the latest generation of antifungal agents, fluconazole and itraconazole.

The effects of ketoconazole on steroid hormone synthesis and on the metabolism of co-administered drugs have a common aetiology; in both cases an inhibitory effect of the drug on cytochrome P-450-mediated enzymes is involved. Since the mode of action of ketoconazole and other azole drugs involves inhibition of the fungal cytochrome P-450-mediated enzyme lanosterol C14-demethylase (YOSHIDA and AOYAMA 1986), it is apparent that novel antifungal agents will need to be highly selective for the fungal enzyme rather than for the various mammalian P-450s which are involved in important physiological pathways and in the systemic clearance of co-administered drugs. This chapter reviews the spectrum of effects of azoles on the various mammalian cytochromes P-450 and describes some of the current research which indicates that the desired degree of selectivity for the fungal enzyme may be attainable.

B. Nature of Cytochrome P-450

Cytochrome P-450 is an ubiquitous haem-containing protein found throughout the plant and animal kingdoms, which acts as a terminal mono-oxygenase in an electron transport chain mediated via NADPH reductase. Although the protein has been extensively studied and reviewed (ORTIZ DE MONTELLANO 1986), its catalytic mode of action appears variable, depending on the substrate being metabolised (GUENGERICH 1988), and is not fully understood. However, the major role of the various P-450s appears to involve the activation of atmospheric oxygen to a reactive form, which subsequently interacts with lipophilic substrates, leading to oxygen insertion by electrophilic attack (see Fig. 1).

The ubiquitous nature of cytochrome P-450 is demonstrated by the fact that more than 50 different forms have been isolated and characterised from tissues of different prokaryotic and eukaryotic species (BLACK and COON 1986). Thus, for example, they are involved in several rate-limiting steps in the steroid cascade, including the lanosterol C14-demethylase enzyme which represents the antifungal target; in several steps in the arachidonic acid cascade; and in the production and metabolism of bile acids. In addition, as previously mentioned, a number of different forms of the protein (for

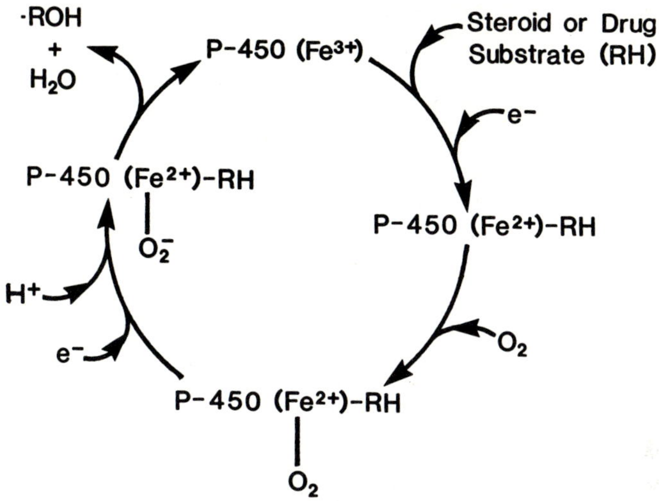

Fig. 1. General scheme of the catalytic cycle of cytochromes P-450

example, there are currently up to 16 in rat liver) are involved in the metabolism of xenobiotics. It is against this background of multiplicity of cytochrome P-450-mediated enzymes in mammalian systems that the selective action of azole compounds for fungal P-450s needs to be judged.

C. Mode of Interaction of Azoles with Cytochromes P-450

The inhibitory effect of the imidazoles and other nitrogen heterocycle-containing compounds on cytochromes P-450 has been known since the early 1970s. Much of the early research work involved investigations of the interaction with hepatic cytochromes P-450. Thus, LIEBMAN (1971) first reported a potent inhibitory effect of 1-arylimidazoles on aminopyrine metabolism in rat liver homogenates. Soon after, WILKINSON et al. (1972) demonstrated the inhibitory effects of N-substituted imidazoles on aldrin epoxidation and N-demethylation of *p*-chloro-*N*-methyl-aniline by rat hepatic microsomes. These workers also showed an apparent correlation between the extent of binding of the imidazole compounds to the microsomes and their inhibitory activity (WILKINSON et al. 1974).

SCHENKMAN et al. (1967) demonstrated that the interaction of nitrogen heterocycles with cytochrome P-450 in rat liver microsomes results in a characteristic visible difference spectrum described as a 'type II' spectrum. This spectrum was confirmed for the imidazole compounds by MAILMAN et al. (1974). The 'type II' spectrum has subsequently been described by these and other workers as indicating the formation of an inhibitory ligand complex

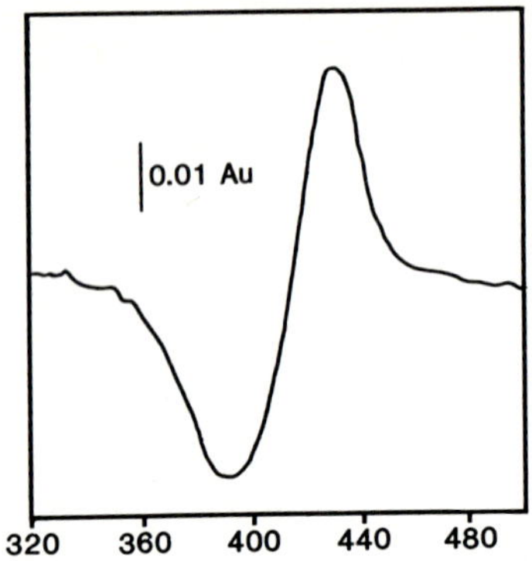

Fig. 2. Characteristic 'type II' difference spectrum of the interaction of azoles with cytochromes P-450. Example shown is the spectrum for ketoconazole (30 μM) interaction with rat hepatic microsomal cytochrome P-450 (1 μM)

between the 'lone pair' nitrogen of the azole moiety and the haem component of the enzyme, converting the enzyme to a low spin or deactivated form of the protein (Kumaki et al. 1978). As illustrated in Fig. 2, most of the azole antifungal agents form this characteristic type II spectrum with cytochrome P-450 (Sheets and Mason 1984).

Recent studies by Yoshida et al. (1986) with purified yeast cytochrome and Ballard (1988) with mouse hepatic microsomes have demonstrated that the binding of lipophilic azoles to cytochromes P-450 is very tight and can be stoichiometric. This high affinity is further supported by several studies (Thompson et al. 1988; Ballard et al. 1988; Rodrigues et al. 1988) which demonstrate that the complex formed between the azoles and the P-450 enzymes following in vivo administration survives the disruption of cells in the preparation of microsomes for in vitro studies.

Several authors, including Lavrijsen et al. (1987), Meredith et al. (1985) and Rodrigues et al. (1987), have attempted to characterise the inhibitory potential of azoles in vitro by titrating the concentration of drug against the size of their difference spectra with microsomes or purified cytochromes P-450 and then using these data to calculate apparent affinity constants. This approach requires caution, however, since as Ballard (1988), Sheets et al. (1986) and Yoshida et al. (1986) have shown at low concentrations all of the drug may be complexed by the protein. Under these conditions, the equilibrium between drug at the binding site and unbound drug, an assumption inherent in binding analysis plots, may not exist. In addition, Hajek et al. (1982) demonstrated that the binding curves for unsubstituted imidazole to purified rabbit cytochromes P-450 were curvilinear, suggesting the presence of more than one binding site on the enzyme. Recently, studies by Shaw et al. (1988), Liebman and Ortiz (1973), Wilkinson et al. (1983) and Ballard et al. (1988) have shown non-linearities in binding plots of several azoles which are consistent with their binding with differing affinities to different hepatic cytochrome P-450s. On the basis of the results of these studies, the use of classic binding plots to characterise the relative affinities of azoles for cytochromes P-450 does not appear to be a reliable means of differentiating between the compounds and can be misleading.

Attempts to characterise the affinity of azoles for cytochromes P-450 by measuring their effects on the rate of formation of the characteristic carbon monoxide complex, used to measure concentrations of the protein (ESTABROOK and WERRINGHOER 1978), appear to be more reliable. Thus, SCHUSTER (1985, 1988) reported that ketoconazole markedly delays the binding of carbon monoxide to cytochrome P-450 in a variety of steroidogenic tissues and liver. Recently, VANDEN BOSSCHE (1987) has shown that itraconazole, a novel triazole antifungal agent, delays the binding of carbon monoxide to fungal cytochrome P-450 significantly longer than ketoconzole does, indicating a higher affinity of the former compound for the fungal protein, and that this is in keeping with differences in their antifungal potency. These researchers were also able to demonstrate major differences in the relative competitive affinities of itraconazole and carbon monoxide binding for the fungal protein and a number of mammalian proteins, supporting evidence from their catalytic studies that itraconazole represents a selective agent.

The determinants of the relative affinities of azoles for different cytochrome P-450s remain unknown. The early work of WILKINSON et al. (1974) and ROGERSON et al. (1977) and the more recent work of BALLARD et al. (1988), examining the binding of series of structurally related imidazole and triazole analogues, have found that the relative field strength of the lone pair nitrogen in the heterocycle and the overall lipophilicity of the molecule are important determinants.

Bearing in mind the problems associated with the accurate determination of classic affinity constants for the azole drugs, the competition assay with carbon monoxide appears to be the most productive way of assessing the affinity of particular azoles for cytochrome P-450 enzymes in vitro and of determining the relative specificity for the fungal enzyme.

D. Effects of Azoles on Mammalian Hepatic Cytochromes P-450

I. In Vitro Metabolism Studies

As mentioned above, WILKINSON et al. (1972) were among the first to demonstrate the inhibitory effects of a homologous series of imidazole derivatives on hepatic microsomal oxidations. Later studies by PALMER and CAWTHORNE (1974), examining the effects of 1-alkylimidazoles on rat hepatic microsomal metabolism of aminopyrine and aniline, by WILKINSON's group (WILKINSON et al. 1974; ROGERSON et al. 1977) examining the inhibition of aldrin epoxidation by aryl- and alkyl-substituted imidazoles, and by LIEBMAN and ORTIZ (1973) examining the effects of 1-arylimidazoles on rat microsomal metabolism of aminopyrine, aniline and acetanilide confirmed that substituted imidazole compounds containing a sterically unhindered lone pair nitrogen were potent inhibitors of cytochromes P-450. These studies indicated that the overall lipophilicity of the molecules and the relative steric hindrance around the liganding nitrogen were important determinants of relative potency as inhibitors.

RAZZOUK et al. (1978) subsequently demonstrated that one of the first generation of lipophilic N-substituted imidazole antifungal drugs, miconazole, was also a potent inhibitor of cytochrome P-450-mediated drug metabolism. They showed differential inhibitory effects of miconazole on the metabolism of benzo[a]pyrene by microsomes from rats induced with phenobarbitone, 3-methylcholanthrene and 2-fluorenylacetamide. This was perhaps also the first indication that azoles could act as selective inhibitors of different forms of cytochrome P-450, since it is recognised that different inducing agents lead to different forms of cytochrome P-450 becoming predominant in microsomes prepared from induced livers.

Later KAHL et al. (1980) also demonstrated differential effects of another first generation imidazole, clotrimazole, and several structural analogues on benzo[a]pyrene and ethoxycoumarin metabolism using microsomes from rats treated with the inducing agents phenobarbitone and 3-methylcholanthrene. Their results indicated that clotrimazole was a more potent inhibitor of control and phenobarbitone-induced microsomes than of the methylcholanthrene-induced enzymes. This apparent selectivity of inhibition for phenobarbitone-inducible P-450s was confirmed for clotrimazole by SCOTT and DREW (1983), who also showed that two other first generation imidazole antifungal agents, econazole and miconazole, followed a similar pattern.

The successful introduction of ketoconazole for the systemic treatment of fungal disease led to a much greater interest in the effects of the azoles on both the steroidogenic and drug-metabolising P-450s, and following the first demonstration of the inhibitory effects of ketoconazole on the metabolism of ethoxyresorufin in benzoflavone-induced rat liver microsomes by SHEETS and MASON (1984), several groups, including KAPETANOVIC and KUPFERBERG (1985), MOSCA et al. (1985), LAVRIJSEN et al. (1987), MEREDITH et al. (1985) and HEUSNER and FRANKLIN (1985), have subsequently examined the effects of ketoconazole and related azoles on rat hepatic cytochrome P-450 using a variety of probe substrates. Much of this work has increased our understanding of the selective nature of the inhibition of the different forms of cytochrome P-450 by different imidazole- and triazole-substituted antifungal agents. Thus, for example, the recent work by RODRIGUES et al. (1987) using purified rat hepatic cytochromes P-450 demonstrated that clotrimazole, miconazole and ketoconazole were more potent inhibitors of ethoxycoumarin metabolism, catalysed by the major phenobarbitone-inducible cytochromes P-450, than reactions catalysed by the major 3-methylcholanthrene-inducible forms.

Several groups have used the androgens testosterone and androstendione as probe substrates to characterise the inhibitory profile of azoles in hepatic microsomes. In many respects the androgens represent ideal probes since they are metabolised by a number of constitutive and inducible forms of P-450 to discrete regio- and stereo-selective products (WAXMAN et al. 1983). Thus, by profiling the effects of the test azoles on the pattern of metabolism of the androgen produced by the microsomes, it is possible to gain rapid information on the relative potencies and selectivity of the compounds as inhibitors of the different forms of P-450 present in the liver.

Using this technique SHEETS et al. (1986) were able to show that whilst clotrimazole and miconazole were equipotent inhibitors of androstenedione-16α-hydroxylation in rat microsomes, a reaction catalysed by the major phenobarbitone-inducible P-450 (WAXMAN et al. 1983), ketoconazole was more than eightfold less potent. All three compounds differed in their potency as inhibitors of the P-450 catalysing 6β-hydroxylation of androstenedione, known to be the major P-450 induced by the steroid pregnenolone carbonitrile in the rat (WAXMAN et al. 1983), with ketoconazole and clotrimazole being fourfold and 20-fold more potent, respectively, than miconazole.

BALLARD et al. (1987, 1988) have used the substrates ethoxyresorufin and testosterone as probes to characterise the inhibitory potential of a series of structurally related imidazole and triazole analogues in non-induced mouse microsomes. These studies have shown for the first time that the determinants of selectivity of azoles for different P-450s include the nature of the azole itself, whether imidazole or triazole, as well as the substitution pattern in the rest of the molecule.

The information emanating from these recent studies with various probe substrates illustrates the selective inhibition exhibited by some compounds and the general inhibition exhibited by others. This highlights the need for close examination of the inhibitory profile of specific azole antifungal agents, since different forms of P-450 are responsible for the metabolism of different drugs. Consequently, the choice of an inappropriate substrate could underestimate the inhibitory potential of an azole or conceivably miss it all together. For example, HOUSTON et al. (1988) demonstrated that although the IC_{50} value for ketoconazole inhibition of total testosterone metabolism in non-induced rat microsomes was relatively high (100 μM), this masked a very potent inhibition of one of the number of forms of P-450, the steroid-inducible form (IC_{50} 0.55 μM), involved in the metabolism of the substrate.

II. In Vivo Drug Interaction Studies

The corollary to the effects of azoles on hepatic cytochromes P-450 outlined in the numerous in vitro studies cited above is that the compounds will have the potential to inhibit the metabolism of drugs which are co-administered in vivo. This was shown to be the case for the experimental aryl- and alkyl-imidazole compounds, with which prolongation of barbiturate sleeping times were observed in rats and mice in the in vivo studies undertaken in support of in vitro findings by LIEBMAN and ORTIZ (1973), WILKINSON et al. (1974) and PALMER and CAWTHORNE (1974). As mentioned previously, however, the first generation imidazole antifungal agents exhibited low systemic availability after oral administration. Consequently, few drug interactions were apparent in clinical studies with these agents, although the use of miconazole infusions has been associated with increased prothrombin times in patients stabilised on warfarin (DERESINSKI et al. 1977).

Several studies with animals using dose levels somewhat higher than those for clinical indications showed that the first generation antifungal imidazoles do have the potential to inhibit the metabolism of co-administered compounds. NIEMEEGERS et al. (1981) demonstrated that ketoconazole as well as clotrimazole and miconazole affected the metabolism of methohexital and acenocoumarol in the rat to varying extents over a range of dose levels. Similarly, BACK and TJIA (1985) showed that the same three antifungals inhibited the hepatic clearance of tolbutamide in the rat. All three compounds exhibited a similar extent of inhibition of the single isozyme responsible for tolbutamide metabolism. This contrasts with the markedly different ED_{50} dose levels for prolongation of methohexital metabolism, indicating that the compounds interact with different P-450s. Other animal studies undertaken with ketoconazole also showed that the drug had differential inhibitory effects on the metabolism of caffeine and aminopyrine in the rat (MEREDITH et al. 1985) and inhibited the metabolism of cyclosporin A in the mouse (ANDERSON and BLASCHKE 1986) and dog (D'MELLO et al. 1986).

Most of these animal studies were carried out at dose levels significantly higher than those used clinically, and the relative clinical importance of the azole drugs as inhibitors of co-administered drugs has awaited studies with ketoconazole in volunteers and patients. Several recent investigations have demonstrated that ketoconazole does affect the metabolism of some co-administered drugs at therapeutic dose levels, although results are somewhat contradictory. D'MELLO et al. (1985) showed a 30% increase in antipyrine half-life following chronic administration of 400 mg ketoconazole. This contrasted with the apparent lack of effect of ketoconazole on antipyrine clearance in the studies carried out by DANESHMEND et al. (1983) and BLYDEN et al. (1986). Similarly, in contrast to the ketoconazole-induced potentiation of warfarin reported by SMITH (1984), the drug was without apparent effect on the metabolism of warfarin in the studies done by BRASS et al. (1982). In a comparative study, BROWN et al. (1985) found that ketoconazole decreased chlorodiazepoxide metabolism in volunteers but had no effect on theophylline metabolism. Other clinical studies with ketoconazole have demonstrated inhibition of cyclosporin metabolism (FERGUSON et al. 1982; DIEPERINK and MØLLER 1982) and methylprednisolone metabolism (GLYNN et al. 1986).

Undoubtedly, some of the anomalies in these studies and differences in the inhibitory effects of ketoconazole reflect the different dose levels used or variations in protocol design. However, another important factor arising out of a consideration of the numerous investigations carried out in vitro (cited above) and results from animal studies is that these effects may reflect the selectivity of inhibition by azoles on the different P-450s involved in the metabolism of the drugs. On this basis it would appear that standard probes used to test for drug interactions, such as antipyrine, may not give a clear definition of the inhibitory potential of test azoles in the clinical situation, since antipyrine is only metabolised by a limited number of cytochromes P-450 (Boobis et al. 1981). The recent approach of Schellens et al. (1988) using a cocktail of test drugs which apparently cover the whole spectrum of human P-450s may represent a better approach.

In keeping with their greater degree of selectivity for the fungal cytochromes P-450 evident in in vitro metabolism studies, the latest generation of triazole antifungal agents appear to have much less effect on the metabolism of co-administered drugs. Houston et al. (1988) showed that fluconazole, a polar bistriazole with selectivity for inhibition of fungal lanosterol C14-demethylase P-450, was markedly less potent an inhibitor of antipyrine metabolism in the rat than ketoconazole; similarly, Awouters and Niemeegers (1983) found that itraconazole did not affect the metabolism of methohexital in rats at dose levels which caused significant inhibition with ketoconazole. These animal studies have been borne out by preliminary studies in human volunteers. Purba and Back (1986) demonstrated that fluconazole does not affect the metabolism of antipyrine or oral contraceptives at therapeutic dose levels, and Heykants et al. (1987) showed that itraconazole does not affect the metabolism of antipyrine in healthy volunteers. Recent reports of an interaction between itraconazole and cyclosporin A (Kwan et al. 1987; Shaw et al. 1987; Trenk et al. 1987) are contradictory, and further confirmatory studies will be required before a clear understanding of its nature emerges.

III. Induction of Cytochromes P-450

One of the characteristic features of cytochrome P-450 proteins is their inducibility by a number of endogenous steroids and xenobiotics (for a review, see Conney 1986). Much of the work investigating the induction of P-450s has been undertaken in laboratory animals, and it is now clear that particular forms of cytochrome P-450 respond to stimuli by specific inducing agents. For example, two classic inducing agents, phenobarbitone and 3-methylcholanthrene, induce different and highly characteristic patterns of P-450s in various species. It is important to realise that these inducing agents also result in the repression of other forms of P-450, and consequently the whole pattern of metabolising enzymes is altered by the inducing agent.

Again the early work with the experimental aryl- and alkyl-imidazoles gave the first indications that azoles were potent inducing agents (Palmer and Cawthorne 1974; Murray et al. 1985; Kaul and Novak 1984). The early studies of Tettenborn (1974) indicated that the imidazole drug clotrimazole shortened hexobarbital-induced sleeping time in the mouse following chronic administration, implying that the antifungal imidazoles were also inducing agents.

It is now evident that not only are the antifungal azoles relatively potent inducing agents but that the specific forms induced vary with the azole administered. Doubling of hepatic cytochrome P-450 concentrations has been demonstrated by KAHL et al. (1980) in the rat following administration of high doses of clotrimazole. Recent studies by BALLARD (1988) have demonstrated a similar degree of induction of a number of specific forms of mouse hepatic P-450s following the subchronic administration of a series of imidazole and triazole antifungal analogues. The induction of specific forms of P-450s by azoles is confirmed in the comparison of the effects of ketoconazole and the topical imidazoles, clotrimazole, miconazole and tioconazole, carried out in the rat by RITTER and FRANKLIN (1987). Results demonstrate that the compounds induced very different patterns of P-450s.

Several authors have attempted to characterise the profile of P-450s induced by the azoles in vitro using the probe substrate techniques outlined above. The work of BALLARD (1988) and RITTER et al. (1987) highlights the difficulties in interpreting results obtained using this approach, since it is apparent that the tight binding of the azoles to the protein survives the preparation of microsomes for in vitro studies. Consequently, several of the P-450s will have significant concentrations of inhibitor remaining complexed at the active site. Under these conditions, catalytic expression may not reflect their true state of induction.

The implications of the induction potential of azole compounds on drug-metabolising enzymes for their clinical utility is debatable, as the induction phenomenon is generally associated with dose levels which are orders of magnitude above those used clinically. However, the use of the first generation imidazoles was associated with the need to modulate the dose levels during chronic treatment to compensate for increased clearance of the drugs due to autoinduction. BURGESS and BODEY (1972) reported a progressive decline in serum concentrations of clotrimazole over an 8-day period following daily administration of 1.5 g q.i.d. The potent inducing potential of clotrimazole in humans was confirmed by SCHOENE et al. (1973), who demonstrated a threefold increase in total hepatic P-450 in one patient receiving 1.5 g daily. It appears likely therefore that azoles, which are potent inducing agents and which are systemically cleared by metabolism, may modulate their own pharmacokinetics or the pharmacokinetics of co-administered drugs when they are administered chronically to patients. On this basis, relative induction potency may represent a further selection criteria for the identification of a suitable clinical agent. That this question is being addressed by modern research approaches to antifungal drug discovery is evident in the recent study by LAVRIJSEN et al. (1987) comparing the induction potential of one of the latest generation of triazole antifungal agents, itraconazole, with that of the imidazoles miconazole and clotrimazole in the rat. The results of this study indicate that the triazoles may have less induction potential than the first generation imidazole drugs.

E. Endocrine Effects of Azoles

I. Mammalian Endocrine System

Hormones are chemical substances secreted into the bloodstream, whose function is to regulate and co-ordinate the activities of different cells. To maintain this function it is essential that the endocrine gland receive constant rapid information on the state of those systems regulated. Various feedback systems operate, and the rate of hormone secretion from the gland is determined by integration of the different signals received. The most simple feedback system is negative feedback. Thus, for example, adrenocorticotrophin (ACTH) from the anterior pituitary acts upon the adrenal gland to stimulate the release of cortisol. Cortisol can then influence its own release by negative feedback at the level of the pituitary and perhaps also at the level of the hypothalamus (Fig. 3). A similar negative feedback system operates to control the luteinising hormone (LH) stimulated secretion of testosterone from the testis.

The way in which a particular hormone exerts a specific effect on its target cell is only partially understood. The hormone must first be recognised by its target cell by interacting with its specific receptor. It may then act on cellular processes by one or more of three major mechanisms: by altering membrane permeability, by activating intracellular signal mechanisms, and by stimulating protein synthesis. For example, ACTH binds to its receptor on the adrenal cell and activates the adenylate cyclase cAMP second messenger system. By a mechanism which is incompletely understood, cAMP then activates the cortisol biosynthetic sequence shown in Fig. 4. Similarly, LH binds to its receptor on the Leydig cell and via the adenylate cyclase cAMP second messenger system activates the biosynthetic pathway leading to the production of testosterone (Fig. 5).

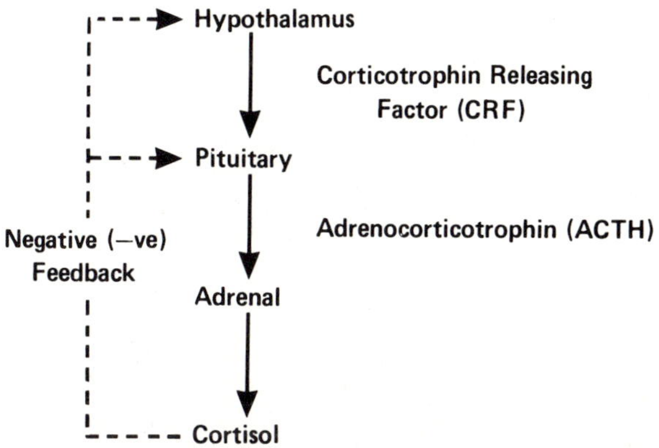

Fig. 3. The control of cortisol secretion from the adrenal gland by negative feedback

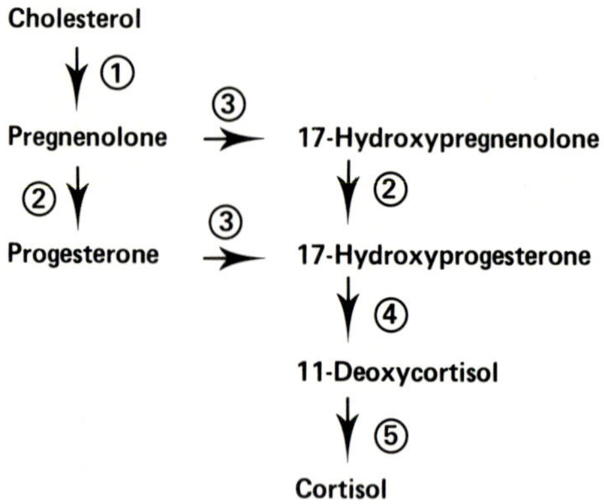

Fig. 4. Biosynthesis of cortisol: (*1*) cholesterol desmolase, (*2*) 5,3β-hydroxysteroid dehydrogenase, (*3*) 17α-hydroxylase, (*4*) 21-hydroxylase and (*5*) 11β-hydroxylase

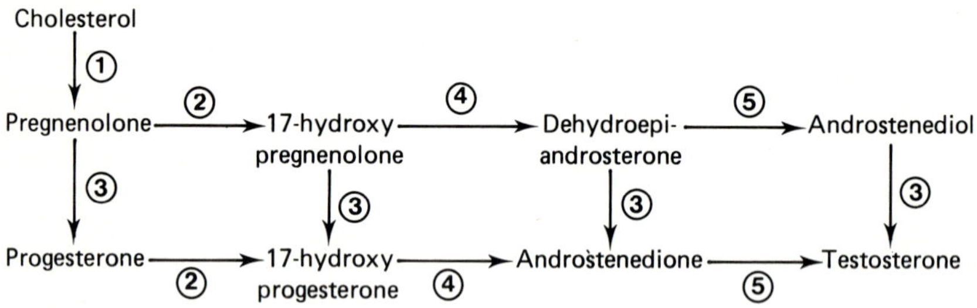

Fig. 5. Biosynthesis of testosterone: (*1*) cholesterol desmolase, (*2*) 17α-hydroxylase, (*3*) 5,3β-hydroxysteroid dehydrogenase, (*4*) C17,20-lyase, (*5*) 17β-hydroxysteroid dehydrogenase

II. Effects of Ketoconazole on Steroidogenic Tissues

Ketoconazole has been shown to suppress both adrenal and testicular steroid secretion in vivo and in vitro. The drug-induced suppression of steroid secretion results from the fact that ketoconazole in common with other imidazole compounds is an inhibitor of cytochrome P-450-catalysed reactions (see Sect. C).

A report by DEFELICE et al. (1981) describing the development of gynnecomastia in two male patients receiving long-term ketoconazole therapy prompted PONT et al. (1982a,b) to study the effects of ketoconazole on steroidogenesis in men. These workers noted that administration of a single therapeutic dose of ketoconazole resulted in a marked but transient reduction in plasma testosterone (PONT et al. 1982a) and significantly blunted the cortisol response to an ACTH stimulation test (PONT et al. 1982b). These findings have subsequently been confirmed by several groups (DE COSTER et al. 1984, 1986; SCHÜRMEYER and NIESCHLAG 1984; SANTEN et al. 1983). In vitro ketoconazole has been shown to be a reversible inhibitor of testosterone synthesis by dispersed Leydig cells (Schürmeyer and Nieschlag 1984; De Coster et al. 1984; Lambert et al. 1986b) and of cortisol synthesis by isolated adrenal cells (Pont et al. 1982b; Lambert et al. 1986b).

In vivo and in vitro in a variety of species including mouse, rat, guinea-pig, dog and humans, ketoconazole has been shown to block adrenal and testicular steroidogenesis between ACTH/LH binding and pregnenolone production (Loose et al. 1983a; Kowal 1983; Engelhardt et al. 1985; De Coster et al. 1986; Lambert et al. 1986b) and C17,20-lyase activity (Santen et al. 1983; De Coster et al. 1984, 1986; Sikka et al. 1985; Kan et al. 1985; Rajfer et al. 1985, 1986; Lambert et al. 1986b; Trachtenberg and Zadra 1988). A further site of action at 11β-hydroxylase has been demonstrated in vitro (Loose et al. 1983a; De Coster et al. 1986) and in vivo (Engelhardt et al. 1985). However, Lambert et al. (1986b), using similar drug concentrations (1.25×10^{-5} M) to those in the study by Loose et al. (0.94×10^{-5} M), failed to observe any inhibitory effect on this enzyme in dispersed guinea pig cells. At high concentrations of ketoconazole ($>2.4 \times 10^{-5}$ M) an additional site of action at 17α-hydroxylase has also been reported (Sikka et al. 1985; Rajfer et al. 1985, 1986; De Coster et al. 1986; Lamberts et al. 1987). However, Loose et al. (1983a) failed to observe inhibition of 17α-hydroxylase even at ketoconazole concentrations up to 5×10^{-5} M. In one study (Sikka et al. 1985) performed in rats on long-term treatment with the drug, inhibition of 17β-hydroxysteroid dehydrogenase activity has been reported. This enzyme is known not to be a cytochrome P-450-dependent enzyme, and confirmation of this finding is awaited.

The clinical data (Santen et al. 1983) and many of the in vitro studies (Schürmeyer and Nieschlag 1984; De Coster et al. 1984; Vanden Bossche et al. 1985; Sikka et al. 1985; Kan et al. 1985) clearly indicate that the most sensitive site of inhibition by ketoconazole is that of the microsomal C17,20-lyase. At therapeutic concentrations (5×10^{-6} M), ketoconazole completely inhibited the late pathway of aldosterone formation in rat zona glomerulosa mitochondria (Sonino and Brownie 1987), and it was suggested that this drug may have a therapeutic application in the management of hyperaldosteronism. High dose ketoconazole treatment has been shown to inhibit partially aldosterone biosynthesis in vivo by inhibiting 11β-hydroxylase (De Coster et al. 1987). However, this inhibition was detected mainly after angiotensin II- or salt-depleted stimulation of aldosterone production. Ketoconazole has no direct effects on pituitary ACTH secretion in vivo or in vitro (Burrin et al. 1986). The increase in plasma ACTH after administration of the drug is due to the operation of the normal feedback system. Similarly, ketoconazole has no direct effect on gonadotrophin release at the pituitary level (Bhasin et al. 1986).

Ketoconazole also depresses ovarian steroidogenesis. Evidence obtained from in vivo experiments using rats indicates that the drug inhibits ovarian aromatase (Watanabe and Menzies 1985, 1986; Malozowski et al. 1986),

17,20-desmolase and 17-ketosteroid reductase (MALOZOWSKI et al. 1986), resulting in depressed ovarian concentrations of progestins, androgens and 17β-oestradiol after administration of single or repeated oral doses. Single dose (400 mg) ketoconazole treatment in healthy human males has been found to lower estradiol levels to 60% of control (DE COSTER et al. 1985).

In summary, various studies have demonstrated that ketoconazole blocks gonadal and adrenal steroidogenesis in humans by inhibiting several cytochrome P-450-dependent enzymes. Recent evidence suggests that cholesterol production in humans is also affected by ketoconazole (KRAEMER and PONT 1986). The drug has been shown to have multiple effects on cholesterol synthesis, directly inhibiting late steps by blocking the conversion of methyl sterols to cholesterol and indirectly suppressing total sterol synthesis via feedback inhibition by sterol intermediates of 3-hydroxy-3-methylglutaryl coenzyme A reductase activity (KRAEMER and PONT 1986). The related imidazole antimycotic clotrimazole had similar effects whereas the imidazole anaesthetic agent etomidate had little impact on cholesterol synthesis. Although serum cholesterol levels are decreased in patients during chronic high dose regimens (TRACHTENBERG and PONT 1984; KRAEMER and PONT 1986), there is no evidence as yet for the potential therapeutic use of ketoconazole in the management of hypercholesterolaemia since the effects of cholesterol precursor accumulation are not known.

III. Other Endocrine Effects of Ketoconazole

In cultured kidney cells inhibition of 24-hydroxylase and 1-hydroxylase by ketoconazole has been demonstrated (LOOSE et al. 1983a; HENRY 1985). Reduced vitamin 1,25-(hydroxy) D levels have been reported in humans receiving ketoconazole (300–1200 mg/day), and some patients receiving the drug for treatment of prostatic cancer have developed hypocalcaemia (WILLIAMS et al. 1986). Dihydrotestosterone and oestradiol binding to sex hormone binding globulin are inhibited by ketoconazole at concentrations in the range of blood levels found in patients on higher therapeutic dosage regimens (GROSSO et al. 1983). It has been suggested that suppression of testicular testosterone synthesis and displacement of oestrogens from sex hormone binding globulin may decrease the androgen/oestrogen ratio of the blood and contribute to the development of the gynaecomastia reported in some ketoconazole-treated patients (DEFELICE et al. 1981).

Using a method based upon the ability of imidazole drugs to inhibit [^{3}H]-dexamethasone binding to hepatoma tissue culture cell cytosol, LOOSE et al. (1983b) demonstrated that ketoconazole and other imidazole antimycotic drugs (e.g. clotrimazole) possess glucocorticoid antagonist activity by virtue of occupancy of the glucocorticoid receptor sites in target tissues. This was the first demonstration of a non-steroidal molecule possessing antiglucocorticoid activity.

IV. Effect of Other Imidazole Antifungal Agents on Steroidogenesis

In vitro inhibition of testosterone production in mouse Leydig cells has also been reported for isoconazole, miconazole, econazole and clotrimazole, while metronidazole and levamisole were without influence (SCHÜRMEYER and NIESCHLAG 1984). In a study of 14 imidazole drugs on rat testicular enzyme activities, AYUB and LEVELL (1987) found the order of decreasing inhibitory effect on 17α-hydroxylase (substrate [^{3}H]-progesterone) was bifonazole > ketoconazole > clotrimazole > miconazole > econazole > tioconazole > isoconazole, and on 17,20-lyase (substrate [^{3}H]-17α-hydroxy-progesterone) was bifonazole > clotrimazole > ketoconazole > miconazole > econazole > tioconazole > isoconazole. However, these imidazole drugs did not inhibit 3β-hydroxysteroid dehydrogenase (HSD) or 17β-HSD activities. A common structural feature of the imidazole drugs having an inhibitory effect was the possession of more than 1 aromatic ring on the imidazole side chain. In contrast, the imidazole drugs having the imidazole ring fused to the benzene ring, i.e. benzimidazoles (astemizole, mebendazole, thiabendazole), and those having an aliphatic side chain on the N1 of the imidazole ring (carbimazole, metronidazole, nimorazole, tinidazole) did not inhibit 17α-hydroxylase, 3β-HSD or 17β-HSD. Some did inhibit 17,20-lyase activity, but only at high concentrations.

In contrast to some other substituted imidazole derivatives, the anaesthetic agent etomidate does not interfere with testicular testosterone synthesis (ALLOLIO et al. 1986), although it is a potent inhibitor of adrenal steroidogenesis (FELLOWS et al. 1983; LAMBERT et al. 1983) and has been implicated in the deaths of critically ill patients (LEDINGHAM and WATT 1983). Neither high dosage (30 mg/h for long-term sedation) nor low dosage (0.26 mg/kg as a single induction dose) had any influence on serum testosterone or LH concentrations in males. It is therefore possible to synthesise clinically useful imidazole derivatives with endocrine actions confined to either the adrenals or testes.

Omeprazole, a substituted benzimidazole and potent inhibitor of gastric acid secretion currently being evaluated in patients with peptic ulcer and Zollinger-Ellison syndrome, inhibited ACTH-stimulated cortisol release from the adrenal in vivo (healthy men) and in vitro (bovine adrenal cells) (HOWDEN et al. 1986). Although substantial inhibition occurred at concentrations higher than plasma levels normally achieved in clinical use, impairment of adrenocortical function may occur in patients on long-term, high-dosage omeprazole treatment for the Zollinger-Ellison syndrome.

N-substituted imidazole derivatives, e.g. clotrimazole and miconazole, have also been shown to inhibit aromatase activity (YAMAMOTO et al. 1987; MASON et al. 1985) making them useful compounds in the treatment of oestrogen-dependent diseases such as breast cancer.

V. New Antifungal Agents

By virtue of structural modification the newer antifungal agents itraconazole and fluconazole, which are both triazoles, exhibit greater specificity as inhibitors of the fungal cytochrome P-450-mediated reactions over mammalian cytochrome P-450-mediated reactions than other azole antifungal agents in clinical use. Both drugs show little or no inhibitory effect on testicular or adrenal steroidogenesis after chronic administration at therapeutic dose levels (VAN CAUTEREN et al. 1987; VANDEN BOSSCHE et al. 1986; SHAW et al. 1987).

VI. Clinical Use of Ketoconazole in Endocrinology

The use of ketoconazole in clinical practice as an antifungal medication has resulted in few endocrine side effects. Even in children receiving long-term (3–52 months), high-dose (10–23 mg/kg daily) ketoconazole for systemic coccidioidomycosis, none required adrenal steroid replacement therapy in times of acute illness or surgery, and none had clinical evidence of adrenal insufficiency (BRITTON et al. 1988). However, a patient with persistent adrenal insufficiency following ketoconazole therapy for blastomycosis has been reported (BEST et al. 1987). Doses much higher than those sufficient for antifungal therapy are required for endocrine effects to become apparent (PONT et al. 1984).

1. Use in Cortisol Overproduction

The ability of ketoconazole to inhibit adrenal and testicular steroidogenesis and to block corticosteroid action at the receptor level led to its trial as an inhibitor of steroidogenesis in cases of cortisol or androgen overproduction. It has been shown to be effective as a treatment for various forms of Cushing's syndrome (CONTRERAS et al. 1985a,b; ANGELI and FRAIRIA 1985; SONINO et al. 1985) including ectopic ACTH production (SHEPHERD et al. 1985; FARWELL et al. 1988). Clinically effective doses have been reported to be between 400 and 1200 mg/day, usually without glucocorticoid replacement, although lower doses (200–400 mg/day) along with dexamethasone replacement have been used to achieve good control in a case of ectopic ACTH production (FARWELL et al. 1988).

2. Use in Androgen Overproduction

High-dose therapy (1200 mg ketoconazole daily) results in long-term suppression of androgen production in patients with prostatic carcinoma (TRACHTENBERG 1984; PONT and TRACHTENBERG 1984; TRACHTENBERG and PONT 1984; HEYNS et al. 1985). However, HEYNS et al. (1985) found that except in the first 2 weeks of treatment, free testosterone levels exceeded those observed in castrated patients throughout a 12-month treatment programme. ENGLISH et al. (1986) demonstrated that a combination of ketoconazole with a gonadotropin-releasing hormone (Gn-RH) analogue resulted in greater suppression of testosterone than either agent alone.

In male rats, long-term treatment has been shown to impair fertility by decreasing sperm number and motility and increasing the number of abnormal sperm (VAWDA and DAVIES 1986). In human subjects after prolonged high dose (800–1200 mg/day) therapy, oligo- and azospermia, impotence and decreased libido have been noted (PONT et al. 1984). Gynaecomastia appears more commonly with lower doses (PONT et al. 1984). It has been suggested that ketoconazole may be a satisfactory treatment for precocious puberty in boys (HOLLAND et al. 1985) and possibly for other conditions characterised by androgen excess. Low doses (200–400 mg/day) have been used with some success in the management of hirsutism (CARVALHO et al. 1985; SONINO et al. 1985).

3. Other Clinical Uses

High-dose therapy (1200 mg/day) has also been used for the treatment of oestrogen-dependent breast cancer (NAMER et al. 1986). However, in one of three patients with breast cancer and in others with prostatic cancer, NAMER et al. (1986) described for the first time thyroid dysfunction as a side effect of ketoconazole treatment. It has recently been suggested that the use of ketoconazole in human malignancies might be worthy of clinical evaluation (ROCHLITZ et al. 1988). It is known to have some activity against human prostate cancer, adrenal cancer and male metastatic breast cancer and has recently been shown to be active in vitro against eight malignant cell lines including human pancreatic carcinoma, human colonic adenocarcinoma and murine leukaemia (ROCHLITZ et al. 1988).

VII. Assessment of Anti-Steroidogenic Biopotency and Site of Action of Antifungal Agents

Potential antifungal agents discovered recently have virtually all been azoles or other sterol synthesis inhibitors. With such compounds additional studies should be performed to assess the toxicological risk with respect to endocrine function, as highlighted by experience with ketoconazole and etomidate. In view of the increasing interest in in vitro systems which allow investigation into the biological effects of drugs and toxic substances without resource to large scale animal experimentation, two systems which are suitable for the rapid assessment of the in vitro anti-steroidogenic potency of drugs affecting adrenal and testicular steroidogenesis have recently been developed (LAMBERT et al. 1985a, 1987). These methods, based on primary dispersions of endocrine cells, have proved of value in testing the biopotency of new and existing compounds (LAMBERT et al. 1985a,b; READER et al. 1985). To date, the anti-steroidogenic effects (expressed as in vitro ED_{50} values) of 19 drugs of different structure and therapeutic action, including the imidazoles ketoconazole and etomidate, have been studied using the dose-related inhibition of cortisol secretion from guinea pig adrenals and of testosterone secretion from mouse Leydig cells.

The relevance of these data to pharmacological effects in vivo is as yet unproven. However, in the absence of clinical or other evidence from animal studies, they may give some indication as to possible in vivo activity. Thus, etomidate, an anaesthetic known to block adrenal steroidogenesis, is present in plasma at a concentration which greatly exceeds (>50 times) its in vitro ED_{50} value 1 min after administration of a single induction dose of 0.3 mg/kg (Doenicke et al. 1982).

Dispersed endocrine cell systems are also suitable for the rapid determination of the enzymic sites of action (Lambert et al. 1984, 1985a,b,c, 1986a,b; Robertson et al. 1985), the reversibility (Lambert et al. 1986b) and kinetics of inhibition and structure-function relationships for the drugs.

F. Conclusions

It is now clear that the various antifungal agents and other drugs derived from imidazole compounds interact with specific enzymes in both the steroidogenic pathway leading to the synthesis of the biologically active steroids cortisol, testosterone, progesterone and oestrogens and with the metabolism of co-administered drugs. These actions are predominantly due to inhibition of the various cytochrome P-450 proteins involved in biochemical pathways. The effects can vary considerably, and changes in the structure of the drugs can radically alter both the potency and selectivity of action of the compound. The ubiquitous nature of cytochrome P-450 and its involvement in a number of biochemical pathways indicates the need for antifungal agents to be highly selective for the lanosterol C14-demethylase P-450 which represents the antifungal target. Thus, the development of in vitro systems such as those described above allows the investigation of the structure-function relationships and selectivity of action of the azoles and could be exploited as a simple first-line screen for unwanted endocrine or drug interaction side effects, as well as in the design of new agents for the treatment of various endocrine disorders. Indeed, it has been the exploitation of a relative lack of selectivity of ketoconazole as an inhibitor of cytochrome P-450 (i.e. the inhibition of cortisol synthesis) which has enabled it to be employed therapeutically in the treatment of Cushing's disease. However, it would have clearly been preferable to have known of the anti-steroidogenic effect of ketoconazole before its clinical use became widespread, rather than discover it as a side effect. The exploitation of in vitro cell techniques will be of great benefit in making this feasible.

References

Allolio B, Stuttmann R, Winkelmann W (1986) Missing effect of etomidate on testosterone secretion in man. Klin Wochenschr 15:86–88

Anderson JE, Blaschke TF (1986) Ketoconazole inhibits cyclosporin metabolism in vivo in mice. J Pharmacol Exp Ther 236:671–674

Angeli A, Frairia R (1985) Ketoconazole therapy in Cushing's disease. Lancet i:821

Awouters FHL, Niemeegers CJF (1983) In vivo study of the possible inhibition and induction of microsomal enzymes by the antimycotic R51211. Janssen Pharmaceutica Preclinical Research Report R51211/4

Ayub M, Levell MJ (1987) Inhibition of testicular 17α-hydroxylase and 17,20-lyase but not 3β-hydroxysteroid dehyrogenase-isomerase or 17β-hydroxysteroid oxidoreductase by ketoconazole and other imidazole drugs. J Steroid Biochem 28: 521–531

Back DJ, Tjia JF (1985) Inhibition of tolbutamide metabolism by substituted imidazole drugs in vivo: evidence for structure activity relationship. Br J Pharmacol 85:121–126

Ballard SA (1988) Interaction of azole antifungal agents with mouse hepatic microsomal cytochromes P-450. PhD Thesis. University of Kent, Canterbury, UK

Ballard SA, Tarbit MH, Burnet FR, Lodola A (1987) Selective interaction of two N-substituted imidazole antifungal compounds with cytochromes P-450 catalysing ethoxyresorufin 0-de-ethylation. Biochem Soc Trans 15:1116–1117

Ballard SA, Lodola A, Tarbit MH (1988) A comparative study of 1-substituted imidazole and 1,2,4-triazole antifungal compounds as inhibitors of testosterone hydroxylations catalysed by mouse hepatic microsomal cytochrome P-450. Biochem Pharmacol 37:4643–4651

Best TR, Jenkins JK, Murphy FY, Nicks SA, Bussell KL, Nesely DL (1987) Persistent adrenal insufficiency secondary to low-dose ketoconazole therapy. Am J Med 82:676–680

Bhasin S, Sikka S, Fielder T, Sod-Moriah U, Levine HB, Swerdloff RS, Rajfer J (1986) Hormonal effects of ketoconazole in vivo in the male rat: mechanism of action. Endocrinology 118:1229–1232

Black SD, Coon MJ (1986) Comparative structures of P-450 cytochromes. In: Ortiz de Montellano P (ed) Cytochrome P-450, structure, mechanism and biochemistry. Plenum, New York, p 161

Blyden GT, Abernethy DR, Greenblatt DJ (1986) Ketoconazole does not impair antipyrine clearance in humans. Int J Clin Pharmacol Ther Toxicol 24:225–226

Boobis AR, Brodie MJ, Kahn GC, Toverud GL, Blair IA, Murray S, Davies DS (1981) Comparison of the in vivo and in vitro rates of formation of the three main oxidative metabolites of antipyrine in man. Br J Clin Pharmacol 12:771–777

Brass C, Galgiani JN, Blaschke TF, Defelice R, O'Reilly RA, Stevens DA (1982) Disposition of ketoconazole, an oral antifungal, in humans. Antimicrob Agents Chemother 21:151–158

Britton H, Shehab Z, Lightner E, New M, Chow D (1988) Adrenal response in children receiving high doses of ketoconazole for systemic coccidiomycosis. J Pediatr 112:488–492

Brown MW, Maldonado AL, Meredith CG, Speeg KV (1985) Effect of ketoconazole on hepatic oxidative drug metabolism. Clin Pharmacol Ther 37:290–297

Burgess MA, Bodey GP (1972) Clotrimazole (Bay b5097): in vitro and clinical pharmacology studies. Antimicrob Agents Chemother 2:423–426

Burrin JM, Yeo TH, Ashby MJ, Bloom SR (1986) Effect of ketoconazole on adrenocorticotrophic hormone secretion in vitro and in vivo. J Endocrinol 108:37–41

Carvalho D, Pignatelli D, Resende C (1985) Ketoconazole for hirsutism. Lancet ii:560

Conney AH (1986) Induction of cytochrome P-450 enzymes: the first Bernard B. Brodie Lecture. Life Sciences 39:2493–2518

Contreras P, Altieri E, Liberman C, Gal A, Rojas A, Ibarra A, Ravanal M, Serum-Ferre M (1985a) Adrenal rest tumor of the liver causing Cushing's syndrome treatment with ketoconazole preceding an apparent surgical cure. J Clin Endocrinol Metab 60:21–28

Contreras P, Rojas A, Costamaillere L, Michelsen H, Pumarino H, Artega E (1985b) Endocrine effects of ketoconazole administration in 10 patients with Cushings syndrome. Proceedings of the 67th Annual Meeting of the Endocrine Society, Baltimore MD, p 112 (Abstract 550)

Daneshmend TK, Warnock DW, Eve MD, Johnson EM, Parker G, Richardson MD, Roberts CJC (1983) Multiple dose pharmacokinetics of ketoconazole and their effects on antipyrine kinetics in man. J Antimicrob Chemother 12:185–188

De Coster R, Beerens D, Dom J, Willemsens G (1984) Endocrinological effects of single daily ketoconazole administration in male beagle dogs. Acta Endocrinol 107:275–281

De Coster R, Caers I, Haelterman C, Debroye M (1985) Effect of a single administration of ketoconazole on total and physiologically free plasma testosterone and 17β-oestradiol levels in healthy male volunteers. Eur J Clin Pharmacol 29: 489–493

De Coster R, Haelterman C, Beerens D (1986) Effects of ketoconazole on the LH-RH induced testosterone biosynthesis in male beagle dogs. Ann Med Vet 130:431–438

De Coster R, Coene MC, Haelterman C, Beerens D, Goeminne N (1987) Effects of high-dose ketoconazole treatment on adrenal mineralocorticoid biosynthesis in dogs and rats. Acta Endocrinol 115:423–431

DeFelice R, Johnson DG, Galgiani JN (1981) Gynecomastia with ketoconazole. Antimicrob Agents Chemother 19:1073–1074

Deresinski SC, Galgiani JN, Stevens DA (1977) Miconazole treatment of human coccidioidomycosis: status report. In: Ajello L (ed) Coccidioidomycosis: current clinical and diagnostic status. Proceedings of the Third International Coccidioidomycosis Symposium, Tucson, Arizona 1976. Symposia Specialists, Miami, pp 257–292

Dieperink H, Møller J (1982) Ketoconazole and cyclosporine. Lancet ii:1217

D'Mello A, Satake M, Toda S, Takaya S, Ptachcinski RJ, Burckart GJ (1986) Cyclosporine-ketoconazole interaction in dogs. Pharm Res 3:Suppl 1545

D'Mello AP, D'Souza MJ, Bates TR (1985) Pharmacokinetics of ketoconazole-antipyrine interaction. Lancet ii:209–210

Doenicke A, Löffler B, Kugler J, Suttmann H, Grote B (1982) Plasma concentration and E.E.G. after various regimens of etomidate. Br J Anaesthesia 54:393–400

Engelhardt D, Dorr G, Jaspers CH, Knorr D (1985) Ketoconazole blocks cortisol secretion in man by inhibition of adrenal 11β-hydroxylase. Klin Wochenschr 63:607–612

English HF, Santner SJ, Levine HB, Santen RJ (1986) Inhibition of testosterone production with ketoconazole alone and in combination with a gonadotropin releasing hormone analogue in the rat. Cancer Res 46:38–42

Estabrook RW, Werringloer J (1978) The measurement of difference spectra: application to the cytochromes of microsomes. Fleischer S, Packer L (eds) Methods in enzymology, vol LII. Academic, New York, pp 212–221

Farwell AP, Devlin JT, Stewart JA (1988) Total suppression of cortisol excretion by ketoconazole in the therapy of the ectopic adrenocorticotropic hormone syndrome. Am J Med 84:1063–1066

Fellows IW, Bastow MD, Byrne AJ, Allison SP (1983) Adrenocortical suppression in multiply injured patients: a complication of etomidate treatment. Br Med J 287:1835–1837

Ferguson RM, Sutherland DER, Simmons RL, Najarian JS (1982) Ketoconazole, cyclosporin metabolism and renal transplantation. Lancet ii:882–883

Glynn AM, Slaughter RL, Brass C, D'Ambrosio RD, Jusko WJ (1986) Effects of ketoconazole on methylprednisolone pharmacokinetics and cortisol secretion. Clin Pharmacol Ther 39:654–659

Grosso DS, Boyden TW, Pamenter RW, Johnson DG, Stevens DA, Galgiani JN (1983) Ketoconazole inhibition of testicular secretion of testosterone and displacement of steroid hormones from serum transport protein. Antimicrob Agents Chemother 23:207–212

Guengerich FP (1988) Cytochromes P-450. Comp Biochem Physiol 89:1–4

Hajek KK, Cook NI, Novak RF (1982) Mechanism of inhibition of microsomal drug metabolism by imidazole. J Pharm Exp Ther 223:97–104

Heel RC, Brogden RN, Carmine A, Morley PA, Speight TH, Avery GS (1982) Ketoconazole: a review of its therapeutic efficacy in superficial and systemic fungal infections. Drugs 23:1–36

Heiberg JK, Svejgaard E (1981) Toxic hepatitis during ketoconazole treatment. Br Med J 283:825–826

Henry HL (1985) Effect of ketoconazole and miconazole on 25-hydroxyvitamin D_3 metabolism by cultured chick kidney cells. J Steroid Biochem 23:991–994

Heusner JJ, Franklin MR (1985) Inhibition of the 'non-classical' antifolate trimetrexate [2,4-diamino-5-methyl-6-(3,4,5-trimethoxy anilino)methyl/quinazole] by drugs containing an imidazole moiety. Pharmacology 30:266–272

Heykants J, Michiels M, Meuldermans W, Monbalin J, Lavrijsen K, Van Peer A, Levron JC, Woestenborghs R, Cauwenbergh G (1987) The pharmacokinetics of itraconazole in animals and man: an overview. In: Fromtling RA (ed) Recent trends in the discovery, development and evaluation of antifungal agents. JR Prous, Barcelona, pp 223–249

Heyns W, Drochmans A, van der Schueren E, Verhoeven G (1985) Endocrine effects of high dose ketoconazole therapy in advanced prostate cancer. Acta Endocrinol 110:276–283

Holland FJ, Fishman L, Bailey JD, Fazekas ATA (1985) Ketoconazole in the management of precocious puberty not responsive to LHRH-analogue therapy. N Engl J Med 312:1023–1028

Houston JB, Humphrey MJ, Matthew DE, Tarbit MH (1988) Comparison of two azole antifungal drugs, ketoconazole and fluconazole, as modifiers of rat hepatic monooxygenase activity. Biochem Pharmacol 37:401–408

Howden CW, Kenyon CJ, Beastall GH, Reid JL (1986) Inhibition by omeprazole of adrenocortical response to ACTH: clinical studies and experiments on bovine adrenal cortex in vitro. Clin Sci 70:99–102

Kahl R, Friederici DE, Kahe GF, Ritter W, Krebs R (1980) Clotrimazole as an inhibitor of benzo(a)pyrene metabolite-DNA adduct formation in vitro and of microsomal mono-oxygenase activity. Drug Metab Dispos 8:191–196

Kan PB, Hirst MA, Feldman D (1985) Inhibition of steroidogenic cytochrome P-450 enzyme in rat testis by ketoconazole and related imidazole antifungal drugs. J Steroid Biochem 23:1023–1029

Kapetanovic IM, Kupferberg HJ (1985) Inhibition of microsomal phenytoin metabolism by nafimidone and related imidazoles. Drug Metab Dispos 13:430–437

Kaul KL, Novak RF (1984) Induction of rabbit hepatic microsomal cytochrome P-450 by imidazole: enhanced metabolic activity and altered substrate specificity. Arch Biochem Biophys 235:470–481

Kowal J (1983) The effect of ketoconazole on steroidogenesis in cultured mouse adrenal cortex tumour cells. Endocrinology 112:1541–1543

Kraemer FB, Pont A (1986) Inhibition of cholesterol synthesis by ketoconazole. Am J Med 80:616–622

Kumaki K, Sato M, Kon H, Nebert DW (1978) Correlation of type I, type II, and reverse type I difference spectra with absolute changes in spin state of hepatic microsomal cytochrome P-450 iron from five mammalian species. J Biol Chem 253:1048–1058

Kwan JTC, Foxall PJD, Davidson DGC, Bending MR, Eisinger AJ (1987) Interaction of cyclosporin and itraconazole. Lancet ii:282

Lake-Bakaar G, Scheuer PJ, Sherlock S (1987) Hepatic reactions associated with ketoconazole in the United Kingdom. Br Med J 294:419–422

Lambert A, Mitchell R, Frost J, Ratcliffe JG, Robertson WR (1983) Direct in vitro inhibition of adrenal steroidogenesis by etomidate Lancet ii:1085–1086

Lambert A, Frost J, Mitchell R, Wilson AV, Robertson WR (1984) On the site of the anti-adrenal steroidogenic effect of etomidate and megestrol acetate. Clin Endocrinol 21:721–727

Lambert A, Mitchell R, Frost J, Robertson WR (1985a) A simple in vitro approach to the estimation of the biopotency of drugs affecting endocrine tissues. J Steroid Biochem 23:235–238

Lambert A, Mitchell R, Robertson WR (1985b) The effect of propofol, thiopentone and etomidate on adrenal steroidogenesis in vitro. Br J Anaesthesia 57:505–508

Lambert A, Mitchell R, Robertson WR (1985c) On the site of action of the anti-adrenal steroidogenic effect of cyproterone acetate. Biochem Pharmacol 34: 2091–2095

Lambert A, Frost J, Mitchell R, Robertson WR (1986a) On the assessment of the in vitro biopotency and site(s) of action of drugs affecting adrenal steroidogenesis. Ann Clin Biochem 23:225–229

Lambert A, Mitchell R, Robertson WR (1986b) The effect of ketoconazole on in vitro adrenal and testicular steroidogenesis. Biochem Pharmacol 35:3999–4004

Lambert A, Mitchell R, Robertson WR (1987) The biopotency and site of action of drugs affecting testicular steroidogenesis. J Endocrinol 113:457–461

Lamberts SWJ, Bons EG, Bruining HA, De Jong FH (1987) Differential effects of the imidazole derivatives etomidate, ketoconazole and miconazole and of metyrapone on the secretion of cortisol and its precursors by human adrenocortical cells. J Pharmacol Exp Ther 240:259–264

Lavrijsen K, Van Houdt J, Thijs D, Meuldermans W, Heykants J (1987) Interaction of miconazole, ketoconazole and itraconazole with rat liver microsomes. Xenobiotica 17:45–57

Ledingham IMcA, Watt I (1983) Influence of sedation on mortality in critically ill multiple trauma patients. Lancet i:1270

Lewis JH, Zimmerman HJ, Benson Gd, Ishak KG (1984) Hepatic injury associated with ketoconazole therapy. Gastroenterology 86:503–513

Liebman K (1971) Studies on modifiers of microsomal drug oxidation. Chem Biol Interactions 3:289–290

Liebman KC, Ortiz E (1973) New potent modifiers of liver microsomal drug metabolism: 1-arylimidazoles. Drug Metab Dispos 1:1495–1499

Loose DS, Kan PB, Hirst MA, Marcus RA, Feldman D (1983a) Ketoconazole blocks adrenal steroidogenesis by inhibiting cytochrome P-450-dependent enzymes. J Clin Invest 71:1495–1499

Loose DS, Stover DP, Feldman D (1983b) Ketoconazole binds to glucocorticoid receptors and exhibits glucocorticoid antagonist activity in cultured cells. J Clin Invest 72:404–408

Mailman RB, Kulkarni AP, Baker RC, Hodgson E (1974) Cytochrome P-450 difference spectra: effect of chemical structure on type II spectra in mouse hepatic microsomes. Drug Metab Dispos 2:301–307

Malozowski S, Mericq V, Cassorla F (1986) Effects of ketoconazole on rat steroidogenic enzymatic activities. Res Commun Chem Pathol Pharmacol 52:403–406

Mason JI, Murry BA, Olcott M, Sheets JI (1985) Imidazole antimycotics: inhibitors of steroid aromatase. Biochem Pharmacol 34:1087–1092

Meredith CG, Maldonado AL, Speeg KV (1985) The effect of ketoconazole on hepatic oxidative drug metabolism in the rat in vivo and in vitro. Drug Metab Dispos 13:156–162

Mosca P, Bohazzi P, Novelli G, Jezequel AM, Orlandi F (1985) In vivo and in vitro inhibition of hepatic microsomal drug metabolism by ketoconazole. Br J Exp Pathol 66:737–742

Murray M, Wilkinson CF, Hetnarski K (1985) Cytochrome P-450 and monooxygenase activity in hepatic microsomes from N-phenylimidazole-treated rats. Toxicol Lett 25:191–198

Namer M, Khater R, Frenay M, Boublil JL (1986) High dose of ketoconazole in the treatment of advanced breast cancers. Bull Cancer 73:89

Niemeegers CJE, Levron JCL, Awouters F, Janssen PAJ (1981) Inhibition and induction of microsomal enzymes in the rat. A comparative study of four antimycotics:

miconazole, econazole, clotrimazole and ketoconazole. Arch Int Pharmacodyn Ther 251:26–38

Ortiz de Montellano P (1986) (ed) Cytochrome P-450: structure, mechanism and biochemistry. Plenum, New York

Palmer ED, Cawthorne MA (1974) The effects of 1-alkylimidazoles on hepatic drug-metabolising enzyme activity. Xenobiotica 4:209–221

Pont A, Trachtenberg J (1984) Hormonal changes in patients on chronic high dose ketoconazole. Clin Res 32:271A

Pont A, Williams PL, Azhar S, Reitz RE, Bochra C, Smith ER, Stevens DA (1982a) Ketoconazole blocks testosterone synthesis. Arch Int Med 142:2137–2140

Pont A, Williams PL, Loose DS, Feldman D, Reitz RE, Bochra C, Stevens DA (1982b) Ketoconazole blocks adrenal steroid synthesis. Ann Int Med 97:370–372

Pont A, Graybill JR, Craven PC, Galgiani JM, Dismukes WE, Reitz RE, Stevens DA (1984) High dose ketoconazole therapy and adrenal and testicular function in humans. Arch Int Med 144:2150–2153

Purba HS, Back DJ (1986) Effect of fluconazole (UK-49,858) on antipyrine metabolism. Br J Clin Pharmacol 21:603P

Rajfer J, Sikka SC, Xie HW, Swerdloff RS (1985) Effect of in vitro ketoconazole on steroid production in rat testis. Steroids 46:867–881

Rajfer J, Sikka SC, Rivera F, Handelsman DJ (1986) Mechanism of inhibition of human testicular steroidogenesis by oral ketoconazole. J Clin Endocrinol Metab 63:1193–1198

Razzouk C, Agazzi-Leonard E, Cumps J, Pondelet F, Mercier M, Roberfroid M (1978) Induction, modification and inhibition of rat liver microsomal benzo(a)-pyrene hydroxylase; correlation with the S-9-mediated mutagenicity of benzo(a)-pyrene. Biochem Biophys Res Commun 85:1007–1016

Reader SCJ, Davison B, Ratcliffe JG, Robertson WR (1985) Measurement of low concentrations of bovine thyrotrophin by iodide uptake and organification in porcine thyrocytes. J Endocrinol 106:13–20

Ritter JK, Franklin MR (1987) Induction and inhibition of rat hepatic drug metabolism by N-substituted imidazole drugs. Drug Metab Dispos 15:335–343

Robertson WR, Reader SCJ, Davison B, Frost J, Mitchell R, Kayte R, Lambert A (1985) on the biopotency and site of action of drugs affecting endocrine tissues with special reference to the anti-steroidogenic effect of anaesthetic agents. Postgrad Med J 61:145–151

Rochlitz CF, Damon LE, Russi MB, Geddes A, Cadman EC (1988) Cytotoxicity of ketoconazole in malignant cell lines. Cancer Chemother Pharmacol 21:319–322

Rodrigues AD, Gibson GG, Ioannides C, Park DV (1987) Interactions of imidazole antifungal agents with purified cytochrome P-450 proteins. Biochem Pharmacol 36:4277–4281

Rodrigues AD, Waddell PR, Ioannides C (1988) Inhibition of the rat hepatic mixed-function oxidases by in vivo administration of clotrimazole. Res Commun Chem Pathol Pharmacol 59:403–406

Rogerson TD, Wilkinson CF, Hetnarski K (1977) Steric factors in the inhibitory interaction of imidazoles with microsomal enzymes. Biochem Pharmacol 26: 1039–1042

Santen RJ, Vanden Bossche H, Symoens J, Brugmans J, De Coster R (1983) Site of action of low dose ketoconazole on androgen biosynthesis in men. J Clin Endocrinol Metab 57:732–736

Schellens JHM, Van Der Wart JHF, Danhof M, Van Der Velde EA, Briemer DD (1988) Relationship between the metabolism of antipyrine, hexobarbital and theophylline in man as assessed by a 'cocktail' approach. Br J Clin Pharmacol 26:373–384

Schenkman JB, Remmer H, Estabrook RW (1967) Spectral studies of drug interaction with hepatic microsomal cytochrome. Mol Pharmacol 3:113–123

Schoene et al. (1973) Unpublished data cited in: Bolt HM, Kappus H (1973) Effect of clotrimazole treatment on the demethylation of mestranol. Hormone Metab Res 5:234

Schürmeyer T, Nieschlag E (1984) Effect of ketoconazole and other imidazole fungicides on testosterone biosynthesis. Acta Endocrinol (Copenh) 105:275–280
Schuster I (1985) The interaction of representative members from two classes of antimycotics – the azoles and the allylamines – with cytochromes P-450 in steroidogenic tissues and liver. Xenobiotica 15:529–546
Schuster I (1988) Potential of allylamines to inhibit cytochrome P-450. In: Fromtling RA (ed) Recent trends in the discovery, development and evaluation of antifungal agents. JR Prous, Barcelona, pp 471–478
Scott J, Drew R (1983) Interaction of imidazole drugs with hepatic cytochrome P-450 dependent enzymes. Clin Exp Pharm Pharmacol 10:679–680
Shaw JTB, Tarbit MH, Troke PF (1988) Cytochrome P-450 mediated sterol synthesis and metabolism: differences in sensitivity of fluconazole and other azoles. In: Fromtling RA (ed) Recent trends in the discovery, development and evaluation of antifungal agents. JR Prous, Barcelona, pp 125–140
Shaw MA, Gumbleton M, Nicholls PJ (1987) Interaction of cyclosporin and itraconazole. Lancet ii:637
Sheets JJ, Mason JI (1984) Ketoconazole: a potent inhibitor of cytochrome P-450-dependent drug metabolism in rat liver. Drug Metab Dispos 12:603–606
Sheets JJ, Mason JI, Wise CA, Estabrook RW (1986) Inhibition of rat liver microsomal cytochrome P-450 steroid hydroxylase reactions by imidazole antimycotic agents. Biochem Pharmacol 35:487–491
Shepherd FA, Hoffert B, Evans WK, Emery G, Trachtenberg J (1985) Ketoconazole. Use in the treatment of ectopic adrenocorticotrophic hormone and Cushing's syndrome in small cell lung cancer. Arch Int Med 145:863–864
Sikka SC, Swerdloff RS, Rajfer J (1985) In vitro inhibition of testosterone biosynthesis by ketoconazole. Endocrinology 116:1920–1925
Smith AG (1984) Potentiation of oral anti-coagulants by ketoconazole. Br Med J 288:188–189
Sonino N, Brownie AC (1987) Inhibition of aldosterone production by ketoconazole in vitro. Med Sci Res 15:853–854
Sonino N, Boscaro M, Merola G, Mantero F (1985) Prolonged treatment of Cushing's disease by ketoconazole. J Clin Endocrinol Metab 61:718–722
Tettenborn D (1974) Toxicity of clotrimazole. Postgrad Med J 50 (Suppl):17
Thienpont D, Van Cutsen J, Van Gerven F, Heeres J, Janssen PAJ (1979) Ketoconazole: a new broad spectrum orally active antimycotic. Experientia 35:606–607
Thompson RG, Rawlins MD, James OFW, Wood P, Williams F (1988) The acute and subchronic effects of ketoconazole on hepatic microsomal monooxygenase in the rat. Biochem Pharmacol 37:403–406
Trachtenberg J (1984) Ketoconazole therapy in advanced prostatic cancer. J Urol 132:61–63
Trachtenberg J, Pont A (1984) Ketoconazole therapy for advanced prostate cancer. Lancet ii:433–435
Trachtenberg J, Zadra J (1988) Steroid synthesis inhibition by ketoconazole: sites of action. Clin Invest Med 11:1–5
Trenk D, Brett W, Jahnchen E, Birnbaum D (1987) Time course of cyclosporin interaction. Lancet ii:1335–1336
Van Cauteren H, Heykants J, De Coster R, Cauwenbergh G (1987) Itraconazole: pharmacologic studies in animals and humans. Rev Inf Dis 9:S43–S45
Vanden Bossche H (1987) Itraconazole: a selective inhibitor of the cytochrome P-450 dependent ergosterol biosynthesis. In: Fromtling RA (ed) Recent trends in the discovery, development and evaluation of antifungal agents. JR Prous, Barcelona, pp 207–221
Vanden Bossche H, Lauwers W, Willemsens G, Cools W (1985) The cytochrome P-450 dependent C17,20-lyase in subcellular fractions of the rat testis: differences in sensitivity to ketoconazole and itraconazole. In: Boobis AR, Caldwell J, De Matteis F, Elcombe CR (eds) Microsomes and drug oxidations. Taylor and Francis, London, pp 63–73

Vanden Bossche H, Bellens D, Cools W, Gorrens J, Marichal P, Verhoeven H, Willemsens G, De Coster R, Beerens D, Haelterman C, Coene M-C, Lauwers W, Le Jeune L (1986) Cytochrome P-450: target for itraconazole. Drug Dev Res 8:287–298

Vawda AI, Davies AG (1986) An investigation into the effect of ketoconazole on testicular function in Wistar rats. Acta Endocrinol (Copenh) 111:246–251

Watanabe H, Menzies JA (1985) Depression of ovarian estradiol-17β following single oral dose of ketoconazole. Res Commun Chem Pathol Pharmacol 48:141–144

Watanabe H, Menzies JA (1986) Effect of single dose ketoconazole on ovarian steroids. Res Commun Chem Pathol Pharmacol 54:271–274

Waxman DJ, Ko A, Walsh C (1983) Regioselectivity of androgen hydroxylations catalysed by cytochrome P-450 isozymes purified from phenobarbital-induced rat liver. J Biol Chem 258:11937–11947

Wenta H (1974) Clinical studies with oral clotrimazole. Postgrad Med J 50 (Suppl):85

Wilkinson CF, Hetnarski K, Yellin TO (1972) Imidazole derivatives – a new class of microsomal enzyme inhibitors. Biochem Pharmacol 21:3187–3192

Wilkinson CF, Hetnarski K, Cantwell GP, Di Carlo FJ (1974) Structure-activity relationships in the effects of 1-alkylimidazoles on microsomal oxidation in vitro and in vivo. Biochem Pharmacol 23:2377–2386

Wilkinson CF, Hetnarski K, Denison MS, Guengerich FP (1983) Selectivity of 1-phenylimidazole as a ligand for cytochrome P-450 and as an inhibitor of microsomal oxidation. Biochem Pharmacol 32:997–1003

Williams G, Kerle DJ, Ware H, Doble A, Dunlop H, Smith C, Allen J, Yeo T, Bloom SR (1986) Objective response to ketoconazole therapy in patients with relapsed prostatic cancer. Br J Urol 58:45–51

Yamamoto TU, Urabe M, Okada H (1987) Inhibitory effect of miconazole on aromatase activity for androstenedione in human placental and ovarian preparations. Bosmoku Gijutsu 36:1379–1385

Yoshida Y, Aoyama Y (1986) Interaction of azole fungicides with yeast cytochrome P-450 which catalyzes lanosterol 14-demethylation. In: Iwata K, Vanden Bossche H (eds) In vitro and in vivo evaluation of antifungal agents. Elsevier, Amsterdam, pp 125–134

CHAPTER 9

Structure-Teratogenicity Relationships Among Antifungal Triazoles

OLIVER P. FLINT and F. THOMAS BOYLE

A. Introduction

Following the observation that the antifungal agent ketoconazole was teratogenic in rats (SYMOENS and CAUWENBERGH 1983), we identified the triazole antifungal ICI 153,066 also as a teratogen in the rat (FLINT and BOYLE 1985). In an effort to elucidate structure-activity relationships, we tested 16 further monotriazoles for in vitro antifungal activity and for toxicity using a simple short-term in vitro test, the micromass teratogen test (FLINT and ORTON 1984; FLINT 1987). The processes of mammalian embryogenesis and cell differentiation are retained in vitro so that an inhibition of cell differentiation is an indication that there may be a potential risk of teratogenicity in vivo (FLINT 1987). Four monotriazoles with widely differing activity in the micromass test were investigated in the rat and good correlation found between in vivo teratogenicity and in vitro inhibition of cell differentiation (FLINT and BOYLE 1985). A correlation was also found between the water-octanol partition coefficient (log P) of the 16 monotriazoles and their in vitro anti-*Candida* and anti-differentiation activities. We have now extended this work to 35 monotriazole and 35 bistriazole compounds in a study which highlights differences between the two structural types and considers the role of substituents in determining teratogenic hazard.

Selected compounds were subsequently tested for teratogenicity in the rat to investigate the significance of the in vitro results.

B. Materials and Methods

All compounds were synthesised at ICI, Alderley Park; structures are indicated in Tables 1 and 2. Log P was determined experimentally by standard methods (MIRLEES et al. 1976) and by calculation based on the methods of FUJITA et al. (1964), HANSCH and LEO (1979) and LEWIS et al. (1983a,b).

Candida albicans B2630 was grown at 37°C in yeast nitrogen base broth in the presence of 3- or 10-fold serial dilutions of the compounds under test. Growth was measured using a nephelometer and compound activity expressed as IC_{50C}, the concentration in nmoles/ml which reduced growth to 50% of that in the control.

For the micromass in vitro teratogen test (described in detail by FLINT and ORTON 1984; FLINT 1987), embryos of 34–36 somites were removed from pregnant Alderley Park (Alpk:APfSD) albino rats 13 days after conception. Forelimbs and midbrains were dissected free, and following enzymatic dissociation, single cell suspensions were adjusted to give 5×10^6 midbrain and 2×10^7 limb cells/ml. Cell suspensions were initially plated out as five 10 µl drops per Falcon Primaria (35 mm) culture dish. After 2 h cells adhered to the substratum, forming micromass cell islands of 6–8 mm diameter. Excess medium containing test compound or vehicle control (0.5% v/v DMSO) was added. Normally there were 7 separate concentrations of test compound, no further apart than one log dose, as well as the vehicle control. Cultures were incubated at 37°C for 5 days in an atmosphere of 5% CO_2/air.

During the 5-day incubation period a proportion of the midbrain cells differentiated as numerous foci of neurones staining darkly with haematoxylin, while limb cells produced foci of mucopolysaccharide-secreting chondrocytes staining blue with alcian blue 8GX. The stained foci were counted as regions of high contrast using an automated image analyser. Counts of differentiated foci were compared in treated and control cultures. IC_{50T} in nmoles/ml of compound inhibiting differentiation by 50% of control values was determined from individual dose-response curves. The product moment correlation coefficients (r) of log P (independent parameter) versus IC_{50C} or IC_{50T} (transformed as 1/log IC_{50}) were calculated. The significance of each correlation coefficient at the 0.5% level was determined from published tables. For a limited number of compounds cytotoxicity was measured using a neutral red assay (GIRLING and FLINT 1984). The cell survival curve for concentration versus cytotoxicity was compared with the concentration versus inhibition of cell differentiation curve to determine whether cell differentiation was inhibited at concentrations which did not affect cell survival. We consider a specific inhibition of mammalian embryo cell differentiation in vitro to indicate some risk of teratogenicity in vivo.

Sighting teratology studies in pregnant Alderley Park rats were done with 7 representative bistriazoles. Rats in groups of 5 were dosed orally over days 6–15 of pregnancy using at least three dose levels of compound, selected so that the top dose either terminated pregnancy or was maternally toxic (statistically significant reduction in weight gain compared with control or death of at least one animal). Rats were killed on day 20 and foetuses examined for any abnormalities. Maternal weight gains, number of foetuses, foetal weights and placental weights were recorded.

C. Results

I. In Vitro Assays

The concentration-response profiles (Figs. 1 and 2) for compound 8 were typical of those observed with all mono- and bistriazoles described in this chapter. Midbrain (CNS) cell survival and differentiation were affected to

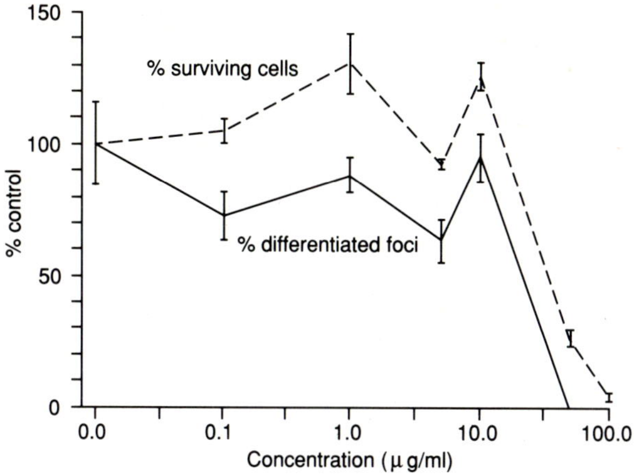

Fig. 1. Differentiation and survival of rat embryo midbrain (CNS) cells exposed to compound 8 for 5 days of culture

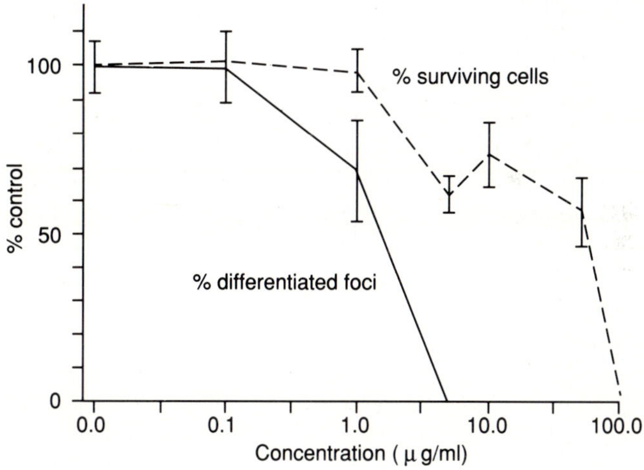

Fig. 2. Differentiation and survival of rat embryo limb (LB) cells exposed to compound 8 for 5 days of culture

similar degrees over all concentrations tested. Limb bud (LB) cell differentiation was typically affected at lower concentrations than those affecting cell survival. In the case of compound 8, the IC_{50} for cell differentiation was approximately 100-fold lower than that for cell survival (Fig. 2).

The IC_{50} for limb cell differentiation (IC_{50T}) was derived from the plotted data for each compound; these data (in nM/ml) are given in Tables 1 and 2 along with the IC_{50}s for anti-*Candida* activity (IC_{50C}) and the log P for each compound. The IC_{50}s for midbrain cell survival and differentiation and limb

Table 1. Monotriazole tertiary alcohols: the effect of substituent type and position on IC_{50T} and IC_{50C}

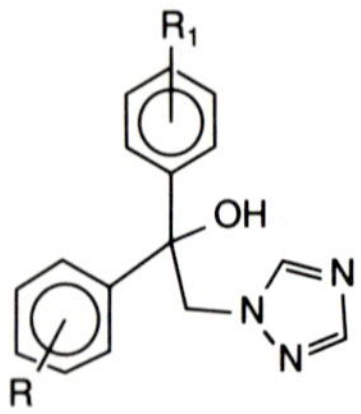

Compound	R	R_1	IC_{50T}[a]	IC_{50C}[a]	log P
1	4CN	4CN	142.70	14.12	−0.49
2	$4NO_2$	$4NO_2$	98.50	10.72	0.09
3	$3NO_2$	H	1.29	123.03	0.37
4	$4NO_2$	H	1.61	0.13	0.37
5	H	H	2.26	3.02	0.65
6	4F	H	2.82	1.23	0.79
7	4F	4F	23.23	0.13	0.93
8	4F	2,4F	6.58	0.08	1.07
9	4Cl	$4NO_2$	2.90	0.08	1.09
10	$4CH_3$	H	1.81	0.21	1.21
11	$2CH_3$	H	14.32	1.26	1.21
12	2,4F	2,4F	19.27	1.58	1.29
13	4Cl	H	13.34	0.56	1.37
14	4F	3Cl	1.26	0.69	1.52
15	2F	4Cl	12.59	0.23	1.52
16	4F	4Cl	3.15	0.22	1.52
17	$3CF_3$	H	0.30	10.23	1.59
18	$2CH_3$	$4CH_3$	7.84	0.89	1.77
19	2,4F	$4CF_3$	48.74	0.12	1.81
20	4F	$2F,4CF_3$	67.80	0.24	1.81
21	$2Cl,5NO_2$	H	3.77	128.82	1.98
22	4Cl	4Cl	14.79	0.15	2.08
23	4F	2Cl	0.005	0.08	2.40
24	$4CF_3$	$4CF_3$	37.38	0.56	2.47
25	4F	2Cl,4F	8.94	0.08	2.54
26	2Cl	4Cl	0.15	0.01	2.97
27	2,4Cl	H	2.69	0.02	2.97
28	4F	2,4Cl	0.57	0.02	3.11
29	2F	2,4Cl	0.06	0.03	3.11
30	4F	2Br	0.17	0.19	3.26
31	2Cl	2,4Cl	0.22	0.16	3.29
32	4Cl	2,4Cl	1.91	0.0027	3.67
33	3Cl	2,4Cl	3.26	0.0026	3.67
34	4Cl	2Br	5.28	0.03	3.80
35	$4OCF_2CF_2H$	H	0.16	0.02	4.17

[a] Figures are in nM/ml.

Table 2. Bistriazole tertiary alcohols: the effect of substituent type and position on IC_{50T} and IC_{50C}

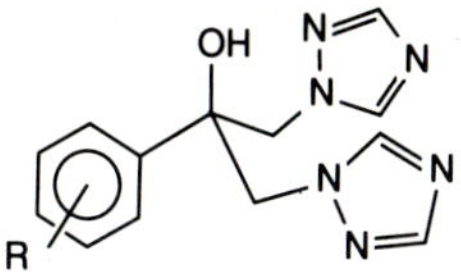

Compound	R	IC_{50T}[a]	IC_{50C}[a]	log P
36	4CN	>1000	31.49	−0.35
37	$4OCH_3$	199.76	268.00	0.20
38	H	166.46	103.58	0.22
39	$2CH_3,4CN$	194.20	87.40	0.23
40	4F	173.42	26.01	0.33
41	2,6F	81.62	107.41	0.44
42	$2CN,4CF_3$	NE	78.44	0.47
43	$2CH_3$	52.94	95.29	0.60
44	2,4,6F	NE	35.46	0.66
45	2,3,5,6F	759.59	87.64	0.78
46	$4CH_3$	352.92	13.76	0.78
47	$4SCH_3$	94.93	90.18	0.90
48	$2CF_3$	88.67	103.45	0.90
49	3Cl	131.25	541.39	0.93
50	4Cl	114.84	3.02	0.93
51	2Cl	85.31	3.05	0.93
52	2Cl,4F	61.96	3.25	0.96
53	4F,4Cl	108.44	1.61	0.96
54	$2CF_3,4F$	177.43	60.05	0.98
55	$4CH = CH_2$	47.24	22.94	1.05
56	$2CH_3,4F$	56.23	100.88	1.10
57	$4OCF_3$	169.33	0.56	1.13
58	$4CF_3$	413.80	3.25	1.15
59	$2OCH_3,4CF_3$	325.77	28.50	1.17
60	$2F,4CF_3$	617.42	1.26	1.29
61	$3F,4CF_3$	477.10	84.19	1.29
62	4[4CNPh]	NE	80.71	1.32
63	$4OCF_2CF_2H$	7.78	77.85	1.44
64	2,4Cl	17.69	0.74	1.53
65	$2Cl,4CF_3$	174.37	0.86	1.85
66	4Ph	NE	13.28	2.22
67	4[2,4FPh]	117.80	18.85	2.46
68	40Ph	NE	2.88	2.73
69	4[4ClPh]	131.28	7.19	2.91
70	4[4ClPhO]	118.83	0.94	3.21
71	2F,4F	130.72	1.97	0.44

[a] Figures are in nM/ml.
NE, not evaluated.

Table 3. Product moment correlation coefficients for IC_{50} versus log P. Values in brackets indicate the approximate probability of the correlation given having arisen by chance

	IC_{50T}/log P	IC_{50C}/log P
Monotriazoles	0.24 ($P > 0.05$)	0.05 ($0.01 > P > 0.001$)
Bistriazoles	0.01 ($P > 0.1$)	0.24 ($P > 0.05$)

cell survival were not considered in the analysis of structure-activity relationships, since limb cell differentiation was the parameter most sensitive to the effect of each compound. The IC_{50}s for limb cell differentiation and anti-*Candida* activity are plotted against log P in Figs. 3–6. Excluding inactive compounds, IC_{50T} and IC_{50C} values ranged over several orders of magnitude – from 0.005 to 759.59 nM/ml and from 0.0026 to 541.39 nM/ml, respectively. Log P values also ranged over several orders of magnitude (−0.35 to 4.17). The median value for monotriazole log P (1.77) was slightly higher than for bistriazole log P (0.96), but there was a considerable overlap of the ranges (Tables 1 and 2). The median values of IC_{50T} were considerably higher for bis- (131.25 nM/ml) than for monotriazoles (3.15 n*M*/ml), as were the median values for bistriazole IC_{50C} (28.50 nM/ml) when compared with monotriazole IC_{50C} (0.19 nM/ml). Correlation coefficients for IC_{50} versus log P are given in Table 3. Taking values of P less than 0.05 as indicative of a statistically significant correlation, only monotriazole IC_{50C} appears to have a strong relationship with log P.

II. In Vivo Teratogenicity

Three monotriazoles (compounds, 2, 28 and 32) and 7 bistriazoles (compounds 50, 51, 57, 58, 60, 64 and 65) with IC_{50T}s ranging from 0.57 to 617 nM/ml were evaluated in the rat for teratogenicity. A high IC_{50T} was taken to be indicative of low potential teratogenicity. The compounds and the results obtained are listed in Tables 4 and 5.

1. Monotriazole Tertiary Alcohols

The in vitro teratogenicity of ICI 153,066 (compound 28, Table 4) was typical of the monotriazole antifungals; dose-related increases in embryo toxicity (number of live foetuses/resorptions) and maternal toxicity (reduced weight gain) were observed in the rat from 5 mg/kg. Soft tissue and skeletal abnormalities were observed at and above 2.5 mg/kg. The number of abnormalities and percentage of foetuses affected increased with dose. At 2.5 mg/kg only cleft palate was observed, while above this dose cranial and facial structures were principally and increasingly involved, leading to microstomia, macroglossia, ablepharia, hydrocephalus, reduction of the lower jaw, loss of the hyoid bone, loss of pinnae and absence of middle ear bones. Limb ab-

Table 4. Maternal and foetal toxicity data for substituted monotriazole tertiary alcohols

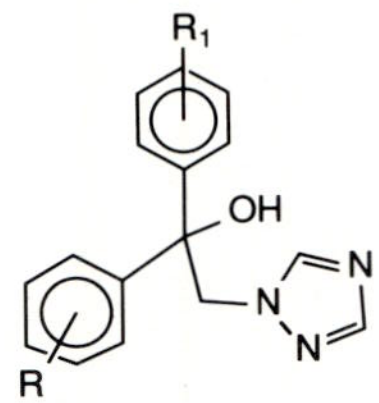

Compound	R	R_1	Dose (mg/kg)	Number dosed	Maternal weight gain[a]	Number of foetuses[a]	Foetal[a] weight	Number of embryos with teratological abnormalities
2	$4NO_2$	$4NO_2$	10	16	92.4	87	99.1	0/158
			25	16	92.5	89	92.2	0/162
28	4F	2,4Cl	5	5	77.8	56.7	83.8	12/38 (32%)
			10	5	68.4	40.3	78.8	21/27 (78%)
32	4Cl	2,4Cl	10	5	87.4	59.7	97.4	0/40
			20	5	57.6	16.0	67.9	0/11

[a] as percentage of control.

Table 5. Maternal and foetal toxicity data for substituted bistriazole tertiary alcohols

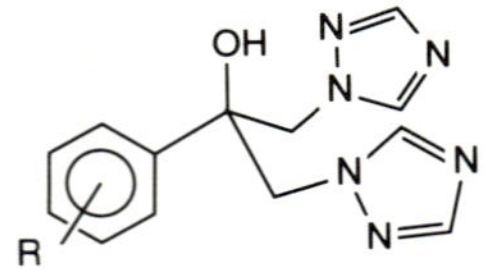

Compound	R	Dose (mg/kg)	Number dosed	Maternal weight gain[a]	Number of foetuses[a]	Foetal[a] weight	Number of embryos with teratological abnormalities
64	2,4Cl	10	10	74.4	69.5	90.2	8/85 (9%)
		25	9	87.9	72.7	77.2	80/80 (100%)
51	2Cl	25	12	102.6	100.9	98.4	9/148 (6%)
		50	10	85.4	66.4	86.6	39/81 (48%)
50	4Cl	25	13	99.1	88.3	96.3	38/141 (27%)
		50	13	81.7	55.1	90.5	33/88 (38%)
57	$4OCF_3$	25	5	90.7	76.0	80.4	0/30
		50	5	58.2	60.0	74.4	0/37
65	$2Cl,4CF_3$	10	5	91.5	71.0	83.5	0/44
		30	5	76.5	67.7	71.2	5/42 (12%)
58	$4CF_3$	50	10	82.0	60.1	90.6	0/66
		100	8	81.8	68.3	87.8	0/67
60	$2F,4CF_3$	50	5	77.6	70.0	73.5	0/44
		100	4	61.2	39.7	64.5	0/20

[a] as percentage of control.
Maternal weight gain over days 0–20 for 58 control rats was 133.57 ± 9.32 g; the average litter size was 12.26 ± 1.35, and the average foetal weight was 3.44 ± 0.12 g.

normalities (loss of digits) were only observed at a dose of 25 mg/kg. ICI 153,066 was therefore teratogenic at a dose (2.5 mg/kg) which was not toxic to the dam, although most teratogenic malformations were observed at maternally toxic doses. The defects are, however, compound-related and not part of the syndrome of abnormalities conventionally associated with drug-related maternal toxicity (KHERA 1984).

2. Bistriazole Tertiary Alcohols

For compounds 64 (2,4Cl, Table 5) and 51 (2Cl), 10 and 25 mg/kg and 25 and 50 mg/kg were the only doses tested. Compound 50 (4Cl) was tested at 25, 50, 100 and 250 mg/kg, but the 100 and 250 mg/kg doses were substantially embryotoxic and did not permit evaluation for teratological abnormalities. Compound 57 ($4OCF_3$) was tested at doses of 25, 50, 75 and 100 mg/kg; 75 mg/kg terminated 8/10 pregnancies, while 100 mg/kg was lethal to 1/5 dams and terminated pregnancy in the survivors. Compound 65 (2Cl, $4CF_3$) was tested at 10, 30 and 100 mg/kg; 100 mg/kg was lethal to 5/5 dams. Compound 58 ($4CF_3$) was tested at 25, 50, 100, 200, 300 and 400 mg/kg in groups of 10 rats; 200 mg/kg was lethal to 5/10, and higher doses were lethal to all dams treated. With compound 60 (2F, $4CF_3$), tested at doses of 1, 2.5, 5, 10, 25, 50, 100 and 125 mg/kg, maternal and embryo toxicity were not observed below 50 mg/kg, but 100 and 125 mg/kg terminated pregnancy in 1/5 and 4/5 cases, respectively.

Cranial and facial anomalies were nearly always found to be associated after exposure to these compounds at teratogenic doses. As with the monotriazoles, these malformations included cleft palate, macroglossia, microstomia, hydrocephalus, ablepharia and agnathia. With compounds 64 and 51, digital anomalies – reduced digital size with compound 51 at 50 mg/kg, and syndactyly with compound 64 at 10 mg/kg – were also observed. Compounds 50, 51 and 64 caused abnormalities at doses which did not significantly affect maternal weight gain or foetal weight and did not cause maternal death. Compound 65 caused abnormalities at 30 mg/kg, but significant dose-related maternal and foetal toxicity were also observed at this and at the lower dose of 10 mg/kg (Table 5). Compounds 57, 58 and 60 did not cause foetal abnormalities at any dose tested, up to and including maternal and foetotoxic doses.

D. Discussion

At the in vitro level, the complexity of a compound-target tissue interaction (in this case fungal or limb bud cell) and the intensity of compound effect depend to a large extent on the concentration of drug in the active phase; the duration of the compound effect is determined by its persistence in sufficient concentration at the receptor site. Rat embryo limb cells are rich in cytochromes P-450 capable of significant metabolic activation (BROWN et al. 1986;

FLINT and BROWN 1987), whereas azole antifungal activity is initiated by the inhibition of the cytochrome P-450-dependent $C_{14}\alpha$-demethylation involved in ergosterol biosynthesis (VANDEN BOSSCHE et al. 1983). It is possible that inhibition of embryo cell differentiation and the antifungal activity of the triazoles are mediated by similar receptor molecules. In the former case the embryo cytochrome P-450 activates the triazole forming a toxic metabolite, and in the latter the triazole binds to the fungal cytochrome P-450, inhibiting its function.

Limited correlations of in vitro potency in a standard environment with in vivo activity against *C. albicans* within tight structural subseries of mono- and bistriazoles have already been reported (BOYLE et al. 1987). Information required to aid structure-toxicity relationships is less often described, because toxicity is normally only assessed in vivo, creating a demand for testing that exceeds the limited available resource of an integrated research programme. Further complicating these analyses, particularly for the azoles, is the host's metabolic capacity (liver/placenta) to modify the structural integrity of the dosed compound. This can markedly affect the levels of bioavailable material, since both inhibition and induction of target/host P-450 systems are the prime locus of intervention. Notwithstanding this, the in vivo teratogenicity of selected monotriazoles has been briefly described, and a correlation found between in vivo teratogenicity and in vitro toxicity using the micromass teratogen test (FLINT and BOYLE 1985).

As part of a continuing programme of antifungal research, the initial monotriazole series has been extended, and a second series of bistriazole molecules has been included. They differ structurally, in their physicochemical characteristics (log P, solubility), and hence would be expected to show markedly different properties.

I. Monotriazole Tertiary Alcohols

Analysis of this more lipophilic series of compounds is complicated by the substitution potential of both aromatic nuclei. For these 35 examples, antifungal activity (*C. albicans* IC_{50C}) shows a highly significant correlation with log P (Fig. 3; $P > 0.01$), whereas inhibition of limb cell differentiation (IC_{50T}) shows little dependency (Fig. 4). Earlier data (FLINT and BOYLE 1985) for a smaller set of 16 compounds had suggested that such a correlation was possible; however, this has not been substantiated following the addition of 19 extra examples to the data set. Since HANSCH (1969) first established a systematic approach to determination of quantitative structure-activity relationships (QSARs), the octanol-water partition coefficient (log P) has been the parameter most often compared with molecular activity(VEITH et al. 1985; HANSCH 1985, 1989; SCHULTZ and RIGGIN 1985; TANII et al. 1986). In the case of this class of azoles, antifungal activity is clearly strongly related to their solubility in lipid cell membranes and affinities for lipophilic intracellular P-450 receptors.

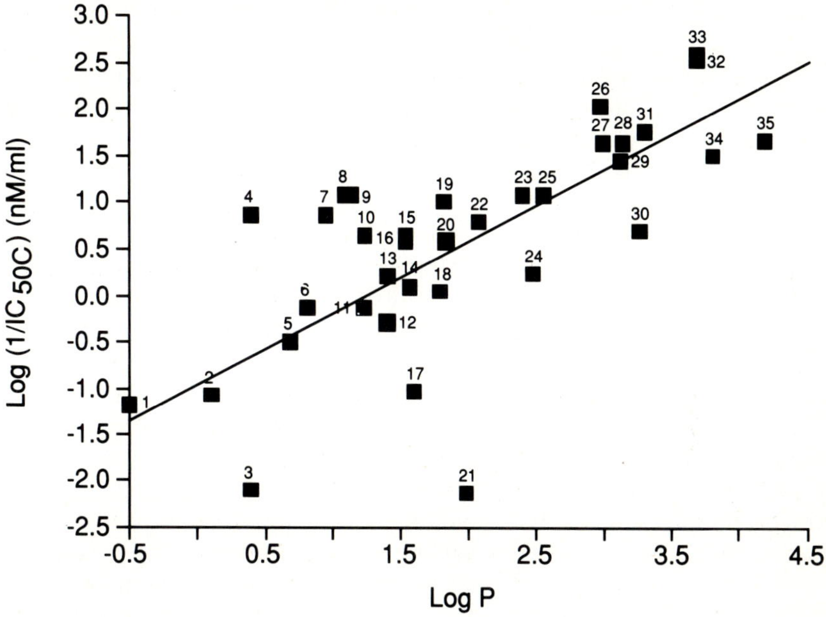

Fig. 3. Effect of log P on monotriazole antifungal activity (IC_{50C})

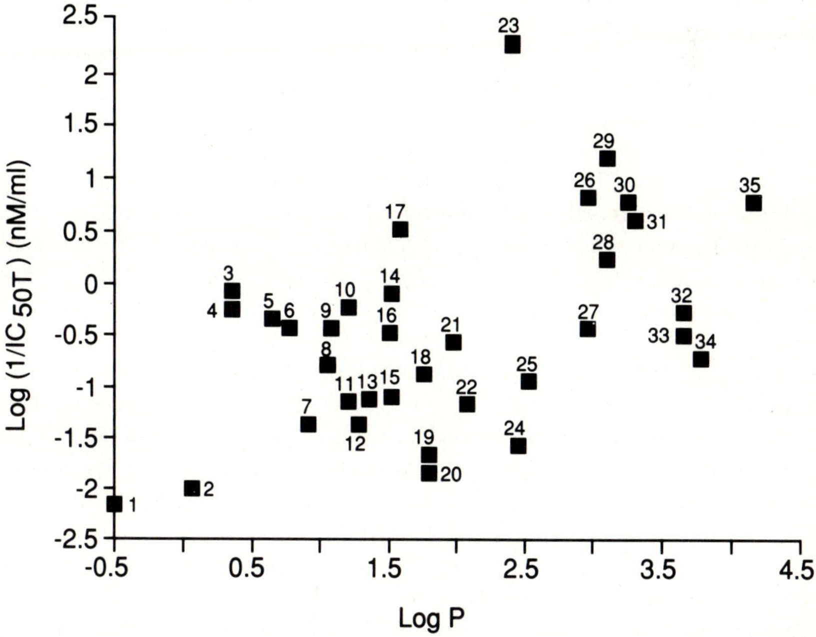

Fig. 4. Effect of log P on monotriazole inhibition of rat embryo limb cell differentiation in vitro (IC_{50T})

Since log P did not generally correlate with IC_{50T}, the monotriazoles were examined for the influence of both substituent type and position. All examples addressing these issues together with their biological data and log P are presented in Table 1. However, before considering this, the following general observations are noteworthy. In the monotriazoles, log P is exquisitely sensitive to changes in steric crowding at the tertiary alcohol centre. The effect is typically illustrated by compounds 22 vs 26 and 32 vs 31, where log P increases of about 0.9 and about 0.4 result from 2-chloro substitution. Presumably, increased crowding or intramolecular hydrogen bonding reduces the ability of the tertiary alcohol to hydrogen bond to bulk water.

Simple monosubstituted monotriazoles (e.g. compounds 4, 6, 11, 13, 27 and 35) show little if any significant change in IC_{50T}. This is irrespective of log P and probably reflects metabolic activation of the unsubstituted aromatic nucleus to the P-450-mediated epoxidase/hydroxylase systems of the embryonic limb cells (FLINT and BROWN 1987). Antifungal activity of this subset of compounds shows the expected increase with log P, except for the 3/5 substituted examples (compounds, 3, 17 and 21) where a much lower activity is observed, probably reflecting a suboptimal fit of these derivatives within the cytochrome P-450 enzyme complex. IC_{50T} for the 4,4′CN (compound 1) and 4,4′NO_2 (compound 2) derivatives with log Ps of around 0 or less clearly show the lowest activity. Relationships between electronic field effects of these substituents and toxicity have been reported (HILLEBRAND et al. 1977; TORANZO et al. 1977; KATIYAR and GUPTA 1982; RICHTER et al. 1983; SCHULTZ and RIGGIN 1985). However, in this case the weak activity in these compounds is more likely due to either the low log P of the molecules or their susceptibility to metabolic attack to produce hydrophilic or ionized molecules (acid, amide or amine). These would in turn not bind easily to a hydrophobic receptor and thus not constitute a toxic threat.

The hypothesis that metabolism of the phenyl ring is necessary for inhibition of embryo cell differentiation and that bulky or metabolically stable *para*-substituents generally prevent this is further substantiated in this series. Compounds 7, 12, 20 and 24, *para*-substituted with fluorine or CF_3, all have high IC_{50T}s compared with their congeners (e.g. compounds 31 and 32). When the subseries of compounds *para*-substituted in one ring and *ortho*-substituted in the second one are compared with their *para*-substituted counterparts (e.g. compounds 31 vs 32, 28 vs 29, 22 vs 26), significant differences in IC_{50T} of one to two orders of magnitude are observed. Clearly metabolic activation of the exposed *para* position increases the potential toxic hazard in these compounds. The *ortho* effect, responsible for profound changes in antifungal efficacy with the bistriazoles, is also apparent in this series but is somewhat more variable in nature. In the more sterically hindered examples 31 (2,4Cl:2Cl) and 32 (2,4Cl:4Cl), much the expected response is observed (IC_{50C} 0.016 versus 0.003 nM/ml), whereas in the less hindered examples 23 (2Cl:4F) and 16 (4Cl:4F) the opposite response is found (IC_{50C} 0.08 versus 0.22 nM/ml).

Three monotriazoles with IC_{50T}s in the range 0.57 (compound 28, ICI 153,066) to 98.5 nM/ml (compound 2) were selected for preliminary in vivo teratology studies.

II. Bistriazole Tertiary Alcohols

This more hydrophilic series of 36 compounds provides a simpler analysis since only one aromatic nucleus is available for substitution. Conventional plots of log P against log in vitro antifungal activity and inhibition of limb cell differentiation for all compounds are shown in Figs. 5 and 6. Statistical analysis confirms the superficial observation that no overall worthwhile correlation exists for either activity ($P > 0.1$ and 0.05 for IC_{50T} and IC_{50C}, respectively). However, they do appear to fall within two subgroups. In the smaller group, comprising 4-substituted aryl and aryloxy derivatives (66–70), it is conceivable that an alternative binding mode is adopted within the cytochrome P-450 enzyme complex, leading to a different structure-activity pattern. The larger group consists of more conventional substituents, and while log P did not generally correlate with either activity, subseries of compounds could be identified which illustrate the consequences of both substituent type and position in the aromatic nucleus on biological activity.

All compounds together with the biological data and log P are presented in Table 2. Bistriazoles are intrinsically poor inhibitors of the growth of *C.*

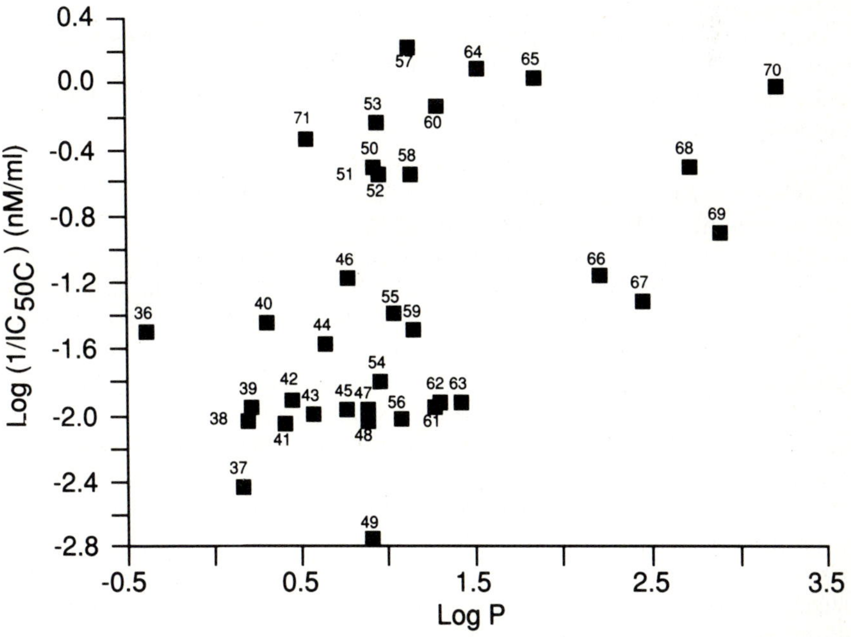

Fig. 5. Effect of log P on bistriazole antifungal activity (IC_{50C})

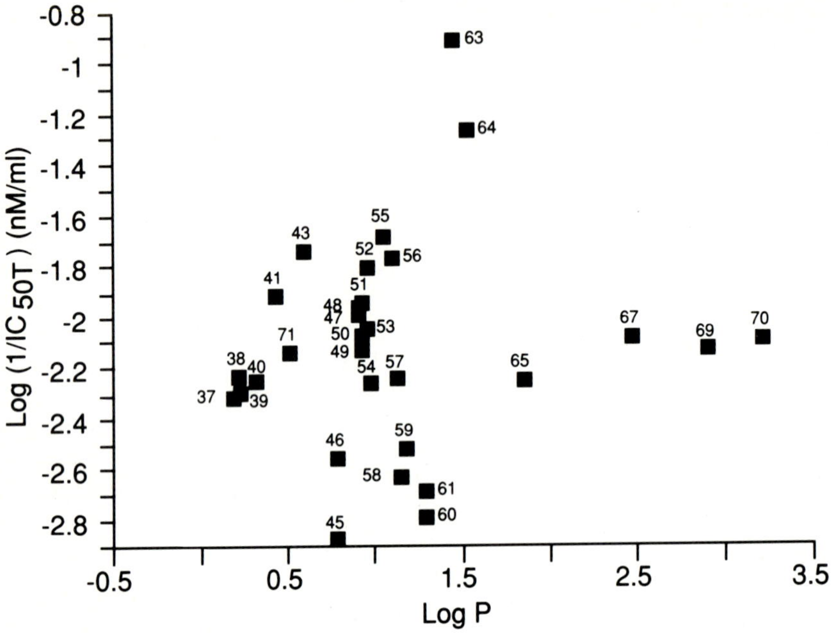

Fig. 6. Effect of log P on bistriazole inhibition of rat embryo limb cell differentiation in vitro (IC_{50T})

albicans and limb cell differentiation in vitro, a property almost certainly due to their hydrophilic character (log P of parent compound 38 is 0.22). *Ortho*/*para* halogen substitution generally increases the activity in both biological systems in parallel, suggesting some commonality in the mechanism of inhibition. However, a major disconnection in this pattern occurs when substitution by metabolically stable carbon or oxygen functionalities is effected. Thus while the $4CF_3$ (compound 58), $4CF_3$,2F (compound 60) and $4CF_3$,2Cl (compound 65) forms continue to give increased potency against *C. albicans*, they are significantly worse inhibitors of limb cell differentiation. On the basis of the reported metabolic capacity of the embryo limb cells and the relatively higher log P in these systems, the hypothesis of metabolic activation of the aromatic ring leading to embryo toxicity was proposed. Both F and CF_3 substituents are known to protect aromatic nuclei from metabolic attack by cytochrome P-450 in hepatic microsomes or hepatocytes (WILEY et al. 1979; NELSON 1982) and would tend to be supported by the observation that the *para* F or CF_3 compounds have higher IC_{50T}s than their congeners. While its IC_{50T} is predictable, compound 59 ($4CF_3$,2-OCH_3) does not fit this pattern; it is significantly worse against *C. albicans*. This observation is consistent with a change in the intramolecular hydrogen bonding of the tertiary alcohol centre (from triazole to methoxy) resulting in a suboptimal conformation of the molecule within the P-450 $C_{14}\alpha$-demethylase complex (MORRIS, personal communication). The strict conformational requirement for P-450 binding leading to good antifungal activity is further substantiated by the results of the 2,6F (compound 41) and 4F,2CF_3 (compound 54) derivatives. Here buttressing by the two fluorines or the bulky CF_3 again leads to poorer inhibitors. For this series, the optimal compound would appear to be the 2F,4CF_3 derivative (compound 60), in which near maximal antifungal activity is linked to a minimal potential for embryo toxicity. Subsequent in vivo studies supported this selection.

III. Correlation Between IC_{50T} and In Vivo Teratogenicity

Attempts to correlate the in vitro potency in the micromass assay with in vivo teratogenicity in the rat impose several extra barriers to expression of the compound-active site interaction. Evidence of high levels of metabolic capacity in the embryo cell have already been referred to. These are further complicated by such factors as rates of absorption, the manner and volumes of distribution, levels of lipid and protein binding, subsequent rate and route of elimination and in this case protection of the foetus by the placenta. An earlier study (Flint and Boyle 1985) did suggest a direct correlation between IC_{50T} and the lowest dose causing abnormalities in the rat foetus for four monotriazoles (ICI 153,066, compound 28; ICI 159,265, compound 2; ICI 166,175 and ICI 163,334). In vitro and in vivo data for the latter two compounds have been omitted from this discussion because their structures were too disparate from the basic monotriazole. Because the mono- and bistriazoles present differing structural and physicochemical characteristics, representative examples from each were subjected to preliminary in vivo teratogenic assessments.

1. Monotriazole Tertiary Alcohols

This series of compounds, which includes ICI 153,066 (compound 28) and its 4,4′ dinitro analogue (compound 2) with IC_{50T}s of 0.57 and 98.5 nM/ml, respectively, was extended by the inclusion of the 4Cl:2,4Cl analogue (compound 32, Table 6). With an IC_{50T} of 1.91 nM/ml we fully expected to see the standard profile of teratology described for ICI 153,066 in the Results section. Interestingly, as with compound 2 at doses up to 20 mg/kg in the rat, this compound was not teratogenic. Significant foetotoxicity at this level prevented dose escalation studies. One is forced to conclude that in this case either a disconnection of the in vitro-in vivo relationship exists, or some mechanism is in place, protecting the developing foetus from toxic exposure. Two clues exist. The higher log P of compound 32 would result in modulated pharmacodynamic behaviour, e.g. higher volume of distribution or protein binding. Perhaps of more importance, however, is that it would also result in an increased metabolic susceptibility of the molecule. 4-Chloro stability to the host's epoxidase/hydroxylase enzyme systems would then give compounds

Table 6. Teratogenicity in vivo/IC_{50T} correlation for monotriazole tertiary alcohols

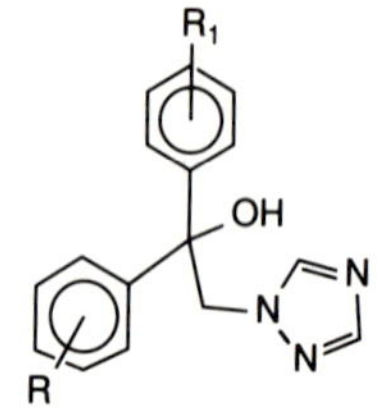

Compound	R	R_1	Lowest teratogenic dose (mg/kg)	IC_{50T} (nM/ml)	Log P
2	$4NO_2$	$4NO_2$	>25	98.50	0.09
28	2,4Cl	4F	2.5–5	0.57	3.11
32	2,4Cl	4Cl	>20	1.91	3.67

Table 7. Teratogenicity in vivo/IC_{50T} correlation for bistriazole tertiary alcohols

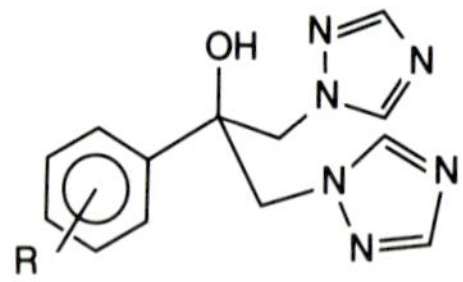

Compound	R	Lowest teratogenic dose (mg/kg)	IC_{50T} (nM/ml)	log P
64	2,4Cl	10	17.69	1.53
51	2Cl	25	85.31	0.93
50	4Cl	25	114.84	0.93
71	2,4,F	NF[a]	130.72	0.44
57	$4OCF_3$	NF	169.33	1.13
65	$2Cl,4CF_3$	NF[a]	174.37	1.85
58	$4CF_3$	NF	413.80	1.15
60	$2F,4CF_3$	NF	617.42	1.25

NF indicates that no teratogenic dose was found up to the first dose showing statistically significant maternal and foetal toxicity.
[a] Although foetal abnormalities were observed with these compounds, they were only seen at doses causing significant maternal and foetal toxicity.

presenting a less toxic threat to the developing foetus. The compound was, however, subsequently shown to be a teratogen in the rabbit at 7.5 and 15 mg/kg.

2. Bistriazole Tertiary Alcohols

Seven compounds were selected for in vivo teratogenicity studies with IC_{50T}s in the range 17–617 nM/ml. These, together with data for the 2,4F analogue (compound 71, fluconazole) are summarised in Table 7; data for fluconazole are taken from TACHIBANA et al. (1987). All compounds tested in vivo with an IC_{50T} below about 115 nM/ml caused dose-related increases in foetal abnormalities at doses at which no maternal or foetal toxicity was observed. The syndrome was similar to that observed with the monotriazoles and is presented in the Results section.

For bistriazoles with an IC_{50T} greater than about 115 nM/ml tested in vivo, two scenarios exist. The first, exemplified by compounds 65 and 71 (IC_{50T}s 174 and 130), showed foetal abnormalities but only at maternal and foetal toxic doses; the second, exemplified by compounds 57, 58 and 60 (IC_{50T}s about 170, 410 and 617 nM/ml), showed no foetal abnormalities up to and including maternal and foetal toxic doses. In these latter examples, particularly compounds 58 and 60, optimum separation of antifungal activity and teratogenicity has been achieved.

E. Conclusions

The purpose of any in vitro-in vivo correlation study is to allow the development of predictive rules which guide and aid the identification of novel chemical structures. In this study, two series of highly active antifungals have been highlighted, and limited overall in vitro-in vivo teratogenicity correlations have been developed. Data have been presented supporting the hypothesis that toxic metabolites produced within the embryonic limb cell may be responsible for the observed teratogenicity. In the bistriazoles, compounds *para*-substituted with metabolically stable substituents (F, CF_3, OCF_3) have been developed which prevent such metabolic activation; these in turn are not teratogenic in vivo. In the monotriazoles the picture is less clear due to the size of the data set.

Log P has a variable effect on both biological responses; in the more hydrophilic bistriazoles, while showing some consistent trends, log P does not correlate overall with either IC_{50C} or IC_{50T}. The monotriazoles correlate well for antifungal potency, but the in vitro micromass assay does not correlate overall with log P. Here again subset analysis allows the identification of substituents and trends which can lead to the generation of antifungal agents of low teratogenic risk. The value of this type of study will only become apparent when the data sets are extended and this type of analysis is applied to other structural series. Perhaps then some of the more subtle trends in structure-teratogenicity relationships can be discussed with confidence.

References

Boyle FT, Ryley JF, Wilson RG (1987) In vitro-in vivo correlations with azole antifungals. In: Fromtling RA (ed) Recent trends in the discovery, development and evaluation of antifungal agents. JR Prous, Barcelona, pp S1:31–S1:41

Brown LP, Flint OP, Orton TC, Gibson GG (1986) In vitro metabolism of teratogens by differentiating rat embryo cells. Food Chem Toxicol 24:737–742

Flint OP (1987) An in vitro test for teratogens using cultures of rat embryo cells. In: Atterwill CK, Steele CE (eds) In vitro methods in toxicology. Cambridge University Press, Cambridge, pp 339–363

Flint OP, Boyle FT (1985) An in vitro test for teratogens: its application in the selection of non-teratogenic triazole antifungals. Concepts in Toxicology 3:29–35

Flint OP, Brown LP (1987) Metabolism of teratogens by mammalian embryos: an in vitro investigation. In: Nau H, Scott WJ (eds) Pharmacokinetics in teratogenesis, vol II. CRC Press, Boca Raton, pp 133–144

Flint OP, Orton TC (1984) An in vitro assay for teratogens with cultures of rat embryo midbrain and limb bud cells. Toxicol Appl Pharmacol 76:383–395

Fujita T, Iwasa J, Hansch C (1964) A new substituent constant, π, derived from partition coefficents. J Am Chem Soc 86:5175–5180

Girling L, Flint OP (1984) Inhibition of embryonic-cell differentiation by teratogens in vitro: quantification using ELISA (enzyme linked immunosorbent assay). Hum Toxicol 3:155–156

Hansch C (1969) A quantitative approach to biochemical structure-activity relationships. Acc Chem Res 2:232–239

Hansch C (1985) The QSAR paradigim in the design of less toxic molecules. Drug Metab Rev 15:1279–1294

Hansch C (1989) Comparative structure-activity relationships. In: Fauchère JL (ed) Progress in clinical and biological research, vol 291, QSAR: quantitative structure-activity relationships in drug design. Liss, New York, pp 23–30

Hansch, C Leo A (1979) Substituent constants for correlation analysis in chemistry and biology. Wiley-Interscience, New York

Hillebrand M, Sahini VE, Volanschi E (1977) Electronic structure of the chlorobenzenes in connection with their biological activity. Buletinul Institutului Politehnic 'Gheorghe Gheorghiu-Dej" Bucuresti 39:27–32

Katiyar M, Gupta SP (1982) Synthesis and fungitoxicity of some 1,3-di-(substituted phenyl) thioureas. Philippine J Sci 3:65–70

Khera KS (1984) Maternal toxicity – a possible factor in fetal malformations in mice. Teratology 29:411–416

Lewis SJ, Mirlees MS, Taylor PJ (1983a) Rationalizations among heterocyclic partition coefficients. Part 1: The π-value of phenyl. Quant Struct Act Relationships 2:1–6

Lewis SJ, Mirlees MS, Taylor PJ (1983b) Rationalizations among heterocyclic partition coefficients Part 2: The azines. Quant Struct Act Relationships 2:100–111

Mirlees MS, Moulton SJ, Murphy CT, Taylor PJ (1976) Direct measurement of octanol-water partition coefficients by high-pressure liquid chromatography. J Med Chem 19:615–619

Nelson SD (1982) Metabolic activation and drug toxicity. J Med Chem 25:753–765

Richter JE, Peterson SF, Kleiner C (1983) Acute and chronic toxicity of some chlorinated benzenes, chlorinated ethanes and tetrachlorethylene to *Daphnia magna*. Arch Environ Contam Toxicol 12:679–684

Schultz TW, Riggin GW (1985) Predictive correlations for the toxicity of alkyl- and halogen-substituted phenols. Toxicol Lett 25:47–54

Symoens J, Cauwenbergh G (1983) Ketoconazole, a new step in the management of fungal disease. Prog Drug Res 27:63–84

Tachibana M, Noguchi Y, Monro AM (1987) Toxicology of fluconazole in experimental animals. In: Fromtling RA (ed) Recent trends in the discovery, development and evaluation of antifungal agents. JR Prous, Barcelona, pp 93–102

Tanii H, Tsuji H, Hashimoto K (1986) Structure-toxicity relationship of monoketones. Toxicol Lett 30:13–17

Toranzo EG, Gillessi T, Mendenhall M, Traiger GJ, Riley PG, Hanzlik RP, Wiley RA (1977) Effect of substituents on arene oxide-mediated liver toxicity among substituted bromobenzenes. Toxicol Appl Pharmacol 40:415–425

Vanden Bossche H, Willemsens G, Cools W, Marichal P, Lauwers WF (1983) Hypothesis on the molecular basis of the antifungal activity of N-substituted imidazoles and triazoles. Biochem Soc Trans 11:665–667

Veith GD, De Foe D, Knuth M (1985) Structure-activity relationships for screening organic chemicals for potential ecotoxicity effects. Drug Metab Rev 15:1295–1303

Wiley RA, Hanzlik RP, Gillesse T (1979) Effects of substituents on in vitro metabolism and covalent binding of substituted bromobenzenes. Toxicol Appl Pharmacol 49:249–255

CHAPTER 10

Formulation

HEINZ HÄNEL and WOLFGANG RITTER

A. Introduction

Once a compound has demonstrated outstanding antifungal activity in laboratory experiments, thought needs to be given to how it might be formulated for clinical use since the nature of the formulation can have a considerable effect on the ultimate efficacy of the compound. It might be thought that oral treatment would present few problems, but with poorly soluble compounds such as griseofulvin or itraconazole, such factors as particle size or solution in a suitable vehicle can have profound effects on the extent to which the compound is absorbed and so exerts its antifungal effects. Most antifungal drugs have limited water solubility, and if the compound is to be administered intravenously to seriously ill patients, a safe and suitable way of formulating the substance in an appropriate vehicle will need to be devised. Recent experience with amphotericin B and liposome formulations has demonstrated how tricks of formulation can reduce potential toxicity without affecting antifungal activity and thus increase the utility of the compound. It is in the area of topical formulation that most scope exists for presenting the compound in a way in which it will reach the fungus, persist until it has done its job and yet not be absorbed into the general circulation in dangerous quantities.

B. Topical Formulations

I. Skin Infections

Topical treatment of fungal infections requires the presentation of the drug in a suitable vehicle. The active constituent must dissolve in the vehicle and diffuse to the upper layer of the stratum corneum in order to penetrate it. The substance may then form a depot in the horny layer or further diffuse into the live epidermis. Here the compound can be metabolised or bound to receptors. Further diffusion leads to the dermis in which the compound again may be metabolised, bound to receptors or diffuse. The active ingredient from there can reach the vascular system. Further diffusion now takes the compound to the fatty tissues which present an additional possibility of forming a depot. In terms of precise definitions, a few mechanisms should be carefully distinguished: adsorption as a physicochemical binding to the skin, absorption as a physicochemical uptake into different layers of the skin, penetration as a general mechanism of going into the skin and permeation as passing through the skin to be taken up by the vascular system (SCHAEFER et al. 1975).

Depending on the class of substance used, the number of hair follicles and sweat glands per unit of surface area may be crucial to penetration. The influence of the vehicle on the extent and rate of penetration is often underestimated. Flux through the skin and the permeability coefficient have been found to be inversely dependent on the drug solubility in the vehicle (SLOAN et al. 1986). This means that each antifungal substance has to be used in specific vehicles of different composition, depending on the site (scalp, trunk, nails, etc.) to which it is to be applied (SCHEUPLEIN and ROSS 1974; WASHITAKE et al. 1975). A number of techniques have been developed to measure penetration rates, but only a few have been found to provide relevant and universally valid results.

1. Penetration Studies

In view of the sparseness of hair on the human skin the excised skin of hairless mice has been widely used for penetration studies. The function of the stratum corneum as a barrier could be verified by separating the epidermis and dermis (FLYNN et al. 1981). However, the possibilities of using the skin of hairless mice are limited due to the fact that the morphology and biophysical properties are very different from those of human skin. After more than 3 days of hydration, the skin of hairless mice exhibits signs of mechanical destruction which leads to a higher penetration rate. In contrast to this, even after several days of hydration, human skin is not damaged in such a way (BOND and BARRY 1988a). There is no correlation either between human skin and hairless mouse skin in the effectiveness of penetration promoters such as azones, dimethyl sulphoxide, oleic acid and polyethylene glycol (BOND and BARRY 1988b). Practical problems have been encountered in studies using the skin of particularly hairy animals. Comparative studies performed with topical administration of radioactive substances to rats, rabbits, pigs and humans showed that pig skin is most similar to human skin as far as penetration is concerned (BARTEK et al. 1972; VAN SCOTT 1972). The skin of hairy animals exhibits a markedly higher permeation rate caused by the number of hair follicles per unit surface area (MARZULLI et al. 1969). Injured skin shows a higher permeation rate than intact skin as demonstrated in a rat model by SCOTT and DUGARD (1986). Topical formulations should be evaluated in normal skin since mechanical damage leads to lack of reproducibility. Abraded skin should only be used if the influence of heavy inflammation is to be investigated (Tables 4,5).

Human skin has been used for a long time as a model system for testing drug formulations. As early as 1951 PINKUS modified the thickness of the stratum corneum by repeated stripping. In vivo studies demonstrated that the loss of keratinized cells served as a stimulus for proliferation (PINKUS 1952). For testing antimycotics, it was possible either to inoculate the adhesive tapes used for stripping (KNIGHT 1973a,b) or to infect the skin itself. The persistence of topical antifungals could be quantitated by prophylactic application to human volunteers subsequently challenged with *Trichophyton mentagrophytes*. An average of 96% of the infections were successful in humans. Stripped stratum corneum layers proved to be a valuable alternative to human trials, except in the case of tolnaftate. This method showed that the penetration characteristics of a particular substance may not be adequately predicted by inoculation studies with stripped stratum corneum.

Excised human skin was widely used for permeation studies because some of the biophysical parameters of these can be directly extrapolated to in vivo conditions (FRANZ 1975; SOUTHWELL and BARRY 1983). As late as 30 h after excision, the kinetics of incorporation of radioactive thymidine were still comparable with those in living skin, indicating its metabolic stability (OEHMICHEN et al. 1988). Penetration studies with radiolabelled oxiconazole were performed by STÜTTGEN and BAUER (1985) using skin obtained at mastectomy and abdominal skin from cadavers. These studies showed that azoles are primarily absorbed via hair follicles. Although the model using excised human skin has been optimised in many ways (BENNETT and BARRY 1986; DITTMAR and JOVIĆ 1980; KINSMAN and COLLARD 1986; KLIGMAN et al. 1987), we have replaced human skin by pig skin because of ethical problems and because of variable reproducibility of results obtained with human skin (DITTMAR 1985). In addition, seasonal differences in the skin of hairy mammals make it difficult to obtain reproducible results (JOHNSON 1977). Due to the relevance of hair follicles to the permeation of some antimycotics, pig skin may also be regarded as a valuable alternative to human skin. REIFENRATH et al. (1984) also found a good correlation between the penetration into pig skin and that into human skin ($r = 0.83$); they recorded similar excretion rates of radiolabelled substances in urine and faeces. Because of this and other research on the similarity of both skin types (BISSETT and MCBRIDE 1985), the optimised method for testing topical antifungals on pig skin in vitro will be described in detail (see DITTMAR and JOVIĆ 1987; HÄNEL et al. 1988).

In conclusion, once percutaneous absorption of an azole antifungal *and* the plasma levels of unchanged drug in the systemic circulation after topical application of a formulation are known in humans, this particular formulation can serve as a reference in animal experiments. Generally, percutaneous absorption in the rabbit is far greater than in other species (SCHALLA and SCHAEFER 1982), and therefore extrapolation of rabbit data to humans without such a standard is impossible. Percutaneous absorption of sulconazole, for example, was 30%–40% in rabbits (BENFIELD and CLISSOLD 1988) and 11%–12% in humans (FRANZ and LEHMANN 1988; BENFIELD and CLISSOLD 1988).

a) Test for Penetration

A layer 3 mm thick of subcutaneous fatty tissue is left on the back of the excised skin of non-scalded slaughtered pigs. After rough shaving, the skin is rolled up with the fatty layer out, wrapped in moist filter paper and deep frozen in airtight plastic bags at −40°C. Comparative studies have shown the freezing procedure to have no adverse effect on permeation kinetics, particularly with pig skin (PITMAN and ROSTAS 1982; PITMAN and DOWNES 1982; SWARBRICK et al. 1982). When required for use, the pig skin is thawed under running water, the layer of subcutaneous fatty tissue is removed with a scalpel and the surface of the skin is thoroughly shaved. Each piece of skin is covered on both sides with filter paper soaked in 99% isopropanol and left to dry for 20–30 min at room temperature. It is then cut into pieces 5 × 3 cm. The pieces of skin are placed on 1% aqueous agar containing 0.01% penicillin, 0.01% streptomycin and 0.01% actidione and kept over-night in a refrigerator at 3°–5°C. On the following morning the pieces of skin are dabbed dry with sterile filter paper. Using instruments sterilised and kept in 70% ethanol, the skin pieces are removed from the agar plates and laid on three layers of sterile filter paper stuck to a dissection board. They are rubbed dry with sterile filter paper and sealed on all four edges with adhesive tape. Using 0.1–0.2 ml in each case, the formulation is applied to the surface and rubbed in with a finger protected with a finger stall; in the case of lacquer formulations a brush is used. During the contact time, the length of which varies depending on the study, the skin pieces are laid on an open water agar plate and placed in an incubator at 29°C. At the end of the contact time, the skin pieces are removed from the incubator, rubbed dry with sterile filter paper and washed four times; the washing procedure consists of dabbing alternately with moist and dry filter paper. The corners of each piece of skin are secured with pins to the dissection board, and each piece is halved with a scalpel so that only the epidermis and the upper part of the dermis is cut through. Both halves are repeatedly stripped using adhesive tape, one half being stripped more than the other. The number of layers of stratum corneum removed increases with the number of stripping procedures done; ten strippings are sufficient to lay bare the living non-hornified layers of the epidermis. The skin pieces are then transferred to water agar plates at room temperature. A 6-week-old culture of *T. mentagrophytes* grown on a malt agar slope is harvested using 0.5 ml water containing 2 drops of 2% Tylose. The turbid suspension is filtered through cotton wool to remove mycelia. One inoculation point made with a platinum wire on an agar plate should contain 50–100 microconidia. Ten inoculation points around 0.8 mm diameter are made with the suspension on each half of each piece of skin. The skin pieces in the water agar plates are placed for 20–30 min under laminar flow to allow the inoculation points to dry. The plates are then closed and incubated at 28°C. Fungal growth is checked every day using a stereoscopic microscope and scored. The extent of growth is a measure of the amount of drug which has penetrated to that particular depth in the skin exposed by stripping. Experiments with human and pig skin and a

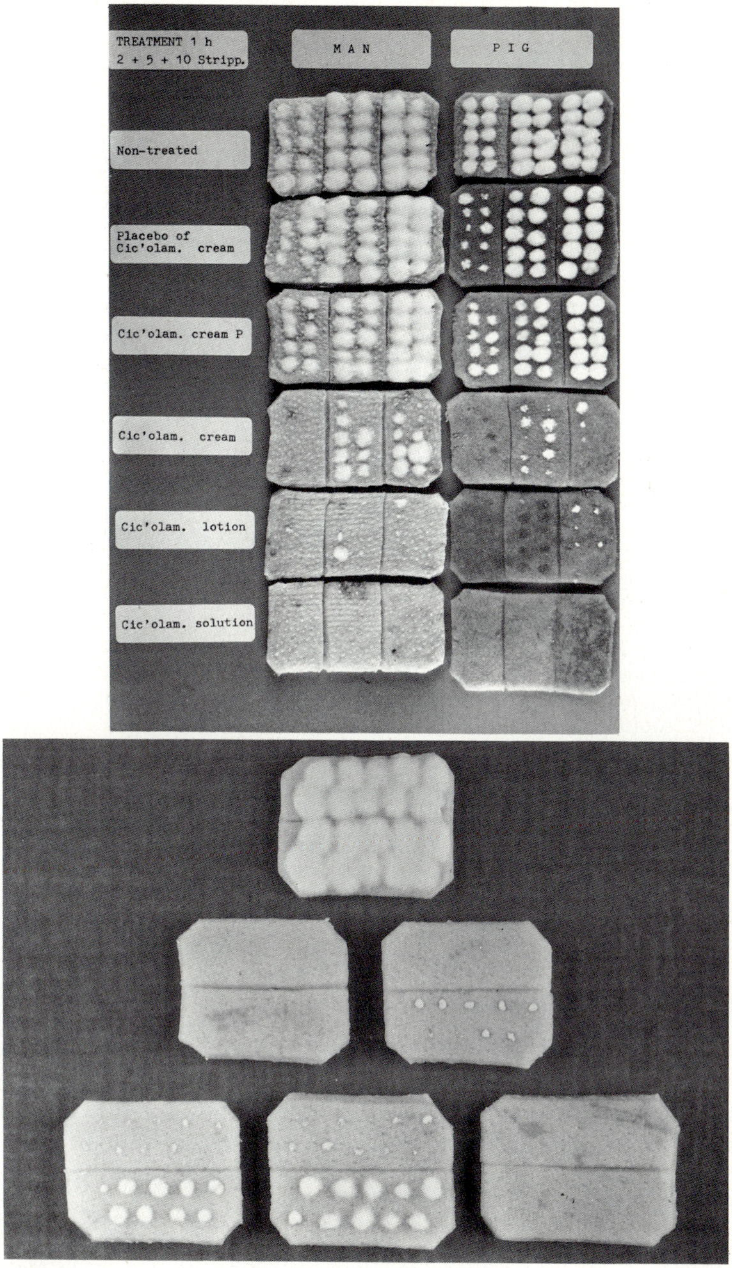

Fig. 1. Skin penetration studies with antifungals. (*top*) Comparison of various formulations of ciclopirox olamine (*Cic'olam*) on human and pig skin; *left side* of each piece of skin stripped twice, the *centre part* 5 times and the *right side* 10 times (after DITTMAR 1985). (*bottom*) Comparison of various antimycotic solutions on pig skin with 1 h treatment; *upper half* of each skin piece stripped twice, *lower half* stripped 6 times; *top row* solvent control; *centre row*, naftifine (*left*), tolnaftate (*right*); *lower row*, oxiconazole (*left*), clotrimazole (*middle*), ciclopirox olamine (*right*)

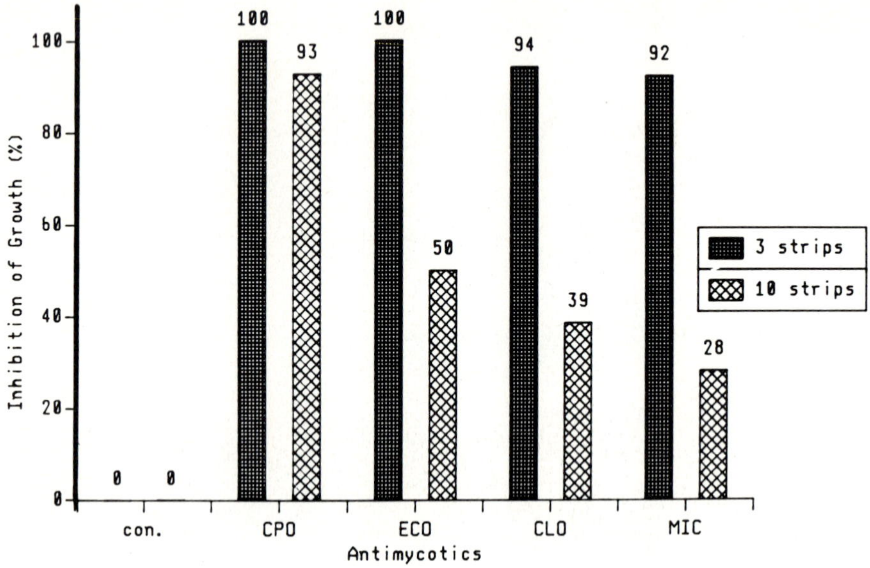

Fig. 2. Inhibitory activity of antifungal creams ciclopirox olamine (*CPO*), clotrimazole (*CLO*) and econazole (*ECO*), each at 1%, miconazole (*MIC*) 2% tested against *Trichophyton mentagrophytes* on pig skin with 3 h exposure, mean of 3 experiments. Modified from Hänel et al. (1988)

number of antifungal preparations are illustrated in Fig. 1. Comparison of growth on treated and untreated skin allows quantitative estimations to be made of penetration of antifungal activity between different formulations of the same compound and between different compounds (Fig. 2).

b) Test for Fungicidal Activity

In a modification of the test just described the pig skin is prepared as previously but is then inoculated with fungi before treatment. After 1–2 days growth, the formulations are applied and rubbed in, or in the case of lacquer formulations are applied with a brush. After a suitable period of exposure the epidermis and part of the dermis are scraped off with a scalpel, homogenised, washed twice with physiological saline by centrifugation to remove the drug and then plated out on malt agar to determine viable counts. As a check for possible residual drug activity following washing of the epidermal homogenate, one drop of the suspension is put on a malt agar plate seeded with *Candida albicans* and incubated at 37°C. Stripping with adhesive tape is not used in this version of the test. Fungicidal effectiveness is evaluated by varying the time of contact of the preparations with the infected skin. Figure 3 illustrates a comparison of a number of lacquer preparations after 2 h exposure and Fig. 4, a comparison of cream formulations with 1 h contact.

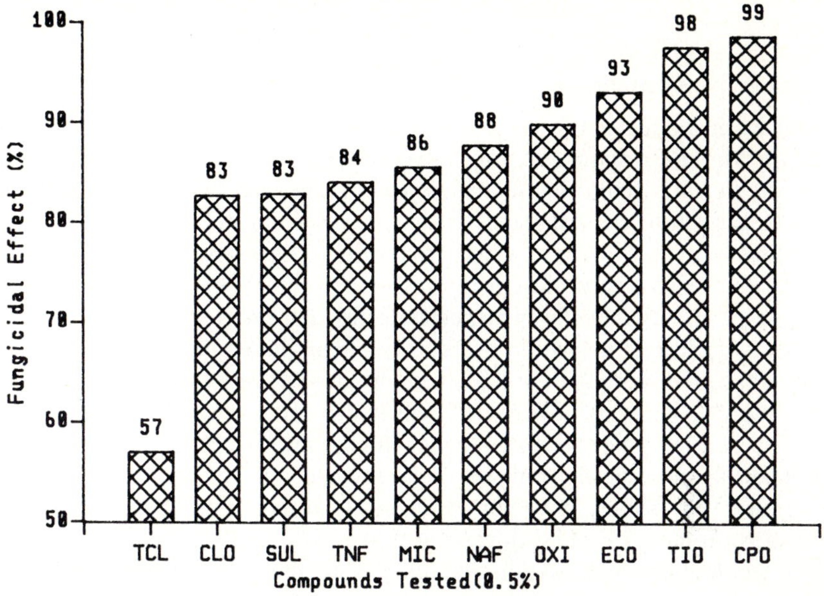

Fig. 3. Fungicidal activity of antifungals in a lacquer formulation tested against *Trichophyton mentagrophytes* on pig skin with 2 h exposure, mean of 3 experiments. *TCL*, tolciclate; *CLO* clotrimazole; *SUL*, sulbentine; *TNF*, tolnaftate; *MIC*, miconazole; *NAF*, naftifine; *OXI*, oxiconazole; *ECO*, econazole; *TIO*, tioconazole; *CPO*, ciclopirox free acid. Modified from HÄNEL et al. (1988)

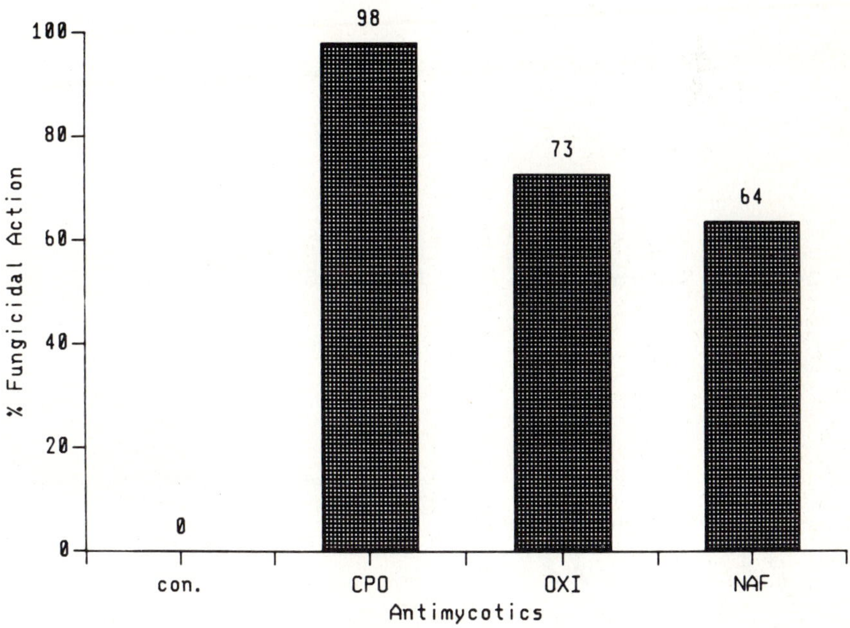

Fig. 4. Fungicidal activity of 1% cream formulations tested against *Trichophyton mentagrophytes* on pig skin with 1 h exposure, mean of 14 experiments. *con*, control; *CPO*, ciclopirox olamine; *OXI*, oxiconazole; *NAF*, naftifine. Modified from HÄNEL et al. (1988)

2. Therapeutic Studies

The classic model for in vivo studies with dermatophytes is the guinea pig (see Chap. 5). The response to topical treatment may be followed clinically or mycologically by culturing hair samples or skin scrapings. Mycological monitoring is open to criticism since traces of compound retained on skin or hair samples can lead to false negative results. There are marked differences between the structure of skin in guinea pigs and humans and between the course of infection in the two species. Thus, the rapid self-healing produced by transepidermal migration of neutrophils in guinea pigs (WENK 1962) and the subsequent desquamation (TAGAMI et al. 1982) are not found in humans. The number of layers of cornified cells which serve as a matrix and substrate for the dermatophytes is much higher in humans (Fig. 5). The tissue changes induced by superficial forms of trichophytosis and microsporosis in guinea pigs are very slight, however, and barely differ from those observed in humans. Some of these differences rather than similarities between guinea pigs and humans may explain anomalies sometimes produced in therapeutic experiments. HARE and LOEBENBERG (1988) treated infections with *T. mentagrophytes* in guinea pigs with 9 azoles and 6 non-azoles applied topically in formulations containing 0.25% active ingredient. Activity of amorolfine, naftifine, terbinafine, tolciclate and tolnaftate was classified as 'great', that of the azoles as 'moderate' or 'slight' while ciclopirox olamine was reckoned to

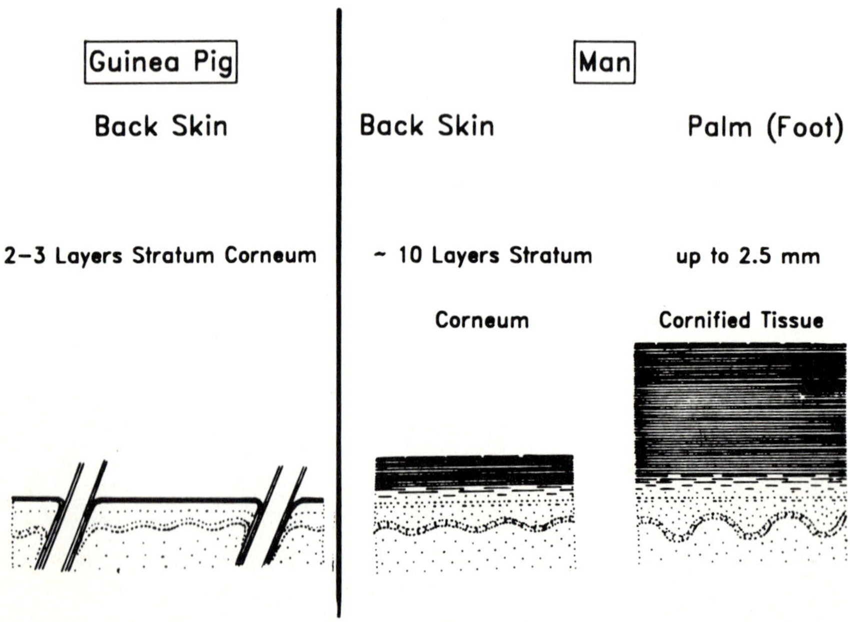

Fig. 5. Comparison of guinea pig skin with human skin; note the different thicknesses of the stratum corneum

Table 1. Guinea pig trichophytosis treated with ciclopirox olamine (CPO)[a]

Specimen	Diameters of bald patch[b] (mm)							
	CPO 2%	CPO 1%	CPO 0.5%	CPO 0.15%	CPO 0.125%	CPO 0.063%	Solvent	No treatment
1	8.2 ± 0.6	4.7 ± 0.8	14.0 ± 1.0	12.3 ± 1.2	15.2 ± 2.4	15.2 ± 0.8	19.8 ± 2.8	19.7 ± 3.1
2	4.3 ± 0.3	5.3 ± 2.3	10.7 ± 3.0	12.7 ± 2.5	17.0 ± 3.0	16.8 ± 3.3	17.2 ± 2.5	19.8 ± 0.4
3	6.3 ± 1.5	6.5 ± 1.3	11.0 ± 1.0	12.0 ± 1.0	16.0 ± 1.0	13.5 ± 1.3	19.0 ± 0	18.7 ± 0.6
4	5.5 ± 0.9	5.8 ± 0.6	9.7 ± 2.1	13.2 ± 2.5	19.8 ± 2.5	17.3 ± 2.9	21.8 ± 1.0	19.8 ± 1.8
5	4.3 ± 1.3	10.0 ± 0.5	11.7 ± 0.6	14.5 ± 1.8	13.8 ± 1.9	18.0 ± 3.5	19.3 ± 5.5	22.7 ± 1.2
6	4.5 ± 1.3	8.2 ± 2.5	13.0 ± 1.5	13.7 ± 2.1	18.2 ± 2.5	16.8 ± 4.5	22.0 ± 2.0	15.5 ± 3.5
n (spots)	18	18	18	18	18	18	18	18
Arithmetic mean (mm)	5.3	6.8	11.7	13.1	16.6	15.9	20.5	19.6
Standard deviation (mm)	1.7	2.3	2.1	1.8	2.8	2.6	2.1	2.8

[a] Twice daily applications on days 3–5 and one on day 6 after inoculation.
[b] measured 24 days after inoculation, means and SD of 3 patches.

be inactive. The results are misleading for ciclopirox olamine because they chose too low a concentration; thus these results do not equate with clinical experience. Double-blind clinical studies showed ciclopirox olamine and clotrimazole to be equally effective (Tarle 1980; Adam et al. 1981). In further clinical studies ciclopirox olamine proved to be equipotent with or slightly superior to tolnaftate (Lozano 1976; Beyer 1981).

Using the guinea pig model, dose-response relationships can be established for compounds which do not persist in the epidermis for a long time. In studies with ciclopirox olamine Dittmar (1975) and Dittmar et al. (1979) established a clear dose-response relationship from 0.063% to 2% ciclopirox olamine dissolved in isopropanol when the response was measured in terms of the diameter of the bald spot 24 days after inoculation (Table 1). With compounds which persist in the epidermis such as allylamines and azoles, it is possible to establish a dose-response relationship when comparing the number of applications; Petranyi (1985) compared naftifine and econazole after 1–7 treatments (Fig. 6). The classes of compounds appear to be quite different as far as mycological evaluation is concerned.

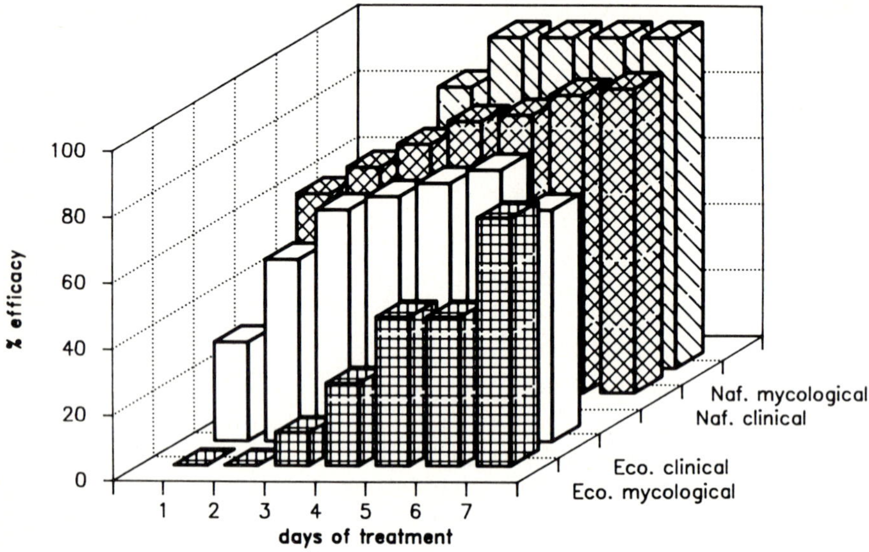

Fig. 6. Comparison of efficacies of 1% naftifine and econazole creams after once daily application for up to 7 days in guinea pigs. Modified from PETRANYI (1985)

The guinea pig model of infection can be used in studies to compare the behaviour of a compound in different vehicles. Table 2 summarises an experiment using the method of DITTMAR (1975). Three inoculation spots on the left side of the animals remained untreated whereas the three on the right side were treated once daily over days 3–7 using 0.3 ml of 1% ciclopirox olamine in two different solvent systems. The diameters of the bald patches were measured on day 24. As can be seen from the table, the infection responded better to the formulation containing aqueous isopropanol and polyethylene glycol than to that containing polyethylene glycol alone.

The fact that a drug will penetrate the skin following topical application does not mean that it will necessarily have therapeutic activity. Griseofulvin, active following oral administration, is not effective topically in treating clinical infections. A 0.5% alcoholic solution applied to the skin led to griseofulvin concentrations in all three levels of the stratum corneum 10–100 times higher than those found following oral administration; moreover, the drug persisted in the skin for 2–5 days after treatment was stopped in concentrations sufficient to kill any fungi present (EPSTEIN et al. 1975). Using experimental infections it was shown that topical griseofulvin had prophylactic activity, but that when given therapetically it failed despite very high levels in the stratum corneum. Studies of RITSCHEL and HUSSAIN (1988) on ointment formulations of griseofulvin indicate a renewed interest in the possible topical use of this drug. Griseofulvin ointments were made containing 23% dimethyl acetamide or diethylene glycol monoethylether. Although the amount of drug that permeated rat skin was 14 times that which permeated human skin,

Table 2. Experimental *Trichophyton mentagrophytes* infection of the guinea pig: influence of different solvents

	A[a] Ciclopirox		B[b] Ciclopirox		C[c] Vehicle	
	Untreated	Treated	Untreated	Treated	Untreated	Treated
n (spots)	45	45	45	45	33	33
Diameter of bald spot (mm)	19.8 ± 2.7	8.4 ± 2.0	19.0 ± 2.6	11.7 ± 3.6	19.9 ± 2.6	19.6 ± 3.0
Percentage Inhibition	57.6		38.4		1.5	

[a] solution A: 1% ciclopirox olamine, 10% polyethyleneglycol (PEG) 400, 35% isopropanol, 54% distilled water.
[b] solution B: 1% ciclopirox olamine, 99% PEG 400.
[c] solution C: vehicle of solution A.

concentrations of griseofulvin in the various layers of human skin after one topical application were far greater than those reported after prolonged peroral administration; no therapeutic data were given.

3. Pharmacokinetic Studies

Among the antifungals, N-substituted derivatives of imidazoles and 1,2,4-triazoles represent the single largest class. Since the advent of clotrimazole and miconazole in the early 1970s, at least eight further azole derivatives have been introduced for the treatment of dermatomycoses. The imidazole and triazole antifungals have pronounced pharmacological and biochemical activities. For safty reasons therefore they have to be examined for the extent of percutaneous absorption. The skin is an effective barrier for the azoles, and percutaneous absorption is generally less than 4% of the dose (Ritter 1988); the only exception is sulconazole with up to 11.3% being absorbed through the skin (Franz and Lehmann 1988). Percutaneous absorption is usually studied after topical application of radiolabelled drug by measuring the fraction of the dose excreted in the urine and faeces. Systemic exposure of the body, however, can also be estimated by determination of plasma levels of the unchanged and active drug, provided a reliable and specific assay procedure with sufficient sensitivity is available. In the following it will be demonstrated how a combination of both approaches was used in the development of several formulations of bifonazole.

Percutaneous absorption of bifonazole through healthy human skin was between 0.6% and 0.8% of the dose applied as a 1% cream or 1% solution and rather greater through inflamed skin; two patients with inflamed skin showed 2.4% and 3.6% absorption (Patzschke et al. 1983). The total dose was 0.2 mg/kg body weight. In the same healthy subjects, bifonazole plasma

Table 3. Bifonazole plasma levels in white New Zealand rabbits after treatment with 1% bifonazole solution once daily at a dose of 3 mg/kg under an occlusive dressing for 6 h: (a) after first treatment, (b) after 15th treatment

(a)

Condition of skin	Sex	Plasma level (ng/ml)				
		0 h	2 h	4 h	7 h	24 h
Intact	m	<1.0	12.0	11.1	8.4	1.0
Intact	m	<1.0	7.7	8.4	4.8	1.0
Abraded	m	<1.0	7.2	8.6	10.4	4.7
Abraded	m	<1.0	9.5	10.2	9.6	3.9
Intact	f	<1.0	7.1	8.5	10.8	7.8
Intact	f	<1.0	7.3	10.2	6.3	2.5
Abraded	f	<1.0	7.9	10.4	13.8	2.8
Abraded	f	<1.0	13.1	5.5	6.7	2.2
Mean ($n = 8$)		<1.0	9.0	9.1	8.9	3.2
± SD		–	2.4	1.8	2.9	2.2

(b)

Condition of skin	Sex	Plasma level (ng/ml)				
		0 h	2 h	4 h	7 h	24 h
Intact	m	3.1	<1.0	6.4	5.5	3.1
Intact	m	3.3	4.0	3.9	6.1	2.8
Abraded	m	11.5	7.4	11.5	7.1	6.2
Abraded	m	2.2	6.7	10.7	13.8	10.8
Intact	f	6.6	7.8	6.0	12.5	8.3
Intact	f	5.6	13.8	7.1	11.3	5.8
Abraded	f	2.4	6.3	7.5	12.0	4.6
Abraded	f	4.2	5.4	6.6	8.3	3.7
Mean ($n = 8$)		4.9	6.5	7.5	9.6	5.7
± SD		3.1	3.8	2.5	3.2	2.8

levels were lower than 1 ng/ml, the limit of detection. In the two patients with inflamed skin, plasma levels were below the 1 ng/ml detection limit with the exception of a 1–2 mg/ml reading at 8 h (RITTER and SIEFERT 1987). Since both the extent of percutaneous absorption and plasma levels in the systemic circulation in humans were available for 1% bifonazole cream and 1% bifonazole solution, these preparations could serve as reference standards in animal studies during the development of further formulations such as powder and gel.

Bifonazole plasma levels in rabbits after topical application of a 1% solution were investigated in conjunction with a study on skin tolerance. The solution was applied to normal or abraded skin at a dose of 3 mg/kg under an occlusive dressing for 6 h. Two hours after the first treatment, bifonazole concentrations in the plasma averaged 9.0 ± 2.4 ng/ml, declining to a mean of

Table 4. Bifonazole plasma levels in rabbits treated once daily for 5 days with 1% bifonazole powder as a suspension under an occlusive dressing for 23 h

Breed	Condition of skin, sex	Bifonazole plasma level (ng/ml)			
		0 h	1 h	4 h	7 h
White New Zealand rabbits	Intact, female	5.6	1.5	<1.0	2.2
		<1.0	2.2	1.3	1.0
		1.9	<1.0	1.3	1.4
	Abraded, female	4.0	<1.0	1.0	1.0
		<1.0	1.1	2.8	4.8
		1.4	1.3	1.3	<1.0
	Intact, male	2.1	2.3	1.7	<1.0
		5.8	<1.0	1.1	2.5
		<1.0	<1.0	<1.0	2.0
	Abraded, male	1.2	1.9	1.0	5.5
		1.9	1.0	1.1	<1.0
		8.8	2.5	2.8	3.7
Great chinchilla rabbits	Intact, female	3.9	1.0	1.0	5.5
		3.9	1.2	1.4	1.0
		5.0	3.4	2.4	1.9
		3.8	2.1	1.7	1.0
		1.1	1.1	3.3	2.3
		1.0	<1.0	3.9	1.9
Mean (N = 18) ± SD		2.9 ±2.3	1.4 ±0.8	1.7 ±1.0	2.0 ±1.5

3.2 ± 2.2 ng/ml at 24 h (Table 3a). After the 15th application, the bifonazole plasma levels were in the same range, with mean trough levels of 4.9 ± 3.1 ng/ml (Table 3b). Nearly the same results were obtained some time later when 1% bifonazole solution served as a reference treatment in the evaluation of percutaneous absorption from some new formulations. It is remarkable that under the conditions of the experiment, no significant differences were observed between plasma levels in rabbits with intact and with abraded skin (Table 3).

Percutaneous absorption of bifonazole after application of 1% powder was studied in white New Zealand rabbits with intact or abraded skin and in chinchilla rabbits with intact skin. The powder was applied at a dose of 3 mg/kg as a suspension once a day under an occlusive dressing for 23 h. After the first application, plasma levels were lower than the detection limit of 1 ng/ml in the majority of the animals; concentrations of 1.3–2.7 ng/ml were found in only 8 of 54 plasma samples taken 4 h and 7 h after application. After the fifth treatment, a steady state was apparently reached because the levels at 0 h on day 5 were not significantly different from those at 7 h after the fifth

Table 5. Bifonazole plasma levels in rabbits after a single topical application of one of three 1% bifonazole formulations at a dose of 3 mg/kg on abraded skin with occlusive dressing for 23 h

Bifonazole Preparation	Animal no.	Bifonazole plasma level (ng/ml)			AUC_{0-7} (ng · h/ml)
		2 h	4 h	7 h	
Gel with surfactant	1	1	3	2	12.8
	2	3	5	6	27.2
	3	3	3	3	16.2
	4	2	1	3	12.1
	5	2	2	2	13.1
	6	3	4	5	22.0
	Mean	2.3	3.0	3.5	17.2
	±SD	0.8	1.4	1.6	6.1
Gel	7	1	2	3	12.9
	8	5	7	7	37.9
	9	<1	1	3	7.2
	10	2	3	4	16.6
	11	1	5	2	17.1
	12	1	1	2	8.2
	Mean	1.8	3.2	4.0	16.7
	±SD	1.7	2.4	1.8	11.2
Solution	13	16	19	11	95.5
	14	14	17	11	85.6
	15	12	18	8	80.5
	16	38	23	11	149.6
	17	16	26	18	125.3
	18	14	12	7	68.8
	Mean	18.3	19.2	11.0	100.9
	±SD	9.8	4.9	3.8	30.6

AUC_{0-7}, area under curve for 0–7 hours.

dose (Table 4). Again the bifonazole levels in the animals with abraded skin did not differ significantly from those with intact skin. In another study in rabbits, bifonazole plasma levels were determined after the topical application of a 1% gel. Two slightly different gel formulations were tested, one with – among other ingredients – 47% water, the second with 10% of the water content replaced by a surfactant. The dose was 3 mg/kg body weight applied to abraded skin under an occlusive dressing for 23 h, and again 1% bifonazole solution served as a reference preparation. Bifonazole plasma levels up to 7 h after treatment with both gel formulations were between 1 and 7 ng/ml; by contrast, levels following application of the 1% solution ranged from 7 to 38 ng/ml (Table 5). Based on the AUC_{0-7}, systemic exposure of rabbits treated with either gel formulation was 5–6 times less compared with those treated with solution.

II. Nail Infections

Fungal infections of the nail present a particular therapeutic challenge. Oral treatment with griseofulvin or ketoconazole is possible, but treatment needs to be prolonged until the affected nail has grown out, and success, particularly with toenails, is by no means assured. EVANS and ROBERTS (1988) have recently achieved remarkable results with 250 mg terbinafine daily by mouth in a short series of patients; 37/39 patients were cured, with an average of 6.8 months to mycological cure, for toenail infections and 3–5 months for fingernails. Because long-term medication, particularly with ketoconazole, may be questioned, topical treatment of nail infections is a desirable alternative. Problems exist, however, in applying medication and keeping it in place and in obtaining sufficient penetration of the infected nail to eliminate infection. Initial attempts at topical medication used simple solutions, e.g. an alcoholic solution of miconazole. Refinements in pharmaceutical presentation have led to a 28% solution of tioconazole (HAY et al. 1985; TULLI et al. 1988) and to nail lacquer formulations containing ciclopirox free acid (8%) or amorolfine (5%). The present section is concerned with methods by which such special topical formulations may be developed and tested in the laboratory. An interesting alternative approach to fungal infections of the nail, particularly applicable in situations in which protracted oral or topical medication is not acceptable, has been described by HAY et al. (1988). Application of a paste formulation containing 40% urea and 1% bifonazole daily for 1 week allows the painless removal of the diseased nail and has resulted in cure rates, which although still far from satisfactory, compare favourably with those obtained with long-term systemic treatment.

Nail growth is continuous throughout life, the length being regulated by breakage or wear. The nail consists of three layers: a thin ventral plate, a thick intermediate plate and a thin dorsal plate. The cells of the dorsal plate are very flat and lack nuclei at an early stage; the thickened plasmatic membranes are connected by tight junctions. The intermediate plate consists of cells which are less flat and still possess cytoplasmic portions. Partial decomposition of DNA in the nuclear fragments still present indicates the better state of preservation of these cells compared with those in the dorsal plate; non-keratinised zones are still found in this layer. The ventral plate consists of only 1–2 cell layers with nuclear residues. The keratinisation which occurs under conditions of pressure and the marked vacuolation distinguish this layer from the dorsal plate.

1. In Vitro Models

In the absence of realistic animal models of nail infection, in vitro systems have been used to study the behaviour of preparations formulated for the treatment of onychomycosis. We use slices of cowhorn (DITTMAR and GRAU 1979) as well as excised human nails for testing the effect of antimycotics against keratinophilic fungi. The water content of the horny material in both models is crucial in extrapolating the results to human onychomycosis.

The core of a cowhorn obtained directly after slaughter is removed, and the horny coat is cleaned with distilled water and smoothed down to a uniform thickness of 0.6 mm. Pieces 5 × 3 cm are then cut and sterilised with ethylene oxide. Further processing is under sterile conditions. The horn slices are kept overnight in distilled water containing 0.05% glucose to compensate for the dehydration caused by drying. A humid chamber consisting of a plastic Petri dish containing 20 ml of 2% water agar is prepared for each horn slice; slices are attached convex side up using an additional 3 ml molten water agar, and covered with the plastic lid to the dish. The slices are treated with the antifungal formulations under test and left for 5 days. The slices are then inverted and the underside inoculated with *T. mentagrophytes*. The inoculum is applied in the form of three rows of inoculation points about 1.5 mm in diameter, each point containing around 100 microconidia. Two glass cover-slips 9 × 18 mm are placed transversally on the inoculated surface and covered with two strips of filter paper soaked in 0.85% saline. The chambers are incubated for 10 days at 28°C, during which time the filter paper strips are kept moist. This is necessary to ensure that the inoculated horn surface is kept humid enough to allow fungal growth to occur. At the end of incubation

a 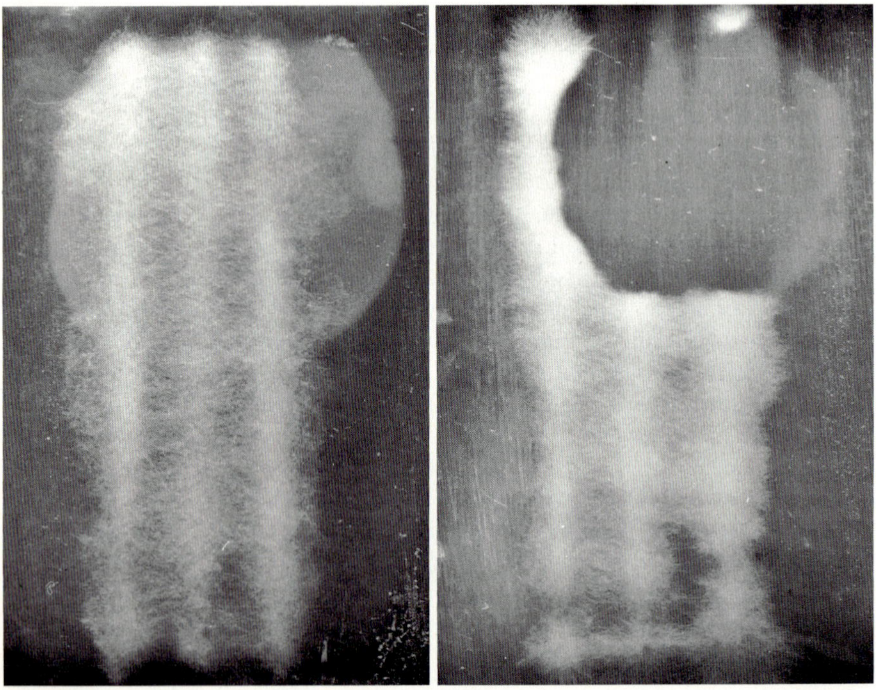 b

Fig. 7a,b. Cowhorn plate with three inoculation lines of *Trichophyton mentagrophytes* and treated on reverse side with cream. **a** Placebo; no inhibition of fungal growth is apparent. **b** Treatment with 1% ciclopirox olamine cream; note absence of fungal growth above the treated area the formulation is wiped off and the fungal growth scored and photographed (Fig. 7). Large scale screening using this method is not possible due to the work involved in smoothing down the horn slices.

More recently we have used another technique, sawing transverse horn slices 0.5 mm thick; these have a keratin arrangement resembling that in the dorsal plate of human nails. Colonisation of the fibres with a vertical orientation resembles that seen in humans when studied by light microscopy. The slices of cowhorn are pretreated as above but are then inoculated with two spots of *T. mentagrophytes* and incubated for 2 days at 28°C. Treatment is applied once daily to the underside of the slice and incubation continued. Effective antimycotics with good penetrating properties are able to arrest growth and even eliminate fungus present on the other side of the slice (Fig. 8).

The use of human nails is problematic because differences in nail thickness, nutritional condition and age of the donors make it almost impossible to compare the results obtained in penetration studies. Using a nail lacquer containing 8% ^{14}C-labelled ciclopirox free acid, ten excised toenails

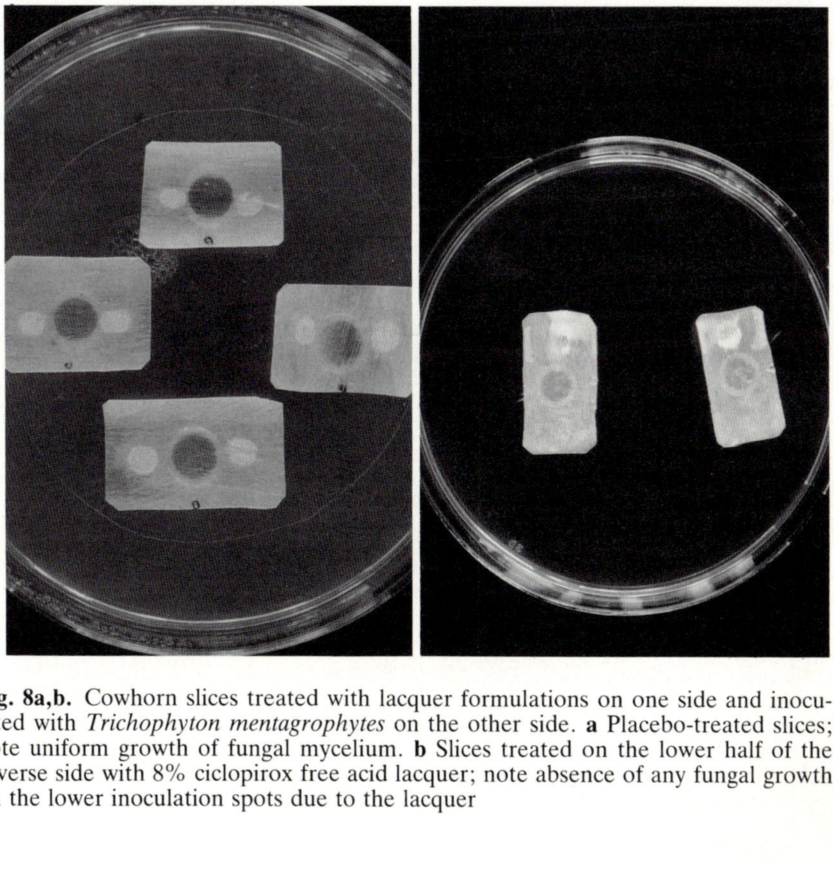

a b

Fig. 8a,b. Cowhorn slices treated with lacquer formulations on one side and inoculated with *Trichophyton mentagrophytes* on the other side. **a** Placebo-treated slices; note uniform growth of fungal mycelium. **b** Slices treated on the lower half of the reverse side with 8% ciclopirox free acid lacquer; note absence of any fungal growth on the lower inoculation spots due to the lacquer

Table 6. Penetration of ciclopirox nail lacquer in human nails (μg/ml)

Nail	1	2	3	4	5	6	7	8	9	10
Incubation time	18 h	18 h	18 h	24 h	24 h	24 h	24 h	48 h	48 h	48 h
Dorsal plate (62 μm thickness)	4102	1780	4708	3639	5957	3565	9967	14245	13970	8189
Upper intermediate plate (240 μm thickness)	1079	130	844	726	538	310	157	1683	1587	1392
Lower intermediate plate-ventral plate (200–600 μm thickness)	1.4	1.3	26.6	6.7	13.7	4.1	6.6	10.1	9.4	73.6

which had been carefully checked for their comparability were treated with 5 mg lacquer per cm^2. After 18–48 h in a humid chamber, the nails were sectioned and analysed (Table 6). The content of ciclopirox free acid increased in the upper layers of the nails after prolonged exposure, whereas penetration into the lower layers seemed to depend on other factors such as brittleness or nutritional condition of the donor. Nevertheless concentrations of ciclopirox free acid above the MICs for dermatophytes were found even in the deepest layers of all nails. The concentrations of radiolabelled miconazole (SCHAEFER and STÜTTGEN 1976) and oxiconazole or econazole (STÜTTGEN and BAUER 1982) dropped by about 1000-fold from the outer to the inner surface of the nail plate. Azole drugs and griseofulvin act mainly as barriers to fungal invasion of the proximal areas of the nail plate (ZAIAS and DRACHMAN 1983).

Water, which accounts for 7%–12% of the nail, is the primary plasticiser (WALTERS and FLYNN 1983). Water flux through the stratum corneum of abdominal skin is ten times less than through the nail (BADEN et al. 1973); other researchers suggest a factor of 1000 when the differences in thickness of stratum corneum and nail are taken into account (WALTERS et al. 1981). As a water-containing tissue, the nail constitutes a membrane; it functions as a hydrogel of highly ionic character. Penetration characteristics of the nail contrast with those of other cutaneous tissues. Thus, the nail prevents hydrophobic rather than hydrophilic substances from penetrating, and classic dermatological penetration enhancers are poorly effective (KLIGMAN 1965; WALTERS and FLYNN 1981). DMSO even reduces the penetration of polar fluids such as methanol and of hydrophobic liquids such as *n*-hexanol. Only substances such as sodium lauryl sulphate or sodium thioglycollate seem to promote the penetration of some substances (WALTERS 1985).

III. Vaginal Infections

For experimental studies on the activity of and absorption from different formulations we have used the rat (see Chap. 5). The rat vagina is 15–20 mm in length, and following the surgical and hormonal pretreatment necessary to render it susceptible to colonisation with *C. albicans*, it has an epithelium consisting of a stratum germinativum with a few cell layers, a stratum granulosum with 4–5 cell layers and a multilayered stratum of cornified cells 8–12 μm thick. The upper layers of the epithelium are shed in flakes. Isolated neutrophils are found in the lamina propria only but not in the epithelium. The layers of cornified cells are not comparable with those found in humans, which are only present for a short period in the cycle and have only 2–3 layers of cells.

Two kinds of effect must be distinguished in therapy with topical preparations. Compounds with transepithelial absorption have a prolonged effect due to their quasi-systemic activity, while compounds which are not absorbed can only exert an effect on the fungi so long as they persist at the site of application. The vehicle in which the antifungal is applied plays a particular role in this context. Many vehicles – extending from 0.2 M hydrochloric acid to different cream formulations – have been tested for suitability. The chemical properties of the antimycotic are crucial in the choice of vehicle. Propylene glycol was often used in the past because it promotes penetration into the layers of cornified cells (MAYER et al. 1978), but it has now been largely abandoned because of the production of toxic eczematous skin reactions (ANDERSEN and STORRS 1982) and intrinsic antimycotic activity which adds to the antimycotic effect of any test compound. We generally use polyethylene glycol 400 (PEG 400) in a dose of 32 μl instilled into the rat vagina to ensure that the observed antimycotic effect results solely from the compound. PEG 400 has good solubilising properties, and heating to 60°C is sufficient to dissolve most hydrophobic substances, e.g. itraconazole. Morphological examination has shown that a 32 μl drop of PEG 400 can spread over the whole vagina and can be detected as a liquid film right up to the neck of the uterus.

1. Absorption Studies

Due to limitations imposed by the stratum corneum of skin, absorption from the vagina in women is greater than absorption through the skin; this is well demonstrated by the azole antifungals (RITTER 1988). Clotrimazole was the first azole to be studied in depth for absorption from the vagina (DUHM et al. 1972). After a single vaginal dose of 100 mg of radiolabelled clotrimazole administered either as a vaginal tablet or as 1% vaginal cream, absorption was found to be in the range of 3%–10% of the dose (PATZSCHKE et al. 1976). In another study in volunteers, clotrimazole plasma levels after vaginal insertion of a 100 mg tablet were lower than 10 ng/ml (RITTER et al. 1982). Based on these data, the clotrimazole vaginal tablet served as a reference formulation during the development of further preparations, e.g. a 3-day treatment schedule with a 200 mg tablet, or single-dose treatment with a 500 mg tablet or 10% vaginal cream. After vaginal application of these formulations, clotrimazole plasma levels were lower than 10 ng/ml (RITTER et al. 1982). On the other hand up to 3 days after the insertion of a 500 mg vaginal tablet with lactic acid, fungicidal levels of clotrimazole could be detected in the vaginal fluid (RITTER 1985). Thus, single-dose treatment of vaginal mycosis with clotrimazole offers the advantage of combining high availability in the vagina with a low availability in the systemic circulation and is a means of solving the problem of patient non-compliance. Just as absorption of clotrimazole from the vagina seems to be independent of the size of the dose, so plasma levels of ketoconazole (ENE et al. 1984) or tioconazole (ARTNER and FUCHS 1983; HOUANG and LAWRENCE 1985) did not rise with increasing dose. By contrast, terconazole plasma levels after a single vaginal dose of 240 mg were about threefold higher than after 80 mg and reached peak levels of up to 35 ng/ml (KENNEDY and FRIEDMANN 1985).

2. Therapeutic Studies

The mouse and rat models of vaginal candidosis (Chap. 5) or the hamster model of HARE and LOEBENBERG (1988) can be used to evaluate the therapeutic potential of different formulations of an antifungal compound. Results, however, need to be treated with some caution. HARE and LOEBENBERG found amorolfine and ten azoles to be active at 0.25% in their system while ciclopirox olamine, amphotericin B and nystatin were among the substances classified as inactive, although they have proved successful in clinical therapy, albeit sometimes in higher concentrations. Azoles, too, may give misleading results in the rat model due to their anti-oestrogenic activity and possibly also due to their anti-bacterial activity which may disturb the ecological equilibrium in the vagina (HANTSCHKE and ZABEL 1979). Oestradiol treatment is necessary to produce a fully cornified epithelium in mice and rats and so render the vagina susceptible to infection with *C. albicans*. Ketoconazole and other azoles, by virtue of their anti-oestrogenic potential, are able to reverse this process, reduce the thickness of the layer of cornified cells to two layers and even allow the appearance of some leucocytes in the vaginal smear. The level of azole necessary to show this anti-oestrogenic effect fully is usually somewhat higher than the therapeutic level, but nevertheless the possibility exists that the apparent efficacy of the compound in the animal model is not due entirely to its antifungal potential.

C. Oral Formulations

Appropriate formulations are necessary for non-absorbable drugs which are used to treat gastrointestinal infections and for potentially absorbable drugs used to treat systemic or superficial infections by the oral route. In the latter case, particularly, the type of formulation can have a profound effect on the degree of absorption and hence therapeutic efficacy.

Nystatin is insoluble in water and is not absorbed from the gut; suspension or tablet formulations have been extensively used in attempts to disinfect the intestinal tract of fungi which may disseminate to give vaginal or systemic infections. Although it is absorbed in mice, amphotericin B is not absorbed to any appreciable extent from the gut of humans, and it can be used in a similar way to nystatin. Lozenge formulations have been devised to treat oral and pharyngeal infections with susceptible yeasts (DEVRIES-HOSPERS and VAN DER WAAIJ 1980), and a similar approach has been taken with clotrimazole.

Among the older systemically active drugs, 5-fluorocytosine has posed no problems due to its solubility in water. By contrast, the efficacy of griseofulvin in the treatment of dermatophyte infections depends very much on the nature of the oral formulation. DAVIES (1980) gives a very comprehensive account of the griseofulvin story. The most important requirement for absorption appears to be particle size; similar blood levels can be achieved in humans following the ingestion of 1 g normal material, 0.5 g micronised griseofulvin (particles around 4 μm in diameter) or 0.25 g ultramicronised griseofulvin (particles predominantly less than 1 μm). It has been suggested that absorption is better if administered in corn oil, in a corn oil/water emulsion or immediately after a fatty meal. There are, however, conflicting views on the effect of lipids on absorption, one view being that rather than solubilising the drug and promoting absorption, lipid slows down intestinal passage, so giving a longer time for absorption to take place. Almost complete absorption is claimed using tablets containing ultramicrosize material dissolved and dispersed in PEG 8000.

With the newer azoles, absorption from the gut presents no problems with fluconazole, which is water soluble to some extent, but lipophilic itraconazole presents an entirely different situation; for experimental use, the drug needs to be dissolved in PEG 200, and for human use a PEG capsule formulation has been developed.

D. Parenteral Formulations

For seriously ill patients, or in situations in which non-absorbable drugs such as amphotericin B are to be used, special formulations need to be developed so that the drug can be given parenterally, usually intravenously. Water-soluble drugs such as 5-fluorocytosine or fluconazole present few problems. Griseofulvin has been dissolved in PEG 300 for experimental intravenous studies in volunteers, while cilofungin is administered in 26% aqueous PEG 300. Miconazole, which has an aqueous solubility of only 0.03%, is formulated with cremophor EL for intravenous medication. Amphotericin B remains the most important candidate for parenteral formulation. Due to its amphipathic character it has limited solubility in water and non-polar solvents. Although soluble in highly polar solvents such as DMSO – which is suitable for some experimental purposes – it is marketed as a sodium deoxycholate complex that forms a colloidal dispersion when hydrated (Fungizone); this is administered by slow infusion using 5% dextrose solution as the carrier.

Amphotericin B remains the ‘gold standard’ among drugs for treating systemic fungal infections. It is, however, a toxic drug. Acute effects of administration include fever, chills, vomiting, nephro- and cardiotoxicity and hypotension, while long-term therapy is associated with hypokalaemia, hypomagnesaemia, anaemia and particularly renal toxicity. The search for active but less toxic analogues has so far been unsuccessful (SCHAFFNER 1987). Sodium supplementation may reduce the risk of nephrotoxicity (BRANCH 1988), although incorporation of high levels of sodium into the actual formulation would probably cause micellar aggregation. In vitro studies suggest that formulation with the mild detergent sucrose monolaurate – which decreases the binding of amphotericin to cholesterol without affecting its binding to ergosterol – may enhance the therapeutic index (GRUDA et al. 1988). Experimental work in rats suggests that amphotericin B administered as an aerosol has activity against progressive pulmonary aspergillosis (SCHMITT et al. 1988). Although this alternative route of administration would not produce nephrotoxicity, only respiratory infections would have any chance of responding, and it is by no means certain how important drug absorption from the lung is, and how this differs between rats and humans. By far the most exciting approach to reducing the toxicity of amphotericin without reducing its activity is by formulation in liposomes.

The first report of the formulation of amphotericin B in liposomes seems to be that of NEW et al. (1981) in connection with experimental studies using a rodent model of a protozoal disease, visceral leishmaniasis. Reports then appeared of efficacy in mice against histoplasmosis (TAYLOR et al. 1982), cryptococcosis (GRAYBILL et al. 1982) and systemic candidosis (LOPEZ-BERESTEIN et al. 1983; TREMBLAY et al. 1984); the first trials in humans were not far behind (LOPEZ-BERESTEIN et al. 1985). These studies all indicated that incorporation into liposomes resulted in a product which had a different tissue distribution and considerably reduced toxicity compared with conventional amphotericin, yet without loss of therapeutic activity. The outcome was that much higher doses of amphotericin could be administered, resulting in an increased therapeutic response; in a trial with 12 cancer patients who were granulocytopenic or immunosuppressed, 8 whose fungal infection had not been controlled by conventional amphotericin showed full or partial remission with little evidence of side effects.

Liposome distribution is primarily to organs rich in reticulo-endothelial cells, including lung, liver, spleen, kidney and bone marrow, so that response to treatment by different fungi will presumably depend on their location within the body. Multilamellar or unilamellar liposomes of different sizes and lipid compositions have been used. In the human trial of LOPEZ-BERESTEIN et al. (1985), multilamellar liposomes made of dimiristoylphosphatidylglycerol and dimiristoylphosphatidylcholine in a molar ratio of 3:7 were used, while in another trial in cancer patients, sonicated and smaller liposomes containing egg phosphatidylcholine, cholesterol and stearylamine in a molar ratio 4:3:1 were employed (SCULLIER et al. 1988). Antifungal action depends on the transfer of amphotericin from the liposome to the fungus, and toxicity on transfer to host tissues; the ease and extent to which this takes place depend on the relative affinities of amphotericin for the lipids of the liposome, fungus and host. Amphotericin has a high affinity for ergosterol, the sterol of the fungal membrane. Inclusion of ergosterol in the liposome results in decreased toxicity to the host but also to decreased antifungal efficacy of the preparation. An interesting development in the liposomal amphotericin story is reported by HOSPENTHAL et al. (1989) who managed to attach antibody specific to *C. albicans* to the surface of the liposome. Studies with infections in mice suggest that antibody-directed liposomes may provide a method of reaching target organisms with reduced toxicity and increased specificity, thus improving the efficacy of the drug. Liposomal amphotericin B is reviewed in greater detail by COUNE (1988) and by WIEBE and DEGREGORIO (1988).

Published studies concerning liposomal amphotericin have all utilised liposomal formulations prepared at the point of use. Widespread application of this undoubted advance in therapy will depend on the development of a suitable, reproducible and stable commercial formulation; the Liposome Company and Squibb appear to be collaborating on just such a development (SCRIP No 1319, June 22nd 1988, p 15). An interesting alternative which appears to have the same advantages of reduction in toxicity without loss of therapeutic activity has been reported by KIRSH et al. (1988), who incorporated amphotericin B in a commercially available and clinically approved emulsion formulation, Intralipid 20%.

References

Adam W, Peil HG, Savopoulos C, Vanderbeke O (1981) Klinische Ergebnisse mit dem Antimykotikum Ciclopiroxolamin. Arzneim-Forsch 31:1360–1365

Andersen KE, Storrs FJ (1982) Hautreizungen durch Propylenglykol. Hautarzt 33: 12–14

Artner J, Fuchs G (1983) Open studies of the efficacy, tolerance, systemic absorption, and vaginal persistence following a single application of tioconazole ointment in the treatment of patients with vaginal candidiasis. Gynäk Rdsch 23 (Suppl 1): 12–19

Baden HP, Goldsmith LA, Fleming BA (1973) A comparative study of the physiochemical properties of human keratinized tissues. Biochim Biophys Acta 322: 269–278

Bartek MJ, LaBudde JA, Maibach HI (1972) Skin permeability in vivo: comparison in rat, rabbit, pig, and man. J Invest Dermatol 58:114–123

Benfield P, Clissold SP (1988) Sulconazole. A review of its antimicrobial activity and therapeutic use in superficial dermatomycoses. Drugs 35:143–153

Bennett SL, Barry BW (1986) The use of human scalp and abdominal skin as in vitro models for percutaneous absorption. In: Marks R, Plewig G (eds) Skin models. Springer, Berlin Heidelberg New York Tokyo, p 245

Beyer M (1981) Ausgewählte Doppelblind-Vergleichsstudien zur Wirksamkeit und Verträglichkeit von Ciclopiroxolaminlösung und -creme. Arzneim-Forsch 31: 1378–1381

Bissett DL, McBride JF (1985) Use of the domestic pig as an animal model of human dry skin. In: Maibach HI, Lowe NJ (eds) Models in dermatology, vol I. Karger, Basel, p 159–168

Bond JR, Barry BW (1988a) Limitations of hairless mouse skin as a model for in vitro permeation studies through human skin: hydration damage. J Invest Dermatol 90:486–489

Bond JR, Barry BW (1988b) Hairless mouse skin is limited as a model for assessing the effects of penetration enhancers in human skin. J Invest Dermatol 90:810–813

Branch RA (1988) Prevention of amphotericin B-induced renal impairment. A review on the use of sodium supplementation. Arch Intern Med 148:2389–2394

Coune A (1988) Liposomes as drug delivery system in the treatment of infectious diseases: potential applications and clinical experience. Infection 16:141–147

Davies RR (1980) Griseofulvin. In: Speller DCE (ed) Antifungal chemotherapy. Wiley, Chichester, pp 149–182

DeVries-Hospers HG, van der Waaij (1980) Salivary concentrations of amphotericin B following its use as an oral lozenge. Infection 8:63–65

Dittmar W (1975) Contribution to the methodology of testing topical antimycotic agents in guinea pig dermatophytosis. Mykosen 18:351–361

Dittmar W (1985) Antibiotikatestung an exzidierter Schweinehaut als Ersatzverfahren für topische Tierversuchs-Prüfmodelle. Abstracts, IXX. Wiss. Tagung Deutschspr. Mykol. Ges. Würzburg, 10–13 Oktober 1985, S 5

Dittmar W, Grau W (1979) Ciclopirox – Eine Substanz mit Aspekten für Mykologie und Kosmetik. Ärztl Kosmetologie 9:209–214

Dittmar W, Jović N (1980) Microbiological penetration studies on ciclopirox and imidazole antimycotics using postmortem skin. Proc. XV Int. Congr. Dermatol., Mexico, 16–21 October 1977. Excerpta Medica Int. Congr. Series No. 451/ Dermatology, Amsterdam, p 730

Dittmar W, Jović N (1987) Laboratory techniques alternative to in vivo experiments for studying the liberation, penetration and fungicidal action of topical antimycotic agents in the skin, including ciclopiroxolamine. Mykosen 30:326–342

Dittmar W, Kellner HM, Petri W, Wagner WH (1979) Resorption von Arzneistoffen von Haut und Schleimhäuten. In: Rietbrock N, Schnieders B (eds) Bioverfügbarkeit von Arzneimitteln. G. Fischer, Stuttgart p 127

Duhm B, Maul W, Medenwald H, Wegner LA, Oberste-Lehn H (1972) Pharmakokinetik nach topischer Anwendung von Bisphenyl-(2-chlorphenyl)-1-imidazolyl-methan-[^{14}C]. Arzneim-Forsch 22:1276–1280

Ene MD, Williamson PJ, Daneshmend TK, Blatchford NR (1984) Systemic absorption of ketoconazole from vaginal pessaries. Br J Clin Pharmacol 17:173–175

Epstein WL, Shah V, Riegelman S (1975) Dermatopharmacology of griseofulvin. Cutis 15:271–275

Evans EGV, Roberts DT (1988) Oral treatment of dermatophytosis of nails with terbinafine, a new allylamine antifungal agent. 28th Intersci Conf Antimicrob Agents Chemother, Los Angeles, Abstr 583, p 211

Flynn GL, Dürrheim H, Higuchi WI (1981) Permeation of hairless mouse skin II: membrane sectioning techniques and influence of alkanol permeabilities. J Pharm Sci 70:52–56

Franz TJ (1975) Percutaneous absorption. On the relevance of in vitro data. J Invest Dermatol 64:190–195

Franz TJ, Lehmann P (1988) Percutaneous absorption of sulconazole nitrate in humans. J Pharm Sci 77:489–491

Graybill JR, Craven PC, Taylor RL, Williams DM, Magel WE (1982) Treatment of murine cryptococcosis with liposome-associated amphotericin B. J Infect Dis 145:748–752

Gruda I, Gauthier E, Elberg S, Brajtburg J, Medoff G (1988) Effects of the detergent sucrose monolaurate on binding of amphotericin B to sterols and its toxicity for cells. Biochem Biophys Res Commun 154:954–958

Hänel H, Raether W, Dittmar W (1988) Evaluation of fungicidal action in vitro and in a skin model considering the influence of penetration kinetics of various standard antimycotics. Ann NY Acad Sci 544:329–337

Hantschke D, Zabel M (1979) Das Verhalten der physiologischen Vaginalflora während antimykotischer Therapie. Mykosen 22:267–273

Hare RS, Loebenberg D (1988) Animal models in the search for antifungal agents. Am Soc Microbiol News 54:235–239

Hay RJ, Mackie RM, Clayton YM (1985) Tioconazole nail solution – an open study of its efficacy in onychomycosis. Clin Exp Dermatol 10:111–115

Hay RJ, Roberts DT, Doherty VR, Richardson MD, Midgley G (1988) The topical treatment of onychomycosis using a new combined urea/imidazole preparation. Clin Exp Dermatol 13:164–167

Hospenthal DR, Rogers AL, Beneke ES (1989) Effect of attachment of anticandidal antibody to the surface of liposomes encapsulating amphotericin B in the treatment of murine candidiasis. Antimicrob Agents Chemother 33:16–18

Houang ET, Lawrence AG (1985) Systemic absorption and persistence of tioconazole in vaginal fluid after insertion of a single 300 mg tioconazole ovule. Antimicrob Agents Chemother 27:964–965

Johnson E (1977) Seasonal changes in the skin of mammals. Symp Zool Soc Lond 39:373–404

Kennedy BK, Friedmann N (1985) Terconazole cream and suppositories: plasma terconazole following vaginal administration. Gynäk Rdsch 25(Suppl 1):26–32

Kinsman OS, Collard AE (1986) Hormonal factors in vaginal candidiasis in rats. Infect Immun 53:498–504

Kirsh R, Goldstein R, Tarloff J, Paris D, Hock J, Hanna N, Bugelski P, Poste G (1988) An emulsion formulation of amphotericin B improves the therapeutic index when treating systemic murine candidiasis. J Infect Dis 158:1065–1070

Kligman AM (1965) Topical pharmacology and toxicology of dimethyl sulfoxide – part 1. J Am Med Assoc 193:796–804

Kligman AM, McGinley KJ, Foglia A (1987) An in vitro human skin model for assaying topical drugs against dermatophytic fungi. Acta Derm Venereol (Stockh) 67:243–248

Knight AG (1973a) Culture of dermatophytes upon stratum corneum. J Invest Dermatol 59:427–431

Knight AG (1973b) Human models for an in vivo and in vitro assessment of topical antifungal compounds. Br J Dermatol 89:509–514

Lopez-Berestein G, Mehta R, Hopfer RL, Mills K, Kasi L, Mehta K, Fainstein V, Luna M, Hersh EM, Juliano R (1983) Treatment and prophylaxis of disseminated infection due to *Candida albicans* in mice with liposome-encapsulated amphotericin B. J Infect Dis 147:939–945

Lopez-Berestein G, Fainstein V, Hopfer R, Mehta K, Sullivan MP, Keating M, Rosenblum MG, Mehta R, Luna M, Hersh EM, Reuben J, Juliano RL, Bodey GP (1985) Liposomal amphotericin B for the treatment of systemic fungal infections in patients with cancer: a preliminary study. J Infect Dis 151:704–710

Lozano MM (1976) Empleo de HOE 296 (Ciclopirox) en micosis superficiales. Semana Med (Mex) 88:10–13

Marzulli FN, Brown DWC, Maibach HI (1969) Techniques for studying skin penetration. Toxicol Appl Pharmacol (Suppl 3):76–83

Mayer A, Szücs L, Török J (1978) Einfluß verschiedener Salbengrundlagen auf den perkutanen Transport eines wasserlöslichen Wirkstoffs in vivo. Pharmazie 33: 284–286

New RRC, Chance ML, Heath S (1981) Antileishmanial activity of amphotericin and other antifungal agents entrapped in liposomes. J Antimicrob Chemother 8:371–381

Oehmichen M, Frasunek J, Zilles K (1988) Kinetics of epidermal cells in skin from human cadavers. Naturwissenschaften 75:319

Patzschke K, Wegner LA, Oberste-Lehn H, Horster FA (1976) Pharmakokinetische Untersuchungen nach topischer Anwendung von Clotrimazol (Canesten^{R}). Münch Med Wschr 118 (Suppl 1):12–15

Patzschke K, Ritter W, Siefert HM, Weber H, Wegner LA (1983) Pharmacokinetic studies following systemic and topical administration of ^{14}C bifonazole in man. Arzneimittelforschung 33:745–750

Petranyi G (1985) Präklinische Evaluation von Exoderil (Naftifin)-I. Experimentelle Untersuchungsergebnisse zum antifungalen Wirkungsprofil. Mykosen 28 (Suppl 1):37–43

Pinkus H (1951) Examination of the epidermis by the strip method of removing horny layers. I. Observations on the thickness of the horny layer, and on mitotic activity after stripping. J Invest Dermatol 16:383–386

Pinkus H (1952) Examination of the epidermis by the strip method. II. Biometric data on regeneration of the human epidermis. J Invest Dermatol 19:431–447

Pitman IH, Downes LM (1982) Cattle and sheep skin permeability: a comparison of frozen and reconstituted skin with that of fresh skin. J Pharm Sci 71:846

Pitman IH, Rostas SJ (1982) A comparison of frozen and reconstituted cattle and human skin as barriers to drug penetration. J Pharm Sci 71:427–430

Reifenrath WG, Chellquist EM, Shipwash EA, Jederberg WW, Krueger GG (1984) Percutaneous penetration in the hairless dog, weanling pig and grafted athymic nude mouse: evaluation of models for predicting skin penetration in man. Br J Dermatol 111 (Suppl 27):123–135

Ritschel WA, Hussain AS (1988) In vitro skin penetration of griseofulvin in rat and human skin from an ointment dosage form. Arzneim-Forsch 38:1630–1632

Ritter W (1985) Pharmacokinetic fundamentals of vaginal treatment with clotrimazole. Am J Obstet Gynecol 152:945–947

Ritter W (1988) Pharmacokinetics of azole compounds. In: Berg D, Plempel M (eds) Sterol biosynthesis inhibitors. Ellis Horwood, Chichester, p 397

Ritter W, Siefert HM (1987) Biological disposition and percutaneous absorption of bifonazole in animals and man. In: Fromtling RA (ed) Recent trends in the discovery, development and evaluation of antifungal agents. JR Prous, Barcelona, p 383–405

Ritter W, Patzschke K, Krause U, Stettendorf S (1982) Pharmacokinetic fundamentals of vaginal treatment with clotrimazole. Chemotherapy 28 (Suppl 1):37–42

Schaefer H, Stüttgen G (1976) Absolute concentrations of an antimycotic agent, econazole, in the human skin after local application. Arzneim-Forsch 26:432–435

Schaefer H, Zesch H, Stüttgen G (1975) Penetration von Medikamenten in die Haut. Hautarzt 26:449–451

Schaffner CP (1987) Amphotericin B derivatives. In: Fromtling RA (ed) Recent trends in the discovery, development and evaluation of antifungal agents. JR Prous, Barcelona, pp 595–618

Schalla W, Schaefer H (1982) Mechanism of penetration of drugs into skin. In: Brandau R, Lippold BH (eds) Dermal and transdermal absorption. Wissenschaftliche Verlagsgesellschaft, Stuttgart, p 41

Scheuplein RJ, Ross LW (1974) Mechanisms of percutaneous absorption: V. Percutaneous absorption of solvent deposited solids. J Invest Dermatol 62:353–360

Schmitt HJ, Bernard EM, Häuser M, Armstrong D (1988) Aerosol amphotericin B is effective for prophylaxis and therapy in a rat model of pulmonary aspergillosis. Antimicrob Agents Chemother 32:1676–1679

Scott RC, Dugard PH (1986) A model for quantifying absorption through abnormal skin. J Invest Dermatol 86:208–212

Scullier JP, Coune A, Meunier F, Brassine C, Laduron C, Hollaert C, Collette N, Heymans C, Klastersky J (1988) Pilot study of amphotericin B entrapped in sonicated liposomes in cancer patients with fungal infections. Eur J Cancer Clin Oncol 24:527–538

Sloan KB, Koch SAM, Siver KG, Flowers FP (1986) Use of solubility parameters of drug and vehicle to predict flux through skin. J Invest Dermatol 87:244–252

Southwell D, Barry BW (1983) Penetration enhancers for human skin: mode of action of 2-pyrrolidone and dimethylformamide on partition and diffusion of model compounds water in alcohols and caffeine. J Invest Dermatol 80:507–514

Stüttgen G, Bauer E (1982) Bioavailability, skin, and nail penetration of topically applied antimycotics. Mykosen 25:74–80

Stüttgen G, Bauer E (1985) Permeation von markiertem Oxiconazol. Vergleich der autoradiographischen mit der Horizontalschnitttechnik an menschlicher Haut. Mykosen 28:138–147

Swarbrick J, Lee G, Brom J (1982) Drug permeation through human skin. I. Effect of storage conditions of skin. J Invest Dermatol 78:63–66

Tagami H, Natsume N, Aoshima T, Inone F, Suehisa S, Yamada M (1982) Analysis of transepidermal leucocyte chemotaxis in experimental dermatophytosis in guinea pigs. Arch Dermatol Res 273:205–217

Tarle SF (1980) Estudo comparativo duplo-cego con ciclopirox e clotrimazol sob as formas de creme no tratamento das micoses superficialis. Rev Bras Med 37:316–321

Taylor RL, Williams DL, Graven PL, Graybill JR (1982) Amphotericin B in liposomes: a novel therapy for histoplasmosis. Am Rev Resp Dis 125:610–611

Tremblay C, Barza M, Fiore C, Szoka F (1984) Efficacy of liposome-intercalated amphotericin B in the treatment of systemic candidiasis in mice. Antimicrob Agents Chemother 26:170–173
Tulli A, Ruffilli MP, De Simone C (1988) The treatment of onychomycosis with a new form of tioconazole. Chimioterapia 7:160–163
Van Scott EJ (1972) Experimental animal integumental models for screening potential dermatologic drugs. In: Montagna W, Bentley JP, Dobson RL (eds) Advances in biology of skin, vol. XII. Appleton Century Crofts, New York, p 523
Walters KA (1985) Penetration of chemicals into and through the nail plate. Pharm Int 6:86–89
Walters KA, Flynn GL (1981) Solvent influences on the transport of homologous chemicals across human nail plate. J Pharm Pharmacol 33:1–6
Walters KA, Flynn GL (1983) Permeability characteristics of the human nail plate. Int J Cosmetic Sci 5:231–246
Walters KA, Flynn GL, Marvel JR (1981) Physiochemical characterization of the human nail plate. I. Pressure sealed apparatus for measuring nail plate permeabilities. J Invest Dermatol 76:76–79
Washitake M, Anmo T, Tanaka I, Arita T, Nakato M (1975) Percutaneous absorption of drugs. IV: Percutaneous absorption of drugs from oily vehicles. J Pharm Sci 64:397–401
Wenk P (1962) Über die Ursachen der Selbstheilung der experimentellen Meerschweinchen-Trichophytie. Trop Med Parasitol 13:201–218
Wiebe VJ, DeGregorio MW (1988) Liposome-encapsulated amphotericin B: a promising new treatment for disseminated fungal infections. Rev Infect Dis 10:1097–1101
Zaias N, Drachman D (1983) A method for the determination of drug effectiveness in onychomycosis. J Am Acad Dermatol 9:912–919

CHAPTER 11

Regulatory Procedures

SARAH C. EARDLEY

A. Introduction

The intention of this chapter is to provide an outline of the regulatory and legislative background to drug development. It is not aimed at regulatory professionals but rather at the research scientist who, while being aware that the pharmaceutical industry is probably the most regulated and restricted of all industries, knows little of the detail of what is involved – or why.

It may seem hard to understand why there is so much regulation of pharmaceuticals when most other products, even potentially dangerous ones, are not subject to similar restrictions. However, although present legislation dates from comparatively recent times, there seems always to have been concern about medicines and their proper control since very early times. Section B gives a short summary of the history of drug legislation and drug development, summarises some of the landmark legislation in the UK and the USA and, in setting today's laws against this historical perspective, tries to answer the question 'Why is drug regulation needed?' Section C describes the parties involved – the regulators and the regulated. Section D then looks at the (very substantial) dossier of information which is now needed to support a marketing application for a new drug. Section E considers some of the implications for a pharmaceutical company in having to provide this information, in time, activities and cost, and Section F describes how the information is processed and reviewed within the regulatory authorities. Section G deals with the somewhat different constraints and regulations which apply to drugs already on the market, particularly the older products. Finally, Section H looks at some of the challenges faced by pharmaceutical companies and their registration departments because of drug legislation.

I have been a registration officer at the UK Headquarters of ICI Pharmaceuticals for some 12 years. Inevitably, therefore, this chapter describes a view of regulatory procedures as seen from a research-based company, from the headquarters of such a company and from the UK. It also emphasises the data requirements and the processes involving marketing applications for new drugs, because that has been my main preoccupation over the past few years. It is not easy to present a universal viewpoint, and other regulatory professionals in other countries and companies might well present different but equally valid descriptions of what regulatory procedures mean to them. However, it is hoped that this personal view from a research-based company is appropriate for a research-based handbook.

B. A Short History and some of the Landmarks in Drug Development and Regulation

I. Early Days

Humans have attempted to cure illness by taking medicines since history began, and throughout all this time there is some evidence of control by governments or other regulatory bodies. The subject has been well reviewed by PENN (1979), and a detailed description of the history of drugs has been given by MANN (1984).

There is hardly any product of the animal, vegetable or mineral kingdoms that has not at some time been reported to have medicinal value, and more than 700 such medicinal products were listed in the Ebers Papyrus around 3500 years ago. Indeed, the ancient Egyptians appear to have had a flourishing medical profession which was supported by public funds and which had to administer treatment in accordance with a written law, composed in yet earlier times by famous Egyptian physicians. Provided that the rules of this law were followed, the physicians were absolved from any charge should the treatment not be successful.

Control of drug quality was the preoccupation of most of the early regulations. For instance, in medieval Muslim countries the manufacture of medicines was controlled quite rigorously. The functions of the Hisba, an office which had been set up in the ninth century to compel observance of codes and regulations, were expanded to embrace the whole conduct of social and economic life. Medicine did not escape, and regulations were made concerning physicians, bone-setters and the syrup makers (who also prepared medicines). The syrup makers' premises could be inspected at any time without warning, and the punishments involved were stringent.

This Islamic example was followed in a number of European countries. In 1140, Roger II, King of the Two Sicilies, promulgated the first known law in Europe for the regulation of medical practice. Under this law, anyone wishing to practice medicine had to present himself before the officials and judges to be examined; the punishment for presuming to practise unofficially was imprisonment. Roger's grandson, the German Emperor Frederick II, also issued a series of laws between 1231 and 1241 which were effective through Italy, France and Germany. Under these laws doctors were forbidden to keep apothecary's shops, as it was recognised that pharmacy required skills separate from those of medicine. Apothecaries were strictly controlled and were required to prepare drugs reliably and of proper quality – this was probably the first European indication of the official pharmacopoeial standards which would develop.

In Britain also, early legislation was concerned mostly with drug quality, to establish the identity of the substance and its freedom from contamination. The earliest written code of quality control was probably the Ordinances of the Guild of Pepperers in 1316. The Pepperers were responsible for the distribution of imported drugs and spices, and the Ordinances forbade the mixing of wares of different quality, the adulteration of bales of goods or the falsification of their weight. Somewhat later the Apothecaries emerged as a separate guild which then divided into those who ultimately became general medical practitioners and those who founded the Pharmaceutical Society and became the pharmacists as we know them today. In 1423 the Physicians and Surgeons of London appointed two apothecaries to inspect the shops of their colleagues for the quality of their goods. The College of Physicians was founded in 1518 by Henry VIII, and in 1540 one of the earliest English statutes on the control of drugs was passed. This empowered the Physicians to appoint inspectors who had the right to search apothecaries' shops for faulty wares, which were to be burnt or destroyed. The Society of Apothecaries was granted a charter by James I in 1617 and also carried out their own inspections.

II. The Development of the Pharmacopoeias

Many ancient writers commented on the problems caused by fraudulent or accidental practices such as the adding of bulk, removal of active constituents and concealment of defects of various drug substances. Pharmacopoeias – authoritative lists of drugs, their preparation and uses – had been known since very early times but lacked the force of legal authority. However, in 1498 the Florentine guild of physicians and pharmacists issued a formulary, the New Compound Dispensary, which was the official and obligatory guide for the apothecaries of Florence, and this is generally regarded as the first official pharmacopoeia in Europe. Other cities followed this example, and similar obligatory formularies were issued in many of the chief cities of mainland Europe in the sixteen century.

In Britain the London Pharmacopoeia was not published until 1618. This pharmacopoeia was to apply not only to London but throughout England as well, making it effective over a much larger political unit than the previous European 'city' pharmacopoeias. In 1864 the first British Pharmacopoeia was published, superseding the three current ones from London, Dublin and Edinburgh. Except for a brief period between 1872 and 1875 the British Pharmacopoeia never achieved status as describing legal enforceable standards, but it was always the presumptive standard for the courts and loomed large in the battle against the adulteration of drugs that started in the early nineteenth century.

Adulteration had been recognised as a problem throughout history, but real controls over it only began when there were standards against which performance could be measured, in the form of official pharmacopoeias, and also sufficiently sophisticated tests to detect it. The development of chemical and physical methodology in the nineteenth century provided some of these weapons, as did the evolution and improvement in microscopy techniques. The first recorded use of the microscope in the identification of a crude drug was in 1847, when Schleiden showed that different forms of sarsaparilla could be distinguished by their microscopic structure. So by the middle of the nineteenth century the weapons to fight adulteration were becoming available, and in 1860 the Adulteration Act became law in Britain. At first it applied only to food and drink but was extended to drugs in 1872. At around the same time, professional organisations were being formed which were very much concerned with the detection and prevention of adulteration. The Pharmaceutical Society was formed in 1841 and the Society of Public Analysts in 1874.

III. The Rise of the Pharmaceutical Industry

The modern era of pharmaceutical development also dates from the nineteenth century. During this time, the active ingredients of several important drugs were isolated for the first time. The first of these was morphine, isolated by Serturner in 1805, and this was followed by other alkaloids such as strychnine, quinine, atropine and codeine. The glycosides digitalin (from foxglove leaves), salicin (from willow bark) and amygdalin (from bitter almonds) were also isolated early in the nineteenth century. At about the same time, in Germany and the UK, efforts at synthesising dyes led to the development of synthetic pharmaceutical products such as phenacetin and antipyrine.

In the UK important work was done by Barger and Dale in the Wellcome laboratories in the 1900s. They looked at the chemistry of the autonomic nervous system and identified the fact that the nervous control of muscles in the body was a chemical effect, that is, that the chemicals moved from one nerve ending to the next taking a message with them. This led to the possibility of altering the behaviour of the body through an understanding of the chemistry involved.

The other important landmarks of the nineteenth century were the development of the cell and germ theories, particularly the work of Pasteur in the 1860s. It was probably the identification of the specific causative agent, in the form of germs, which allowed a German physician, Paul Ehrlich, to lay the foundations of modern chemotherapy in the 1890s. Ehrlich had the concept of the 'magic bullet', that pharmaceutical research should be directed towards finding chemical agents which would be taken up by and kill the target germ but be tolerated by the host organism.

All these developments – ranging from Pasteur's germ theory to the work of the early physiologists and Ehrlich's concept of targeting the disease-causing organism – led to a much better understanding of the biochemistry of the human body, the sort of things that could go wrong with it, and how they might be put right by administering specific pharmaceutical compounds. And it was this new understanding which led on to the therapeutic explosion of the 1930s, starting with the development in 1933 of sulphanilamide.

IV. Self-Medication, Patent Medicines and Secret Remedies

It is important to realise that in early times ordinary people had much less recourse to a physician than they do today. Doctors were not always available, particularly in the country, and the poor could not usually afford them anyway. Until the nineteenth century the active principle of most cures and medicines came from plants, many of which were widely available. From early times there had been country men and women who gathered and sold herbs, and who not only used them but handed down their knowledge through the successive centuries.

In the reign of Henry VIII, the Royal College of Physicians and the Society of Apothecaries were trying to bring about better standards of medical and pharmaceutical practice and succeeded in getting the Medical Act of 1512 passed. This restricted the practice of medicine to licenced persons. However, 30 years later a further Act was passed which, after castigating the surgeons for 'minding only their own lucres and nothing the profit or ease of the diseased' went on to recognise 'divers honest persons... endowed with the knowledge of the nature, kind and operations of certain herbs' and made it lawful for 'every person, being the King's subject, having knowledge and experience of the nature of herbs, roots and waters...to practice and use any herb or herbs...according to their cunning, experience and knowledge'.

This Act of 1542, while allowing honest herbalists to practice their craft, also opened the door to unlicensed healers of many other sorts, and because of this later became known as the 'Quack's Charter'. And indeed, quacks, people boasting of medical knowledge or skill that they did not possess or offering wonderful remedies or devices without basis and with intent to defraud, seem always to have been with us. They certainly flourished in Victorian times in the UK, and in the late nineteenth and early twentieth centuries the medical profession became very concerned with the exploitation of the public by those who sold patent medicines. The British Medical Association analysed some of these medicines and in 'Secret Remedies, what they cost and what they contain' (BMA 1909) made the findings public, comparing the cost of the ingredients with the sales price, and the contents with the claims made. This led to a formal investigation by a Parliamentary Select Committee whose report was published in 1914, and which pointed out that:

> for all practical purposes British law is powerless to prevent any person from procuring any drug or making any mixture, whether potent or without any therapeutical activity ...advertising it as a cure for any disease or ailment...and selling it under any name...for any price he can persuade a credulous public to pay.

This report (SCPM 1914) contained important and far-reaching recommendations for the control, sale and advertisement of patent and proprietary medicines. Unfortunately, the report was ordered to be printed on August 4th, 1914, and the onset of the First World War at that time almost certainly delayed the establishment of effective drug regulatory control in the UK. However, some of the proposals made then now seem to underlie the provisions of the Medicines Act in force in the UK today.

V. Poisons and Dangerous Drugs

Some control over the sale of dangerous and poisonous substances had been taken in the eighteenth century, when the Gin Acts recognised the responsibility of the Government to prevent adulteration and abuse of what was in effect a drug. The Arsenic Act was passed in 1851 – arsenic was by then widely available as a rat poison and seed dressing and for various industrial processes, and the authorities became worried about poisonings from it.

The first professional register of chemists or druggists was established by the Pharmacy Act of 1852, and the subsequent Pharmacy Act of 1868 was the first serious attempt to control the labelling and selling of poisons – poisons were divided into two schedules and the seller was obliged to label them as 'poison' and with the name and address of the seller, who had to be a registered chemist or pharmacist. However, there was still no restriction of the sale of poisons or dangerous drugs to prescription by a medical practitioner only. Not until the Defence of the Realm Regulations of 1917 was the supply of certain drugs such as barbitone, cocaine and morphine limited to those for whom a physician had prescribed them. In 1920 the Dangerous Drugs Act was the first of a long series of Acts which over the years have controlled the supply and prescription of dangerous and narcotic drugs.

VI. The Therapeutic Substances Act

The increasing use of potent biological substances and the extension of immunisation in the early twentieth century led to questions of standardisation of such preparations and of the competence of manufacturers. Control of biological substances was difficult to contain within a pharmaceutical monograph because the purity and potency of these substances could not be measured by chemical means. The Therapeutic Substances Act of 1925 aimed to regulate the manufacture and sale of such substances, to provide standards to which they must conform and to regulate their labelling and sale. The Act applied to substances such as vaccines, sera, toxins and anti-toxins, antigens, insulin and pituitary hormone. The Act provided for a licensing system and factory inspections by the Licensing Authority. The manufacturer had to keep records of sale, and the container had to identify both the manufacturer and the batch. For the UK, the beginning of modern concepts of safety and efficacy can be seen in this Act.

VII. Thalidomide and After

Although there had been concern about the safety of some drugs and there had been recommendations that an independent body be established to assess drug safety, nevertheless little drug legislation was in force in most countries until the 1960s. The one notable exception to this was the USA. Before the 1960s, in all other countries, a drug manufacturer could market a new medicine without pre-marketing approval. Most reputable companies did in fact carry out preclinical and clinical testing, but the amount and quality of testing was probably very variable. Certainly, the safety evaluation of drugs by animal testing was still evolving and at an early stage when compared with the testing done today. Although it had been known that chemical substances could act as teratogens in mammals, little or no testing of new drugs for their effect on the embryo was undertaken by most companies.

Thalidomide was developed and placed on the market in 1956 in the FRG and was widely sold there and in other countries as a tranquilliser, sleeping pill and as a treatment for 'morning sickness' in pregnancy. It sold well and was regarded as a safe and effective medicine. Starting in 1959 there were reports of a rise in incidence in the FRG of an unusual malformation of the limbs of newborn babies. Unfortunately, it took several years before it became clear that it was the thalidomide taken by the mothers of the babies during pregnancy that had caused their skeletal deformities – and by that time several thousand 'thalidomide babies' had been born around the world.

In most countries the thalidomide tragedy was the catalyst which speeded up or brought into being the regulatory process for drugs as we would recognise it today. While legislation and guidelines for testing and approval are constantly evolving, in most countries the establishment of an independent body for assessing drugs prior to marketing and the legislation governing drug approval date back to the immediate post-thaliomide era (see Table 1).

VIII. Evolution of Regulatory Procedures in the USA

Regulation and drug development in the USA has been well reviewed by WARDELL and LASAGNA (1975). In the USA, as in Europe, before the twentieth century most food and drug controls were directed against impure and adulterated foods. Much of the development of the science of pharmacy in the nineteenth century was concerned with attempts to standardise and improve the quality of prescription drugs. However, there were some safety considerations – for instance, there were concerns about the therapeutic use of frankly toxic substances, such as hydrocyanic acid in the treatment of pulmonary tuberculosis. Some questions of efficacy also arose because of the concerns about the false claims made for patent medicines. In 1906 the Pure Food and Drug Act was passed, and while this was primarily concerned with food, it also controlled the labelling (but not advertising) of any substance used to affect disease. The Act made no legal distinction between prescription

Table 1. Main regulatory authorities and dates when their registration laws were enacted

Country	Regulatory authority	Main statutory basis for regulation
Australia	Commonwealth Dept of Health	Therapeutic Goods Act 1966 and amendments
Belgium	Ministry of Public Health	Royal Decree of July 1969 and amendments
Canada	Dept of National Health and Welfare, Health Protection Branch	Food and Drugs Act, Food and Drugs Regulations and amendments
Denmark	National Health Board	Medicines Act June 1975 and amendments
France	Ministry of Social Affairs and Employment, Dept of Pharmacy and Medicine	Public Health Code, Book V, Articles 601, 602 of Feb 1959, modified 1967
FRG	Drug Institute Federal Health Office	Law on Trade in Medicaments, August 1956 (the Drug Law) and amendments
Italy	Ministry of Health	Health Laws 1265 (1934), 519 (1973), 833 (1976), ministerial decrees of July and August 1977.
Japan	Ministry of Health and Welfare	Pharmaceutical Affairs Law 1960 and amendments
Norway	Medicines Control Authority	Law no 5, 1964, and amendments Pharmaceutical Specialities Regulations 1979
Sweden	National Board of Health and Welfare	Drug Ordinances of 1962 and 1963 and amendments
Switzerland	Intercantonal Office for Control of Medicaments	Intercantonal Convention on Control of Medicaments 1971
UK	Dept of Health	Medicines Act 1968, and statutory instruments enacted under the Act
USA	Food and Drug Administration, Center for Drugs and Biologics	Federal Food, Drug and Cosmetic Act 1938, amended 1962 and 1984 regulations codified under title 21 of Code of Federal Regulations

and non-prescription drugs, but any drugs included in the United States Pharmacopoeia or the National Formulary had to meet their standards for composition.

Although the 1906 Act was shown to have many weaknesses and loopholes, until the 1930s drug control in the USA had seemed essentially a problem of protecting the public against quacks, preventing misleading labelling and prohibiting the sale of drugs that were known to be dangerous. The regulations were still not much concerned with safety or with efficacy. Until the advent of sulphanilamide, which heralded the pharmaceutical revolution in the early 1930s, new drugs had posed few problems because there were so few of them. Sulphanilamide was quickly followed by a whole family of sulpha drugs targeted on a wide range of infectious diseases. The discovery of the antibacterial action of the sulphonamides in 1933 and the isolation of penicillin in 1939 revolutionised medical treatment and the pharmaceutical industry.

By the beginning of the 1940s medical science's expanding knowledge of the disease processes and their causes and of the mechanisms of drug action and their effects on specific organs was beginning to have a major impact on the drugs being produced for general use. For instance, in the years prior to 1935 an average of only six new products appeared annually in the US Pharmacopoeia. In comparison, in the period 1935–1970, new products constituted an average of nearly 40% of the annual listings. It was in this setting of the explosive growth of new drugs that the concern of the regulatory authorities with safety as opposed to quality was prompted, as in Europe, by a disaster.

In order to produce a liquid form of sulphanilamide one of the drug companies developed an elixir in 1937. Unfortunately the solvent they chose, ethylene glycol, was toxic, and there were 107 deaths – many of them young children – before it was realised that the solvent was a poison. The elixir sulphanilamide disaster brought to light the specific dangers that might be associated with new drugs and the need to test them for safety. The US Government acted swiftly, and in 1938 the Food, Drug, and Cosmetic Act was signed. This extended the government's control over advertising and labelling and required new drugs to obtain approval for safety before being marketed. However, the Food and Drug Administration (FDA) had as yet no control over how much preclinical testing was done prior to first use in humans and was not empowered to concern itself specifically with a drug's efficacy. These latter controls were added in 1962 when the Kefauver-Harris amendments to the FDA regulations required an investigational new drug (IND) submission prior to clinical testing and also required new drug applications (NDAs) to include substantial evidence for efficacy as well as safety.

IX. Summary

Legislative and regulatory controls have evolved parallel to – and generally in response to – developments (or disasters) in medical and pharmaceutical science. From the earliest times the major concerns were the detection and prevention of adulteration of herbs and then drugs. To these were added in the nineteenth and early twentieth centuries the need to suppress false and outrageous claims for nostrums and patent medicines. There were concerns about the safe handling of recognised poisons. But only in comparatively recent times and following the explosive growth of the pharmaceutical industry which started in the 1930s have the concerns and controls moved from purity to safety and finally to efficacy and the manner in which drugs are used.

C. Who Is Involved? The Regulators and the Regulated

There are very few countries in the world in which drugs can be sold without restriction – most countries have a regulatory authority which is responsible for registering drugs and controlling the use of drugs in that country. ICI, for instance, makes drug registration applications in around 100 countries. Of these, about 25 require the full dossier of data to be submitted for a new drug. The rest, generally the countries with smaller government agencies which are not set up to review a full dossier, require proof that the drug is already on sale in major markets and usually accept summary data.

A list of the major drug regulatory authorities is shown in Table 1, together with the name and date of the law which provides the main basis for regulation. Although, as discussed in the previous section, there have been laws about drugs since early times, nevertheless it is worth noting that in most cases the main legislation dates from the late 1960s or early 1970s – that is, shortly after the thalidomide episode.

Although the names are different, it can be seen that the regulators are usually part of the national Ministry of Health. The process of review of data on new medicines will be described in more detail later, but in general the dossiers are first reviewed by the professional (medical and pharmaceutical) secretariat of the regulatory authority. Their evaluation reports then go to a committee which is independent of the government, for instance the various Advisory Committees in the USA or the Committee on Safety of Medicines in the UK. The independent committees make their recommendations, which are usually accepted, back to the Ministry of Health, which is responsible for issuing a licence for the new medicine. There is one multi-national authority, the Committee for Proprietary Medicinal Products (CPMP), which can deal with marketing applications among the member countries of the European Community. This committee and the process of drug approval by the CPMP are sufficiently important and also sufficiently complex that they are described separately. There are also some less formal associations of countries with similar interests, such as the Scandinavian countries in the Nordic pact.

Who are the regulated? Who needs to get marketing approval for their medicinal products? And, indeed, what is a medicinal product? Although the legislation in different countries varies in presentation, format and degree of detail, in fact the definition of a medicinal product or 'therapeutic substance' is very similar in most countries. A therapeutic substance is defined as a substance which is administered to humans or animals for the purpose of treating, preventing or diagnosing disease, for contraception, for inducing anaesthesia or for otherwise preventing or interfering with normal physiological functions. (This is a summary of the wording from the UK Medicines Act, Section 130.)

It is generally the company which discovers and develops the new drug that puts together the dossier of information on it, but legally either they or the manufacturer or the seller of the product (if these are different) can apply for marketing approval.

D. Data Requirements for a New Drug

What does the dossier of data for a new drug contain? While there are differences in emphasis between the requirements of the main regulatory authorities, they are nevertheless broadly similar and address the same range of issues. The regulatory authority is concerned with ensuring that:

- New drugs are evaluated for safety and for efficacy in their proposed use
- New drugs meet specified standards for pharmaceutical quality
- The prescribing information informs but does not mislead physicians or patients

There are other considerations about drugs once they are on the market and older drugs, and these are considered in a later section.

The main concerns here are therefore safety, efficacy and quality, and drug legislation requires that the pharmaceutical manufacturer supply the regulatory authority with the following three types of data:

- Experimental data on animal pharmacology (efficacy data) and on a wide range of animal toxicity tests (safety data)
- Complete data on the human pharmacology studies and on all clinical trials carried out (efficacy and safety data)
- Scientific and technical data about the synthesis, analysis and chemistry of the new drug, and the manufacture, composition, analysis and stability of the formulated product (quality data)

The data requirements vary according to the type of drug, and clearly the amount of testing needed for a drug which will only have limited or occasional exposure to humans (e.g. an anaesthetic) will be less than that required for a drug which will be given continuously and long term (e.g. an antihypertensive or an antifungal drug).

A summary list of the data requirements for a chronically administered drug based on current EEC guidelines is displayed in Table 2. Although this is a simplified version of the detailed requirements, it can be seen that a very large amount of information is asked for these days.

E. The Regulatory Process: Pre-Submission

What are the implications to a pharmaceutical company of the data requirements for a new drug? What does it mean in terms of time scale, activities and cost? And how is a marketing application put together?

Table 2. Data requirements for a new drug

Pharmaceutical data

Data on the active agent

- Specification, and the analytical methods relating to each clause of the specification.
- Nomenclature and description.
- Manufacture and synthetic route.
- Quality control during manufacture.
- Development chemistry (evidence for chemical structure, validation of analytical methods)
- Impurities resulting from synthesis or breakdown during storage, and the analytical methods used to detect them.
- Batch analysis: analytical results for the batches used in development, and for the reference standard.
- Data validating the analytical methodology.

Data on the formulated drug product

- Specification, and the analytical method relating to each clause.
- Composition of sales and clinical trial formulations.
- Development pharmaceutics (the rationale and supporting data for choice of composition and ingredients)
- Manufacturing formula and process, and the in-process checks and controls.
- Data validating the analytical methodology.

Stability data

- Data on several batches of active agent and formulated drug product under various storage conditions, and the proposed shelf lives.
- The analytical methodology, and validation of this method as stability-indicating.

Toxicological and pharmacological data (preclinical studies)

Pharmacodynamic studies

- Actions relevant to the proposed use:
  - Data establishing the mechanism of the main pharmacological action preferably in well-validated experimental models.
  - Evidence of activity by the proposed route of administration, and comparison with standard drugs in the same therapeutic class.
- Other actions demonstrated or sought:
  - Data from screening tests in a wide variety of physiological systems (e.g. cardiovascular, central nervous, gastro-intestinal) to establish the pattern of activity.
- Interactions:
  - Data on interactions with other drugs which might be co-administered.

Pharmacokinetic and metabolism studies

Data indicating the pattern and time course of absorption, distribution, biotransformation and excretion of the active drug, and if possible its metabolites. These studies should be conducted in the animal species used in the toxicological and reproduction studies.
Doses and routes of administration should be related to the proposed clinical use. Some pregnant animals should be studied, to assess what level of drug the animal foetus has been exposed to.

Acute toxicity studies

- Single dose studies in two mammalian species.

Chronic Toxicity studies

Repeated dose studies in two mammalian species, one a non-rodent (usually rat and dog).
Generally 1-, 6-, and 12-month studies will be needed.

Table 2. (Continued)

Three dose levels, the lowest relating to the proposed human dose, the highest to give some target organ toxicity.

Foetal toxicity and fertility

Teratogenicity studies in two species, one a non-rodent.

Fertility study in one species, dosing from before mating and through pregnancy, with some females allowed to litter and rear progeny.

Peri- and post-natal study in one species, dosing from gestation through parturition to weaning.

Mutagenicity

A battery of tests designed to study the potential to damage genetic material. This is a relatively new and changing requirement but at present includes tests for: gene mutation in bacteria, and in eukaryotic systems; chromosomal aberrations in mammalian cells in vitro; genetic damage in vivo.

Carcinogenicity

Studies in two species, generally mouse and rat, and generally over 2 years.

At three dose levels, the lowest a small multiple of the proposed therapeutic dose and the highest designed to produce some toxic effect such as a 10% weight loss.

Human pharmacological and clinical data requirements

Clinical pharmacology studies

Pharmacodynamic studies demonstrating the mode of action and dose response relationships in humans.

Pharmacokinetic studies in healthy volunteers, patients relevant to the therapeutic indication, patients at increased risk (the elderly, children, people with renal or hepatic failure).

The studies need to demonstrate the way the drug is metabolised in humans, and the bioavailability of the proposed formulation.

Clinical trials

The trial programme must demonstrate the therapeutic efficacy and the safety of the drug in humans.

Efficacy:

The minimum requirement is for two controlled studies, for each indication and in the target population, demonstrating either statistically significant improvement over placebo or similar efficacy to a comparator drug which is already recognised as effective.

Safety:

The patients in all the clinical trials must have been carefully monitored for all adverse events, and this includes both major and minor adverse reactions reported and clinical laboratory measurements.

For a chronically administered drug, data from at least 1000 patients in total, including 100 patients treated for more than year, would be expected.

Safety data from patients at increased risk (the elderly, children, patients with renal or hepatic failure) would also be expected.

Prescribing information

I. The Activities and the Time Scale

Let us look first at some of the activities required prior to a marketing application, and their timing. Typical activities for a research-based company are summarised in Fig. 1 and can be broken down broadly into two main

	Discovery Phase 2-4 years	Development Phase Safety 2-4 years Clinical trial 3-6 years
Pharmacology	Observed activity; General pharmacological screening, confirm activity	Detailed animal pharmacology
Animal toxicity	Preliminary toxicity	Acute toxicity Chronic toxicity Reproductive toxicity Carcinogenicity
Kinetics and metabolism	Preliminary work	Detailed absorption, distribution, metabolism and excretion studies Human bioavailability studies
Human pharmacology and clinical trials		Approval for human trial Volunteer studies Open studies Initial controlled studies Large scale clinical studies to prove safety and efficacy
Pharmaceutical and process development	Early formulation development, stability	Chemical process devt Quality control methods Develop formulations Early stability tests Develop sales formulation Plant design Stability studies Establish manufacturing process
Regulatory		Regulatory advice on development programme Clinical trial application Review preclinical and clinical reports Assemble marketing application Submit

Fig. 1. Summary of activities and time scale for development of a new drug

phases – the research and discovery phase and the development phase. The discovery phase covers the activities through early screening of a new chemical entity for activity, toxicity, etc. to its adoption as a 'candidate new drug'. The development phase covers all the subsequent activities through preclinical (animal) and clinical testing to the submission of the marketing application. So far as the regulatory process goes, the Regulatory Affairs or Registration people are involved with a new drug from the time it enters the development phase right through to the marketing application and beyond.

In the first part of the development phase the activities lead up to approval for trials in humans. The detailed animal pharmacological screening will be done and also the acute toxicity tests, the 1-month toxicity tests and the two teratology tests. These, together with details of the drug compound's chemistry and proposed formulation, make up the package of data which, if satisfactory, will allow first use in humans. The pharmacology indicates that the compound may be active in humans, and the safety data suggests that there is a satisfactory margin between the proposed therapeutic dose and the dose which might give rise to any toxicity. Countries differ more in their data requirements for clinical trial approval than they do in their requirements for marketing approval, for instance as to whether they want full or summary data, whether volunteer studies need authorisation, and how long it takes to gain approval. Some countries require only notification of the proposed trials, some allow them to start after a set time if there have been no objections, and some require prior approval of all trials. A summary of various differences in a few of the more important countries for clinical trial work is shown in Table 3. This is by no means an exhaustive list, but it does show that the degree of control exerted over clinical trials varies considerably from country to country. In those where the control by the regulatory authority is limited, there may well be more onus placed on the clinical investigator and on the hospital ethical committee to make a careful review of the clinical trial protocol and the data. There is a requirement in most countries to supply the investigator with a 'Clinicians Brochure' or 'Data for Clinical Investigators'. This is a document containing a summary of the preclinical and clinical information in order to ensure that the investigator is familiar with the data on the product.

Once human trials start, the development phase moves into the second stage in which many and varied activities lead towards the marketing application. The long-term toxicity studies and the rest of the reproductive toxicology studies are completed, and reports on them are usually submitted to the regulatory authorities to allow approval of larger scale clinical studies, and longer term dosing in humans. The metabolism studies are completed. The clinical trials progress through volunteer studies and small open studies in patients (phase I) and initial controlled studies (phase II) to the large scale clinical studies which will provide proof of efficacy and safety (phase III). The Pharmaceutical and Process Development Departments work on optimising formulations of the new drug for performance and stability and scaling up the processes from the laboratory to pilot plant to full scale production. All the information which has been carefully checked and written up over this 3–6 year period comes to the registration officer responsible for making the marketing application, first for review and then as a final report.

II. The Cost

The development costs for new drugs (excluding drug discovery investment) will vary and depend on such factors as the type of drug, the country in which development takes place and the ratio of successful to unsuccessful products. However, average costs in the mid 1970s were thought to be around £10 million and by the mid 1980s were generally estimated to be £100 million or more – for each successful new drug. This is because the scale of the work required has increased, as shown below, and also because the quality of control required has changed. It is beyond the scope of this chapter to discuss Good Laboratory Practice (GLP), Good Clinical Practice (GCP) and Good Manufacturing Practice (GMP) in any detail, but undoubtedly the advent of these codes of practice in the three main areas of preclinical, clinical and pharmaceutical work has both improved the quality of the data recorded and added greatly to the cost of acquiring those data.

Table 3. Summary of data requirements and timing for clinical trial approval

Country	Type of data required	Summary or full data	Approval for volunteer studies needed	Timing to trial approval	Comment
Australia	Pharmaceutical Preclinical Clinical	Full + special summaries	Yes	Trial may start after 12 weeks if no objections	
Belgium	Pharmaceutical + Trial protocol	Summary	Yes	4–6 weeks	
France	Notification (but full data to French expert)	Full	Yes	Trial may start after 30 days if no objection to expert's opinion	Data not reviewed by Ministry but by expert
FRG	Preclinical Clinical	Full	No distinction between types of trial	Approval not needed	Data deposited but not reviewed unless problem occurs
Italy	Pharmaceutical Preclinical Clinical	Full	Yes	Around 12 months	
Sweden	Pharmaceutical Preclinical Clinical	Full	Yes	Around 12 months	
UK	Pharmaceutical Preclinical Clinical	Summary	No	Trial may start after 30 days if no objection	
USA	Pharmaceutical Preclinical Clinical	Full	Yes	Trial may start after 30 days if no objection	

Table 4. Increase in size of ICI's marketing applications since 1965

Product	Date of application	No of volumes	No of pages
Inderal	1965	4	406
Nolvadex	1973	7	647
Tenormin	1975	12	2793
Zoladex	1986	75	11000 approx.
Corwin	1987	240	37000 approx.

III. The Scale of the Marketing Application

Since the 1960s the amount of data required to be included in a marketing application has increased enormously. Table 4 shows the size of five applications made by ICI between 1965 and 1987. These were for new chemical entities, and all were intended to be used for long-term dosing in humans. The size of the earliest (Inderal) amounted to only 400 pages while that of the latest (Corwin) was nearly 100 times greater at 37000 pages. There are several reasons for the increase. Firstly, as experience and knowledge in the area of animal safety evaluation have evolved, a requirement has grown for more preclinical tests, over a longer term, using more animals per group. On the human side, too, experience has shown that while testing in small numbers of patients might provide proof of efficacy, it is not sufficient for safety. It is now recognised that in order to show a reasonable benefit-to-risk balance, trials of a new drug must be conducted in quite large numbers of the intended patient population and also in specific 'at risk' populations who may metabolise the drug differently, such as the elderly and renally or hepatically impaired patients. Finally, there is now a requirement for regular and careful monitoring, in both animal and human studies, of a large number of clinical laboratory parameters. Some of the major regulatory authorities ask for all these data, at all time points and for each individual, to be listed in the application, and these individual clinical laboratory data may well contribute more than half of the total number of pages in the final application.

IV. Compiling the Marketing Application

The registration officer has been involved with the new drug throughout its development. Indeed, he or she has an important role to play in the early and middle stages in trying to ensure that the development programme is adequate for future as well as current regulatory requirements. However, without doubt the heaviest workload comes in the months leading up to the submission of the marketing application for a new drug.

The registration officer sees and reviews draft reports on all the work outlined in Table 2. When each final report has been completed and signed off by the department responsible for the work, a good clear copy is received and kept in a safe place. The reports may be issued over a period of up to 10 years, and by the time the last one is received for a major new drug, the application may well run to more than 200 volumes and 30 000–40 000 pages. Because of the expanding size of modern applications it has been essential for registration departments to develop systems to cope with compiling, checking, printing and binding an application. In ICI, a Systems and Documentation Unit has been created within the Registration group, and this unit has a dedicated printing facility with well-trained staff so that a good quality of printing can be maintained. Each volume is carefully checked before printing and a one in ten sample of the printed copies are also checked for print quality and data integrity before binding starts.

The logistics involved with just a single application can be formidable. For instance, the application for Corwin, submitted in 1987 and for which the full dossier ran to 37 000 pages and 240 volumes, was printed for all the major markets at the same time. Not all markets took the full dossier; some took an abridged version from which individual clinical laboratory data had been omitted. However, the print-run for most volumes was 65, and altogether around 10 000 volumes and one and a half million pages were printed. The applications for each country had to be kept separate; some had to be bound and some left unbound because they would be put into special binders for a particular country later. Some needed special treatment – for instance, every single page of the full dossier had to be notarised for the Italian submission. Because of the number of volumes, the application was divided into around twenty consignments, and each consignment was bound, boxed and labelled for despatch before the next one was printed.

V. Structuring the Marketing Application

The constant increase in size of marketing applications has caused concern to both pharmaceutical companies, who have to put the information together, and to regulatory authorities, who have to review it. It is obviously essential that such a large amount of information is presented and structured in a way which does allow the reviewers to find their way around it. However, the best way of doing it is not always all that obvious. The information has come from many sources, is presented in a number of different styles and has been gathered together over a period of some years. More importantly, most major regulatory authorities have their own regulations or guidelines as to how they want the information presented, and some of these formats are not compatible with each other. Some countries ask for both an evaluation of as well as a summary of the key information, while others wish only to have a factual summary without any evaluation. And, finally, there are two quite different ways in which reviewers can approach the reviewing process: starting from the summaries and working down towards the detailed information, or starting with the detail and then working back up to the summaries. The majority of countries in Europe choose the first approach, but some important authorities such as the USA and Australia tend to use the second. The ideal structure of the dossier for the two approaches is not necessarily the same.

This is an important topic, particularly for international companies who are aiming to submit applications in all their major markets at much the same time, and a lot of thought and discussion has gone into the concept of an 'international dossier' and how this should best be presented. The aim of the international dossier is that a single set of definitive documents can be produced which can then be used, in whole or in part, to make up a marketing application for any country. The dossier has to be constructed so that it will suit those countries who rely mostly on summary data as well as those who place the greatest emphasis on individual reports. It is probably fair to say that many companies are still working on the fine detail of the structure of their International Dossier, but there is a fair measure of agreement on the broad outline. There should be a modular approach, and the information should be organised into several levels of detail which can be thought of as forming a pyramid. The concept has been well described by SNODDY et al. (1985) from the point of view of a major USA company and is illustrated in Fig. 2.

There are five levels of detail, with short summaries (or, alternatively, expert reports as described in the next section) forming the peak of the 'pyramid' of information. The next layer down is formed by detailed summaries of the preclinical and clinical work. The third layer is all the separate reports on the animal and human studies. The fourth layer is made up of the appendices containing the listings of individual animal and human data, particularly the clinical laboratory values, from these studies. The final layer contains further tabulations of individual values taken from the clinical case record forms, the case record forms themselves and perhaps other raw data and archived material.

The concept of the modular approach is that it would be possible to make a cut at any of points A–D and still have a complete and free-standing application. For instance, many European countries do not in the first instance want to see the appendices with individual data, and a cut at point C would be appropriate. Their application would then consist of expert reports plus comprehensive summaries plus the separate study reports. Other countries, such as Australia, want the appendices, and their cut-off point would be D. For the USA the application is made up of all the information, and although not everything in the bottom layer would be submitted initially, it would be available on demand. At the other end of the scale, the 'second wave' countries take summaries only, as described below, and their cut-off point would be B. The important point about being able to take different slices from the same pyramid is that, whatever the level of detail needed, the information is accurate and is consistent with that supplied to other countries.

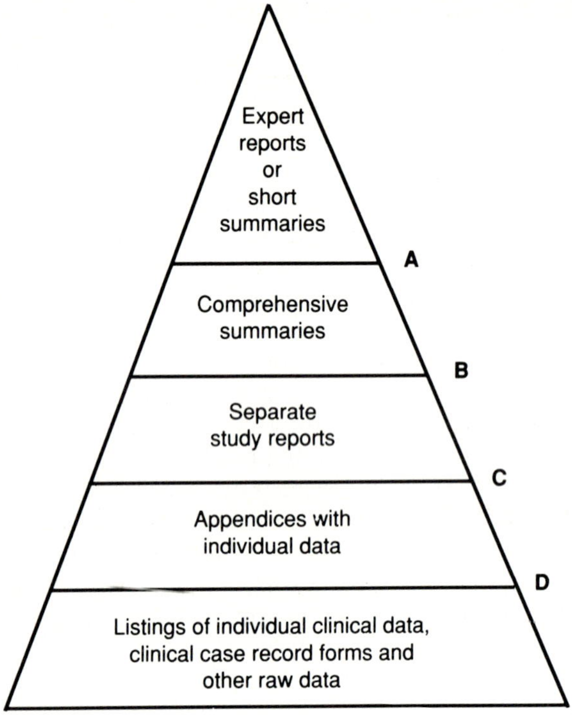

Fig. 2. Outline of structure of an international dossier

VI. Expert Reports

A number of European countries, such as the FRG and France, have always asked for 'expertises', or appraisals written by independent experts, as part of the marketing application. This approach has also been followed by the European Community when the Committee for Proprietary Medicinal Products (CPMP) formulated its requirements for a multi-national application within the Community. All EEC countries have now incorporated the CPMP guidelines within their own national regulations. The precise format, length and style of these expert reports is something that has changed and evolved over the past few years and is still evolving. A detailed discussion of expert reports is beyond the scope of this chapter and would in any case soon be out of date. However, the concept behind the expert reports is that they should be a concise and accurate summary of the key data in each of the three areas (pharmaceutical, preclinical and clinical), and that they should also contain a critical, detached and independent evaluation of those data, their adequacy and presentation, and that they should aim to highlight any perceived problems. They may be written either by a suitably qualified person within the pharmaceutical company or by an independent expert outside the company.

For most EEC countries they are the most important part of the application, and good expert reports are the key to a speedier review because they help the reviewer by highlighting the important issues.

VII. 'Second Wave' Countries

The 'second wave' of countries has been mentioned above. Essentially, these are all the countries in which registration applications have to be made but which are not included in the first wave of applications to the major regulatory authorities. The great majority of the first wave countries take the full dossier of information, or at least a substantial slice of it, as described in Part V above. In contrast, the great majority of the second wave countries ask for proof that the new drug has been approved in at least one major country, preferably the country in which the pharmaceutical company has its headquarters, and then generally only wish to review summary data. Because of the requirement for proof of marketing, in the form of an 'export certificate' from the country of origin, the second wave of applications is generally made about 12–18 months after the first wave. The distinction between first and second wave countries may differ a little between pharmaceutical companies, perhaps depending on where they are based, but a list of both categories as currently used by ICI is shown in Table 5.

F. The Regulatory Process: Post-Submission

What happens when a marketing application arrives at a regulatory authority? What process does it have to go through before a new drug can be approved or rejected? And how long does it take? This section looks at the process within a health authority, as typified by the UK Department of Health, and also at the process within a supra-national authority, the CPMP.

I. Processing of a Marketing Application Within the UK Department of Health

A summary of the process is shown in Fig. 3. The company prepares the appropriate number of copies of the submission. At the present time this is 6, but it has changed over the years – it used to be more than 20, so that a full copy of the application could be sent to each member of the Committee on Safety of Medicines, the independent review committee. All the volumes are boxed up and labelled in sets so that they can be more easily identified on arrival at the Department of Health. For a new drug there are probably enough boxes to fill quite a large van, and they are in fact despatched by secure courier to make sure that they do not get lost on the way. At the Department of Health, the boxes are given a Department of Health label. A postcard acknowledging the application is sent to the company. The appli-

Table 5. List of countries where ICI makes registration applications, divided into 'first' and 'second' waves

First wave countries	*Second wave countries*
Argentina	Hong Kong
Austria	Hungary
Australia	India
Belgium	Indonesia
Brazil	Iran
Canada	Iraq
Denmark	Ivory Coast
Finland	Jordan
France	Kenya
FRG	Kuwait
Greece	Lebanon
Holland	Liberia
Iceland	Libya
Italy	Luxembourg
Japan	Malaysia
Mexico	Malta
New Zealand	Mauritius
Norway	Morocco
Portugal	Mozambique
Rep. of Ireland	Nicaragua
South Africa	Nigeria
Spain	Oman
Sweden	Pakistan
Switzerland	Panama
UK	Paraguay
USA	Peru
	Philippines
Second wave countries	Poland
Algeria	Qatar
Angola	Rumania
Bahrain	Saudi Arabia
Bangladesh	Singapore
Bolivia	South Korea
Bulgaria	Sri Lanka
Chile	Sudan
Columbia	Surinam
Costa Rica	Syria
Curaçao	Taiwan
Cyprus	Tanzania
Czechoslovakia	Thailand
Dominican Rep.	Tunisia
Ecuador	Turkey
Egypt	Uganda
El Salvador	United Arab Emirates
Ethiopia	Uruguay
Ghana	USSR
Gibraltar	Yemen Arab Republic
Guatemala	Yugoslavia
Guyana	
Honduras	

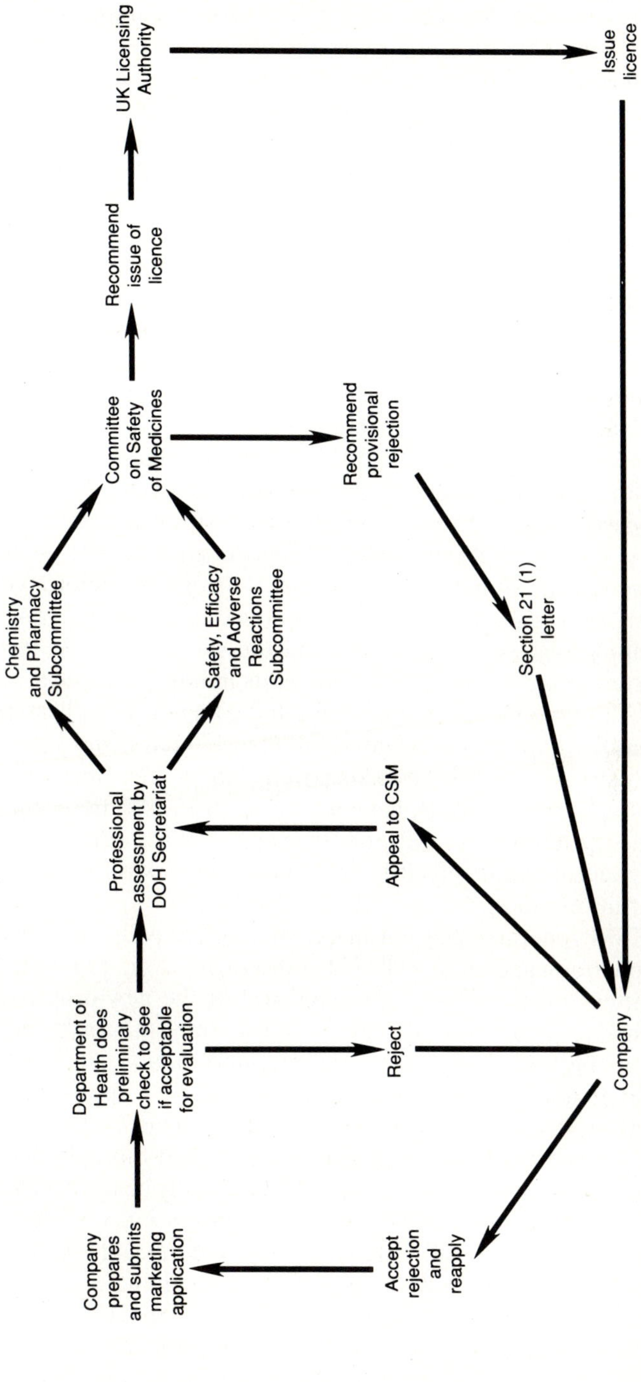

Fig. 3. Processing of the marketing application within the UK Department of Health

cation is registered, and a special file is opened. A preliminary check is made, probably of the summaries and list of contents only, to see whether or not the application is acceptable for evaluation. If it has important omissions or other major problems, e.g. with presentation, it can be rejected at this stage and returned to the company for amendment. If it is accepted for evaluation then the pharmaceutical data will be sent to the Pharmaceutical Secretariat, and the preclinical and clinical data to the Medical Secretariat, to await review. The pharmaceutical reviewer will be a pharmacist, and the medical reviewer will be medically qualified, although they will not necessarily be an expert in the particular clinical area covered by the application.

The reviewer's evaluation reports first go to two subcommittees of the Committee on Safety of Medicines (CSM). The pharmaceutical review goes before the Chemistry and Pharmacy subcommittee, and the reviews of the preclinical and clinical data go before the Safety, Efficacy and Adverse Reactions subcommittee (SEAR). The members of these subcommittees and of the CSM are independent of the Department of Health and are distinguished people, many of them from academic life, who are chosen for their expertise in different specialist areas. They will consider the application and the reviewers' evaluation reports and make a recommendation to the CSM as to whether the application should be approved or rejected.

The application, the evaluation and the subcommittees' recommendations are considered by the CSM at one of its monthly meetings. Under EEC guidelines the time from acknowledging the company's application until the CSM's consideration should be not more than 120 days, and the UK Department of Health tries very hard to keep to this timetable. Because of the large number of applications which have had to be processed in recent years, this places a heavy burden on both the reviewers and the committee members, who are given comparatively little time to work their way through a very large amount of information.

The CSM generally, but not invariably, agrees with the subcommittees' recommendations and may well add some of its own. For instance, if the subcommittees have recommended approval of the new drug but there are minor concerns about specific safety issues, they may ask for additional warnings to be added to the prescribing information. It is important to understand that a new drug is not given a blanket approval: rather, the committees have to consider the balance of the benefit that a new therapy may bring against any risks that may be perceived. If this risk: benefit ratio is thought to be favourable, then the drug will probably be approved, but within the context of being prescribed for the proven indication(s) in the appropriate patient population, and with stated warnings and precautions to try to minimise any possible risks. Any constraints to prescribing are handled by the prescribing information text (the 'Data Sheet' in the UK) which must be agreed between the CSM, the Department of Health and the pharmaceutical company. The final agreed wording of the Data Sheet text is very important because this is the information which the company is required to send to every physician who might prescribe the drug, and it also forms the basis for all advertising and promotion.

If the CSM recommends approval, and when the final prescribing text has been agreed, the recommendation comes back to the Licensing Authority (technically, the Minister of Health) who is responsible for issuing the Product Licence. Once the product Licence has been received, the company is free to sell and promote the product. If, on the other hand, the CSM recommends rejection, the Department of Health issue a formal letter to the company (called a Section 21.1 letter because that section of the UK Medicines Act covers the rejection of licence applications). The company may accept the decision and will probably hope to resubmit the application when they have amended it with additional information answering the committee's queries or criticisms – or they may contest the decision and make an appeal to the CSM. Th appeal will be backed by written arguments and will probably be decided at a formal hearing.

The process outlined here is fairly simple and straightforward, and if a new drug is indeed approved at the first meeting of the CSM then the approval process from application to issue of licence may take around 8–10 months. In practice, however, the passage of a new drug application through the regulatory authority is not always that smooth, and there may be one or more rejections and amended applications before approval is finally gained. Since each amended application has to go through much of the process as the original application, each pass through the system may take another 8–10 months, and this is why it may take 18 months, 2 years or even longer for some applications to be approved.

II. The Committee for Proprietary Medicinal Products

The concept and philosophy behind the CPMP scheme is that there should be harmonisation between the EEC member states in drug legislation and approvals. Clearly, if each member state makes an independent and separate review of the same new drug application, at much the same time, as they have been doing in the past, then there has been much duplication of effort. If the main, detailed review can be undertaken by one country, and the results of that evaluation made available to the other countries before their own review, then resources within the reviewing authorities will be better utilised, and the reviewing process more consistent.

The European Community issued its first directives in 1965, and it must be said that progress towards harmonisation was rather slow in the early years, but it is now speeding up as we approach 1992 and the achievement of the single European Market. Initially the countries had rather different approaches to registration, sometimes different concerns about new drugs and certainly different regulations and guidelines to work to. In addition, the medical culture and disease profile is not the same in all countries, so that a new drug which is seen to be useful and effective in one may not be so

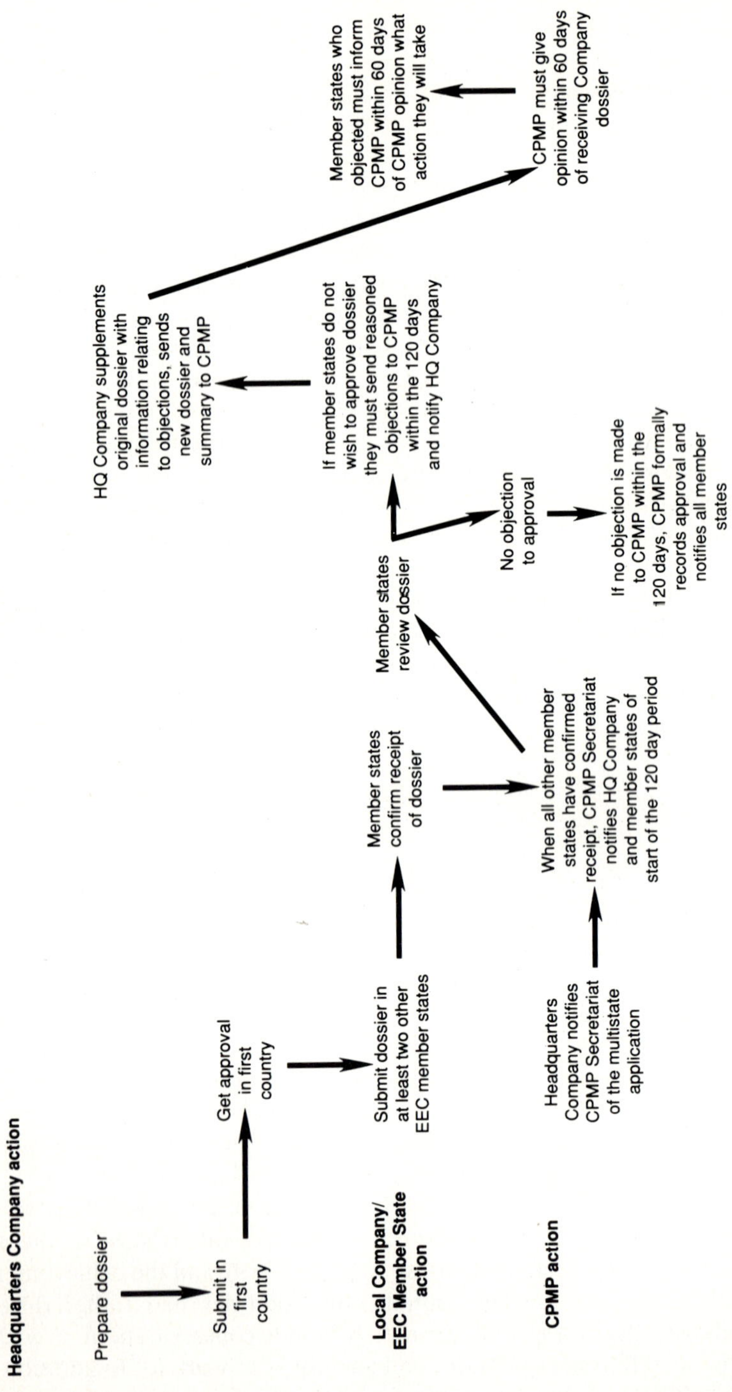

Fig. 4. Processing of the marketing application within the Committee for Proprietary Medicinal products (CPMP)

acceptable in another. Many of these differences are now disappearing, and most EEC countries have now incoporated the EEC guidelines within their own drug legislation and guidelines.

An outline showing how marketing applications are processed within the CPMP is shown in Fig. 4. Because a number of countries are involved, rather than just one, the process is inevitably fairly complex. The company prepares the dossier on a new drug, submits it to the regulatory authority in one country (usually that in which the company's headquarters is based) and obtains approval there. The dossier can then be submitted to other EEC member states, and the CPMP secretariat is notified that a multi-state application is being made. The regulatory authorities in the member states check the dossier and confirm its receipt to the CPMP secretariat. Only when all member states have made this formal acknowledgment does the CPMP notify the headquarters company and the member states of the start of the 120-day period within which they have to review the dossier. If there have been no objections, the CPMP makes a formal record of the approval and notifies all the member states of the EEC. If, however, any member state does not wish to approve the new drug, for the proposed indications and with the proposed prescribing information, they must send reasoned objections to the CPMP within the 120 days and also notify the headquarters company of the objections. The company must now supplement their original dossier with arguments or new information relating to the objections which have been made, and this new dossier is sent to the CPMP. Another 'clock' now starts running, because the CPMP must give their opinion about the approvability of the new drug within 60 days of receiving the dossier. This opinion is not binding on the member states but in practice is likely to be accepted by the majority of them. The member states who objected must now inform the CPMP, within 60 days of receiving the opinion, of what action they will take – i.e. whether they will approve the drug or not.

It can be seen that this is a long and complicated process, and it does take quite a long time for a new drug application to go through all the different stages. Although there are the three set periods of 120, 60 and 60 days, in practice the total process takes a good deal longer than this. Although the dossier submitted in the EEC member states is essentially the same as that submitted in the first country, it has to be amended to take account of any changes agreed with the first regulatory authority, and it also takes time for the local companies to do any necessary translations, for instance of the expert reports. If there are objections and the headquarters company has to supplement the original dossier with new information, this also takes time because summaries, etc. may have to be rewritten. Experience to date has been that no single application so far has ever received unanimous approval without reference to the CPMP for an opinion. Finally, although the member states who objected are supposed to tell the CPMP within 60 days whether they will approve the drug, in practice many of them take up to a year or more to do this. If you add the 1–2 years that it may take to gain approval in the first country, it is clear that the whole process may take 4 years or more. So although the concept of the CPMP process is attractive, and there may be savings of reviewers' time and resources, at the present time the process does not necessarily bring about speedier approvals for the company.

III. The Regulatory Process in 'Second Wave' Countries

Apart from the major regulatory authorities who review the full dossier on a new drug, there are about 75 countries who have regulatory processes of some kind and who require pre-marketing approval for drugs. The processes in these countries vary quite widely, from those who make a careful review of the data received to those in which registration approval is a formality. Factors such as whether the new drug will be manufactured locally and the proposed price can be important. The time taken varies from a few months to a few years. Over the past few years quite a number of these countries have taken measures to control the over-large number of drugs which are already available on their markets, some of them of doubtful efficacy and some, local counterfeit copies of the more expensive imported drugs. The authorities have tried to control the ineffective products by instituting new registration laws and requiring companies to make registration applications for all their drugs – those already on the market as well as their new drugs. This probably is the best, or the only, way in practice for some countries to eliminate unnecessary or unsafe drugs. However, because of the limited scale of the reviewing resources in these countries, such a re-registration scheme has often tended to overload the system and led to long queues of applications waiting to be processed. Control of the counterfeiting of products has been tried by insisting on special pack identification markings. Sometimes the new laws aim to be a close copy of those from a larger and more sophisticated regulatory authority, and while this should give a better quality of review, at the moment it remains to be seen how well the laws can be made to work with more limited expertise and resources. Although the process may seem relatively simple and straightforward when compared with the major regulatory authorities, because of cultural and language differences registration in many of the second wave countries has never been easy, and it is unlikely to become easier as time goes by.

G. Regulatory Processes for Marketed and Older Products

The description of regulatory procedures in this chapter has largely concentrated on new drugs. However, it is important to know that the story does not end once a drug is put on the market. Indeed, it is likely that registration officers spend most of their time servicing products that are already on sale. Some of the main areas of activity are shown below.

I. Supplementary Applications

The first application for a new drug will often cover only an initial major clinical indication. As information on the drug increases and perhaps also as medical knowledge or thinking changes, then further registration applications will be made. These applications may be as large as, or even larger than, the original application, and secondary indications may turn out to be more useful or important than the first. An example of this from the ICI range of products would be Inderal, which was first introduced in 1965 primarily as a treatment for arrhythmias. It was not realised at the time that beta-blockers were effective in hypertension, and the more important indications for Inderal, such as hypertension and angina, were not added for some years.

New applications are also made for improved formulations of a product, perhaps when a more stable formulation is developed, or a more bioavailable one or a sustained release form.

II. Drug Review Programmes

As discussed in Section B, most regulatory authorities did not require pre-marketing approval until the 1960s. When they did introduce their new legislation, most countries allowed drugs which were already on the market to continue to be sold. Some of these older drugs were superseded by newer therapies as time went by and were withdrawn from sale, but many were still seen to have some usefulness. This means that even in the 1980s there were many drugs on the market whose efficacy and safety had not been tested and documented to the same standards as the newer drugs. Most countries therefore instituted a drug review programme which required companies to submit dossiers of safety, efficacy and qualify information on their older products. For instance, the EEC requires its member states to review all older products by 1990, and in the UK this led to the Committee on Review of Medicines (CRM) being set up. This is an independent committee similar in set-up to the CSM but responsible for the review of older products.

The review programme has placed a heavy burden on the regulatory authorities, who have had to cope with reviewing all the extra applications. Although these applications are not as detailed as a new drug application, there have been many thousands of them, and they have had to be reviewed to a strict timetable. Many pharmaceutical companies, too, who have had to assemble dossiers on a large number of older products, have had to dedicate a significant amount of effect to it. For some older products, the amount of effort which would be needed to put the information together has not been justified by their current or expected sales, and their licence has been allowed to lapse.

III. Maintaining the Consistency of Prescribing Information

International pharmaceutical companies who sell their products in many countries have to ensure that the information supplied about their products in one country is consistent with that given in others. In order to accomplish this, many companies have now introduced a standard basic text which includes all the essential prescribing information for a product and insist that the text in all countries be consistent with this. For a new drug, consistency between texts should be made easier because they have at least started from the same base. Even here, however, some authorities may ask for additional statements or warnings, such as class statements for a particular type of drug. They may approve some indications and not others, or may insist on a lower starting dose to be used. The format used for prescribing texts can differ markedly between countries, and some are much more detailed than others. So even from the start the prescribing texts for a product will not be precisely the same in all countries, although they should not be inconsistent.

Maintaining the consistency of the prescribing text for an older product can be more difficult because the various countries may have started off with more differences in format and detail initially, and as time goes by changes may be introduced in one country but not in others, usually at the request of the regulatory authorities. Some indications will be more important in some countries than others, new formulations will be introduced in some countries but not others, and so the texts can evolve differently with time. Finally, many of these texts will be translations into the local language and have to be translated back before they can be checked for consistency.

ICI has approximately fifty products and sells the majority into most of the one hundred markets that have regulatory requirements. Whenever a supplementary application is made for a product, a dossier will be prepared for each market, and these will usually be slightly different because of different application forms, etc. If a country introduces new registration requirements or says that all drugs must be re-registered, then many new dossiers must be prepared for that one country. Whenever there is a change in prescribing information for any product, then all countries must be informed and sent the supporting information. Not all markets or all products are active at once, of course, but at any one time there will be hundreds of active files and dossiers being updated, and this represents a substantial part of the workload for a registration group.

H. Discussion

As we saw in Section B, there have always been concerns about drugs, and laws and codes attempting to control their use go back as far as the ancient Egyptians, more than 3000 years ago. Legislative controls have evolved parallel to developments in pharmaceutical and medical science. Until quite recently, most drugs were herbal in origin, and the main concerns were about gross contamination or adulteration of these herbal products. Real control of quality only became possible, however, in the second half of the nineteenth century when there were in place both official standards against which purity could be measured (the pharmacopoeias) and sufficiently sophisticated and accurate testing methodology. The modern era of pharmaceutical development also dates from the nineteenth century when the different threads of developments in synthetic chemistry, physiology and microbiology came together and led on to the therapeutic explosion of the 1930s. During this century many of the regulatory controls have been introduced as a result of, or accelerated by, specific disasters such as those caused by the elixir of sulphanilamide or by thalidomide. We have moved quite quickly from the situation in the 1950s, in which there was probably not enough regulation of new drug products, to the present position in the 1980s where there is so much regulation that it threatens innovation.

There are many challenges faced by pharmaceutical companies and their registration departments because of today's drug legislation, and it may be worth enumerating some of these. One of the most obvious is that the greatly increased amount of testing required, both preclinical and clinical, means that more of the research and development budget now must go on development, and less of it can be allocated to original research. One result of the increased testing has been the greatly increased size of the marketing application dossier. As we have ssen, in ICI these have grown almost 100-fold since the 1960s and have reached almost unmanageable proportions, both for the companies who have to assemble them and for the regulatory authorities who have to review them. Indeed, a number of authorities have said that they are not able to handle the full dossier with all the individual animal and human data, even though their regulations say that these data must be included. The cost of developing a new drug has probably risen tenfold since the 1970s and is now so great that only one which will be prescribed for a large patient population and remain prescribable over many years is likely to recoup its development costs. It is very difficult for a pharmaceutical company to develop drugs to treat uncommon diseases or diseases which only occur in a small number of countries, because they cannot afford to do so.

Another result of the increased demands for testing is the much longer time that the development programme takes. When mandatory testing began in the 1960s, the tests might have taken 1–2 years. Now, as illustrated in Fig. 1, they are likely to take at least 10 years. The regulatory requirements will almost certainly have changed, perhaps quite substantially, during this time, so the pharmaceutical company is always shooting at a moving rather than a fixed target. The development programme planned at the beginning will have to be continually updated and amended. It is not unknown for authorities to publish new guidelines for testing and expect them to be complied with almost immediately, but a company submitting a dossier around that time may in fact have done some of the tests 10 years previously.

As discussed in Section E, most pharmaceutical companies which are planning to register a new product in several major markets at the same time aim to produce an international dossier which can be used in all countries. The intention is that some countries will take the whole dossier while others may omit some of the detailed appendices, but all authorities will be reviewing essentially the same information. One of the challenges for the company is to prepare the dossier in such a way that it is possible to take only part of it and still have an intact and free-standing entity that is consistent and representative of the whole. Also, some authorities review from the 'top down' and others from the 'bottom up', so the dossier has to be prepared in such a way that either of these approaches is possible. Because the dossiers are required to be extensively cross-referenced, for instance between the summaries and the separate reports and between the reports and the appendices, this is not as easy as it might sound.

Section E also describes expert reports; this is an area which has cost most pharmaceutical companies registering drugs within the EEC considerable effort and difficulty. The formats required for the three expert reports (pharmaceutical, preclinical and clinical) has been fairly strictly laid down at any one time, although the CPMP has changed the guidelines from time to time. This has sometimes meant that companies have worked to one format, only to find that by the time they had made their application a different one was required. The correct number of pages, initially set at no more than 25 for each report, was demanded by some authorities while others were equally insistent that they required more detail and a longer report. Indeed, it may be difficult for a company to make a good summary and a reasoned evaluation of a 30 000 page clinical dossier in only 25 pages. Perhaps the main challenge, however, is that in the expert reports the company is asked to present a detached and even critical evaluation of their own development programme and their presentation of it in the dossier. In practice it may be difficult for the external expert to spend sufficient time to gain a full understanding of the data base, particularly in a new disease area. It may be equally difficult for an internal company expert, who might have been closely associated with the development programme and the assembly of the dossier, to have the required detached and critical viewpoint.

The challenge of maintaining consistent and up-to-date prescribing information has been discussed in Section G. International pharmaceutical companies give high priority to doing this, but the difficulty of achieving it should not be underestimated. Every change has to be notified to each regulatory authority, and in many of the smaller countries the authorities are not really set up to cope with a lot of little changes. Often, because of the time it takes for registration or re-registration applications to be approved in these countries, a product file may be stuck in the system for months if not years, and it will not be possible to make any further amendment to it until it has emerged. When a very technical text is translated into a language such as Farsi or Korean or other languages which are not easily translated at company headquarters, and then translated back again for checking, it can be difficult to know whether they are incorrect or simply poorly translated.

In summary, it can be seen that the need to meet the many and varied drug regulatory requirements from all the different countries does present a unique challenge for pharmaceutical companies and, specifically, for their working registration officers. After 20 years of very active change and growth, it could be expected or hoped that drug legislation would have reached a plateau and enter a more settled phase. This seems unlikely. Changes are still taking place within the EEC regulations, particularly with respect to the 'high technology' products. Indeed, regulations everywhere are going to have to deal with new classes of products, such as those made by genetic engineering. In the USA the strong feelings of consumers that they have a 'right to know' and the Freedom of Information Act which allows them access to quite a lot of the information submitted on new drugs is going to be in conflict with pharmaceutical companies' needs to protect their intellectual property. There are moves to find alternatives to animal testing, and if progress is made then there could be years of discussion ahead in the area of preclinical safety evaluation. There are increased expectations, however unrealistic, that companies can enlarge and improve their safety testing in human patients to a level at which they are sure of a product's safety. So there is, if anything, an acceleration of change in the regulatory scene at the present time, and certainly it is unlikely ever to become static.

Names quoted thus – 'Inderal' – are trademarks, the property of Imperial Chemical Industries PLC.

References

British Medical Association (1909) Secret remedies: what they are and what they contain. British Medical Association, London

Mann RD (1984) An equiry on historical principles. MTP Press, London

Penn RG (1979) The state control of medicines: the first 3000 years. Br J Clin Pharmacol 8:293–305

Select Committee on Patent Medicines (1914) Report of the Select Committee on Patent Medicines. HMSO, London

Snoddy CS, Michalak RA, Kaufman LS (1985) The pyramid concept. Drug Information J 19:27–33

Wardell WM, Lasagna L (1975) Regulation and drug development. American Enterprise Institute, Washington

CHAPTER 12

Clinical Trials

THOMAS C. JONES and JOHN J. STERN

A. Introduction

The process of applying or administering a drug to humans, either healthy volunteers or patients, under careful observation by research physicians and directed at answering questions about the drug, is referred to as the conduct of clinical trials. Although most people would agree with this definition, one must predict that few other statements regarding aspects of clinical trials would result in uniformity of opinion. Indeed, if one were to place a value judgement on the conduct of clinical trials, such as whether they are good, or important, or necessary, or scientifically based, or unethical, vigorous disagreements would immediately emerge. Therefore, in this chapter we will only touch on a few aspects of clinical trials relevant to the study of antifungal drugs. For a general review of clinical trials numerous other texts should be consulted (e.g., BURLEY and GLYNNE 1985; SPRIET and SIMON 1985; World Health Organization 1975; CIOMS 1983). We have attempted to place this presentation in perspective by discussing briefly in the first section why clinical trials are used in the development of new antifungal drugs.

The principles and organization of clinical trials of antifungal drugs follow the general approach to drug development for all drugs. These are reviewed in subsequent sections of this chapter. The procedure is designed to achieve maximum protection for healthy volunteers and patients, while attempting to identify the efficacy and tolerability of a new drug as rapidly as possible. Some would say that clinical trials have only one purpose: to protect patients and society against useless and unsafe drugs. Therefore, although we set out to find efficacy and tolerability, we are in reality trying to prove the inefficacy and poor tolerability of the drug. If we are unable to demonstrate these negative drug features, the short drug development process leading to rejection of further drug development is turned into a rather long one of 3–5 years while the drug is reluctantly accepted. This frustrates many investigator clinicians who become enthusiastic about the usefulness of a drug during its early testing, become critical of the pharmaceutical industry and regulatory agencies for inefficiency, bureaucracy and incompetence, but forget that the primary goal of the whole process is the opposite of what they want, i.e., drug rejection not drug acceptance. Occasionally, owing to tremendous pressure, such as has been recently seen in attempts to find treatments for AIDS, modifications of the system are tried, but such attempts are often ineffective because they are at variance with the reason clinical trials exist in the first place.

In this chapter we also review special difficulties in the design of clinical trials in serious disease states, such as systemic mycoses and particularly AIDS. Special clinical trials in these diseases are done in part to short cut some of the problems raised in the preceding paragraph. Such studies resolve some ethical issues of comparative drug trials, but they often end with incomplete data for reaching sound clinical judgements. How to achieve the best balance of these points is a major part of the clinical trial process.

To complete this review of clinical trials, we present special issues of statistical analysis, protocol preparation, good clinical practice, and study summation. We have been highly selective in our presentation in this area, but we hope we have focused on certain points which will allow clinical trials with divergent goals to each have a firm basis in accepted trial procedure. This brings out the point that trials of drugs in humans may have different purposes which lead to varied trial designs. To state that only one design is correct and the others are faulty would be inaccurate. However, if simple procedures of study preparation, conduct, and summation are followed, then the varied goals of clinical trials can be accepted as reasonable. If, however, these procedures are not followed, the investigators involved deserve the criticism and lack of scientific enthusiasm their studies evoke.

B. Why Clinical Trials Exist

Clinical trials would be unnecessary if new drugs were sufficiently harmless and tests for human safety sufficiently standardized, since the effects of drug use could simply be observed after the drug was made available in the community. In addition, if placebo effects did not occur and if efficacy was easily recorded by the patient and clinician, then proof of efficacy prior to release of a drug into the community would not be necessary. We would simply rely on the physician and patient to judge, as they used the drug, its efficacy and the ratio of any risks (side effects) to benefits. Since none of the above statements applies to most drugs (i.e., drugs are harmful), there are no standard reliable tests of human drug safety, there are placebo effects, and efficacy may be hard to judge, clinical trials are necessary.

This situation, however, has placed investigative clinicians in important ethical and legal dilemmas which are reviewed but not resolved in weekly journal publications. One of the most recurring themes is that if an open-labelled drug trial is done and the effects of the drug are impressive, then a double-blind, placebo-controlled study of the same drug would deny known effective therapy to a group of patients (placebo treated). These patients may then complain of the unethical nature of their treatment to appropriate review bodies, and attempt to receive financial compensation in court by legal means for their mistreatment. The only way to avoid this dilemma is to avoid open-labelled, uncontrolled trials as much as possible. The results, whether negative or positive, are potentially misleading, since no control group exhibits the natural course of the disease, and if perceived as positive, the above-cited ethical and legal concerns may prematurely influence the scientific questions to be answered in subsequent clinical trials research.

Another theme of importance in clinical trials is how informed is the volunteer or patient who gives 'informed' consent for the clinical trial? It is agreed now that all studies require such an informed state; however, the patient is usually not tested on the degree to which he or she is informed. In some countries the informed consent can only be signed by a witness who believes the information has been received. In other countries informed consent would have to be redefined because individuals are not technically free to make a choice about whether or not they participate in a study. This is because the definition of 'self' may not be separable from 'tribe', 'village', or 'social group'. Thus, some other person, such as a village elder, may be responsible for the individual's medical decision. The difficulty of applying Western style methodology in a patient population with a distinctly different culture need not mean abandoning all attempts to conduct trials abroad. Through cooperation with community leaders and local health officials, and adherence to the ethical principles defined in the Helsinki Declaration and the Nuremberg Code, these studies remain possible (BARRY 1988). Each clinical trial investigator must face the issue whether the patient is properly informed or not in order to proceed with the trial in an ethical manner.

In most pharmaceutical companies it is estimated that only one in eight drugs survives the clinical research process. This usually means that seven have been demonstrated to be ineffective, without therapeutic advantage over existing drugs, or unsafe. For the drug company this usually entails a significant financial loss because of preclinical research investment; however, it is a loss budgeted in the existing realities of drug development. What happens to the eighth drug is the real subject of this chapter. This one must go through the process of clinical trials that allows the drug to be registered in scores of countries around the world. Although the various regulatory authorities determine the direction of this process, it must be clear to all that no pharmaceutical company would invest its time and finances in a drug it perceived could not be registered.

From this viewpoint one can conclude that clinical trials have two important purposes: (a) to reject, at the earliest possible stage of development, ineffective or harmful drugs and (b) to ensure that the remaining compounds can satisfy regulatory concerns in numerous countries about the drug's use in treating human disease. Careful balance of these purposes is what makes clinical trials research a vital part of the basic aspects of medical science not simply a mechanical process of applied technology or a routine process of regulatory documentation.

C. General Principles in the Study of Antifungal Drugs

I. Evaluation of Drug Efficacy in Epidermal and Mucosal Mycotic Infections

The clinical evaluation of an antifungal drug is made complex by the numerous different fungi that can infect various anatomic sites. On the other hand, the procedure for evaluating drug efficacy in epidermal and mucosal infections is simplified by the rather standard clinical trials designs, the relatively low level of complexity of statistical analysis, and the ease in determining the success or failure of the drug. The marked fluctuations in patient signs and symptoms which occur in some diseases are usually not a problem in evaluating the effects of an antifungal drug on cutaneous mycoses.

There are two important criteria for measuring drug efficacy in the treatment of dermatomycoses: (a) Tests for the presence of the fungi must be positive at the beginning of the therapy under study, become negative by the end of treatment, and remain negative at a follow-up visit; (b) signs and symptoms must decrease and then disappear coincident with the negative mycological tests. The first criterion must be present before attention to the second is meaningful. That is, if the fungal cultures and tissue microscopic survey remain positive, there can be little attention paid to the change in signs and symptoms, since the drug must be termed an antimicrobial failure. On the other hand, if negative cultures and tissue microscopy are not associated with rapid resolution in signs and symptoms, the drug has limited usefulness no matter what eventual cause for this apparent paradox is identified. Therefore, the clinical design for evaluating antifungals must include a careful system for quantitating, summarizing, and observing the response of the mycological and the clinical signs and symptoms to the experimental drug. Once this is done, the clinical protocols, case report forms, monitoring, and study analysis become routine. One may add to the analysis more sophisticated measures, such as the rate at which cultures or signs revert, or design studies to evaluate carefully relapse or reinfection rates, but these will not be substitutes for the basic issue of the number of patients showing drug success or failure.

The development of an antifungal drug requires identifying the groups of fungi which most commonly cause fungal disease in humans and then devising formulations most suitable for the safe and effective treatment of the different fungi. It has become customary to describe superficial fungal infections not by their microbial cause but by the anatomical site of infection. This has justification since the response to therapy is often dependent more on the infection site than on the genus and species of the causative fungus. There are five main sites of significant fungal infection:

1. Infection of the body, referred to as tinea corporis, tinea cruris (infection of skin in the groin), tinea pedis (plantar infection type of the feet) and tinea manuum (infection of the hands).

2. Interdigital infections of the feet, referred to as tinea pedis (interdigital or athlete's foot type).
3. Infection of the hair of the scalp and the scalp itself (tinea capitis).
4. Infection of the finger or toe nails, tinea unguium or onychomycosis.
5. Infection of the mucosal surfaces, most commonly by yeasts causing oral thrush and vaginitis.

To evaluate a new antifungal drug completely each of these sites of infection should be studied. This is so common an approach to antifungal therapy that a dermatologist may refer to a drug as being effective in tinea cruris rather than saying it is effective against the most common cause of infection at this anatomical site, *Trichophyton rubrum*. However, as many causative organisms as possible should be studied in order to define the antimicrobial spectrum of the new drug.

Among the major issues in the analysis of data during evaluation of antifungal drugs are:

1. What is the meaning of the mycological diagnostic test?
2. How can the signs and symptoms best be evaluated?
3. What is the significance of and best way to evaluate relapse or reinfection?

These three issues must be constantly considered during clinical trial preparation as well as during data analysis and presentation.

1. What Is the Meaning of the Mycological Test?

Two kinds of mycological test are usually done in the evaluation of fungal disease: microscopy for fungal elements and culture. Both of these are important, since culture alone does not ascertain whether the organism is present in large quantities (i.e., if it is present only as a contaminant), and microscopy alone does not allow identification of the organism. In addition, diagnosis from skin scrapings alone could prove difficult for less experienced technicians. In some diseases, such as pityriasis versicolor, microscopy is of vital importance, since culture is not used in the diagnosis of this condition. In addition, the presence of fungicidal or fungistatic drugs in the skin could transiently influence culture but would not alter microscopy of the fungal elements. One organism, *Microsporum canis*, is of particular interest, since it can be cultured from normal hair for several weeks after cure of an associated skin infection. It then disappears spontaneously from the hair. If one relied only on culture and did not wait long enough after treatment, a cured patient would be rated a failure because the culture was positive from the nearby hair contamination of the culture. Fortunately, studies of the two methods of mycological evaluation have shown 85% concordance in patients with fungal disease, although microscopy is often positive for a week after the organism fails to grow on culture. Awareness of these features of mycological testing is important in the evaluation of antifungal studies.

2. How Can Signs and Symptoms Best be Evaluated?

Three mechanisms have been utilized to summarize statistically the clinical results of antifungal therapy.

(a) Each of a number of signs and symptoms is rated with a score from 0 to 3 depending on whether the sign or symptom is absent, mild, moderate, or severe. This score is used to rate progress in the various variables. As many as seven or eight such variables may be listed, but usually three are the major contributors to the disease: erythema, desquamation, and pruritus (itching). These signs and symptoms can separately be followed in evaluating response to therapy. The first two are more reliable for assessing the disappearance of the microbe and healing than the last, since pruritus has many causes, including drug reaction and healing itself. In addition, pruritus is a subjective rather than an objective parameter.

(b) The sum of scores of all signs and symptoms yields a summation picture of the severity of the patient's illness. This allows comparison of the study groups for homogeneity, and it provides a summary view of the healing process for comparative and statistical purposes. The sum of scores may identify a problem in study design. For example, the mean sum of scores for pityriasis versicolor infections prior to therapy may be 2, rather than 7 as often recorded for tinea corporis infections. This is simply a numerical record confirming that the former is a mild skin disease even in its severest form. This recognition makes it clear that reduction in signs and symptoms in pityriasis versicolor would be difficult to quantitate, i.e., only presence or absence of disease can be observed.

(c) The scores for clinical signs and symptoms can be combined with mycological testing in an overall evaluation to determine whether a patient is completely cured, mycologically cured with minimal signs and symptoms, improved, or mycologically and symptomatically a drug failure. This system, though arbitrary, is a mechanism for evaluating the most important feature in drug testing, the overall outcome of treatment.

3. What Is the Significance of and Best Way to Evaluate Relapse or Reinfection?

Only a follow-up evaluation can determine whether cure is permanent. Unfortunately, a number of issues other than the value of the experimental drug may play a role. A primary question to be answered is, how long must therapy be given in order to prevent relapse of infection after the drug is discontinued? When one is using a fungistatic drug such as griseofulvin, one must treat until all the diseased tissues have been removed by body repair mechanisms. In the case of nail infections, this may take 6–12 months until the infected and damaged nail has been removed by the growth of healthy nail. The time required when a fungicidal drug is used is unknown. This can, however, be studied by varying the treatment period and ensuring careful and complete follow-up. Causes of relapse or reinfection other than ineffective drug therapy must be excluded. One cause of reinfection, particularly when topical therapy is used, is reinfection from untreated, asymptomatic, yet infected areas of skin. One cannot regard as ineffective a drug that was not applied to all areas of the infected skin. Another cause of reinfection is from untreated, infected family members. The presence of such infections in the family must therefore be documented as a part of the patient's history. The period of follow-up is also of importance in determining whether relapse of infection or reinfection has occurred. Normal skin requires 4 weeks to renew itself. One could have high concentrations of an antifungal drug in the skin in the first few weeks, but by 4 weeks relapse would be evident. On the other hand, the longer one waits the more likely is reinfection from a family member or other environmental source to occur. For these reasons 2–4 weeks is the usually accepted minimum duration for a follow-up check of mycological and clinical cure. Since fungal infections tend to be recurrent in susceptible people, an important parameter of drug efficacy is its ability to prevent this process. Therefore, even very long follow-up periods of from 6 months to 1 year are recommended in an effort to record the effect of a new drug on recurrence. If a drug is effective in preventing this process it can be assumed that relapse of disease from inapparent sites of infection on the patient himself was the cause of his previous chronic, recurrent disease, not reinfection from the environment.

II. Evaluation of Drug Efficacy in Systemic Mycoses

Evaluating drug efficacy in patients with systemic mycoses, particularly in the setting of AIDS, requires a multi-level assessment of the patient (DISMUKES 1988). AIDS patients infected with *Cryptococcus neoformans*, *Histoplasma capsulatum*, or *Coccidioides immitis* usually have no hope of ever completely eradicating the organism from their body. Because of the particular refractoriness of these infections in AIDS patients, evaluation of efficacy must involve not only the rapidity with which a new antifungal agent sterilizes a patient's infected tissues, but also how quickly a patient begins to feel better. For example, in AIDS patients suffering from crypotococcal meningitis, resolution of headache, nausea, vomiting, or signs of increased intracranial pressure, and the rapidity with which a patient feels well enough to leave the hospital are as important as sterilization of the cerebrospinal fluid. Drug efficacy studies involving AIDS patients or others with serious systemic mycoses must include not only specific microbiological data but also an assessment of the patient's functional status, such as the quality of life. While measuring the quality of life may be difficult in comparison with microbiological and traditional clinical evaluation, recent attempts have been made to measure a patient's subjective physical and social well-being. These measurements will be an important new area of evaluation of antifungal therapy of systemic mycoses in future clinical trials (WIKLUND et al. 1986).

III. Documentation of Drug Tolerability During Topical Application

Before a topically applied drug can be used in comparative clinical trials it must be tested in standard studies in volunteers for: irritation potential in normal and damaged skin, sensitization potential, and photoirritation or photosensitization. The methods for conducting these studies are recorded well elsewhere (Phillips et al. 1972). In summary, skin irritation is evaluated by repeated application of the topical drug to the skin over several weeks and assessing erythema, edema, or pruritus. Sensitization is evaluated by re-exposing volunteers to the agent 2 weeks after repeated skin applications. Photoirritation is evaluated by exposing drug-treated skin to ultraviolet light and observing evidence of enhanced irritation compared with controls. When these tests show no significant drug-induced effects, the drug may be used in clinical trials.

During all clinical trials with topical agents patients are asked to record adverse events. The presence of erythema, itching, dryness, or other signs or symptoms is recorded at the time of summation of all patient data. When possible a series of patch tests for sensitization are used to document a sensitization reaction. Patches will contain the vehicle base alone, the drug alone, or combinations of the two. This is helpful in confirming the presence of a sensitization reaction. A major difference between the analysis of drug-induced irritation in healthy volunteers and in patient trials is that in the latter the disease itself may produce signs and symptoms similar to those of drug irritation. That is, irritation may result from drug inefficacy in treating the condition rather than represent an adverse event of drug use. Careful attention to this potential artifact in drug evaluation requires the use of patch testing, properly controlled trials, and good documentation of the details of each adverse event.

IV. Documentation of Drug Tolerability During Oral or Intravenous Drug Use

As indicated in the Introduction, a major purpose of clinical trials is the careful assessment of whether a new drug leads to unacceptable adverse events. In antifungal drug therapy the approach to assessment of tolerability follows standard procedures. These include: careful dose-ranging tolerability studies in volunteers under careful observation, the documentation of each adverse event recorded by the patient during the trial, and detailed analysis of hepatic, renal, and hematopoietic blood tests done frequently during use of the drug in comparative clinical trials.

Antifungal drugs have a rather poor track record of adverse events, as seen by the gastrointestinal effects of griseofulvin, the renal toxicity of amphotericin B, and the hepatic and endocrine effects of the azoles. Therefore, careful attention to these parameters must be an important part of the evaluation of any new drug. The registration file for the drug will list each adverse event and abnormal biochemical or hematologic test. In addition, each pharmaceutical company now conducts careful postmarketing surveillance for serious adverse events in order to detect evidence of drug intolerance. This is done in recognition of the fact that clinical trials are conducted in rather carefully defined settings, using rather small numbers of reliable patients, and for short periods of treatment; thus, certain adverse events may be missed (IDÄNPÄÄN-HEIKKILÄ 1985). Determination of safety in patients with serious systemic mycoses is particularly complex in AIDS patients because they often have one or more coexisting infections in addition to their underlying HIV infection, and many of these patients are taking a bewildering number of concomitant medications such as zidovudine, pentamidine, INH, rifampin, etc. in addition to the investigational agent being evaluated in a particular trial. This pharmacological stew may pose a great challenge to the investigator attempting to evaluate drug toxicity and drug-drug interaction.

In an attempt to identify an offending, potentially toxic agent in this situation, large numbers of patients must be enrolled to ensure even distribution in each part of the study of patients taking the unknown agent. If the study is not sufficiently large to rely on randomization to distribute the patients evenly, the researcher should stratify according to a particular concomitant medication (such as AZT) in order to assign equal numbers of patients to each part of the study. When ethically justified, the investigator should also make every effort to rechallenge a patient who has developed an unexplained clinical abnormality in the course of the study. If possible, biopsy material of the affected organ, e.g., liver, skin, or bone marrow, should be obtained when evaluating potential drug toxicity. These biopsy specimens can provide the additional information necessary to determine the precise cause for a clinical abnormality.

D. Organization of Clinical Trials for the Treatment of Dermatomycoses

Clinical trials follow the same organizational pattern in the testing of antifungal drugs as they do in the evaluation of any drug. Tests are first done in healthy volunteers to investigate and document pharmacodynamic and pharmacokinetic features and to gain any evidence of drug intolerance (phase I), then efficacy of the drug action in one or two clinical indications plus the appropriate dose and duration for drug use are determined (phase II), finally carefully controlled clinical trials are done to prove efficacy and to identify adverse events in adequate numbers of patients (phase III). After the drug is marketed, special studies are carried out to refine understanding of the use of the drug (phase IV). The following includes a brief overview of the type of studies in these stages of clinical development of an antifungal drug, with selected comments concerning special points.

I. Tolerability and Pharmacokinetic Assessment in Healthy Volunteers (Phase I)

Usually at least two studies are done to study and document pharmacokinetics and tolerability; single administration of varied doses and then multiple administration of various doses usually for a number of weeks depending on the planned duration of drug use in subsequent trials (Federal Register 1987). The doses used are determined from the no-toxic-effect levels observed in animal toxicology studies and initial data on the doses required to achieve efficacy in animals.

II. Open-Label Efficacy Trials (Phase I)

As indicated previously, open-label uncontrolled trials should be very limited in number and size. Their purpose is to determine whether the pharmaceutical company should invest considerable time and money in the development of the drug. With this in mind, the most challenging part of the clinical design is to be certain that patient selection has been correct so that proper conclusions can be reached. This means that patients with too severe a disease should be avoided since dose and duration are not yet defined, patients with mild, self-healing disease should be avoided since a false picture of efficacy will emerge, and only small numbers of patients should be treated so that the proper studies are not subsequently prejudiced by the availability of excessive, uncontrolled efficacy data.

III. Dose Finding and Duration Finding Studies (Phase II)

These studies are of particular interest in the clinical trials of antifungal drugs. Since one is dealing with an antimicrobial agent, several features unique to this pertain. One needs the appropriate concentration of drug in the appropriate tissue for the appropriate time to have the maximum fungicidal or fungistatic effect. Therefore, each drug, depending on qualities of tissue distribution, tissue elimination, and antifungal properties, will exhibit different dosage and duration requirements. For example, the drug dose optimal for terbinafine could only be tested after the shortest duration of drug therapy possible was determined, since with a well-tolerated drug, short duration of treatment is more important than the dose. In the use of clotrimazole for topical treatment of vaginal candidosis, the change from 10 days of therapy to 1 day required a ten fold increase in drug dose. These examples simply emphasize the fact that in antimicrobial drug therapy, drug dose and duration are interdependent. In addition, dose and duration will vary depending on the site of infection, even when the disease is caused by the same microbe. For example, treatment of chronic tinea pedis, plantar type due to *Trichophyton rubrum* may take 4–6 weeks; the same organism in the groin will require a shorter treatment, while in the toenail longer treatment will be necessary.

IV. Exploring Drug Efficacy and Tolerability in Various Diseases (Phase III)

At this stage one starts to gain the solid data from pivotal studies in proving (to the drug company, regulatory authorities, and clinicians) whether the new drug is worth considering for use in advancing patient health care or not. These studies should all be randomized, double-blind, placebo or comparative drug controlled following the most rigorous criteria of good study design, patient selection, monitoring, and data summation. For most new antifungal drugs, studies will have to be done with a topical preparation or an oral preparation in each of the primary dermatomycoses for which the drug will be claimed as efficacious. For an international registration file this will usually include at least two double-blind, placebo-controlled trials and one large, multicenter trial comparing the new drug with existing marketed drugs having the same indication (FARLEY 1988). Sufficient studies will have to be done so that at least 1000 patients have been treated with the new drug.

V. Evaluation of Special Features of the Drug: Profiling Studies (Phase IV)

After the new drug has been registered for use in various countries the process of refining its use by adjustments in dosc or duration of therapy, new formulations such as slow-releasing forms, and postmarketing adverse events surveillance are done. These are a necessary part of the clinical trials process since new information about a drug can be obtained by careful observation of its use in each patient.

E. Special Aspects of Clinical Trials in the Treatment of Systemic Mycoses

The traditional deliberate and comprehensive approach to licensing of new antimicrobials has been seriously challenged by the requirements of study in severe systemic mycoses. This has occurred because systemic mycoses are relatively rare and because they are associated with immunologic unresponsiveness by the patient, making them of life-threatening severity. In diseases such as disseminated coccidioidomycosis, histoplasmosis, and blastomycosis the task of organizing clinical trials with appropriate sample sizes is particularly difficult. In the USA this challenge has been met in part by the formation of the Mycoses Study Group (MSG) sponsored by the NIH. However, in other countries attempts to document the effects of a new antifungal drug have usually required extrapolating from a very small experience in one or two health care centers. There is little opportunity to change this situation. Therefore, a pharmaceutical company interested in evaluating a new drug usually must rely on specialists who have had detailed clinical trial experience in each of the systemic mycoses. This at least allows for a common pattern of trial design. The most confusing situation occurs when a new investigator claims dramatic drug effects using a unique trial design which may require years to validate.

The second complication of the study of systemic mycoses is that patients have disease of life-threatening severity due to immunologic unresponsiveness either induced by widespread infection or by other conditions such as malignancy or AIDS. The special situation of the occurrence of systemic mycoses in AIDS is discussed below. However, even in the study of mycoses associated with wide-spread disease or malignancy, placebo-controlled trials are usually impossible, making historical data of critical importance. This means the center must have available careful records concerning the natural history of the disease as well as the effects of other drugs. Absence of such records may considerably mislead the evaluation of the new drug. Whenever possible, milder forms of the disease should be studied in a randomized, controlled manner to complement the data collected on the drug's efficacy in more severely ill patients.

Because of the inevitable and rapid demise of most AIDS patients and the unsatisfactory existing therapy, there exists great pressure both from the public and within the medical community to produce and release potential therapeutic agents more rapidly than before. In the past several years, the FDA has stated that it has made a commitment to complete its review of agents of potential benefit to AIDS patients more quickly – shrinking the several years' process down to 6 months (National Academy of Sciences 1988). This pressure has also led the FDA to allow terminally ill AIDS patients access to promising new drugs still under study in controlled clinical trials. These drugs have been termed Investigational New Drugs or 'Treatment IND.' (MONACO and GOTTLIEB 1987). The treatment IND permits a drug sponsor to make available a new substance if there is no satisfactory alternative agent available.

The FDA believes the Treatment IND to be the best compromise in reconciling the competing interests of the desperately ill and of scientific prudence by making available potentially life-saving agents prior to completion of the clinical trials, without interfering with the execution of carefully planned studies. Zidovudine (AZT) was released under a prototype Treatment IND. Trimetrexate, a new treatment for *Pneumocystis carinii*, was also granted Treatment IND status in February 1988.

The scientific community can sympathize with the concerns of those who protest that even the Treatment IND program is too restrictive, given the desperate needs of AIDS patients. The reality of AIDS, however, does not change the reality of science; to unleash untested drugs will neither benefit the terminally ill now nor serve the interests of the community at large in the future. Incomplete studies are destined to yield inaccurate and misleading results and defeat the intended purpose of the clinical trial. These errors may also substantially increase the cost of an already expensive process of bringing a new drug to the market (now estimated to be approximately $120 million) and have the potential to delay the ultimate licensing of the agent.

In the special cases of the testing of cancer drugs or in testing drugs in AIDS patients, terminally ill patients are used instead of healthy volunteers in phase I studies, and investigators search for evidence of the agent's effectiveness as well as tolerability. These phase I trials are referred to as 'pilot trials,' and like typical phase I trials they are usually open-label, noncomparative studies; thus, any data suggesting efficacy can only be compared with experience from historical controls. Successfully completed phase I trials are followed by the second phase, which includes carefully controlled studies using either historical, case-control, or randomized prospective methods. These trials are intended to yield additional information about an agent's safety and effectiveness for a particular indication. Phase II trials often include up to several hundred patients. These studies, particularly when historical controls are used, may yield erroneous information. Illnesses may be diagnosed at an earlier stage during the study than in previously treated patients, the patients may have new concomitant illnesses besides the one being focused on, they may be receiving other newer drugs (such as AZT), and ancillary care may have improved over time. Historical controls provide a comparison of the experience of patients who have suffered from a particular illness in the past and received treatment with Drug A with patients currently suffering from that same illness who have received treatment with Drug B. The advantage of the historical control is that it does not expose additional patients to the continued use of ineffective therapy when a new effective drug may be available. The disadvantage, as numerous studies have pointed out, is the tendency for historical control studies to embellish or overestimate the potential usefulness of the new investigational agent (Sacks et al. 1982).

Even when the studies have been corrected for a particular study bias involving AIDS patients (e.g., an imbalance in the number of homosexual versus intravenous drug abusers, level of CD4 cells, concomitant use of zidovudine [AZT], etc.), the results are unlikely to yield a truly clean comparison (Feinstein 1983). Even under the best of circumstances, historically controlled studies are bound to be less credible than prospective parallel-group comparative studies.

Although the FDA has recorded that it will make every effort to reduce the period of time it takes to review new therapies, the entire three-phase investigational process must also be condensed to meet the challenge of AIDS.

Making an effort to use either prospective or historical controls during phase I trials (rapid escalation of drug dose) in clinically ill patients may enable the maximal tolerated and effective dose of the drug to be determined more rapidly. Investigators have developed this kind of 'telescoped' phases I and II trial during the past several years, and it is now becoming the method of choice for investigating new AIDS drugs. The recently completed, open-label clinical trial of the new azole, fluconazole, as a suppressive agent in

AIDS patients with cryptococcal meningitis is an excellent example of a phase I–II dose escalation trial done in patient volunteers (STERN et al. 1988; SUGAR and SAUNDERS 1988). This study provided both early safety data and pharmacokinetic information on fluconazole in AIDS patients while providing some suggestive evidence of the clinical utility of this agent in cryptococcal disease. Because this was an open-label, noncomparative trial, the data suggestive of clinical efficacy were based on historical controls treated with amphotericin B and were of limited value. Nevertheless, incorporating aspects of a phase I–II trial into one study enabled sufficient data to be obtained in ill AIDS patients to proceed in 18 months to a large multicenter phase III comparative study in which fluconazole is currently being compared with amphotericin B in a prospective randomized study.

Because of the complexity of antifungal drug trials and because of the relatively low numbers of patients with serious systemic mycoses, the NIH have sponsored for the past 10 years the MSG, a working group of mycology investigators. The group meets annually to develop standard protocols for research in the field and assist researchers in antifungal therapy to coordinate their studies. They organize many of the phase III multicenter collaborative trials and have developed detailed charts and computer programs to sift through and evaluate the mass of data in an effort to avoid potential conflicts among researchers who may disagree about what conclusions to draw from their studies. This group of investigators of the effects of antifungal drug therapy currently plays a major role in designing and implementing many of the antifungal studies in both AIDS and non-AIDS patients.

F. Statistical Issues in the Conduct of Clinical Trials

The use of proper statistical planning and analysis of clinical trials is at the foundation of all appropriate studies. This is so true today that even the reporting of studies for registration of a drug has been changed from two separate reports, a statistical one and a clinical one, to a combined clinical/statistical study report. This simply reflects the fact that no clinical statement can be made about the study of a drug without the statistical support for it. This chapter is not the appropriate vehicle for a review of the medical use of statistics. The reader must review other texts devoted to this issue (BAILAR and MOSTELLER 1986; KOCH and EDWARDS 1988; BULPITT 1983). We will address here only several of the most important aspects of the use of statistics in the evaluation of the efficacy of an antifungal drug, including: (a) descriptive versus categorial analysis, (b) randomization and assessment of sample size for achieving meaningful results (i.e., power), (c) multicenter studies, and (d) statistically significant versus medically significant results.

The confirmation analysis of a clinical trial lies in the statistics applied to the one to three parameters that clearly define the overall effects of a drug on the course of the fungal disease. Analyses of this type must be stated clearly in the study protocol before the study begins, and they must be the only parameters referred to at the end of the study that support or reject the efficacy of the drug. Their number must be very limited, or otherwise the study design has not been properly constructed. In the case of treatment of dermatomycoses the two acceptable parameters are the comparison of positive to negative mycological tests and the overall combined treatment results, i.e., effectively treated versus ineffectively treated patients. All other statistical analyses are descriptive or exploratory and are used to allow the reader to evaluate clinical statements and perhaps to identify new questions for further trials but do not contribute to the overall outcome of the study. Examples of such analyses are the P values which allow one to say, 'Cultures became negative significantly faster (i.e., at week 1 of treatment) when drug A was used compared with drug B,' or 'Signs and symptoms were significantly better controlled at week 3 of treatment by drug A compared with drug B.'

Randomization of patients into treatment groups is the best method for obtaining comparable groups in a clinical trial. When sufficiently large numbers of patients are enrolled, various co-factors such as age, sex, concomitant illnesses or medications, degree of debilitation, etc. will be assigned in approximately equal numbers to the two parts of the study. Randomization removes physician bias in choosing a particular therapy. Prospective, randomized trials also have limitations. Unless the patient groups are sufficiently large, randomization may not ensure even distribution of modifying factors. In these smaller studies, efforts should be made to identify prognostic variables carefully and build into the protocol a method for stratifying these features equally into each treatment group.

The size of the sample of patients to be studied is one of the most important issues in clinical trials design. When we set up a clinical trial designed to observe whether a drug is more effective than placebo or another active drug, we set out to reject the null hypothesis that they are equal. We have agreed that if the confirmatory parameters decided upon show a percentage change sufficiently large between the two groups for the chances of this occurring at random to be less than 1 in 20, then we have rejected the null hypothesis and shown a significant difference between the two groups. We could still be wrong (type I error), but the clinical trials community has accepted this potential error as a reasonable one. We then simply consult standard tables to tell us the appropriate sample size to reject the null hypothesis if we expect a 30% cure rate in one group and an 80% cure rate in another. A more difficult problem in study design is to select the appropriate sample size to prove that the new drug is equal to existing therapy. Here the question, how equal is equal? defines the number of patients required. If we say two drugs are equal in efficacy, was the sample size large enough to identify with a probability of 95% a difference of 50%, 25%, 10%, or 5% if it had existed? For each of these degrees of certainty another, larger number of patients is required in the study. To state that two drugs are similar when inadequate sample sizes were used is the type II error in statistical analysis (FREIMAN et al. 1978).

The problem in clinical trials is that rather small numbers of patients, perhaps in several trials, will provide the confidence that we have not committed a type I error, but hundreds even thousands of patients will be required to ensure that a type II error has not occurred. The only resolution of this problem in clinical trials is to be sure that proper attention to sample size has been paid prior to start of the study, and that statements after the study to the effect that if drug A and B are not different ($P > 0.05$) they must be equal are avoided. In addition, studies designed to prove drug A is equal to drug B should be approached with caution on account of the large investment in time and money involved.

When multicenter studies are required, special attention must be given to the possible effects of each center on the clinical trials results (FLEISS 1986). This special attention is referred to as the treatment-by-center interaction analysis. The problem here is straightforward: if two centers show highly significant effects, enough to yield a significant result to the multicenter pooled results, but eight other centers show no effects or even the opposite results, the multicenter study is considered flawed. The best prevention of such flawed studies is the careful selection of centers using similar methods, a well-organized investigator meeting prior to start of the study, and careful monitoring during the study to be sure one center is not following different procedures. The best summation of results of multicenter trials is the presentation of all data center by center, so that the reviewer can easily conclude whether special treatment-by-center effects did or did not affect the overall study results.

Even when statistical significance is observed in clinical trials, the question of medical significance remains. Each study will require discussion of the medical relevance of statistical observations. Some of the variations between statistical and medical significance will be easily resolved; however, some cannot be. These can only be prevented by appropriate study design, including proper sample size (not too large resulting in excessive heterogenicity, and not too small leading to potential type II statistical errors), reasonable numbers of exploratory (descriptive) analyses, and careful discussion of the results at the summation of a study. For example, a statistically significant reduction in SGOT values during a study which started with values in the normal range probably has no medical significance and is most probably due to changes in the baseline of normal values at the laboratory. On the other hand, increases of SGOT values in only a few patients in a study of 100 patients will not be statistically significant but is a very important and medically significant observation. In this context it is best to remind ourselves that the statistical analytical process is but a tool for clear thinking about a study; it is not a substitute for careful review of the medical issues involved in evaluating a new drug in the treatment of human disease.

G. Selected Issues in Protocol and Investigator Brochure Preparation, Good Clinical Practice Implementation, and Final Study Report Documentation

I. Protocol and Investigator Brochure Preparation

Many investigators may not be aware that two documents are an integral part of the clinical trial and the drug registration process. These are the clinical trial protocol and the brochure of background data for use by the investigator. Both of these documents are a part of the material submitted for review by the hospital ethics committee, and both are later submitted to regulatory authorities for proof that proper clinical trials procedure has been followed. The investigator brochure must contain the background data on why the drug is being tested, that is, its contribution to medical care, its background pharmacology, animal toxicology, and pharmacokinetics in humans. Then, depending on the stage of development, all clinical data collected until the time of the most recent revision of the brochure are included. This, of course, means that the brochure must be updated at regular intervals, perhaps once each year.

The protocol becomes almost a legal document in the drug registration process. If there is any deviation from the stated goals, inclusion/exclusion criteria, or evaluation procedures of the protocol, the document must be amended. A deviation from a protocol by an investigator will at least require detailed documentation and justification in the final report and may invalidate the study for registration. An investigator recently decided that microscopy for fungi was just as reliable as culture after the causative organism had been originally identified and that neither microscopy nor culture was required after a skin lesion was completely healed. He may have been entirely correct; however, the protocol stated otherwise and the study was therefore worthless, although well conducted from the viewpoint of the investigator.

The protocol must also state how statistical analysis will be done and particularly whether review of the results prior to the end of the study will be done, i.e., interim analysis. There are important ethical reasons for having an interim analysis, such as to have as few patients as possible receive a placebo or ineffective drug. If interim analysis is to be done it must be a part of the original protocol, otherwise the sponsor or the investigator may be accused of trying to manipulate the results of the study in some way. It also must be clear that when an interim analysis is done which was not clearly planned in the protocol, the significance levels for drug efficacy required at the end of the study are changed (usually doubled) for each interim analysis. For this reason, since changing significance levels increases the study size and duration, interim analysis should be considered only when it is absolutely necessary.

II. Good Clinical Practice Implementation

Good clinical practice (GCP) simply refers to a set of procedures that lead to confirmation that clinical trials have been run in accordance with the best tradition of clinical investigative research. This means that the Tokyo amendment of the Helsinki convention has been adhered to, that informed consent has been properly obtained, that clinical investigators have been properly chosen and their expertise for conducting a clinical trial documented, that proper ethical review has been obtained from the hospital or clinic involved, that monitoring of the study is done appropriately, and that all aspects of the protocol, drug delivery, accountability, and final study reports are well documented and available for review. The pharmaceutical company invests a great deal of effort to ensure that GCP is followed. However, this documentation process cannot replace the philosophical process that each member of the clinical trials team must achieve, that is, that a clinical trial must be conducted in an informed, ethical, and well-documented manner.

III. Final Study Report Documentation

The final clinical statistical report of each clinical trial becomes the primary summary document for submission to any authority concerning the results of a clinical trial. The report includes a summary of the efficacy and tolerability of the drug, plus appendices containing the original study protocol and amendments, case report forms, and the listings and tables of all statistical analyses. This document should be agreed to by each investigator in the study and should then be the source for data to be submitted for publication in medical journals. When all studies are prepared for submission to regulatory authorities, these clinical/statistical reports of each study are summarized in a clinical data summary which is the primary clinical document for claiming that a drug should be made available for use by physicians. When new drug applications (NDA) are delayed or rejected it is often because one or more of these reports are inadequate to support the claims of efficacy and tolerability which are made.

H. Summary and Conclusions

Clinical trials have become essential parts of the process of identifying effective and safe drugs for use by patients in the reversal of diseased states. We have presented the reasons why such trials must exist, even though we must always be able to respond to ethical and legal questions about them. We have outlined the standard procedures for progressing through the process of studying and documenting that a new drug is effective while insuring the minimum risk to volunteers or patients. We have discussed the special problems of conducting clinical trials in patients with serious diseases, such as the systemic mycoses. Finally, we have reviewed selected aspects of statistical analysis, document preparation, and use of (GCP) guidelines. We conclude that clinical trials design, conduct, and summation is a dynamic science of clinical investigative medicine. When done properly, it can be viewed as a creative process of tremendous aid to the task of making available to society new and safe therapeutic measures.

References

Bailar JC, Mosteller F (1986) Medical uses of statistics. N Engl J Med Books, Boston

Barry M (1988) Ethical considerations of human investigation in developing countries: the AIDS dilemma. N Engl J Med 319:1083–1086

Bulpitt CJ (1983) Randomized, controlled clinical trials. Martinus Nijhoff, The Hague

Burley DM, Glynne A (1985) Clinical trials. In: Burley DM, Binns TB (eds) Pharmaceutical medicine. Edward Arnold, London, pp 70–109

CIOMS (1983) Safety requirements for the first use for new drugs and diagnostic agents in man. Council for International Organization of Medical Sciences, Geneva

Dismukes WE (1988) Azole antifungal drugs: old and new. Ann Int Med 109:177–179

Farley D (1988) How FDA approves new drugs. ASM News 54:666–670

Federal Register (1987) Document 87–6064. March 19

Feinstein AR (1983) An additional basic science for clinical medicine: III. The challenges of comparison and measurement. Ann Int Med 99:705–712

Fleiss JL (1986) Analysis of data from multiclinic trials. Controlled Clin Trials 7:267–275

Freiman JA, Chalmers TC, Smith H, Kuebler RR (1978) The importance of beta, the type II error and sample size in the design and interpretation of the randomized control trial. N Engl J Med 299:690–694

Idänpään-Heikkilä JF (1985) Adverse events and post-marketing surveillance. In: Burley DM, Binns TB (eds) Pharmaceutical medicine. Edward Arnold, London, pp 126–148

Koch G, Edwards S (1988) Biopharmaceutical statistics for drug development. Marcel Dekker, New York

Monaco GP, Gottlieb MG (1987) Treatment INDs: research for hire? JAMA 258: 3296–3297

National Academy of Sciences (1988) Confronting AIDS, update 1988. Institute of Medicine, National Adademy Press, Washington DC

Phillips L, Steinberg M, Maibach HI, Akers WA (1972) A comparison of rabbit and human skin response to certain irritants. Toxicol Appl Pharamcol 21:369–382

Sacks H, Chalmers TC, Smith H (1982) Randomized versus historical controls for clinical trials. Am J Med 72:233–240

Spriet A, Simon P (1985) Methodology of clinical drug trials. Karger, Basel

Stern JJ, Hartman BJ, Sharkey P, Rowland V, Squires KE, Murray HW, Graybill JR (1988) Oral fluconazole therapy for patients with acquired immunodeficiency syndrome and cryptococcosis: experience with 22 patients. Am J Med 85:477–480

Sugar AM, Saunders C (1988) Oral fluconazole as suppressive therapy of disseminated cryptococcosis in patients with acquired immunodeficiency syndrome. Am J Med 85:481–489

Wiklund I, Lindvall K, Swedberg K (1986) Assessment of quality of life in clinical trials. Acta Med Scand 220:1–3

World Health Organization (1975) Guidelines for evaluation of drugs for use in man. Technical Report Series 563, Geneva

Section III. Clinical Usage

Introduction

JOHN F. RYLEY

The ultimate aim of those involved in the discovery and development of new antifungal drugs is to provide more effective and acceptable treatment for the unfortunate victims of fungal attack (as well as to generate more profit for their sustaining organisations!). The basic purpose of this section is not to teach clinicians how to do their job – though hopefully clinicians reading it will be stimulated to think again about their current attitudes and approaches to fungal diseases. Rather, I have sought for chapters that highlight the limitations of presently available treatments and that indicate directions in which further research is required. Clinical feedback is essential if research management is to be supportive and basic researchers realistic in their endeavours. Marguerite ROBERTS has written from her very down-to-earth experience of dermatology in a number of our local hospitals in the Manchester area (Chap. 13), and my long-standing friend Jack SOBEL has highlighted some of the problems he faces in a hospital situation when confronted with the more refractory forms of fungal vaginitis (Chap. 14).

Alan SUGAR received his training in infectious diseases in California and is now putting it into practice on the eastern seaboard of the USA. I find his contribution (Chap. 15) particularly interesting since he highlights not so much the deficiencies of currently available antifungal treatments but rather the problems associated with quick and accurate diagnosis – so difficult with systemic fungal diseases and yet so essential if appropriate therapy is to be given. When David SPELLER's *Antifungal Chemotherapy* appeared in 1980, not only was the era of orally active azole drugs just beginning, AIDS and its fungal complications were not yet recognized. Much of the pioneering work on HIV infection has been done at the Pasteur Institute in Paris, and I am particularly grateful therefore to one of its members, Bertrand DUPONT, for writing on fungal infections and AIDS (Chap. 17), even though his contribution was submitted in French!

Although it has been my aim that this book should not be product-orientated, it seemed appropriate to review the current situation with the older antifungal drugs, which in spite of their age and the advent of newer remedies have a vital part to play in current clinical practice; Donald ARMSTRONG has grown up with these drugs and could thus call on his vast experience in writing Chap. 18. Outstanding among the newer remedies are the orally active azoles. I am grateful to my friend Dick GRAYBILL for taking time off from his orchid growing – as well as his more professional duties – to describe a bird's eye view of the possibilities and limitations of the currently available products in this exciting class as we enter the 1990s (Chap. 19). Although the majority of the newer antifungals are azoles, two promising compounds emerging from the developmental stage into clinical usage are not azoles and seem to merit special attention. Tom JONES and Annemarie POLAK and their colleagues deal, therefore, with these unique compounds, terbinafine and amorolfine, in Chaps. 20 and 21.

CHAPTER 13

Clinical Usage – A Dermatologist's Viewpoint

MARGUERITE M. ROBERTS

A. Introduction

Fungal infections occur worldwide, and different types of infection assume importance according to the frequency with which they cause disease within a particular setting. From the dermatological viewpoint fungal diseases may be grouped as:

1. The superficial mycoses, comprising dermatophyte and yeast infections. These are the most common form of fungal disease. Yeast infections include candidosis and pityriasis versicolor. A sub-group of non-dermatophyte superficial infections due to *Scopulariopsis*, *Hendersonula* and *Scytalidium* is included, and some other infections of hair, nail and skin are discussed.
2. The subcutaneous mycoses, comprising chronic fungal infections such as mycetoma and sporotrichosis.
3. The systemic mycoses, which include opportunistic infections, are dealt with elsewhere and do not generally come within the domain of the dermatologist.

In the beginning of this chapter a general description of conditions falling within the first two categories above will be presented. Specific treatments for the condition under discussion will be given at the end of each section. In the second part of the chapter a more general approach to therapy will be discussed with emphasis on the problems that need to be considered and overcome if treatment of this increasingly important group of disorders is to advance.

B. The Superficial Mycoses

I. Dermatophyte Infection

1. Aetiology and Epidemiology

Since dermatophytes have a predisposition for keratin, involvement of skin, hair or nails, or any combination of these, may occur. Anthropophilic, zoophilic and geophilic groups of dermatophytes are recognised according to their preference for human, animal or soil habitat, but all may cause the

Table 1. Dermatophyte species causing human infection

Species	Anthropophilic	Zoophilic	Geophilic
Microsporum	*M. audouinii*	*M. canis*	*M. fulvum*
	M. ferrugineum	*M. distortum*	*M. gypseum*
	M. langeronii	*M. equinum*	
	M. rivalieri	*M. nanum*	
		M. persicolor	
Trichophyton	*T. concentricum*	*T. equinum*	
	T. gourvilii	*T. mentagrophytes* var. *erinacei*	
	T. mentagrophytes var. *interdigitale*	*T. gallinae*	
	T. megninii	*T. mentagrophytes* var. *granulare*	
	T. rubrum	*T. quinckeanum*	
	T. schoenleinii	*T. simii*	
	T. soudanense	*T. verrucosum*	
	T. tonsurans		
	T. violaceum		
	T. yaoundei		
Epidermophyton	*E. floccosum*		

human infection known as ringworm. Examination of morphological characteristics allows further division into *Microsporum*, *Trichophyton* and *Epidermophyton* species (see Table 1).

Many of the common dermatophytes are seen worldwide, e.g. *Trichophyton rubrum* and *T. mentagrophytes*, but certain species are more limited in their distribution, e.g. *T. simii* to India, *Microsporum ferrugineum* to Japan, Asia, Africa and Eastern Europe, or *T. soudanense* to Africa (JOHNSON and ROSENTHAL 1968). However, immigrants from these countries may bring the disease with them into the host country (RIPPON and MEDENICA 1964; RIPPON and MALKINSON 1968; VANBREUSEGHEM 1968). Climatic factors, vegetation and soil provide varying situations, and an increase in worldwide travel has led to the introduction of new species. Environmental factors are of importance in the distribution of certain species, e.g. *M. audouinii* in urban populations or *T. verrucosum* in rural communities.

The risk of contracting ringworm infection in certain occupations such as mining is well recognised (GENTLES and HOLMES 1957; GOTZ and HANTSCHKE 1965), and the increased use of leisure centres with saunas and swimming pools is likely to lead to a rising incidence of infection unless preventative measures are undertaken (GENTLES and EVANS 1973; GENTLES et al. 1974). There is a reservoir of infection in the animal population, and types of infection seen will vary in different parts of the world.

2. Clinical Features

Dermatophyte infection, often known as ringworm or by the Latin term tinea, may present on the skin as dry scaly annular lesions with a tendency to peripheral spread, sometimes accompanied by pustule formation. Central clearing of the lesions is due to the development of natural resistance to the infection. Flexural involvement may result in maceration. Onychomycosis, defined as any fungal infection of the nail plate, may in dermatophyte infection present as yellow or white discoloration with crumbling of the keratin. Distal involvement of the nail plate may spread proximally, or a more diffuse change known as superficial white onychomycosis may occur. On the scalp or other hairy areas, circular scaly lesions with broken-off hairs may be indicative of dermatophyte involvement, or the inflammatory state known as kerion, which often results in scarring, may occur. In infection with *Microsporum* species or with *T. schoenleinii*, fluorescence under Wood's light is present.

The extent to which these features may be present in the individual case is variable but may allow likely prediction of the species involved. For instance, diffuse erythema and scaling of palms and soles, often associated with nail involvement, is characteristic of *T. rubrum* infection, whereas the scaly concentric rings of tinea imbricata are due to *T. concentricum*. Certain types of infection are more likely to result in kerion formation, e.g. *T. verrucosum* or *T. mentagrophytes* which are both zoophilic species. Yellow cup-shaped crusts or mats of hyphae (scutula) on the scalp due to *T. schoenleinii* characterise the clinical condition known as favus, and scarring alopecia may result. Other family members may become infected in this often long undiagnosed condition.

3. Differential Diagnosis

Many skin conditions may mistakenly be thought to be fungal in aetiology. If treatment is to be effective it is essential that a correct diagnosis is made. Psoriasis, which is an inherited condition, may involve the skin, scalp and nails. In the chronic discoid variety, well-defined, red, scaly plaques with silvery scales occur typically on the extensor aspect of the limbs and on the lumbosacral region. Sometimes the plaques show central clearing, but the scaling is unlike that of a fungal infection. Other acute or more extensive generalised forms of psoriasis cause less diagnostic confusion. In localised pustular psoriasis of palms and soles, well-defined scaly plaques with scattered, overlying, sterile pustules and brown crusts occur. Nail abnormalities may be present without skin involvement and include pitting, yellow discoloration, distal subungual thickening and onycholysis, in which the nail lifts distally from the nail bed. Scalp involvement may occasionally result in hair loss if thick plaques are present, but no broken hairs are evident.

In seborrhoeic dermatitis, itchy, often moist, eczematous changes occur, especially in proximal flexures; the central chest and back may be affected, and diffuse fine scaling of the scalp occurs without hair loss unless involvement is severe. Irregular pitting and transverse ridging of the nails is seen in eczema, and there is adjacent skin involvement at some stage in the condition. Pompholyx, an acute type of eczema, presents as tiny vesicles along the sides of fingers or toes. Occasionally much larger blisters called bullae occur on palms or soles. Sometimes a pompholyx reaction on the fingers may be associated with a fungal infection of the feet.

In alopecia areata, a condition associated with organ-specific autoimmune disease, characteristic 'exclamation mark' hairs occur at the edge of the circular bald areas, and eventual hair growth is likely. Erythrasma, a bacterial infection due to *Corynebacterium minutissimum*, occurs as a brownish, finely scaly eruption in the flexures or toe webs. Coral pink fluorescence occurs under Wood's light, and bacteriological examination will confirm the diagnosis.

4. Laboratory Diagnosis

Confirmation of the clinical diagnosis of a dermatophyte infection should be obtained by direct microscopic examination of infected material from the active spreading part of the lesion using a potassium hydroxide preparation and by culture on Sabouraud medium. This is particularly important where there is widespread skin involvement or if nails or scalp are infected, since lengthy treatment may be required, especially for nail infection, and it is difficult to confirm the diagnosis once treatment has commenced. The presence of another skin condition such as eczema does not rule out the possibility of secondary fungal infection. Sometimes microscopy may be positive but culture negative, particularly with some toenail infections. The presence of spores in infected hairs, whether within the hair shaft (endothrix) or without (ectothrix), will give a clue as to the likely causative agent with direct microscopy alone. Species identification on culture leads to prognostic implications. For instance, *T. rubrum* nail infection is notoriously difficult to eradicate whereas *Epidermophyton floccosum* infection of the groin responds easily to treatment. In long-term management, serial testing is helpful to ensure mycological as well as clinical cure in difficult cases. In the assessment of the epidemiological status of particular infections, laboratory diagnosis is mandatory. Where topical steroids have been used inadvertently, laboratory diagnosis of infection may be difficult to prove, but cessation of steroid therapy results in increased inflammatory changes in the skin, and fungal hyphae may then be found more easily (MARKS and DAWBER 1972).

5. Treatment

Localised skin infection, including toe web involvement, is treated by topical means. The imidazole group of preparations provides a cosmetically acceptable treatment when compared with benzoic acid compound ointment BPC (Whitfield's ointment) which is greasy. In the past, paints such as magenta (Castellani's paint) or gentian violet have been advocated, but they have now been withdrawn because of a recent report of carcinogenicity in mice (Food Advisory Committee UK 1987). In practice, there seems little to choose between the efficacy of various imidazole preparations, but sulconazole may be better absorbed and has the advantage of a once daily application (LASSUS et al. 1983). The length of treatment required may be several weeks, depending upon the extent of involvement, site and particular sensitivity of the species.

Where there is widespread skin, scalp or nail involvement, systemic therapy is indicated. Griseofulvin given in adequate doses (10–25 mg/kg daily) for a sufficient number of months will cure the majority of infections. Toenail infections, especially those due to *T. rubrum*, are particularly difficult to treat by oral griseofulvin alone, since treatment with this fungistatic drug is required for 1 or 2 years, and even then the relapse rate may be as high as 60% (DAVIES et al. 1967). Factors such as poor drug absorption and failure to maintain adequate drug levels within the nails are responsible. Avulsion of grossly infected nails, removal of the infection by drill or burr (NOLTING et al. 1975; BARAN and HAY 1985) or chemical dissolution by urea paste (WHITE and CLAYTON 1982) – the last a more acceptable approach as far as the patient is concerned – may produce a higher cure rate when combined with oral therapy (see Chap. 10). A recent topical nail preparation which combines tioconazole and undecylenic acid (Trosyl) may produce improvement in nail disease without the need for oral therapy (JEVONS and LEES 1985), but in more resistant cases, oral griseofulvin plus Trosyl nail lotion applied locally may be useful (HAY et al. 1987). Nail lacquers containing ciclopiroxolamine or amorolfine are being developed and appear to be effective.

If penicillin hypersensitivity is present with risk of cross-reaction to griseofulvin, oral imidazoles, especially the newer drugs itraconazole and fluconazole, offer a good alternative, although success rates with the earlier ketoconazole are comparable to those achieved with griseofulvin in adequate dosage (LEGENDRE and STELZ 1980; ROBERTSON et al. 1980; HAY and CLAYTON 1982). Terbinafine, an allylamine, is interesting because of its novel structure and mode of action in dermatophyte infection. Clinical assessment of this drug is at an early stage, but results look very promising indeed (see Chap. 20).

Chronic dermatophyte infection due to anthropophilic species may cause problems in certain areas. *M. audouinii* was a problem in Europe, but this infection is now rare in this area. *T. tonsurans* is particularly prevalent in the USA and Latin America, where failure to respond to treatment is due to inadequate immunity. Detection of cases and adequate programmes to eradicate infection take low priority in some of the countries involved. In favus, infection with *T. schoenleinii* may persist because of defective cell-mediated immunity in spite of the active inflammatory response.

Chronic tinea corporis due to *T. rubrum* may occur rarely in Europe. *T. concentricum* is difficult to eradicate in endemic areas, since relapse and reinfection are common. Chronic *T. rubrum* infection of the hands and feet, as well as the nails, may be associated with other diseases (HAY 1982) but is found in a high proportion of griseofulvin-unresponsive patients in whom evidence of defective cell-mediated immunity is found. In all these instances of chronic, apparently resistant disease, the newer imidazole drugs and terbinafine may provide a better chance of cure. Estimation of the minimal inhibitory concentration for the available drugs may help to determine the best chance of success, since resistance to treatment, though rare, should always be considered as a potential reason for treatment failure.

II. Superficial and Mucocutaneous Candidosis

1. Aetiology and Epidemiology

This yeast infection is commonly caused by *Candida albicans* but other species of *Candida* such as *C. parapsilosis* or *C. guilliermondii* may be important in a pathogenic role. Yeasts of this genus are found worldwide and flourish in hot humid situations. *C. albicans* is a commensal of the alimentary tract (Cohen et al. 1969; Rebora et al. 1973b; Odds 1979), but this and other *Candida* species may be found on the skin surface adjacent to body orifices (Noble and Somerville 1974). Superficial infections of the skin and mucous membranes are frequent, but serious systemic illness can occur where appropriate conditions exist. Infection by *Candida* spp. on the skin occurs in moist areas such as the flexures, nail folds or the angles of the mouth, and certain conditions may predispose to the development of infection (see Table 2).

Table 2. Predisposing factors in the development of candidosis

Ill-fitting dentures	
Broad-spectrum antibiotics	
Certain occupations	Cooks, housewives, bartenders
Circulatory conditions	Raynaud's phenomenon
Immunological disorders	
Endocrinological disorders	Diabetes mellitus Hypoparathyroidism Cushing's syndrome
Haematological conditions	Iron deficiency

2. Clinical Features

The accentuation of skin folds at the angles of the mouth as a result of ill-fitting dentures will predispose to the development of angular stomatitis, although other conditions such as the use of broad-spectrum antibiotic therapy may precipitate an episode due to overgrowth of *Candida* when other organisms are suppressed. The moist, macerated skin provides an ideal environment for *Candida* superinfection. Similarly, macerated body folds or intertrigo, often associated with obesity, result in erythematous areas with overgrowth of *Candida* species. Satellite papules or pustules are typical. As with dermatophyte infection, the presence of other dermatological conditions such as psoriasis, napkin dermatitis or eczema, as well as the frequent use of topical steroids in these patients, may produce sufficient damage to allow *Candida* to gain a foothold (BEARE et al. 1968). It is particularly important to exclude diabetes if oral or genital candidosis causing pruritus ani or pruritus vulvae should occur. Occasional finger web maceration usually as a result of a deformity due to a problem such as rheumatoid arthritis may result in a condition known as erosio interdigitalis blastomycetica. Gram-negative bacterial infection often coexists in this situation (COHEN et al. 1969; REBORA et al. 1973a).

Chronic paronychia is an infection of the nail folds due to *Candida* species, although on occasion bacterial infection may occur concurrently and may even be the initial event (MARTEN 1959; WHITTLE et al. 1959; BARLOW et al. 1970). Erythema and a shiny bolstered appearance of the involved nail folds is characteristic. There may be loss of cuticle and an associated nail dystrophy known as onychomycosis, with white or greenish discoloration. Pus may sometimes exude from the nail fold. *Candida* infection with distal nail involvement may occur as a sharply defined area starting at the nail tip and proceeding proximally.

Where immunity is impaired, chronic muco-cutaneous candidosis with persistent severe involvement of the mucosal surfaces, skin and nails may occur. In long-standing skin lesions, the involved areas often show gross hyperkeratosis, or a marked tissue inflammatory reaction produces a granulomatous change. The scalp may be similarly involved. Genetic and clinical criteria are used for classification purposes (HIGGS and WELLS 1973; VALDIMARSSON et al. 1973).

In group 1 there is a primary defect of cellular immunity, and the candidosis seems to be directly related to this defect. Systemic infections with many organisms including *Candida* occur, but bacterial infections are probably more important. In group 2, candidosis occurs in early childhood, and yeast infection predominates. The prognosis is usually better in this group. Defects in immunity may be demonstrated, and in several patients autosomal recessive or dominant inheritance may be present. In this group some of the patients show extensive, severe, cutaneous involvement with granuloma formation, and there may be evidence of systemic candidosis and serious infection from other causes. In other patients endocrinological factors may predispose. In a late-onset variety, myopathies and fibromata have been recorded (MAIZE and LYNCH 1972; KIRKPATRICK and WINDHORST 1979; PALESTINE et al. 1983), and there may be some association with AIDS or underlying malignancy. These patients show defects of cell-mediated immunity (GATENBY et al. 1980).

3. Differential Diagnosis

Differential diagnosis of flexural candidosis includes seborrhoeic dermatitis and psoriasis. These conditions have been discussed in a previous section

(B.I.3). Angular stomatitis might be confused with a contact dermatitis reaction to toothpaste, lip licking or with atopic eczema in which a rash around the mouth, particularly in young patients, is not infrequent. Evidence of distal flexural eczema or a family history of atopy will help to differentiate atopic eczema. Vitamin deficiency should also be considered in cases of angular stomatitis.

Acute paronychia, or "whitlow", is a painful, acutely inflammatory condition of the nail fold with abscess formation due to staphylococcal infection. Other chronic nail infections due to fungal infection such as *Scopulariopsis*, *Fusarium*, *Hendersonula* or *Scytalidium* need to be distinguished, but although the adjacent skin, particularly in the toe webs, may be involved in some cases, culture will confirm the diagnosis. *Pseudomonas* infection causes a green discoloration of the nail and will be isolated on culture. Sometimes this organism may coexist with *Candida* species in nail fold infection (BARLOW et al. 1970). Psoriasis and eczema of the nails may be associated with evidence of disease elsewhere. Other dermatological conditions causing leukonychia, or white nails, may be inherited or acquired and also need to be differentiated.

4. Laboratory Diagnosis

Confirmation of diagnosis is obtained by culture of skin, nail scrapings or pus on Sabouraud medium at 37°C and subsequent laboratory identification to determine the species by the germ tube method and API test.

In the past it had always been stated that only *C. albicans* can cause a pathogenic infection, but it is now recognised that other species of *Candida* may be important in the causation of clinical problems. It is even possible for more than one *Candida* species to be isolated from different sites in the same patient. It is, therefore, important to distinguish between the species for epidemiological reasons. Whether a difference in response to treatment may develop is difficult to predict. Other factors such as the development of resistance to treatment and the immunological status of the patient are important when determining the likely response to treatment.

5. Treatment

In the management of superficial and subcutaneous candidosis the underlying mechanism for infection in the individual patient needs to be considered. Remedial measures to deal with any such problems should be undertaken if feasible. Where there is involvement of skin adjacent to an orifice, treatment of both areas is essential to ensure that the infection is completely eradicated. Any infected partners need to be treated to reduce the risk of re-infection.

Improvement of angular stomatitis with provision of new dentures is simple, but reduction of obesity to lessen the risk of intertrigo or change in the working environment for patients with chronic paronychia is often not possible in practice. Systemic problems resulting in superficial *Candida* infection may be difficult or impossible to resolve. This means that the chance of relapse or re-infection may be considerable in some instances, even if infection is apparently treated adequately at any one time.

Topical treatment alone is often sufficient to deal with infection in flexural areas, including the angles of the mouth, and some nail infections. The polyene antibiotics, amphotericin B, nystatin, natamycin, candicidin and pimaricin, are all poorly absorbed but are very effective topically. Amphotericin B or nystatin can be given orally for associated mouth, gastrointestinal or anal infection, but absorption is then only 5%–10%. No spontaneously occurring resistance to these drugs has been reported.

The imidazole group of drugs can all be used topically for candidosis of the skin, and significant resistance is rare. Vaginal preparations may now be effective after single-dose treatment where genital involvement is present. The combination of tioconazole and undecyclenic acid as a nail lotion may be useful, particularly in cases of distal nail involvement in which penetration of keratin is necessary. Systemic therapy with the imidazoles ketoconazole, itraconazole or fluconazole is required in mucocutaneous candidosis and is combined with other therapy to restore T-cell function (KIRKPATRICK and SMITH 1974) such as transfer factor (PABST and SWANSON 1972) or lymphocyte grafting (LEVY et al. 1971; VALDIMARSSON et al. 1972). Other influences such as iron deficiency need to be corrected. In these cases topical therapy has only a limited role. 5-Fluorocytosine is a very useful drug for systemic candidosis but should not be used topically because the development of resistance is common.

The length of treatment required for individual cases is dependent upon the sites involved, host factors of resistance and immunity and environmental factors including hygiene. Most intertriginous infections respond well within 2 weeks, but genital disease combined with skin involvement is more resistant. In chronic mucocutaneous candidosis, other support measures as well as an effective drug regime are necessary to achieve any degree of success (HIGGS and WELLS 1973; HAY 1981).

III. Pityriasis Versicolor

1. Aetiology and Epidemiology

The infection is due to the yeasts *Pityrosporum orbiculare* or *P. ovale*. *Pityrosporum* spp. are found as commensal organisms on the skin (ROBERTS 1969), but if present in sufficiently large numbers in predisposed individuals, they may develop into the more pathologically active hyphal form known as *Malasezzia furfur*. The condition occurs more commonly in younger age groups, though it is rare in childhood. In tropical climates up to 30% of the population may be affected (MARPLES 1965), whereas in temperate climates approximately 1% have pityriasis versicolor (National Health Survey 1978). Patients on immunosuppressive therapy, including steroids, are more prone to develop the infection (Boardman and Malkinson 1962). The organism is a lipophilic yeast, and use of topical products containing coconut oil will increase the incidence of *Pityrosporum* species on the skin (Roed-Petersen 1980; Dave et al. 1987).

2. Clinical Features

Finely scaly circular areas, which may coalesce where extensive involvement is present, occur predominantly on the trunk or proximal parts of the limbs. Other sites, including face and neck, may be affected occasionally. The involved areas may be of variable hue ranging from white to pale pink to brown. Depigmentation of the skin is a typical feature due to production of dicarboxylic acid by the yeast. Competitive inhibition of tyrosinase may have a direct effect on hyperactive melanocytes (Nazarro-Porro et al. 1978).

3. Differential Diagnosis

A petaloid form of seborrhoeic dermatitis may be seen on the trunk, but there is likely to be evidence of eczematous change elsewhere. Pityriasis rosea is a self-limiting condition of unknown aetiology, generally lasting up to a period of 6 weeks. The annular scaly herald patch is followed a few days later by a more generalised eruption on the trunk and proximal limbs. The lesions are oval with a crenated scale and tend to follow dermatomal lines. In patients in whom there is widespread depigmentation, vitiligo may be considered, but this condition, associated with the organ-specific group of disorders and due to non-functioning melanocytes, shows no scaling.

4. Laboratory Diagnosis

Direct microscopy of an ink/potassium hydroxide preparation from infected material (Cohen 1954) showing yeast cells and short angular hyphae is usually sufficient to confirm the diagnosis, and culture of this lipophilic yeast is rarely considered to be necessary in the standard laboratory situation.

5. Treatment

Any method used must aim to treat the entire condition, otherwise relapse will occur. Topical therapy with selenium sulphide shampoo (Selsun) applied neat overnight and washed off the following morning and repeated 1 and 6 weeks later is highly effective. Zinc pyrithione could be used in a similar manner (Faergemann and Fredriksson 1980). Other preparations such as sulphur and salicylic acid ointment or Whitfield's ointment are helpful but unpleasant to use because they are greasy, may cause a burning sensation and require daily treatment. The imidazole topical agents usually need to be applied twice a day for at least 3 weeks to ensure mycological as well as clinical cure. There is probably little to choose between the currently available drugs.

A short course of oral ketoconazole for a few days will clear the infection and is used in some centres (HAY and MIDGLEY 1984), but it can be hard to justify this treatment with its potential risk of hepatic damage (VAN TYLE 1984). Itraconazole and fluconazole may become more widely used because of their lower risk of side effects. The advantage of an oral drug is treatment of the entire rash, whereas with topical treatments some areas may be missed. Many patients find the residual depigmentation cosmetically undesirable, and a course of ultraviolet light therapy is sometimes given. PUVA (psoralen + UVA) treatment, however, hardly seems appropriate in most patients.

IV. Less Common Superficial Fungal Infections of Nails

1. Aetiology and Epidemiology

On occasion, other non-dermatophyte superficial infections may present in the dermatology clinic (see Table 3).

Table 3. Opportunistic fungal infections of nails

Site	Type of infection	Causative agent
Nail	Onychomycosis (nail plate invasion)	*Scopulariopsis brevicaulis* *Acremonium* sp. *Fusarium* sp. *Aspergillus* sp. *Pyraenochaeta* sp. *Botryodiplodia theobromae* *Curvularia lunata*
Skin or nail	Tinea-like lesions or onychomycosis	*Hendersonula toruloidea* *Scytalidium hyalinum*

Many of the fungi causing onychomycosis are saprophytic moulds which may invade nails already damaged by trauma, ischaemia or disease. Sometimes, a dermatophyte may produce the initial nail injury, and the two fungi then co-exist. *Scopulariopsis brevicaulis*, however, may invade a previously undamaged nail. *Hendersonula toruloidea* is a plant pathogen found in tropical areas, particularly the Caribbean, Africa and the Indian subcontinent. The clinical diagnosis is often made outside the country of origin (MOORE 1978). *Scytalidium hyalinum* is also a saprophytic organism and presents comparable clinical features when it adopts a pathogenic role.

2. Clinical Features

Sco. brevicaulis most frequently causes a dystrophy of the great toenail, but other nails may be involved. Clinical features resemble ringworm infection, but the brown spores of the fungus may produce a similar discoloration of the nail. Other fungi such as *Acremonium* spp. or *Fusarium* spp. may produce superficial white onychomycosis. In infection with *Aspergillus* sp. a green or black discoloration of the nail plate can occur and is dependent upon the particular species present. Both *H. toruloidea* and *Scy. hyalinum* produce a clinical picture indistinguishable from that of ringworm infection of the hands, feet and nails. In some cases of *Hendersonula* infection, brown discolouration of the nail may be present. Paronychia may occur in the presence of both *Hendersonula* and *Scytalidium* infections but may be an independent infection rather than casually related.

3. Differential Diagnosis

These nail infections have to be differentiated from other fungal infections due to dermatophyte and *Candida* species. The colour of the nail may give a clue as to the possible aetiological agent. Chronic paronychia due to *Candida* infection is very much commoner than *Hendersonula* or *Scytalidium* infection. Other causes of nail dystrophy including psoriasis or eczema must be considered, but evidence of these diseases could exist elsewhere, and negative culture results will be helpful where the diagnosis is in doubt.

4. Laboratory Diagnosis

Microscopic examination of a potassium hydroxide preparation may show variation in hyphal width and more irregularity than that seen with dermatophyte hyphae. Culture of the infecting fungus on several inoculation sites on Sabouraud medium is likely to indicate a clinically significant isolation, but care should be taken to exclude the presence of a co-existent infection with *Candida* or dermatophyte species. Growth on Sabouraud medium at 28°C both with and without cycloheximide is necessary, since this chemical will inhibit growth of some fungi.

5. Treatment

Avulsion of the infected nail is often the treatment of choice in the absence of an effective topical treatment, but if a dermatophyte infection coexists, then oral griseofulvin will be required as well. None of the above non-dermatophyte infections respond to griseofulvin treatment. *H. toruloidea* and *Scy. hyalinum* are sensitive to imidazoles in vitro, but topical treatment with occlusion is disappointing, although recent nail varnish preparations which allow greater penetration of the topical medicament should be more useful. Oral ketoconazole is not beneficial. Whitfield's ointment may be effective where there is adjacent skin infection. In other nail infections a similar problem is evident. Imidazoles do not seem to be very helpful, while 1% natamycin in dimethyl sulphoxide has been used in *Scopulariopsis* infection. Infection may be recurrent, especially where there is underlying disease of the nail due to trauma or ischaemia.

V. Less Common Superficial Fungal Infections of Skin and Hair

1. Aetiology and Epidemiology

Tinea nigra due to *Exophiala werneckii* occurs most frequently in Central and South America and in the Caribbean. Piedra, which is a fungal infection confined to the hair shaft, occurs in two forms. Black piedra due to *Piedraia hortae* and found in the tropics, especially Central and South America and Indonesia, may infect monkeys as well as humans. White piedra due to *Trichosporon beigelii* occurs in temperate regions in the Orient, America and Europe. This infection may also be present in horses and monkeys.

2. Clinical Features

H. toruloidea and *Scy. hyalinum* may cause skin infection and have been discussed above (Sect. B.IV).

Tinea nigra presents as smooth, brown or black, non-scaly patches, most often on the palms although other parts of the body can be affected. In black piedra dark, adherent, gritty nodules composed of the fungus occur on hairs in the scalp, beard, moustache or pubic areas. The hairs break easily because the fungus grows into the shaft. White piedra infects axillary and pubic hair and also the beard area. Soft, white or light-brown nodules may coalesce, but the mass of fungus is easily detached from the infected hair.

3. Differential Diagnosis

The black colour of tinea nigra and clinical absence of scaling will differentiate the condition from pityriasis versicolor. Pigmented naevi, Addison's disease and the pigmented lesions seen in pinta and sometimes in syphilis need to be excluded clinically. Pruritus and the distinctive appearance of nits will distinguish pediculosis from piedra.

4. Laboratory Diagnosis

In suspected cases of tinea nigra a potassium hydroxide preparation of epidermal scales will show septate hyphae and budding cells. Culture on Sabouraud medium is slow but yields white or grey yeast-like colonies. Morphology is very variable.

In piedra examination of infected hairs under the microscope is diagnostic. *Piedraia hortae* is a slow growing, dark fungus, and microscopy may reveal asci and ascospores. The creamy colonies of *T. beigelii* grow best at 37°C on Sabouraud medium.

5. Treatment

Whitfield's ointment will have some effect on *Hendersonula* and *Scytalidium* skin infections and also on tinea nigra. Thiabendazole preparations are also effective in the latter condition. In piedra shaving the infected hair will produce a rapid cure, but Whitfield's ointment should be applied thereafter to prevent recurrence. White piedra responds to amphotericin B lotion. Imidazoles are of no benefit.

VI. Otomycosis

1. Aetiology and Epidemiology

This chronic inflammatory disease of the external ear is caused by *Aspergillus* spp. (especially *A. niger*), *C. albicans*, and by *Mucor*, *Rhizopus* and *Penicillium* species. Other common yeasts and moulds may cause disease on occasion, but bacterial infection is often the primary event.

Otomycosis can occur worldwide, but fungal isolates from an apparently normal external ear are more common in tropical regions. An assessment of the possible pathogenic role of an isolate has to be made with knowledge of the particular clinical situation. Trauma and maceration of the external auditory meatus, e.g. from swimming, may be predisposing factors.

2. Clinical Features

The features of redness, scaling, itch and possible pain in the external ear are common to all cases of otitis externa. Serous discharge may be present, and in advanced cases of otomycosis, a mass of white material due to fungal overgrowth is evident.

3. Differential Diagnosis

Other causes of otitis externa such as seborrhoeic dermatitis, eczema, psoriasis or bacterial infection need to be excluded.

4. Laboratory Diagnosis

Light growth of a fungus on culture is not significant, but heavier growth in the absence of bacterial pathogens may be more important, especially if there is considerable fungal material on direct microscopy of the specimen.

5. Treatment

Careful ear toilet is mandatory. Nystatin powder has been used to treat *Aspergillus* and *Candida* infection, but this leaves more debris for removal. Clotrimazole lotion has been used more recently. Treatment of any underlying bacterial infection will often remove the conditions which favour fungal growth.

C. The Subcutaneous Mycoses

I. Mycetoma

1. Aetiology and Epidemiology

The term mycetoma is used to denote any tumour due to fungal infection. This group of infections is caused by a variety of unrelated fungi which are found on plants or in the soil, mainly in tropical and subtropical areas (Mariat 1963). Patients have been described in Europe and America (Anning et al. 1958; Murray et al. 1964), but the infection has usually started in the tropics in these instances. Trauma is necessary to provide a portal of entry for fungal spores, and therefore most cases occur in male agricultural workers, especially those who work barefoot. Subcutaneous infections of this type are not common but are difficult to treat and tend to be very chronic. In those parts of the world in which the infections are most commonly seen, the morbidity of the condition can pose a problem both for the patient and the local community.

Mycetomata are classified according to the appearance of 'grains' which are composed of microcolonies of the causative fungus or actinomycete filaments found within the lesion (Mahgoub and Murray 1973). Actinomycetes are bacteria producing filamentous hyphae, and this type of infection which often produces systemic disease will not be dealt with to any great extent in this chapter (see Table 4).

Table 4. Aetiological agents of mycetomata

Disease	Causative agent
Eumycotic mycetomata yellow/white grains	*Pseudoallescheria boydii* *Acremonium* sp.
brown/black grains	*Madurella mycetomatis* or *grisea* *Exophiala jeanselmii* *Leptosphaeria senegalensis* *Pyrenochaeta romeroi* *Neotestudina rosatii* *Curvularia lunata*
Actinomycotic mycetoma yellow/white grains (sulphur granules)	*Actinomycete* sp. *Nocardia* sp. *Streptomycete* sp.
red grains	*Actinomadura pelletieri*

2. Clinical Features

The clinical features are not specific for the particular fungus present. In the typical case of mycetoma, a firm painless nodule appears frequently on the foot (Madura foot). The inflammatory response within the lesion causes liquefaction, necrosis and sinus formation. Grains are found within the subcutaneous tissue and sinuses and are relatively indestructable due to the presence of cement in the outer wall of the grain (FINDLAY and VISMER 1974). When inflammation is severe enough, there may be destruction of underlying bones or joints.

3. Differential Diagnosis

Osteomyelitis of bacterial origin and botryomycosis where there is chronic inflammatory disease of bacterial origin in the subcutaneous tissues resulting in a tumour similar to mycetoma can arise in the differential diagnosis. Tuberculosis must always be considered.

4. Laboratory Diagnosis

Culture from a biopsy specimen or of material obtained from an appropriate lesion may yield the causative agent. In particular, tuberculosis should be excluded. Direct microscopy of crushed grains will show multiple fungal hyphae or actinomycete filaments. Culture on different media is necessary to cover the range of possible fungi which might be responsible for the mycetoma. Serology can be helpful in some instances.

5. Treatment

Actinomycosis is due to bacterial infection and responds to massive doses of penicillin given for a sufficient length of time. Other antibiotics suitable for treating gram-positive bacterial infection can be used, but penicillin is the therapy of choice.

In patients with true fungal mycetoma, surgery is often necessary and may well be the best measure in localised cases, since results with chemotherapy tend to be disappointing. Ideally, the drug used should be the appropriate one for the fungus isolated and based on in vitro testing of sensitivity. In practice, it may be difficult to isolate and identify a fungus, although every effect should be made to obtain grains for culture. Serology may be unhelpful, and in vivo activity of a drug may not correlate well with in vitro testing. Drugs that can be used include amphotericin B, the systemic imidazole group, griseofulvin and streptomycin combined with either dapsone or sulphamethoxazole-trimethoprim. Nevertheless, chemotherapy should always be attempted, although long-term usage in the face of progressive disease should be resisted, and surgical measures should then be adopted.

II. Chromomycosis

1. Aetiology and Epidemiology

This condition is a chronic fungus infection of the subcutaneous tissues caused by a group of dematiaceous fungi. This group includes *Fonsecaea (Phialo-*

phora) pedrosoi, *F. (P.) compacta*, *P. verrucosa*, *Cladosporium carrionii* and *Wangiella dermatitidis*. These are saprophytic organisms on soil or organic matter, and trauma by a wood splinter for instance is the normal portal of entry into humans. The disease is found worldwide but is most common in Central and South America and in Africa. The condition can occur in children but is most frequent in male agricultural workers.

2. Clinical Features

Painless warty nodules appear especially on the legs and feet. Occasionally, ulceration may be an early feature, but secondary ulceration of the large hyperkeratotic masses is very frequent. If there is secondary infection, then itching and pain may be present. Satellite lesions produced as a result of scratching may spread via the lymphatics and in chronic cases elephantiasis may eventually occur. Haematogeneous spread is rare.

3. Differential Diagnosis

Blastomycosis, which is a chronic systemic disease caused by *Blastomyces dermatitidis*, primarily affects the lungs, but in the disseminated form skin lesions can occur. However, the central healing of the lesions with a tendency to flat scar formation and the presence of peripheral spreading warty nodules forming a serpiginous border has to be differentiated from chromomycosis. The causative organism can be isolated from abscesses at the margin of the lesion.

Cutaneous tuberculosis and leishmaniasis can be distinguished by culture, by examination of smears from the tissues in the latter condition and by histological study. Skin testing may also be helpful. Hyperkeratotic papular lesions in the tertiary phase of syphilis and yaws need to be differentiated in both these instances. Culture, histology and serology will be required.

4. Laboratory Diagnosis

Direct examination of a potassium hydroxide preparation or of a biopsy section will show deeply pigmented, thick-walled, sclerotic cells, and culture on Sabouraud medium with antibiotic at 26°C for about 3 weeks will provide confirmation of the diagnosis. Histologically the reaction is granulomatous with isolated abscess formation.

5. Treatment

For early localised lesions, surgical removal by excision or destruction by means of cryotherapy, cautery or diathermy is the treatment of choice. The need for early diagnosis is therefore evident. Local infiltration of lesions with amphotericin B has been used (Costello et al. 1959), but a combination of 5-fluorocytosine with ketoconazole seems to have been more successful (Silber et al. 1983). It is probably better to combine 5-fluorocytosine with another drug to reduce the risk of resistance which might occur when 5-fluorocytosine is used alone (see also Chap. 19 concerning the use of itraconazole).

III. Sporotrichosis

1. Aetiology and Epidemiology

This fungal infection involves the lymphatics and subcutaneous tissues and is caused by *Sporothrix schenckii*, which is a dimorphic yeast. The fungus exists in mycelial form as a saprophyte in the soil, on plants and on various plant materials. The yeast form exists in animal tissue. The condition occurs in both temperate and tropical zones but is particularly seen in mining areas of South Africa. The incidence and possibly the geographical distribution is dependent on climatic conditions, and the presence of high humidity and temperatures between 16°C and 22°C favours saprophytic growth. The fungus grows on decaying vegetable matter, and minor trauma is usually responsible for the development of infection in humans. The use of infected timber in mines is sometimes responsible for outbreaks of this infection; if the timber is treated before being taken underground, this is likely to eliminate the possibility of an epidemic (FINDLAY 1970).

2. Clinical Features

In the most common type of sporotrichosis lesions, spread is via the local lymphatics from the primary wound. The initial lesion, which normally occurs on an exposed area of skin such as the arm, is a nodule or pustule which quickly ulcerates. Thereafter, secondary nodules develop along the line of the lymphatics draining the area. These nodules also tend to ulcerate and are joined by hard lymphatic cords. Sometimes more localised infections with nodular, ulcerated or even verrucous lesions occur. Plaque formation may indicate a high degree of immunity. On rare occasions haematogenous spread may occur and then any organ in the body may be involved. It seems likely that the immunological response of the host will determine the form which the infection will assume in a particular individual.

3. Differential Diagnosis

Sporotrichosis has to be considered in any granulomatous condition particularly if this follows injury. The localised lymphatic form of the condition is, however, highly characteristic clinically. In particular, atypical mycobacterial infection must be considered in the differential diagnosis. Histological examination and culture, where appropriate, and skin testing or serology under certain conditions will help to confirm the diagnosis.

4. Laboratory Diagnosis

Diagnosis of the condition is dependent on culture, since direct microscopy of clinical material is of little value, and histology is not always helpful. It is necessary to take the material for culture from intact lesions. To be certain of the diagnosis, both forms of the fungus need to be demonstrated. The mycelial form will grow on Sabouraud agar with cycloheximide at 26°C, whereas the yeast form requires brain-heart infusion agar at 37°C. Histology, if helpful, may show a granulomatous reaction with asteroid bodies.

5. Treatment

In the localised type of sporotrichosis, potassium iodide in large doses by mouth together with intravenous sodium iodide if required need to be continued for about a month after apparent clinical cure and form the treatment of choice for the cutaneous type. However, if patients are extremely ill or if iodide therapy is unsuccessful, then amphotericin B intravenously will be required (SMITH et al. 1981) (see also Chap. 19 concerning the use of itraconazole).

Thermotherapy can be effective in localised cases (MACKINNON and CONTI-DIAZ 1962). Intravenous and oral imidazole drugs have been used, but they seem to be less effective than potassium iodide. In some patients 5-fluorocytosine or amphotericin B was injected intralesionally.

IV. Phaeohyphomycosis

1. Aetiology and Epidemiology

This is a condition caused by dematiaceous, brown pigmented fungi including *Exophiala jeanselmii* and *Wangiella dermatitidis*. The organism is implanted from an external source, and infection occurs both in temperate and tropical areas (ICHINOSE 1971), particularly in agricultural workers. It is likely that there will be an increasing number of such cases reported in immunosuppressed patients.

2. Clinical Features

Subcutaneous or intramuscular infection occurs, and there is development of a tender nodule which may become cystic. There is considerable thickening of the overlying epidermis. The condition rarely spreads elsewhere.

3. Differential Diagnosis

It is unlikely that the diagnosis will be made clinically, and other causes of solitary tender cysts or tumours should be excluded by biopsy or excision.

4. Laboratory Diagnosis

Brown hyphae and budding cells are seen on microscopy of the granulomatous tissue.

5. Treatment

Excision of the lesion is the only treatment reported to be successful.

V. Lobomycosis

1. Aetiology and Epidemiology

This is a rare condition due to the fungus *Loboa loboi*, seen mainly in Latin America. It is likely that injury provides the portal of entry for the fungus.

2. Clinical Features

The granulomatous reaction forms keloidal skin lesions which generally remain quite localised without undue upset to the health of the patient. Chronic lesions tend to be crusted and fungating.

3. Differential Diagnosis

The condition has to be differentiated from chromomycosis which it closely resembles.

4. Laboratory Diagnosis

The fungus has not been isolated on culture but can be seen as chains of budding cells on microscopic examination of a potassium hydroxide preparation.

5. Treatment

Excision of localised lesions is the only treatment available.

VI. Zygomycosis (Phycomycosis)

1. Aetiology and Epidemiology

A disseminated form of the condition caused by *Mucor*, *Absidia* and *Rhizopus* species occurs in patients with diabetes mellitus, leukaemia or other severe illnesses. Subcutaneous zygomycosis occurs in two forms, namely basidiobolomycosis caused by *Basidiobolus haptosporus* and rhinoentomophthoromycosis due to *Conidiobolus coronatus*. Basidiobolomycosis occurs in tropical and subtropical zones especially East and West Africa and South-East Asia. The fungus is associated with decaying vegetable matter but is also found in the gastrointestinal tract of frogs, toads and lizards. Rhinoentomophthoromycosis occurs particularly in Africa, though it has been reported in the Caribbean and South America. The causative agent *C. coronatus* also occurs in the soil or on decaying vegetable matter.

2. Clinical Features

Basidiobolomycosis occurs as a subcutaneous swelling on the limbs particularly of children. There is no ulceration, and the lesions remain firm. In rhinoentomophthoromycosis there is involvement of the nasal mucosa, sinuses and subcutaneous tissues of the face including the nose.

3. Differential Diagnosis

Histological and mycological examination is required. Lymphatic oedema and erysipelas need to be excluded clinically, and malignant lymphoma will be evident on histological examination.

4. Laboratory Diagnosis

Both *B. haptosporus* and *C. coronatus* grow on Sabouraud medium without cycloheximide at 37°C. Examination of the morphological characteristics will confirm the diagnosis.

5. Treatment

The more severe generalised form of Zygomycosis will often only be recognised at autopsy, but the subcutaneous variety will usually respond to potassium iodide orally.

VII. Rhinosporidiosis

1. Aetiology and Epidemiology

This is a chronic granulomatous mycosis caused by *Rhinosporidium seeberi*. It is endemic in India and Sri Lanka, but patients have been described in Africa and elsewhere.

2. Clinical Features

Enormous fungating lesions with a cauliflower-like appearance and a vascular surface can occur on any mucosal area. The lesions may be pedunculated. The nasopharynx and soft palate are particularly likely to be involved, and there may be some obstruction to breathing. The condition lasts for years but is not contagious.

3. Differential Diagnosis

In the genital area the lesions have to be differentiated from warts, condylomata and haemorrhoids. The pink/purple colour and friable consistency of the fungal lesions are characteristic.

4. Laboratory Diagnosis

R. seeberi has not been isolated on culture. Sporangia are seen on the surface of the polyps by the naked eye as well as on histological examination. On microscopy, the single, thick-walled cysts may be packed with numerous endospores.

5. Treatment

Excision is the treatment of choice to eradicate this fungus infection.

D. Present Therapeutic Practice and Future Needs

I. Introduction

Several factors influence the success of a particular approach to therapy. These principles are referable to treatment in general but are here applied to the problems associated with therapy for fungal disease. Differing requirements depend to some extent on the superficial or subcutaneous nature of the infection. There are a number of topical and systemic treatments available for the management of dermatophyte and superficial yeast infections, but there are circumstances in which these treatments may fail or be unsuitable for a particular situation. There is less to offer in the way of therapy for some of the other uncommon, non-dermatophyte, superficial infections.

Management of the subcutaneous mycoses poses a much greater problem, since therapeutic approaches are limited or non-existent, and surgical measures may often be required. Because particular infections are rare in some parts of the world, less attention has been focussed on problems of epidemiology where such mycoses are rife. In the development of drugs to combat such conditions, the cost factor is obviously of paramount important in the production of a marketable product.

II. Choice of Preparation

1. Introduction

When considering the type of treatment to be used in an individual patient, the nature of the causative agent, sites to be treated and suitability of available products to gain most benefit in terms of treatment efficacy are important. The risk of side effects has to be weighed against the gravity of the clinical situation, and drug interactions have to be considered. When the diagnosis of a particular fungal infection is made, available treatments are quite clearly defined, but under certain conditions the choice may be limited.

2. The Superficial Mycoses

When a dermatophyte infection is localised to the groins, toe webs or a relatively circumscribed area of glabrous skin, then topical therapy will suffice. It is likely that the patient will use this if the area is uncomfortable, especially if there is groin involvement. Toe web infections are treated solely by topical means, either by one of the imidazole preparations, tolnaftate or Whitfield's ointment, since a much higher dose of griseofulvin than that normally prescribed is necessary to cure such an infection. Although a powder preparation would seem reasonable for use in the toe webs, this creates more debris, and creams or lotions are more acceptable from the patient's point of view. Cream bases are easy to use in flexural areas such as the groin or on hairy sites and are cosmetically more acceptable than ointments.

If there is widespread skin, scalp or nail involvement, oral therapy is indicated. Griseofulvin is the drug of choice at present, because although there is a potential risk of many side effects, in practice these are not a great problem. However, where there is penicillin hypersensitivity with the risk of cross-reaction, an alternative has to be found. Ketoconazole has been used, but it is hard to justify for localised toenail infection, and removal of the diseased nail plus use of tioconazole/undecylenic acid nail lotion may be better. The newer imidazoles, itraconazole and fluconazole, can be used on a named patient basis. Terbinafine seems likely to be an acceptable alternative to griseofulvin without the hepatotoxic effects of ketoconazole. As far as the patient is concerned, the long-term treatment necessary to clear chronic tinea unguium may not be justified.

Treatment of nail infections due to opportunistic infections such as *Fusarium* or *Acremonium* and to pathogens such as *Scopulariopsis*, *Hendersonula* or *Scytalidium* is limited. Removal of the diseased nail and then treatment with a topical imidazole preparation, possibly with occlusion, may be attempted.

In *Candida* infection, topical therapy with an imidazole preparation is most frequently used, although older drugs such as nystatin or amphotericin B can have a place, especially if there is an adverse effect with imidazole usage. In addition, oral therapy is required in angular stomatitis and pruritus ani due to candidosis, and a pessary preparation which may be either nystatin or an imidazole can be used for pruritus vulvae. The imidazole preparations have the advantage of a shorter duration of treatment. In chronic mucocutaneous candidosis use of an oral imidazole drug is essential, and in certain cases 5-fluorocytosine may be added. Treatment with amphotericin B may well be required.

Systemic therapy for pityriasis versicolor is advocated in some centres because of the difficulty of ensuring adequate treatment by topical means. It is easier for the patient to take a week's course of oral therapy than to treat large areas of skin with selenium sulphide shampoo or Whitfield's ointment. Both these preparations are messy and potentially irritant. With the imidazole creams a 3-week course of treatment is required. Itraconzole or fluconazole orally may be justified where the lesions are extensive.

3. The Subcutaneous Mycoses

In these conditions the range of treatment is limited to systemic therapy which is clearly defined, assuming that the causative agent can be accurately identified (C I–VII) and that an appropriate drug is available. Side effects of the drugs used may cause difficulties, and there is often uncertainty as to whether an effective dose is reaching the site of disease. More options exist for mycetoma, but the nature of the condition may mean that the result of treatment is disappointing, even if the minimum inhibitory concentration of the available drugs is assessed.

III. Factors Influencing Treatment Failure

1. Lack of Compliance

It is well recognised that patients do not take treatment regularly, regardless of whether topical or systemic therapy is provided. Many patients are averse to the use of internal therapy in any form, and this may be particularly relevant in the management of relatively localised dermatophyte infection on the soles of the feet, for instance, where discomfort may be minimal, but topical therapy may be insufficient. In other instances in which topical therapy may suffice, the preparation may not be used because it is not practical to apply it during working hours, and after work treatment may simply be forgotten. Where treatment is lengthy, as in chronic tinea infection of the nails, the slow progress may dishearten the patient. If side effects occur and especially if there is interaction with other drugs which the patient is taking, then the therapy is all too readily discarded.

2. Host Factors

The question of drug absorption is important, particularly with regard to internal therapy. Some cases of apparent griseofulvin-resistant dermatophyte infection may be due to poor drug absorption even if the drug is taken with food as recommended. With topical therapy, ease of absorption in different body sites may be relevant. For instance, the absorption rate in flexural areas is enhanced by maceration.

Problems with liver disease may limit the use of drugs such as the imidazoles, and although the new preparations (itraconazole and fluconazole) seem to be safe, clinicians will tread warily for some time until confidence in this group has been restored. In situations which may be life-threatening, for example severe mucocutaneous candidosis, there will be no reservations about the use of such drugs. Renal disease may affect the rate of clearance of a drug or its metabolites and thus increase the risk of side effects.

Where host resistance is compromised or defective, even apparently satisfactory treatment may fail. This applies to such conditions as mucocutaneous candidosis, leukaemia, patients on life-support systems or those with AIDS. Resistance to infection is related to the presence of innate immunity such as serum factors, for example unsaturated transferrin, which may be inhibitory to the growth of certain fungi, or acquired immunity, in which specific antibodies may be demonstrated, particularly in some chronic infections such as favus. The appearance of specifically activated T cells is necessary in the recovery process.

3. Fungal Pathogenicity

Unless host factors of lowered resistance to infection are present, some break in the host's surface is necessary to allow the fungal spores to enter. This may occur as a result of trauma or some preceding infection, especially of bacterial origin. If the underlying process including bacterial infection remains, then treatment of the fungus infection alone will be insufficient. If two fungi coexist as in some nail infections with, for example, *T. rubrum* and an opportunistic fungus such as *Fusarium*, both organisms need to be eradicated.

Some fungi such as dermatophytes are pathogenic when in contact with humans, but there are differences in the extent to which individual species will produce disease. The physical properties of some fungi with spores resistant to temperature change and with thick, impenetrable or impervious walls may mean that only a limited number of drugs are available to treat such infections. This is particularly relevant when managing the chronic subcutaneous mycoses.

4. Drug Factors

Drug resistance to currently available medication is rare. Where there are problems with griseofulvin and the imidazoles, it is more likely that host factors play a part in the effectiveness of treatment in a particular situation. In addition, interaction with other drugs that the patient is currently taking may reduce the efficacy of therapy. It is common for 5-fluorocytosine resistance to develop in the treatment of candidosis, and combination therapy with another drug such as one of the imidazoles may help to delay or prevent this possibility.

In the treatment of the subcutaneous mycoses, the defence mechanism of the invading fungus such as the thickness of the cement wall in mycetoma grains or the phase in the life cycle at which the available drugs attack the fungus are important. If the host produces a considerable granulomatous or scarring tissue reaction, this may reduce the efficacy of drug absorption at the disease site, assuming that transport of the drug to the appropriate area is actually achieved.

Occasionally, allergy to the drug used may cause problems, for instance, the development of a rash with griseofulvin in a patient allergic to penicillin. Side effects of the particular drug may limit its use.

5. Inadequate Treatment

It is important to establish the diagnosis accurately to assess the factors responsible for a particular disease state. Treatment failure may be due to a combination of inadequate drug dosage for a sufficient length of time, failure to consider host factors, environmental conditions leading to rapid reinfection and emerging resistance of a fungus to the drug prescribed. In certain cases such as chronic mucocutaneous candidosis, multiple drug therapy as well as measures to improve the underlying immunological problem are important. In pityriasis versicolor topical treatment may fail because some infected areas are missed when the drug is applied. In mycetoma it is necessary to establish the nature of the underlying infection, but if the drug does not penetrate to the site of the infection, treatment will be inadequate, even though the dose given may seem to be sufficient. In some patients with subcutaneous mycoses such as phaeohyphomycosis, lobomycosis or rhinosporidiosis, there are simply no drugs available to deal with the problem, and surgery is the only option.

6. Epidemiological Factors

Although dermatophyte infections are not considered to be of great significance by the population in general, there is an appreciable morbidity which may have social as well as economic consequences. This is particularly relevant when the disease is widespread, for instance, tinea imbricata which is endemic in South-East Asia, the West Pacific and South America, or in chronic tinea infections in miners (Gentles and Holmes 1957; Gotz and Hantschke 1965). Infections by saprophytes or plant pathogens such as *Hendersonula* or *Scytalidium* may cause infections which resemble tinea, but unless culture is undertaken the diagnosis may be missed and such patients classed as treatment failures when griseofulvin is unsuccessful.

The subcutaneous mycoses generally tend to occur in Latin America, India, Africa or the Caribbean and are not common. They are difficult to treat because they are relatively unresponsive to present therapy. Considerable tissue destruction may occur, and this will have an effect on the potential work capacity of the individual. As travel to these countries becomes more general, the frequency with which such diseases are brought back to the host's country will increase. Early recognition is essential so that appropriate treatment can be instituted as soon as possible.

IV. Future Requirements

Although considerable progress in the management of fungal disease has occurred over the past few years, there is need for more powerful chemotherapeutic agents, particularly in some of the rarer subcutaneous mycoses. Ideally, these drugs should be fungicidal rather than fungistatic, since host factors such as lowered immunity will be overcome more effectively with the former approach. In clinical terms, there is probably no great requirement for further topical therapy. Research should be concentrated on the development of systemic therapy, both oral and parenteral, and chemicals with a different basic structure from those currently available would provide greater scope for success. Since transport of a drug in sufficient concentration is so important, solubility factors and methods of reducing the tissue and fungal factors which mitigate against efficient drug delivery should be explored further.

Immunological methods of overcoming infection may have some place, especially in some of the more chronic dermatophyte infections, candidosis or mycetoma. Development of vaccines, particularly to deal with disease in animal reservoirs, may be relevant.

In summary, although the range of available treatments is increasing, particularly for superficial fungal infection, some facets require further research, and the challenge of more effective treatment for the subcutaneous mycoses remains.

References

Anning, La Touche, Hunter (1958) Madura foot (mycetoma), North of England Dermatological Society (case report). Br J Dermatol 70:309

Baran R, Hay RJ (1985) Partial surgical avulsion of the nail in onychomycosis. Clin Exp Dermatol 10:413–418

Barlow AJE, Chattaway FW, Holgate MC, Aldersley T (1970) Chronic paronychia. Br J Dermatol 82:448–453

Beare JM, Cheeseman EA, Mackenzie DWR (1968) The association between *Candida albicans* and lesions of seborrhoeic eczema. Br J Dermatol 80:675–681

Boardman CR, Malkinson FD (1962) Tinea versicolor in steroid treated patients. Arch Dermatol 85:44–52

Cohen MM (1954) A simple procedure for staining tinea versicolor (*M. furfur*) with fountain pen ink. J Invest Dermatol 22:9–10

Cohen R, Roth FW, Delgardo E, Ahearn DG, Kalser MH (1969) Fungal flora of the normal human small and large intestine. N Engl J Med 280:638–641

Costello MJ, DeFoe CP, Littman ML (1959) Chromoblastomycosis treated with local infiltration of amphotericin B solution. Arch Dermatol 79:184–193

Dave VK, Roberts MM, Butterfield W (1987) Pityriasis versicolor and sunscreens containing coconut oil. Lancet ii:685–686

Davies RR, Everall JD, Hamilton E (1967) Mycological and clinical evaluation of griseofulvin for chronic onychomycosis. Br Med J 3:464–469

Faergemann J, Fredriksson T (1980) An open trial of the effect of a zinc pyrithione shampoo in tinea versicolor. Cutis 25:667–669

Findlay GH (1970) The epidemiology of sporotrichosis in the Transvaal. Sabouraudia 7:231–236

Findlay GH, Vismer HF (1974) Black grain mycetoma: a study of the chemistry formation and significance of the tissue grain in *Madurella mycetomi* infection. Br J Dermatol 91:297–303

Food Advisory Committee UK (1987) Carcinogenicity in mice produced by crystal violet. Fd, AC/Rep/4. HM Stationery Office, London

Gatenby P, Basten A, Adams E (1980) Thymoma and late onset mucocutaneous candidiasis associated with a plasma inhibitor of cell-mediated immune function. J Clin Lab Immunol 3:209–216

Gentles JC, Evans EGV (1973) Foot infections in swimming baths. Br Med J 3: 260–262

Gentles JC, Holmes JG (1957) Foot ringworm in coal-miners. Br J Indust Med 14:22–29

Gentles JC, Evans EGV, Jones GR (1974) Control of tinea pedis in a swimming bath. Br Med J 2:577–580

Gotz H, Hantschke D (1965) Einblicke in der Epidemiologie der Dermatomykosen im Kohlenbergbau. Hautarzt 16:543–549

Hay RJ (1981) Special symposium on dermatological therapy: II. Infections and infestations, management of chronic mucocutaneous candidosis. Clin Exp Dermatol 6:515–519

Hay RJ (1982) Chronic dermatophyte infections. I. Clinical and mycological features. Br J Dermatol 106:1–7

Hay RJ, Clayton YM (1982) Treatment of chronic dermatophyte infections – the use of ketoconazole in griseofulvin treatment failures. Clin Exp Dermatol 7:611–617

Hay RJ, Midgley G (1984) Short course ketoconazole therapy in pityriasis versicolor. Clin Exp Dermatol 9:571–573

Hay RJ, Clayton YM, Moore K (1987) A comparison of tioconazole 28% nail solution versus base as an adjunct to oral griseofulvin in patients with onychomycosis. Clin Exp Dermatol 12:175–177

Higgs JM, Wells RS (1973) Chronic muco-cutaneous candidiasis: new approaches to treatment. Br J Dermatol 80:179–190

Ichinose H (1971) Subcutaneous abscesses due to brown fungi. In: Baker RD (ed) The pathologic anatomy of mycoses. Springer-Verlag, Berlin Heidelberg New York, pp 719–730

Jevons S, Lees L (1985) In: Trosyd (Tioconazole) Pfizer Kent, clinical experience. A monograph. Academy Professional Information Services Inc, New York, pp 22–28

Johnson JA, Rosenthal SA (1968) Superficial cutaneous infection with *Trichophyton soudanense*. Arch Dermatol 97:428–431

Kirkpatrick CH, Smith TK (1974) Chronic mucocutaneous candidiasis: immunologic and antibiotic therapy. Ann Int Med 80:310–320

Kirkpatrick CH, Windhorst DB (1979) Mucocutaneous candidiasis and thymoma. Am J Med 66:939–945

Lassus A, Forstrom S, Salo O (1983) A double-blind comparison of sulconazole nitrate 1% cream with clotrimazole 1% cream in the treatment of dermatophytoses Br J Dermatol 108:195–198

Legendre R, Stelz M (1980) A multi-center double blind comparison of ketoconazole and griseofulvin in the treatment of infections due to dermatophytes. Rev Infect Dis 2:586–591

Levy RL, Huang S-W, Bach ML, Bach FH, Hong R, Ammann AJ, Bortin M, Kay HEM (1971) Thymic transplantation in a case of chronic mucocutaneous candidiasis. Lancet ii:898–900

MacKinnon JE, Conti-Diaz IA (1962) The effect of temperature on sporotrichosis. Sabouraudia 2:56–59

Mahgoub ES, Murray IG (1973) In: Mycetoma. Heinemann Whitefriars Press, London

Maize JC, Lynch PJ (1972) Chronic mucocutaneous candidiasis of the adult. A report of a patient with an associated thymoma. Arch Dermatol 105:96–98

Mariat F (1963) Sur la distribution geographie et la repartition des agents des mycetomes. Bull Soc Pathol Exot Filiales 56:35–45

Marks R, Dawber RPR (1972) In situ microbiology of the stratum corneum. Arch Dermatol 105:216–221

Marples MJ (1965) Fungi inhabiting the skin: *Pityrosporum* and other yeasts. In: Ecology of human skin. Thomas, Springfield Chap. 23, pp 407–427

Marten RH (1959) Chronic paronychia. A mycological and bacteriological study. Br J Dermatol 71:422–426

Moore MK (1978) Skin and nail infections caused by non-dermatophyte filamentous fungi. Mykosen (Suppl 1):128–132

Murray IG, Dunkerley GE, Hughes KEA (1964) A case of madura foot caused by *Phialophora jeanselmii*. Sabouraudia 3:175–177

National Health Survey (1978) Skin conditions and related need for medical care among persons 1–74 years, United States 1971–1974. U.S. Dept of Health Education and Welfare DHEW Pub No (PHS) 79–1660 Office of Assoc Sec for Health. National Center for Health Statistics, Hyattsville

Nazarro-Porro M, Passi S, Morpurgo G, Breathnach AS (1978) Effect of dicarboxylic acids on Harding-Passey melanoma. J Invest Dermatol 70:235

Noble WC, Somerville DA (1974) In: Microbiology of the skin. WB Saunders, London

Nolting S, Fegeler K, Ludwig G, Plischewski K (1975) Behandlung der Tinea unguium und Nachuntersuchungsergebnisse seit Einführung des Griseofulvins. Mykosen 18:11–15

Odds FC (1979) In: Candida and candidosis, Ch 5. University of Leicester Press, Leicester

Pabst HF, Swanson R (1972) Successful treatment of candidiasis with transfer factor. Br Med J 2:442–443

Palestine RF, Su WPD, Wesegang TJ (1983) Late onset chronic mucocutaneous and ocular candidiasis and malignant thymoma. Arch Dermatol 119:580–586

Rebora A, Marples RR, Kligman AM (1973a) Erosio interdigitalis blastomycetica. Arch Dermatol 108:66–68

Rebora A, Marples RR, Kligman AM (1973b) Experimental infection with *Candida albicans*. Arch Dermatol 108:69–73

Rippon JW, Medenica M (1964) Isolation of *Trichophyton soudanense* in the United States. Sabouraudia 3:301–302

Rippon JW, Malkinson FD (1968) *Trichophyton simii* infection in the United States. Arch Dermatol 98:615–619

Roberts SOB (1969) *Pityrosporum orbiculare*: incidence and distribution on clinically normal skin. Br J Dermatol 81:264–269

Robertson MH, Hanifin JM, Parker F (1980) Oral therapy with ketoconazole for dermatophyte infections unresponsive to griseofulvin. Rev Infect Dis 2:578–581

Roed-Petersen J (1980) Tinea versicolor and body lotions. Acta Derm Venereol 60:439–440

Silber JG, Gombert ME, Green KM, Shalita AR (1983) Treatment of chromomycosis with ketoconazole and 5-fluorocytosine. J Am Acad Dermatol 8:236–238

Smith PW, Loomis GW, Luckasen JL, Osterholm RK (1981) Disseminated cutaneous sporotrichosis. Arch Dermatol 117:143–144

Valdimarsson H, Moss PD, Holt PJL, Hobbs JR (1972) Treatment of chronic mucocutaneous candidiasis with leucocytes from HL-A compatible sibling. Lancet i: 469–472

Valdimarsson H, Higgs JM, Wells RS, Yamamura M, Hobbs JR, Holt PJL (1973) Immune abnormalities associated with chronic mucocutaneous candidiasis. Cell Immunol 6:348–361

Vanbreuseghem R (1968) *Trichophyton soudanense* in and outside Africa. Br J Dermatol 80:140–148

Van Tyle JH (1984) Ketoconazole: mechanism of action, spectrum of activity, pharmacokinetics, drug interactions, adverse reactions and therapeutic use. Pharmacotherapy 4:343–373

White MI, Clayton YM (1982) The treatment of fungus and yeast infections of the nail by the method of chemical removal. Clin Exp Dermatol 7:273–276

Whittle CH, Moffatt JL, Davis RA (1959) Paronychia or perionychia: aetiological aspects. Br J Dermatol 71:1–11

CHAPTER 14

Therapeutic Considerations in Fungal Vaginitis

JACK D. SOBEL

A. Introduction

Vaginitis due to fungi is almost always due to *Candida* spp. and less frequently to *Torulopsis glabrata* (ODDS 1988). Rarely, patients with *Saccharomyces cerevisiae* are reported. *Candida* vaginitis continues to plague women throughout the world, and in most countries it is the most common cause of vaginitis. This is particularly the case in those countries with hot subtropical and tropical climates. In the USA, *Candida* vaginitis is the second most common cause of vaginal infection, surpassed only by bacterial vaginosis (Centers for Disease Control 1979). Although not a reportable disease, several evaluations indicate that the incidence of *Candida* vaginitis has increased as a result of a variety of exogenous factors including abuse of antibiotics, etc. Several epidemiological studies have recently been published which discuss pathophysiological aspects of *Candida* vaginitis (SOBEL 1988). This review will focus mainly on therapeutic aspects of vulvovaginal candidosis, including the use and abuse of antimycotic agents, as well as identifying the more controversial aspects of therapy:

1. Should one treat asymptomatic vulvovaginal candidosis?
2. Oral versus topical therapy of acute *Candida* vaginitis.
3. Single dose versus conventional duration therapy of acute *Candida* vaginitis.
4. Can topical azoles be used in the first trimester of pregnancy?
5. In recurrent vulvovaginal candidosis:
   a) Should one treat the asymptomatic male sexual partner?
   b) What is the role of concomitant oral nystatin therapy?
   c) What is the role if any of the glucose tolerance test?
   d) Selection of maintenance prophylaxis regimen (topical versus systemic).
6. Status of antifungal susceptibility tests in selecting therapy.

B. Therapeutic Principles

The practitioner is now faced with a vast, possibly overwhelming array of antimycotics including both topical and oral agents. Given this enormous range of products, how does the practitioner select a therapeutic regimen?

Perhaps the most important advance in therapy for *Candida* vaginitis has been the recognition that no single agent or regimen is appropriate for all patients. Several factors should influence both the agent selected as well as the route of administration and duration of therapy:

1. Duration of present attack
2. Severity of signs and symptoms
3. Anatomical distribution of inflammation (vulvitis)
4. Past history of chronic or recurrent *Candida* vaginitis
5. Patient preference
6. History of local hypersensitivity reaction to topical imidazole
7. Patient compliance
8. Mixed infection
9. Pregnancy
10. Likelihood of a resistant microorganism

The clinician should attempt to individualize therapy based upon the severity of signs and symptoms, duration of clinical manifestations, and whether the attack is an occasional, infrequent episode or represents a frequent recurrence or chronic problem. These factors, together with other patient considerations including pregnancy status, likelihood of patient compliance, and patient's preference, influence the route of administration, choice of agent, and duration of therapy. It goes without saying that therapy should never be given without first confirming the diagnosis of fungal vaginitis. Regrettably, only too often is the diagnosis made over the telephone or in the doctor's office without pelvic examination. This practice is to be condemned and cannot be justified because of the lack of specificity of the signs and symptoms of vaginitis.

The ideal antimycotic agent suitable for all patients with *Candida* vaginitis is not yet available. In particular, recalcitrant cases and pregnancy constitute the major therapeutic challenge. The characteristics of the ideal antimycotic agent for *Candida* vaginitis are listed:

1. Single dose or short course
2. Oral agent
3. Lack of local and systemic side effects and toxicity
4. Rapid action
5. Fungicidal
6. Safe in pregnancy
7. Minimal effect on normal bacterial flora of vagina
8. Inexpensive
9. Reduced recurrence rate

Although many of the newer agents, especially the imidazoles and triazoles, achieve remarkable efficacy, problems remain in identifying the ideal antimycotic. The limiting factors other than pregnancy in many respects reflect problems with host defence mechanisms, particularly in those women with chronic and frequently recurring episodes (SOBEL 1988).

I. Topical Agents for Acute Candida Vaginitis

Antimycotics are available for local use as creams, lotions, aerosol sprays, vaginal tablets, suppositories, and coated tampons. There is little to suggest that formulation of the topical antimycotic influences clinical efficacy, and for the most part the patient's preference should dictate which vehicle is used to deliver local therapy. Extensive vulvar inflammation dictates local application of vulvar cream. Antifungal agents that have been used in the topical treatment of *Candida* vaginitis are listed:

Polyenes	*Azole derivatives*	*Miscellaneous agents*
Amphotericin B,	Butoconazole,	Boric acid,
candicidin, hamycin,	clotrimazole,	chlordantoin,
mepartricin,	econazole,	copper oxine,
natamycin, nystatin,	fenticonazole,	cyclopiroxolamine,
trichomycin.	isoconazole,	flucytosine,
	miconazole,	hydrargaphen,
	oxiconazole,	nifuratel,
	terconazole,	povidone-iodine,
	tioconazole.	phenylomorpholine.

1. Polyenes

Nystatin creams and vaginal suppositories have been used extensively for almost 3 decades (ISAACS 1973). Conventional therapy consists of nystatin suppositories 100 000 units daily for 14 days or twice daily for 7 days. The average mycological cure rate is approximately 75%–80%. Other topical polyenes such as amphotericin B, mepartricin, and trichomycin appear at least as effective as nystatin; natamycin is perhaps slightly less so (CSONKA 1967; CORKILL and MCCARTHY 1972; MCNAIR et al. 1978; ODDS 1988). In this group only nystatin is available in the USA.

2. Azoles

The various azole derivatives appear to achieve slightly higher clinical and mycological cure rates than the polyenes, in the order of 85%–90% (DROEGEMUELLER et al. 1984; BRADBEER and THIN 1985; ADAMSON et al. 1986; BREWSTER et al. 1986; ODDS 1988). Although multiple comparative studies have been performed comparing the clinical efficacy of the various azoles, there remains little evidence of substantial superiority of one over the others. Unfortunately, the various studies have often had major differences in design, including the standardization of the inclusion criteria, which take into consideration the severity and duration of infection. Moreover, pregnant

Table 1. Azole therapy of vaginal candidosis

Drug	Formulation	Dosage
Butoconazole	2% cream	5 g at bedtime × 3 days
Clotrimazole	1% cream	5 g at bedtime × 7–14 days
	10% cream	5 g, single application
	100 mg vaginal tablet	1 tablet at bedtime × 7 days
		2 tablets at bedtime × 3 days
	500 mg vaginal tablet	1 tablet once
Miconazole	2% cream	5 g at bedtime × 7 days
	100 mg vaginal suppository	1 suppository at bedtime × 7 days
	200 mg vaginal suppository	1 suppository at bedtime × 3 days
	1200 vaginal suppository	1 suppository once
Econazole	150 mg vaginal tablet	1 tablet at bedtime × 3 days
Fenticonazole	2% cream	5 g at bedtime × 7 days
Tioconazole	2% cream	5 g at bedtime × 3 days
	6.5% cream	5 g at bedtime, single dose
Terconazole	2% cream	5 g at bedtime × 3 days

women should not be compared with non-pregnant women, and women with infrequent infections should not be compared with women with chronic infection or those with frequent recurrences. Another major defect in the majority of studies is the short duration of follow-up, rarely extending for more than 14 days after completion of therapy. Recommended regimens for the various topical azole agents are listed in Table 1.

The newest addition to the therapeutic armamentarium is terconazole (VAN CUTSEM et al. 1983). Terconazole is a lipophilic triazole agent which like the imidazoles inhibits fungal cytochrome P-450s involved in ergosterol biosynthesis (VANDEN BOSCHE 1985). It differs from the imidazoles by the presence of a nitrogen atom in the ring nucleus which appears to enhance binding to the fungal cytochrome P-450s. In addition, it has other characteristicis that enhance its antifungal activity, including a greater affinity for cytochrome P-450 and inhibition of chitin synthetase. In clinical studies, terconazole is at least as effective as miconazole and clotrimazole, and some trials indicate possibly more rapid relief of vulvovaginal symptoms (KJAELDGAARD and LARSSON 1985; LITSCHGI 1985; NAHMANOVICI 1985).

Topical azoles are remarkably free of local and systemic side effects; nevertheless, the initial application of topical agents is not infrequently accompanied by local burning and discomfort. There appear to be some differences among the various azole topical agents in this respect; in particular, some studies indicate that tioconazole (STEIN et al. 1986) and miconazole are especially associated with burning. In preliminary studies terconazole appears to have a low incidence of local side effects (GREENWAY 1988). In contrast, although vaginal therapy rarely results in systemic complications, recently a flu-like syndrome was reported in FRG in association with a high dosage (160 mg vaginal suppository) of terconazole (MOEBIUS 1988). Similar reactions have been noted with 80 mg and 40 mg pessary presentations, and the product has been temporarily suspended from the FRG market (SCRIP No 1367, p 20, 1988).

II. Status of Short Course Topical Therapy

Treatment duration of topical antimycotic therapy has been the subject of many published clinical trials in *Candida* vaginitis. ODDS (1979) analyzed statistically the data from large numbers of published trials of topical vaginal antifungals. He concluded that treatment duration of the order of 2 weeks was superior to shorter courses, not in relation to immediate clinical response but in terms of mycological eradication and recurrence of vaginal yeast pathogens. GOUGH (1979) subsequently concluded, however, that at least for topical miconazole the total dose of antifungal used was as important as the duration of treatment in terms of mycological cure. It is apparent that in the above retrospective analyses of clinical studies, neither researcher was able to control for severity and duration of signs and symptoms. From a practical point of view, it seems reasonable to select a longer duration and higher dose regimen for patients with more recalcitrant and chronic infection. For the average patient seen by the clinician, Gough's conclusion appears to be supported by both clinical experience and controlled studies. This is especially relevant when one considers the known deterioration in patient compliance with long courses of topical antifungal therapy (MASTERTON et al. 1976).

Accordingly, there has been a major trend towards shorter treatment courses with progressively higher antifungal doses, culminating in single-dose therapeutic regimens. In several clinical trials, both short courses and single-dose regimens have been shown to be effective for most of the azole and polyene antifungals (BREUKER et al. 1986; LOENDERSLOOT et al. 1985; ADAMSON 1988; VAN DER MEIJDEN et al. 1986; BROWN et al. 1986; BREWSTER et al. 1986).

Although single-dose and short (3-day) courses of therapy imply a short duration of treatment, this is somewhat misleading since the formulation of these agents together with the high doses used result in the persistence of active compounds in inhibitory concentration for several days. This has been well documented for clotrimazole, e.g. a single administration of a 500-mg suppository achieves measureable local therapeutic inhibitory concentrations for at least 2–3 days (RITTER 1985). Similar information is available for miconazole (ODDS and MACDONALD 1981) and isoconazole (TAUBER et al. 1984). Plasma levels of antifungals are very low, resulting in extremely few systemic toxic effects and indicating that antifungal action is virtually entirely local.

Although numerous studies show that single-doses therapy is usually effective, anecdotal evidence suggests that individual failures are by no means uncommon. Studies in patients with severe and more intractable infection have not as yet been undertaken. It should be remembered that the natural history of *Candida* vaginitis is such that the spontaneous clinical cure rate is approximately 15%–20% (PROOST et al. 1972; ISAACS 1973); in some placebo-controlled studies it has been as high as 50%–60%, reflecting the mild degree of symptoms/signs in some patients enrolled in these studies. It seems reasonable to use single-dose therapy in patients with infrequent episodes of mild to moderate severity in pregnant and nonpregnant women.

III. Oral Systemic Agents for Candida Vaginitis

Orally active agents include ketoconazole, itraconazole, fluconazole, and flucytosine. Most of the published data deals with the first introduced imidazole, ketoconazole. Ketoconazole has now been tested in multiple studies throughout the world and in conventional doses of 400 mg daily for 5 days results in clinical and mycological cure rates similar if not minimally superior to the results obtained with topical imidazoles (BINGHAM 1984; BLOCH and SMYTHE 1985; ODDS 1988). The same can also be said for itraconazole and fluconazole, although these agents have not as yet been subjected to the same extensive study and scrutiny. One can summarize the comparative efficacy of the systemic azoles in comparison with the topical azoles by stating one can anticipate a clinical and mycological cure rate with topical azole therapy of 84%–90% and a marginally higher cure rate of 85%–95% with systemic therapy (ODDS 1988). The therapeutic advantages in terms of the final outcome are therefore not great. A practical advantage of oral therapy is the avoidance of the inconvenience and messiness associated with topical therapy. TOOLEY (1985) investigated patients' subjective preferences for different vaginal antifungal preparations. Of 1710 patients questioned, 28% preferred topical creams, 14% hard suppositories, 10% soft pessaries, and 47% oral formulations. They also preferred single-dose therapy to longer courses of treatment.

Any therapeutic advantage of oral therapy must be weighed against the potential side effects and toxicity associated with systemic treatment. It is abundantly clear that oral therapy is contraindicated during pregnancy. Ketoconazole therapy is accompanied by mild nausea and vomiting and other gastrointestinal upsets in about 10% of patients (SOBEL 1986). Rarely, anaphylaxis is also reported to occur. The major concern with ketoconazole use is the risk of hepatotoxicity, which is estimated to occur in approximately 1 in every 10000–15000 women treated (LEWIS et al. 1984). Although toxic hepatitis is usually rapidly reversible when the agent is stopped, rare fatalities have been reported. These potential side effects have diminished the enthusiasm for the widespread use of oral antimycotic agents, especially in patients with mild to moderate disease.

The triazole itraconazole has been shown in animal models to be at least 5 times more potent than ketoconazole in the treatment of experimental

Candida vaginitis (CAUWENBERGH 1987). Its greater in vitro antifungal activity allows lower daily doses, and higher tissue levels relative to corresponding plasma levels result in abbreviated courses of oral administration. Schedules initially recommended were 200 mg daily for 3 days (total dose 600 mg) and more recently 200 mg b.i.d. for 1 day (CAUWENBERGH 1987). Single-day therapy resulted in clinical and mycological cures of 85% and 79%, respectively, at 1 week, and 83% and 81%, 1 month after completion of treatment. A factor favoring the successful therapy was the observation of itraconazole levels in vaginal tissue persisting at therapeutic concentrations for at least 2 days after the end of therapy (LAROSA et al. 1986). Several investigators (PEETERS et al. 1986; SANZ SANZ and DEL PALACIO HERNANZ 1987) have shown similar good results with itraconazole prescribed over 3 days. To date, side effects and toxicity have been less frequent than those observed with ketoconazole, but experience is currently still limited. No adrenal or endocrine side effects have been reported, and there are no definite published reports of clinical hepatitis.

Fluconazole is the newest bistriazole to be studied in vulvovaginal candidosis (RICHARDSON et al. 1985). Its mechanism of action is similar to that of ketoconazole and itraconazole, but it has unique pharmacokinetic advantages in that it is less prone to metabolic degradation with an elimination half-life of more than 20 h (HUMPHREY et al. 1985) and possesses higher tissue penetration capacity. In preliminary studies a single oral dose of 150 mg of fluconazole resulted in excellent clinical and mycological results comparable to that achieved with other systemic forms of azole therapy (BRAMMER 1988; INTERNATIONAL MULTICENTRE TRIAL 1989). Early results suggest that fluconazole is safe and well tolerated.

C. Chronic and Recurrent Vulvovaginal Candidosis

Whereas the majority of women diagnosed with acute symptomatic *Candida* vaginitis have infrequent episodes, often with an obviously recognizable precipitating factor, a minority suffer from chronic and recurrent vaginal yeast infection. There are no accurate figures with regard to the magnitude of the latter group, although no busy practitioner will deny having several such patients in the practice. There has been considerable confusion in the literature primarily because of a lack of a clear concise definition of what constitutes recurrent disease. A definition which appears reasonable is that of at least four mycologically proven symptomatic episodes in the previous 12 months and also requires exclusion of other common vaginal pathogens.

The clinical features, both subjective and objective, are identical in all groups of women with *Candida* vaginitis. The management of recurrent *Candida* vaginitis is extremely problematic. In order to understand the fundamentals of therapy of this difficult-to-treat group, pathogenic mechanisms of recurrent vulvovaginal candidosis should be reviewed.

I. Pathogenesis of Recurrent Vulvovaginal Candidosis

Several endogenous and exogenous factors are associated with repeated bouts of candidal vaginitis:

Host factors
Pregnancy
Uncontrolled diabetes mellitus
Estrogen, corticosteroids (? oral contraceptives)
Antibiotics
Tightfitting and synthetic clothing, panty hose, etc.
Local allergy (commercial douches, perfumes)
Idiopathic, acquired antigen-specific immunodeficiency (CMI)

Micro-organism
Resistance to antimycotic agents
Switching colonies

The most important factor of all is repeated courses of physician-prescribed broad spectrum antibiotics. The use of tight-fitting clothing, nylon and poorly ventilated underclothing may in some women predispose to infection by increasing local perspiration and the local surface temperature. Similarly, local hypersensitivity or allergic reactions to perfumed toilet paper, commercial douche materials, and heavily chlorinated water (swimming pools) may cause local reactions which set the stage in women already colonized with yeasts for the development of frank symptomatic vulvovaginitis. In the majority of women suffering from recurrent or chronic vulvovaginal candidosis (VVC), no predisposing factors can be identified in spite of careful questioning (SOBEL 1985, 1986).

In the past, repeated infections were attributed to frequent vaginal reinfection from a persistent intestinal reservoir. In one study (MILES et al. 1977), *Candida* organisms were recovered on rectal culture in 100% of women with recurrent VVC. This has been the basis for the widely used approach of long-term therapy with oral, nonabsorbable nystatin. This hypothesis has been criticized in the past few years. Several investigators have found much lower concordance between rectal and vaginal cultures in patients with recurrent vaginitis (ODDS 1982; BERTHOLF and STAFFORD 1983; O'CONNOR and SOBEL 1986). Vaginitis recurs frequently in the absence of simultaneously positive rectal cultures. Two controlled studies using oral nystatin treatment, which reduces intestinal yeast carriage, failed to prevent symptomatic recurrence of vaginal candidiasis (MILNE and WARNOCK 1979; VELLUPILLAI and THIN 1977). Furthermore, some women have persistent intestinal yeast carriage and fail to develop vaginal colonization. Nevertheless, in spite of mounting criticism, the possibility of persistent gastrointestinal tract carriage being a source of vaginal reinfection cannot be entirely dismissed, especially since strain typing reveals that the majority of *Candida* isolated simultaneously from the rectum and vagina are identical strains (MEINHOF 1982; O'CONNOR and SOBEL 1986).

A role for sexual transmission has similarly not been confirmed. Penile skin colonization with *Candida* is present in approximately 20% of male partners of women with recurrent vaginal candidosis (RODIN and KOLATOR 1976; THIN et al. 1977; DAVIDSON 1977). Usually asymptomatic, the microorganisms are most commonly found in uncircumcised males in the vicinity of the coronal sulcus. Asymptomatic male genital colonization is four times more common in male sexual partners of infected women (RODIN and KOLATOR 1976). Strain typing techniques indicate that infected partners usually carry identical strains (O'CONNOR and SOBEL 1986).

In spite of the aforementioned circumstantial evidence, the contribution of sexual transmission to the pathogenesis of infection remains unknown. Based upon the prevalence of positive penile cultures, the role of sexual spread appear extremely limited, and hence routine therapy of male partners, even those of women with recurrent VVC, is unlikely to reduce recurrence rates substantially. No single controlled study has shown that treatment of males prevents recurrence in females. Recently, positive *Candida* cultures of prostatic ejaculate revealed an additional small reservoir for male partners of women with recurrent VVC (HOROWITZ et al. 1987; OGUNBANJO 1988). Even including these numbers, the majority of males remain culture negative, and therapy of the partners to date has not been beneficial. It is conceivable that therapy of male partners in order to be effective should be systemic and not topical, but this remains conjecture. Anecdotal evidence is available that anogenital and particularly orogenital contact may transmit infection; however, adequate documentation is lacking.

The rapidity with which negative vaginal yeast cultures become positive during systemic antibiotic therapy together with the observation that within 30 days of successful topical antimycotic therapy of VVC vaginal cultures once more turn positive in 20%–25% of women strongly support the hypothesis that vaginal relapse is responsible for recurrent vaginal infections (ODDS 1979). Typing studies show identical strains in more than two-thirds of recurrences (O'CONNOR and SOBEL 1986). According to this theory, during clinically successful topical therapy of vaginitis, symptomatic relief is accompanied by a drastic reduction in the number of viable yeasts in the vagina. Small numbers of the microorganisms persist, however, within the vaginal lumen in numbers too small to be detected by a conventional vaginal swab. ODDS (1982) has emphasized the insensitivity of the swab in detecting small numbers of yeasts in suspension. It is also conceivable that small numbers of *Candida* might sojourn temporarily within superficial cervical or vaginal mucosal cells only to reemerge some weeks or months later (GARCIA-TAMAYO et al. 1982).

Whatever the source of the vaginal recolonization, it is apparent that the primary acquired abnormality in women with recurrent *Candida* vaginitis appears to be an inability of these patients to tolerate recolonization of the lower genital tract. This includes a failure of local vaginal defense mechanisms to prevent transformation from the dominant blastospore phase of the yeast observed in asymptomatic carriers to the more virulent germinated organisms seen in symptomatic vaginitis. Similarly, higher counts of yeasts are present during symptomatic vaginitis.

As yet, no clear explanation exists for the failure of local host defense mechanisms to prevent the transformation from carrier to symptomatic status. Women with recurrent vaginitis have not been shown to have defective local immunoglobulin synthesis or titers (WALDMAN et al. 1972; GOUGH et al. 1984). Similarly, no defect in quantitative or qualitative phagocytic or complement function has been identified. While it is tempting to suggest that an altered or defective natural vaginal bacterial flora may permit or facilitate yeast proliferation and germination, evidence to support this concept is lacking, although one study did document reduced counts of lactobacilli in women with acute *Candida* vaginitis (AUGER and JOLY 1980). Recent evidence suggests that women with recurrent vaginitis have an acquired *Candida* antigen specific defect in cell-mediated immunity (HOBBS et al. 1977; SYVERSON et al. 1979; MATHUR et al. 1980; WITKIN et al. 1983). It has been postulated that a subpopulation of lymphocytes or a serum factor induces suppression of local genital tract mucosal lymphocytes or effector cells (MATHUR et al. 1980; WITKIN et al. 1983). Studies by WITKIN (1986) provide an attractive hypothesis of selective acquired immunodeficiency in women with recurrent *Candida* vaginitis. Once more the fundamental observation is that of in vitro impaired T-lymphocyte response only in response to *Candida* antigen; a normal proliferative response to mitogens and other non-*Candida* antigens is present in these patients with recurrent infection.

II. Treatment of Recurrent and Chronic Candida Vaginitis

The first step the clinician should take is to identify and eradicate possible underlying or predisposing causes. Uncontrolled diabetes must be mastered if any chance of clinical success is to be achieved. Similarly, the use of corticosteroids, other immunosuppressive agents, and hormones such as estrogens should be halted where possible. Although most women with recurrent and chronic *Candida* vaginitis have long since abandoned the use of oral contraceptives, consideration should be given to stopping the use of birth control tablets. In my experience (SOBEL 1984) it was not found to be either beneficial or even necessary to discontinue low-dose estrogen oral contraceptive use when long-term antimycotic agents were prescribed. Similarly the yield of performing a glucose tolerance test in otherwise asymptomatic healthy premenopausal women to diagnose latent or chemical diabetes mellitus is extremely low and is not worthwhile (SOBEL 1984). Most women with recurrent VVC already avoid tightfitting clothing and synthetic underwear. Douching with commercial preparations and vinegar is of no value and should be discouraged. Unfortunately, in the majority of women with recurrent or chronic VVC, no underlying or predisposing factor can be identified (SOBEL 1985, 1986).

In the past, when physicians were faced with women with recurrent VVC they usually resorted to a method based on patient self-diagnosis and early initiation of self-treatment with topical therapy. The patient is given a repeat prescription and institutes therapy with the first appearance of recurrent symptoms. In some women with two or three attacks per year this approach may be successful, using short courses of topical therapy. The majority of this recalcitrant group of women, however, require a long-term maintenance-suppressive-prophylaxis regimen. Several studies have confirmed the success of maintenance regimens using oral ketoconazole or topical clotrimazole and miconazole in significantly reducing the frequency of symptomatic episodes of vaginitis during long-term prophylactic therapy (DAVIDSON and MOULD 1978; SOBEL 1985, 1986; BALSDON and TOBIN 1988). Because of the duration of therapy, the convenience of oral treatment is apparent, and the best suppressive prophylaxis has been achieved when maintenance oral ketoconazole was administered (SOBEL 1986). In this study ketoconazole was initially administered at a dose of 400 mg daily for 14 days to achieve both resolution of symptoms and negative mycological status (SOBEL 1986). Thereafter, patients were randomized to receive daily placebo tablets, cyclical ketoconazole therapy 400 mg daily with the onset of menses for 5 days over a 6-month period, or daily ketoconazole 100 mg for 6 months. Women receiving placebo had an extremely high recurrence rate, and over 70% had a symptomatic mycological proven recurrence within 6 months, the mean time to recurrence being less than 2 months. Women receiving cyclical prophylaxis suffered relapses at less than half the rate of the placebo group, and the mean time to recurrence was more than doubled. The best results were obtained in women receiving low-dose daily ketoconazole therapy, with only a 5% recurrence rate.

The benefits of successful suppressive therapy must be weighed against the potential toxicity of oral therapy. In all four above-mentioned reports of successful maintenance prophylaxis, including topical therapy, cessation of antifungal prophylaxis was associated with resurgence of symptomatic infection in approximately half the women studied. The mechanism of successful prophylaxis, particularly with low-dosage ketoconazole which results in subinhibitory vaginal concentrations only, is by no means clear. Possible explanations include a direct fungistatic effect, inhibition of germ tube formation, direct effect of ketoconazole on the vaginal epithelium (KINSMAN and COLLARD 1986), and finally effects on the bacterial flora and immune system. DENNERSTEIN (1986) reported a reduced rate of recurrence in chronic VVC in 15 patients during a 3-month period of depot medroxy-progesterone acetate therapy. This isolated report of success with progesterone requires confirmation. The rationale for progesterone therapy is that it creates a state of relative estrogen deficiency.

Not all long-term maintenance regimens have been successful in suppressing recurrence of *Candida* vaginitis. Monthly clotrimazole 500 mg vaginal suppositories proved only marginally superior to placebo (SOBEL et al. 1989). The maintenance therapy must be given at a frequency sufficient to prevent vaginal regrowth or recolonization of *Candida* organisms. An alternative approach to long-term maintenance anti-*Candida* therapy for recurrent vaginitis is the use of hyposensensitization with laboratory prepared *Candida* antigen. In a small and limited uncontrolled study, ROSEDALE and BROWNE (1979) achieved encouraging results. The status of concomitant oral therapy with oral nystatin as adjunct therapy is discussed below.

Finally, in dealing with women patients with chronic or recurrent VVC it is necessary to emphasize the importance of reassurance, support, and counselling. Chronic vaginitis results in chronic dyspareunia, and inevitably sexual and marital relations suffer, often irreversibly. Women should be reassured that today virtually all chronic infections can be adequately controlled, if not cured.

III. Resistance to Antimycotic Agents

Antimycotic resistance plays a very small role in treatment and should not be considered at all in patients with infrequent occasional episodes of *Candida* vaginitis. It has become a more relevant issue in women with chronic and recurrent VVC, especially when patients fail to improve on conventional therapy. Even under these circumstances, other factors are more likely to explain failure of the clinical and mycological response, including lack of compliance and the presence of mixed infections, especially bacterial vaginosis and focal vestibulitis syndromes. Nevertheless, occasional patients are seen in whom fungal vaginitis occurs due to (relatively) resistant yeast species. In a busy vaginitis clinic, we encounter such rare patients two or three times a year. They are usually infected with *Saccharomyces cerevisiae* or certain strains of *Torulopsis glabrata* or *C. tropicalis*. These organisms in general have higher MICs to azoles, flucytosine, and even amphotericin B. Susceptibility testing should be reserved for these rare cases only. When resistance is documented, therapy should be selected on the basis of susceptibility tests. Patients exhibiting resistance to one azole usually, but not always, demonstrate cross-resistance to other azoles including the newer imidazoles and triazoles. Azole resistance is, however, not associated with cross-resistance to polyenes and flucytosine (5-fluorocytosine), and they can be used topically or rarely systemically. HOROWITZ (1986) described 15 symptomatic patients with recurrent VVC due to *C. tropicalis* in whom relapses followed topical or systemic azole therapy. These patients subsequently responded to topical flucytosine in a dosage of 1000 mg per application administered daily as a topical vaginal cream for 7 nights. Unfortunately, susceptibility tests of antifungal agents were not performed, and the role of antifungal resistance in the chronic and recurrent infections was not clearly established. The use of topical application of flucytosine is to be discouraged, other than in exceptional cases, to avoid the risk of the large scale emergence of flucytosine-resistant *Candida* organisms (SELIGMAN 1974; SPELLER and WARNOCK 1976).

Concern in this regard has been raised with the use of long-term maintenance regimens of imidazoles and triazoles in women with recurrent and chronic VVC. In the only long-term longitudinal study conducted, O'CONNOR and SOBEL (1986) failed to detect the emergence of clinically significant resistance in isolates obtained from patients receiving long-term ketoconazole. Moreover, the use of ketoconazole was not associated in this study with selection for non-*albicans Candida* strains in the vaginal and rectal isolates obtained during the follow-up period. This observation is in contrast to observations in leukemia patients receiving prophylactic oral ketoconazole in whom rectal isolates showed a tendency for selection of *T. glabrata* isolates.

D. Acute Vaginitis in Pregnancy

Management of *Candida* vaginitis during pregnancy is more difficult, since the clinical response tends to be slower and recurrences more frequent (LANG et al. 1956; WALLENBURG and WLADIMIROFF 1976; MCNELLIS et al. 1977; LINDEQUE and VAN NIEKERK 1984). In general, most topical antifungal agents are effective, especially when prescribed for longer periods, i.e. 1–2 weeks. Although absorption of topical antifungals is minimal, the potential risk of vaginal antimycotic therapy to the developing fetus during the first trimester of pregnancy must be seriously considered and weighed against the benefit derived by the patient. Similarly, the safety of topical imidazoles administered to women in the first trimester with regard to risk of spontaneous abortion needs additional study (ROSA et al. 1987). Longer duration of therapy may be necessary to eradicate yeast infection. Recently, however, high single-dosage therapy with clotrimazole was shown to be effective in pregnancy and may be considered for the initial therapeutic attempt.

E. Management of Sexual Partners of Women with Vulvovaginal Candidosis

As mentioned above this issue continues to fuel controversy. Partners of women with occasional episodes need no therapy. With regard to the partners of patients with recurrent and chronic disease, the issue remains unsettled. Studies of male partners reveal increased frequency of penile and urethral colonization, but only of the order of 20% (fourfold increase when compared with control males). This has been the basis of the argument against sexual transmission since no more than 20% of women with recurrent infections could be explained on this basis (O'CONNOR and SOBEL 1986). If one adds recent studies looking not only at penile and urethral cultures but adding urine, oral, and seminal ejaculate cultures, one can identify another 20% of male partners with positive tests (HOROWITZ et al. 1987). In fact in one recent study an exceptionally high percentage rate of male partners had positive semen cultures (OGUNBANJO 1988). The other argument against sexual transmission has been the failure to prevent recurrent disease in patients following treatment of their male partners. There have been multiple studies reaching the same conclusion (BUCH and CHRISTENSEN 1982; BISSCHOP and MERKUS 1986; CALDERON-MARQUEZ 1987). However, virtually all the studies involved treating males with topical therapy, and hence the failure to reduce recurrence may reflect failure to eradicate oral (orogenital sex) or semen ejaculate sources of *Candida*. A careful long-term prospective study is required of oral systemic azole therapy administered to male partners with confirmation of post-therapy negative cultures (urine, semen, oral, penile, urethral) before the matter can finally be put to rest.

F. Therapeutic Caveats in Vulvovaginal Candidosis

The treatment of asymptomatic vulvovaginal candidosis infection remains controversial. Most clinicians do not recommend therapy since this would entail treatment of thousands of women for what is often a transient colonization state. Nevertheless, under certain circumstances it appears reasonable to treat asymptomatic infection. Asymptomatic colonization is usually detected in women undergoing routine gynecologic examination including Papanicolaou smears. However, before deciding not to advocate topical therapy, closer questioning of 'asymptomatic' women often reveals symptoms which the patient had come to accept as 'normal'. This includes mild but tolerable pruritus and the need to use daily minipads for a chronic vaginal discharge. Only after treatment with an antimycotic and eradication of vaginal yeasts does the patient appreciate what a 'normal' state really is.

A prophylactic course of antimycotic therapy may be appropriate in asymptomatic women with a past history of recurrent *Candida* vaginitis when faced with a course of oral broad-spectrum antibiotic. Similarly, treatment of asymptomatic infection at term in pregnant women is reasonable to reduce the risk of neonatal oral thrush.

Mixed vaginal infections including VVC are not uncommon. In my experience (unpublished data) at least 10% of women presenting with symptomatic vaginitis at the Wayne State University Vaginitis Clinic have mixed infections involving the simultaneous presence of at least two vaginal pathogens. Most frequently, the mixed infections involve bacterial vaginosis and *Candida* vaginitis. Clinical and laboratory features of both pathologic processes are present to varying degrees. Depending upon the clinical picture and the determined dominant clinical process, the clinician can decide to treat the dominant process only or treat all pathogens simultaneously. In the latter situation it is advisable to use a different route of administration of therapy for each pathogen, for example, oral metronidazole together with a topical azole antimycotic, etc. Less commonly, bacterial vaginosis and trichomoniasis occur simultaneously, as may trichomoniasis and VVC.

Not all patients presenting with symptoms of vaginitis and a positive vaginal culture for *Candida* sp. have in fact an infectious process caused by the isolated *Candida* microorganisms. Under these circumstances *Candida* may be an innocent bystander or vaginal commensal responsible for vaginal colonization only. In particular, vulvitis due to contact hypersensitivity reactions, *Herpes simplex* infections, idiopathic vestibulitis, and vulvar dystrophies are frequently misdiagnosed as intractable chronic VVC, prompting repeated courses of topical antimycotics which only aggravate the symptoms. When vulvar or vaginal cultures are in fact positive for *Candida* sp. under these circumstances, a trial of oral ketoconazole is often useful as a diagnostic test, since persistence of symptoms over the next few days in the presence of now negative vaginal yeast cultures excludes the yeast as a cause of symptoms. It should be emphasized that all topical antimycotics can induce transient local burning and irritation, but occasionally more persistent hypersensitivity reactions result in chronic vestibular symptoms.

The role of repeated courses of topical antimycotics in disrupting the vaginal bacterial flora is largely unknown. It has been suggested that the unexplained increased incidence in bacterial vaginosis, an entity characterized by a major upheaval in the vaginal flora, could in part be related to abuse of topical antimycotics. This remains conjecture at present but appears worthy of investigation. Topical antimycotics are widely abused by physicians and patients alike, and apart from psychological dependence, these products do have the potential to alter normal bacterial flora. Similarly, topical antimycotics have been suspected as contributing to the syndrome of idiopathic vestibulitis or focal vulvitis (vulvodynia). Once more no data supporting this hypothesis exist.

The issue of oral nystatin therapy in VVC is sufficiently controversial as to merit additional consideration. This widespread practice has existed for many years and is targeted primarily at women with chronic and recurrent VVC in an attempt to reduce yeast counts in the gastrointestinal tract and prevent vaginal reinfection or reinoculation from the adjacent perianal area. The merits of the gastrointestinal reservoir theory and the criticism of this concept are reviewed elsewhere (Sobel 1988). Oral nonabsorbable nystatin therapy has not in several controlled studies been shown to reduce recurrent symptomatic *Candida* vaginitis. One recent multicenter study did suggest short-term benefits, but unfortunately the longitudinal follow-up was relatively brief (Nystatin Multicenter Study Group 1986). Currently available data do not support the use of oral nystatin together with or following conventional antimycotic therapy.

G. Summary

The availability of a large armamentarium of antimycotic agents has greatly facilitated the treatment of VVC. The new antimycotics available, both for the oral and topical routes, have at the same time created new dilemmas since new modalities and too many options often serve to confuse the general practitioner. With the wide spectrum of available agents and more importantly newer regimens, the physician is finally in a position to select carefully an agent and regimen optimal for the individual patient. Selecting a regimen is just as critical as choosing the antimycotic. This refers to the route of administration, formulation, and duration of therapy. Advances in therapy made possible by the introduction of newer, more potent antimycotics are in no small way the result of diligent basic science and clinical research into the pathogenesis of VVC. With clinical cure rates approaching and often exceeding 90%, any additional progress in the future will depend more upon the basic science research investigator than the pharmaceutical industry.

References

Adamson GD (1988) Three day treatment of vulvovaginal candidosis. Am J Obstet Gynecol 158:1002–1005

Adamson GD, Brown D, Standard JV, Henzl MR (1986) Three day treatment with butoconazole vaginal suppositories for vulvovaginal candidosis. J Reprod Med 31:131–132

Auger P, Joly J (1980) Microbial flora associated with *Candida albicans* vulvovaginitis. Obstet Gynecol 55:397–401

Balsdon MJ, Tobin JM (1988) Recurrent vaginal candidosis: prospective study of effectiveness of maintenance miconazole treatment. Genitourin Med 64:124–127

Bertholf ME, Stafford MJ (1983) Colonization of *Candida albicans* in vagina, rectum, and mouth. J Fam Pract 16:919–924

Bingham JS (1984) Single blind comparison of ketoconazole 200 mg oral tablets and clotrimazole 100 mg vaginal tablets and 1% cream in treating acute candidosis. Br J Vener Dis 60:175–177

Bisschop MPJM, Merkus JMWM (1986) Co-treatment of the male partner in vaginal candidosis: a double blind randomized control study. Br J Obstet Gyn 93:79–81

Bloch B, Smythe E (1985) Ketoconazole in the treatment of vaginal candidosis. S Afr Med J 67:178–179

Bradbeer CS, Thin RN (1985) Comparison of econazole and isoconazole as single dose treatment for vaginal candidosis. Genitourin Med 61:396–398

Brammer KW (Multicenter Study Group) (1988) Treatment of vaginal candidiasis with a single oral dose of fluconazole. Eur J Clin Microbiol Infect Dis 7:364–367

Breuker G, Jurezok F, Lenaerts M, Weinhold E, Krause U (1986) Single-dose therapy of vaginal mycoses with clotrimazole vaginal cream 10%. Mykosen 29:427–436

Brewster E, Preti PM, Ruffman R, Studd J (1986) Effect of fenticonazole in vaginal candidiasis: a double-blind clinical trial versus clotrimazole. J Int Med Res 14:306–310

Brown D, Henzl MR, LePage ME, Tsao LL, Isu AE, Walker KAM, Adamson ED, Droegmuller W (1986) Butoconazole vaginal cream in the treatment of vulvovaginal candidiasis. Comparison with miconazole nitrate and placebo. J Reprod Med 31:1045–1048

Buch A, Christensen ES (1982) Treatment of vaginal candidosis with natamycin and effect of treating the partner at the same time. Acta Obstet Gynecol Scand 61:393–396

Calderon-Marquez JJ (1987) Itraconazole in the treatment of vaginal candidosis and the effect of treatment of the sexual partner. Rev Infect Dis 9:S143–S145
Cauwenbergh G (1987) Itraconazole: the first orally active antifungal for single-day treatment of vaginal candidosis. Curr Ther Res 41:210–214
Centers for Disease Control (1979) Non-reported sexually transmitted diseases. Morbid Mental Wkly Report 28:61
Corkill BM, McCarthy NJ (1972) Comparative trial of fungilin (amphotericin B) and pimafucin (natamycin) pessaries in the treatment of vaginal candidiasis. Med J Aust 2:33–34
Csonka GW (1967) Comparison of amphotericin B and nystatin pessaries in *Candida* infections. Br J Vener Dis 43:210–211
Davidson F (1977) Yeasts and circumcision in the male. Br J Vener Dis 53:121–122
Davidson F, Mould RF (1978) Recurrent genital candidosis in women and the effect of intermittent prophylactic treatment. Br J Vener Dis 54:176–183
Dennerstein GJ (1986) Depot-Provera in the treatment of recurrent vulvovaginal candidiasis. J Reprod Med 31:801–803
Droegemueller W, Adamson DG, Brown D, Cibley L, Fleury F, Lepage ME, Henzl MR (1984) Three day treatment with butoconazole nitrate for vulvovaginal candidiasis. Obstet Gynecol 64:530–540
Garcia-Tamayo J, Castillo G, Martinez AJ (1982) Human genital candidosis. Histochemistry, scanning and transmission electron microscopy. Acta Cytol (Baltimore) 26:7–14
Gough D (1979) The influence of dosage and duration of administration of miconazole on the cure and relapse of candidal vaginitis. R Soc Med Int Congr Symp 7:15–20
Gough PM, Warnock DW, Richardson MD, Mansell NJ, King JM (1984) IgA and IgG antibodies to *Candida albicans* in the genital tract secretions of women with or without vaginal candidosis. Sabouraudia 22:265–271
Greenway JL (1988) The scope and speed of therapeutic responsiveness in U.S. clinical trials: the efficacy of terconazole creams. In: Sobel JD (ed) Clinical perspectives: terconazole, an advance in vulvovaginal candidiasis therapy. McGraw-Hill, New York, pp 105–117
Hobbs JR, Brigden D, Davidson F, Kahan M, Oates JK (1977) Immunological aspects of candidal vaginitis. Proc R Soc Med 70(Suppl 4):1–14
Horowitz BJ (1986) Topical flucytosine therapy for chronic recurrent *Candida tropicalis* infections. J Reprod Med 31:821–824
Horowitz BJ, Edelstein SW, Lippman L (1987) Sexual transmission of *Candida*. Obstet Gynecol 69:883–886
Humphrey MJ, Jevons S, Tarbit MH (1985) Pharmacokinetic evaluation of UK-49,858, a metabolically stable triazole antifungal drug in animals and humans. Antimicrob Agents Chemother 28:648–653
International Multicentre Trial (1989) A comparison of single-dose oral fluconazole with 3-day intravaginal clotrimazole in the treatment of vaginal candidiasis. Br J Obstet Gynecol 96:226–232
Isaacs JH (1973) Nystatin vaginal cream in monilial vaginitis. Ill Med J 143:240–241
Kinsman OS, Collard AF (1986) Hormonal factors in vaginal candidiasis in rats. Infect Immun 53:498–504
Kjaeldgaard A, Larsson B (1985) Single-blind comparative clinical trial of short-term therapy with terconazole versus clotrimazole vaginal tablets in vulvovaginal candidosis. Curr Ther Res 38:939–944
Lang WR, Stella JG, Benchakan V (1956) Nystatin vaginal tablets in treatment of candidal vulvovaginitis. Obstet Gynecol 8:364–367
Larosa E, Cauwenbergh G, Cilli P, Woestenborghs R, Heykamps J (1986) Itraconazole pharmacokinetics in the female genital tract: plasma and tissue levels in patients undergoing hysterectomy after a single dose of 200 mg itraconazole. Eur J Obstet Gynecol Reprod Biol 23:85–89
Lewis JH, Zimmerman HJ, Benson GD, Ishak KG (1984) Hepatic injury associated with ketoconazole therapy: analysis of 33 cases. Gastroenterology 86: 503–513

Lindeque BG, Van Niekerk WA (1984) Treatment of vaginal candidiasis in pregnancy with a single clotrimazole 500 mg vaginal pessary. S Am Med J 65:123–127
Litschgi M (1985) Assessment of clinical efficacy and tolerability of terconazole 240 mg vaginal suppositories. Gynackol Rundsch 25(Suppl 1):59–66
Loendersloot EW, Goormans E, Weisenhaan PE, Barthel PJ, Branolte JH (1985) Efficacy and tolerability of single-dose versus six-day treatment of candidal vulvovaginitis with vaginal tablets of clotrimazole. Am J Obstet Gynecol 152: 953–955
Masterton G, Henderson JN, Napier IR, Moffet M (1976) Vaginal candidosis. Br Med J 1:712–713
Mathur S, Melchers JT III, Ades EW, Williamson HO, Fudenberg HH (1980) Antiovaria and anti-lymphocyte antibodies in patients with chronic vaginal candidiasis. J Reprod Immunol 2:247–262
McNair AL, Gough DA, Emanuel MB (1978) The assessment of an antimycotic in the day to day functioning of venerology clinics. Br J Clin Pract 32:20–24
McNellis D, McLeod M, Lawson J, Pasquale SA (1977) Treatment of vulvovaginal candidiasis in pregnancy: a comparative study. Obstet Gynecol 50:674–678
Meinhof WL (1982) Demonstration of typical features of individual *Candida albicans* strains as a means of studying sources of infection. Chemotherapy 28(Suppl 1): 51–55
Miles MR, Olsen L, Rogers A (1977) Recurrent vaginal candidiasis. Importance of an intestinal reservoir. JAMA 238:1836–1837
Milne JD, Warnock DW (1979) Effect of simultaneous oral and vaginal treatment on the rate of cure and relapse in vaginal candidosis. Br J Vener Dis 55:362–365
Moebius UM (1988) Influenza-like syndrome after terconazole. Lancet ii:966– 967
Nahmanovici C (1985) Treatment of vaginal candidosis with three 80 mg terconazole vaginal suppositories: results of a multicenter study in France. Gynakol Rundsch 25(Suppl 1):52–58
Nystatin Multicenter Study Group (1986) Therapy of candidal vaginitis: the effect of eliminating intestinal *Candida*. Am J Obstet Gynecol 155:651–654
O'Connor MI, Sobel JD (1986) Epidemiology of recurrent vulvovaginal candidiasis: identification and strain differentiation of *Candida albicans*. J Infect Dis 154: 358–363
Odds FC (1979) Candidosis of the genitalia. In: Odds FC (ed) *Candida* and candidosis. Leicester University Press, Leicester, pp 101–112
Odds FC (1982) Genital candidosis. Clin Exp Dermatol 7:345–351
Odds FC (1988) Candidosis of the genitalia. In: Odds FC (ed) *Candida* and candidosis, 2nd ed. Baillière Tindall, London, pp 124–135
Odds FC, MacDonald F (1981) Persistence of miconazole in vaginal secretions after single applications of the antifungal: implications for the treatment of vaginal candidosis. Br J Vener Dis 57:400–401
Ogunbanjo BO (1988) Isolation of yeasts from male contacts of women with vaginal candidosis. Genitourin Med 64:135–136
Peeters F, Van der Pas H, Proost J, Janssens D, Snauwaert E, Van Cutsem J, Cauwenbergh G (1986) Itraconazole (R51211) a new orally active triazole derivative for treatment of vaginal candidiasis. Curr Ther Res 39:496–504
Proost JM, Maes-Dock FM, Nelis MO, Van Cutsem JM (1972) Miconazole in the treatment of mycotic vulvovaginitis. Am J Obstet Gynecol 112:688–692
Richardson K, Brammer KW, Marriott MS, Troke PF (1985) Activity of UK-49,858, a bis-triazole derivative, against experimental infections with *Candida albicans* and *Trichophyton mentagrophytes*. Antimicrob Agents Chemother 27:832–835
Ritter W (1985) Pharmacokinetic fundamentals of vaginal treatment with clotrimazole. Am J Obstet Gynecol 152:945–947
Rodin P, Kolator B (1976) Carriage of yeast on the penis. Br Med J 1:1123–1124
Rosa FW, Baum C, Shaw M (1987) Pregnancy outcomes after first-trimester vaginitis drug therapy. Obstet Gynecol 69:751–754

Rosedale N, Browne K (1979) Hyposensitisation in the mangement of recurring vaginal candidiasis. Ann Allergy 43:250–253
Sanz Sanz F, Del Palacio Hernanz A (1987) Randomized comparative trial of three regimens of itraconazole for the treatment of vaginal mycoses. Rev Infect Dis 9:S139–S142
Seligman SA (1974) Treatment of vulval candidiasis with 5-fluorocytosine. Br Med J 3:173–174
Sobel JD (1984) Recurrent Vulvovaginal candidiasis. What we know and what we don't. Ann Int Med 101:390–392
Sobel JD (1985) Management of recurrent vulvovaginal candidiasis with intermittent ketoconazole prophylaxis. Obstet Gynecol 65:435–460
Sobel JD (1986) Recurrent vulvovaginal candidiasis. A prospective study of the efficacy of maintenance ketoconazole therapy. N Engl J Med 315:1455–1458
Sobel JD (1988) Epidemiology and pathogenesis of vulvovaginal candidosis. Ann NY Acad Sci 544:547–558
Sobel JD, Schmitt C, Meriwether C (1989) Clotrimazole treatment of recurrent and chronic *Candida* vulvovaginitis. Obstet Gynecol 73:330–334
Speller DCE, Warnock DW (1976) Vaginal candidosis. Br Med J 2:107
Stein GE, Gurwith D, Mummaw N, Gurwith M (1986) Single dose tioconazole compared with three day treatment with clotrimazole in vulvovaginal candidiasis. Antimicrob Agents Chemother 29:969–971
Syverson RE, Buckley HR, Gibian J, Ryan GM Jr (1979) Cellular and humoral immune status in women with chronic *Candida* vaginitis. Am J Obstet Gynecol 123:624–627
Tauber A, Rach P, Lachnit U (1984) Persistence of isoconazole in vaginal secretion after single application. Mykosen 27:97–101
Thin RN, Leighton M, Dixon MJ (1977) How often is genital yeast infection sexually transmitted? Br Med J 2:93–94
Tooley PJH (1985) Patient and doctor preferences in the treatment of vaginal candidosis. Practitioner 229:655–660
Van Cutsem J, Van Gerven F, Zaman R, Janssen PAJ (1983) Terconazole – a new broad-spectrum antifungal. Chemotherapy 29:322–331
Vanden Bossche H (1985) Biochemical targets for antifungal azole derivatives: hypothesis on the mode of action. Curr Top Med Mycol 1:313–351
Van der Meijden WI, Vander Hoek JCS, Staal HJM, Van Joost T, Stolz E (1986) Double-blind comparison of 200 mg ketoconazole oral tablets and 1200 mg miconazole vaginal capsule in the treatment of vaginal candidosis. Eur J Obstet Gynecol Reprod Biol 22:133–138
Vellupillai S, Thin RN (1977) Treatment of vulvovaginal yeast infection with nystatin. Practitioner 219:897–901
Waldman RH, Cruz JM, Rowe DS (1972) Immunoglobulin levels and antibody to *Candida albicans* in human cervicovaginal secretions. Clin Exp Immunol 10:427–434
Wallenburg HCS, Wladimiroff JW (1976) Recurrence of vaginal candidosis during pregnancy: comparison of miconazole and nystatin treatments. Obstet Gynecol 48:491–494
Witkin SS (1986) Inhibition of *Candida*-induced lymphocyte proliferation by antibody to *Candida albicans*. Obstet Gynecol 68:696–699
Witkin SS, Yu IR, Ledger WJ (1983) Inhibition of *Candida albicans* – induced lymphocyte proliferation by lymphocytes and sera from women with recurrent vaginitis. Am J Obstet Gynecol 147:809–811

CHAPTER 15

An Infectious Disease Specialist's Viewpoint

ALAN M. SUGAR

A. Introduction

Systemic mycoses, once thought to be rare, exotic diseases, are more frequently being recognized as agents of serious infections in a diverse and emergent group of patients. Opportunistic fungal infections represent a significant cause of morbidity and mortality in the immunocompromised patient (MEUNIER-CARPENTIER et al. 1981; GOLD 1984; MEUNIER 1987; CAIRNS 1988). The more common fungi, *Candida*, *Aspergillus*, and *Cryptococcus*, are not, however, the only agents responsible for this surge in the prevalence of mycotic disease. The organisms responsible for the 'endemic mycoses', *Blastomyces dermatitidis*, *Coccidioides immitis*, *Histoplasma capsulatum*, and *Paracoccidioides brasiliensis*, are infecting large numbers of immunologically normal individuals who live in, or who have visited, the endemic areas. *H. capsulatum* and *Co. immitis* also are being increasingly recognized as causing refractory and usually fatal disease in immunosuppressed patients, especially those with the acquired immunodeficiency syndrome (AIDS) (DERESINSKI and STEVENS 1975; BRONNIMANN et al. 1987; SALZMAN et al. 1988; JOHNSON et al. 1986). In addition, other fungi (e.g., *Fusarium*, *Penicillium*, *Trichosporon*, see Table 1) once thought to be relatively avirulent have been shown to produce systemic invasive disease (ANAISSIE et al. 1988; WALLING et al. 1987; DENG et al. 1988). Sporotrichosis, chromoblastomycosis, and eumycetoma represent invasive mycotic infections occurring in different parts of the world and with varying frequencies.

As a result of the evolving epidemiology of the mycoses, clinicians must recognize the protean clinical manifestations of the different fungal diseases, some of which may be uncommonly seen, consider them in the differential diagnosis, perform appropriate diagnostic evaluations, and select the best antifungal agent to treat the infection. Since the various medically important fungi can involve virtually any organ, physicians from all medical and surgical specialities must include these diseases in the differential diagnosis in the appropriate clinical setting.

Against this backdrop of the increasing importance of the mycoses in clinical practice, advances in the development of new and useful antifungal agents have finally been realized. Improvements in the spectrum of activity, toxicity profiles, and routes of administration have been made. The details

Table 1. Unusual fungi isolated from immunocompromised patients

Alternaria	*Pseudallescheria*
Fusarium	*Saccharomyces*
Geotrichum	*Scopulariopsis*
Kluveromyces	*Trichophyton*
Penicillium	*Trichosporon*

of these new agents have been summarized in this volume and elsewhere (FROMTLING 1987; IWATA and VANDEN BOSSCHE 1986). In stark contrast to the remarkable progress in antifungal drug research and development, introduction of newer techniques that improve the accuracy and rapidity of diagnosis of fungal infections has lagged behind. Diagnosis of invasive mycoses still depends on combined evidence of histopathologic tissue invasion and culture of organisms from the infected sites. Successful routine application of modern rapid serologic immunoassays for the detection of circulating antibodies or antigens has not been achieved; the problems of differentiating colonization from infection have remained too complex for current methods to separate these overlapping clinical situations. Many times empiric treatment must be initiated for fungal infections that may never ultimately be definitively diagnosed. Because of the lack of clinically useful progress in the diagnosis of most of the important mycoses, there is an ever widening gap between the ability to identify accurately those patients with invasive fungal infections and to choose from the available therapeutic options. The purpose of this chapter is to provide an infectious diseases physician's perspective of developments in the antifungal field and how these are reflected in the clinical management of patients with invasive fungal diseases.

B. The Problem

Systemic mycoses have become a major factor in the morbidity and mortality of immunocompromised patients (GOLD 1984; MEUNIER 1987; CAIRNS 1988). With the increasing use of aggressive chemotherapy for malignancy, transplantation of organs, and supportive care of patients with a variety of medical and surgical illnesses, the importance of fungal infection in these patients has become clear. In addition to the more well-known agents causing systemic infection in the neutropenic population, a larger and expanding list of unusual fungi has been compiled, reflecting the opportunistic nature of many of these microorganisms previously thought to be harmless (Table 1). With the advent of AIDS, consideration of the problems posed by *Candida* and *Cryptococcus* has become routine. Thus, the clinician is faced with the difficulties inherent in the diagnosis of both common and uncommon fungal infections, even before having to make appropriate therapeutic decisions.

In the usual clinical situation, the presentation of systemic fungal infection is nonspecific. Fever and systemic signs of inflammation may or may not be present. Local signs of infection also may be unreliably present, depending in large part on the immunologic status of the patient. Occasionally, a patient may present with a lesion, such as in the skin, which can be biopsied and in which fungal elements can be demonstrated. A lesion in the retina can be presumptively identified as due to *Candida* (HENDERSON et al. 1981), especially in those with intravenous catheter-related candidemia. A distinctive myositis/cutaneous symptom complex has also been identified in neutropenic patients with systemic candidosis (ARENA et al. 1981). However, most of the patients one would usually suspect of having a systemic fungal infection will have no easily identifiable constellation of symptoms or signs that will accurately identify the presence or absence of mycotic infection. Moreover, it is virtually impossible to make a specific etiologic diagnosis on the basis of the clinical presentation. Thus, we must rely heavily on obtaining appropriate cultures and good laboratory technique in isolating fungi from clinical material and ultimately making the appropriate identification. As antifungals with a specifically narrow spectra of activity become available for clinical use (e.g., cilofungin), the precise identification of the etiologic agent becomes of paramount importance so that appropriate therapeutic decisions can be made.

C. Diagnosis

It is beyond the scope of this chapter to provide an in-depth discussion of the details of methods for the rapid diagnosis of the different medically important mycoses; summaries have been written to direct the interested reader to the primary sources (BENNETT 1987; DE REPENTIGNY and REISS 1984). Rather, a general overview of the current approaches and the clinical utility of these methods will be presented.

The gold standard for the diagnosis of invasive mycotic infection is the demonstration of the organism in tissue. This necessitates biopsy of clinically involved organs. The most easily accessible is the skin, but most patients with systemic fungal infections do not develop cutaneous manifestations of their disease. Thus, biopsy of other organs (e.g., lung, brain) may be required to demonstrate the presence of the organism. It is well documented, for example, that up to 80% of patients with biopsy-proven invasive candidosis will have negative blood cultures (EDWARDS 1985). In contrast, many patients with candidemia will have transiently positive blood cultures and no evidence of systemic, invasive disease. Similarly, patients with positive sputum cultures for *Aspergillus* may or may not have pulmonary aspergillosis. Certainly, the neutropenic patient with cavitary lung lesions and *Aspergillus* growing in the sputum will be treated as though the fungus is responsible for the pulmonary lesions. However, definitive proof still requires a lung biopsy with demonstration of hyphae invading the lung tissue. The combination of a positive culture and histologic evidence for tissue invasion confirms the diagnosis of virtually all systemic mycoses. The primary problems of this approach to diagnosis are that it requires an invasive biopsy and time for the organism to grow in culture in the laboratory. Very often it is impossible to perform surgery on critically ill immunocompromised patients, so biopsy may be out of the question. Moreover, if one waits until the cultures are positive to initiate antifungal therapy, the infection may progress so far that therapy would be started too late to have a salutary effect. Thus, effort aimed at developing serologic assays have received priority, but results have not been particularly encouraging.

Of the opportunistic mycoses, the vast majority of laboratory work concerns *Candida* and *Aspergillus* (KAHN and JONES 1986; MATTHEWS et al. 1984; BAILEY et al. 1985; DE REPENTIGNY et al. 1985; SABETTA et al. 1985; DUPONT et al. 1987; TALBOT et al. 1987; DRUTZ 1986), although some notable attempts have been forthcoming with other less common pathogens, e.g., *Trichosporon* (MCMANUS and JONES 1985). The assays are designed to detect antibody, circulating antigens, or fungal metabolites and have been tested in experimental models of candidosis or aspergillosis and in actual human disease and can be performed within a matter of hours. While the most significant advances have been made in detecting specific antibodies directed to certain well-defined *Candida* antigens (e.g., MATTHEWS et al. 1984; BURNIE 1987; MATTHEWS and BURNIE 1988; GREENFIELD et al. 1988), for the most part, serologic assays have not proved to be clinically useful in distinguishing patients with invasive disease as opposed to those merely colonized by the organisms. The problem of separating uninfected patients, those colonized, those with mucosal disease (in the case of *Candida*), and those with bona fide systemic disease has not yet been overcome, and prospects do not appear promising. However, if results from one group can be reproduced and confirmed, selective determination of IgG responses to specific *Candida* antigens may be helpful in identifying patients with invasive candidosis (MATTHEWS et al. 1984; MATTHEWS and BURNIE 1988). The detection of circulating *Aspergillus*-derived antigen in the serum or urine (TALBOT et al. 1987; DUPONT et al. 1987) has been demonstrated and, if these studies are confirmed, may provide some help in the identification of patients with invasive aspergillosis.

Using a different approach, several groups have utilized DNA fingerprinting techniques to compare *Candida* isolates recovered from one or more patients (OLIVO et al. 1987; MASON et al. 1987; SCHERER and STEVENS 1987). This approach seems to be well suited for epidemiologic studies but has yet to have an impact on our ability to make an early diagnosis of invasive candidosis. If virulence can be correlated with specific electrophoretic patterns or if specific DNA sequences can be detected in the blood of infected patients, this technology may offer some help in determining whether patients are infected or merely colonized.

D. Therapy

Reviews of the indications for the use of the routinely employed antifungals and the details of their administration are readily available (BENNETT 1981; MEDOFF and KOBAYASHI 1980), and the details will not be reiterated here. Rather a brief overview of one physician's approach to antifungal therapeutics will be presented. The choices now available to clinicians that must be made to ensure the best possible treatment regimen will become obvious.

The antifungal chemotherapeutic era began in the 1950s with the introduction of amphotericin B. Until the introduction of ketoconazole, almost 30 years later, amphotericin B was the 'gold standard', the drug of choice for virtually all systemic mycoses. It still remains the drug against which all other agents are compared. The use of amphotericin B in general relies on the empiric observations accumulated since it was released for use. Because of the many difficulties inherent in conducting appropriate clinical studies, comparisons of the efficacy and toxicity of amphotericin B vis-á-vis other agents have not been made. It is precisely because of the relative rarity of many of the mycoses that entry of all possibly eligible patients into studies performed at central research centers should be strongly encouraged. This will permit the evaluation of specific drugs in as many patients as possible, thereby enhancing the likelihood of detecting important therapeutic effects of the investigational agents.

In most hospital-based clinical settings, amphotericin B is the drug of choice for treating systemic mycoses. In intensive care units, this will usually mean therapy directed against different species of *Candida*. In units caring for patients with hematologic malignancies who become neutropenic during the course of chemotherapy or bone marrow transplantation, *Candida*, *Aspergillus*, the agents of mucormycosis, and the rare opportunists (some of which are listed in Table 1) are of greatest concern. Amphotericin B is the most reliable currently available drug for these indications. However, amphotericin B alone may not provide adequate therapy in many critically ill patients (GOLD 1984). Some investigators recommend the addition of flucytosine to the regimen at the start of therapy (GOLD 1984; KARP et al. 1988; GOERING et al. 1988). Others are more concerned with the marrow suppressive effects of flucytosine and would hesitate to use this drug until later, if at all, during the course of therapy. The recommended doses of amphotericin B vary, depending on the general condition of the patient and the specific mycosis. For example, 0.5–0.6 mg/kg daily is commonly used in treating candidosis, but doses up to 1.5 mg/kg daily may be employed in treating aspergillosis or mucormycosis.

Amphotericin B is also the clear choice for use in treating immunocompromised patients with one of the 'endemic' mycoses. This is particularly true for patients with AIDS and reactivation coccidioidomycosis or histoplasmosis. It is especially disconcerting that while results of amphotericin B therapy in these patients are usually not satisfactory, ketoconazole or one of the new azoles has not been particularly successful either. Thus, new approaches and more effective drugs are required for treating mycoses in severely immunosuppressed patients.

Perhaps the most ominous development in antifungal therapeutics is the appearance of fungi resistant to available drugs. Relative resistance of the Mucorales to amphotericin B has always been evident. However, the isolation of *Candida* from patients receiving, and not responding to, amphotericin B has been more frequently reported (e.g., DICK et al. 1980, 1985; POWDERLY et al. 1988). The reasons that strains of *Candida* develop resistance during a course of therapy are not entirely clear, but clinicians are left with few options in such a situation. There have not yet been studies of alternative treatment regimens in patients infected with amphotericin B-resistant *Candida* species. Thus, should another drug be added to the amphotericin B (e.g., flucytosine, rifampin, tetracyclines), or should miconazole or another azole be used instead? Answers to these questions are not known, and more experience with treating these resistant isolates will be needed before recommendations can be made.

Another area of conflict is that of the role of combination therapy in the treatment of patients with different mycoses. For example, in vitro studies suggest that combinations of amphotericin B with flucytosine, rifampin, or tetracyclines may exert synergistic effects on *Aspergillus* and *Candida* (EDWARDS et al. 1980; LEW et al. 1977). Experimental mycoses have also been treated with some success with these combination regimens (POLAK et al. 1982; ARROYO et al. 1977). The results of such an approach in human infections are difficult to ascertain, and the literature is largely anecdotal. However, some investigators justify the use of combination therapy, given the poor results of amphotericin B alone in many fungal infections.

There is some controversy concerning the proper role for flucytosine in treating systemic mycoses. Most investigators would agree that the combination of flucytosine with amphotericin B provides the best chance for cure of cryptococcal meningitis (BENNETT et al. 1979; DISMUKES et al. 1987). However, questions remain as to the dose of amphotericin B that should be used and on the total duration of therapy (SUGAR and LEVITZ 1988). In addition, it has become very clear that flucytosine is not well tolerated by patients with AIDS. The combination of decreased bone marrow reserve, the effects of zidovudine (AZT), and the bone marrow suppressive effect of flucytosine acts to produce unacceptable toxicity in most AIDS patients. The other use of flucytosine, which may be supplanted after the water-soluble azoles are approved, is in the treatment of urinary tract candidosis. Because of the well-known problems with the development of resistance of *Candida* to flucytosine, urinary tract catheters should not be used in patients who are to receive flucytosine for upper or lower urinary tract candidosis. Since very high urinary concentrations of flucytosine are achieved following oral administration of the drug, resistance does not usually develop during therapy of renal or bladder candidosis. However, flucytosine alone is not recommended when treating other forms of invasive candidosis.

Finally, there may be some role for flucytosine in treating patients with chromoblastomycosis, although some of the newer azoles may be as effective. Because of the relative rarity of these diseases, controlled randomized trials are unlikely to be done, and the opinion of investigators with experience in using the different drugs to treat these chronic infections should be sought.

The first parenterally administered imidazole, miconazole, has no well-defined role in antifungal treatment regimens. The reasons for this are multi-factorial and instructive. Miconazole has been used in candidosis and in various forms of coccidioidomycosis and in patients with different underlying conditions. However, because of the possible effects of reporting bias, i.e., successfully treated cases may appear preferentially in the literature, it is virtually impossible to know how this drug compares with amphotericin B. Miconazole must be given frequently and has toxicity that can rival that of amphotericin B in severity. Perhaps the most significant problem with understanding its proper use is the lack of randomized studies designed to compare its efficacy and toxicity with that of amphotericin B. The introduction of a potentially useful drug into medical practice with essentially no evidence of its comparative worth to standard therapy serves to underline the difficulties in this field in performing such clinical trails and emphasizes the problems that must be tackled with the newer agents that are ready for study in humans, so that these drugs will have clearly defined clinical indications.

The availability of several azoles (e.g., itraconazole, fluconazole), lipopeptides (e.g., cilofungin), allylamines (e.g., terbinafine), and other agents will exacerbate many of the problems confronting physicians who care for patients with mycoses (e.g., difficulties in making rapid and accurate diagnoses, interpretation of in vitro susceptibility test results, determination of duration of therapy). However, clinicians will have unprecedented options from which to choose when managing these patients. Clinical investigations of the new agents have begun and have acted as catalysts, forcing researchers to design protocols which will contribute information not only concerning drug efficacy and toxicity but which will also define the natural history and clinical manifestations of rigorously defined disease. For example, candidemia may reflect a transient phenomenon or a manifestation of serious invasive disease. On the other hand, positive blood cultures are not a requirement for the diagnosis of invasive candidosis. In clinical studies of new agents, precise definitions of disease and carefully framed categories of response to therapy must be employed to ensure that the data obtained from these trials will be interpretable. Without the need for assessing the roles of the newer antifungal drugs, satisfactory comparative clinical studies would most likely not be done. Thus, one result of the development of new antifungals and the need for therapeutic comparisons is that a more rational and less empirical approach to antifungal therapy should emerge.

A discussion of the field of antifungals would not be complete without some acknowledgement of the confusion engendered by in vitro susceptibility testing, especially since physicians appreciate the importance of these tests in directing therapy of patients with bacterial infections. Simply stated, in vitro antifungal susceptibility testing has not yet been standardized, and no evidence has been presented to suggest that in vitro results from any laboratory or any assay have a role in helping the physician to decide on an appropriate antifungal drug. Therefore, the absolute minimum inhibitory concentration (MIC) is of no use in patient care. Research laboratories with experience in in vitro antifungal susceptibility testing may be able to create relative scales of susceptibility using well-defined reference strains tested in parallel with the clinical isolates (CALHOUN et al. 1986; GALGIANI et al. 1987). Whether these results have clinical significance is debatable. Recent reports suggest that relative susceptibility to amphotericin B as measured by in vitro techniques may correlate with clinical outcome (POWDERLY et al. 1988). Thus, in vitro susceptibility testing research continues, but its ultimate value has yet to be determined.

With the production of virtually unlimited supplies of recombinant human cytokines, such as interferon, tumor necrosis factor (TNF), and granulocyte monocyte colony stimulating factor, the possibilities for use of these biological response modifiers as adjuncts in the treatment of mycoses should be considered. Experimental data provide a basis for the participation of cytokines in the host response to certain mycoses (e.g., blastomycosis, candidosis, coccidioidomycosis, cryptococcosis, histoplasmosis) (WU-HSIEH and HOWARD 1987; BRUMMER et al. 1985, 1988; BRUMMER and STEVENS 1987; DEEPE et al. 1986; BEAMAN et al. 1983), but their role as therapeutic agents remains undefined. Certainly in chronic infections such as coccidioidomycosis and histoplasmosis, evaluation of these compounds is of considerable interest. In seriously immunocompromised patients, the use of cytokines in therapy may be problematic, since host cells may not be able to respond to the cytokine because of the underlying condition or effects of immunosuppressive therapy, or the cytokines might exacerbate the underlying disease. The scientific foundation has been laid for the study of the clinical utility of these agents, and studies over the next several years should shed light on their possible roles in clinical practice.

E. Prospect for Vaccines

Two major examples of vaccines for the prevention of fungal diseases can be cited as indicative of the state of the art with respect to the mycoses. A vaccine for the prevention of coccidioidomycosis has been tested in humans, and several vaccine preparations for preventing candidosis in experimental models have been reported (KHARDORI et al. 1986; SHARMA et al. 1986; LEVY et al. 1981, 1983).

The large multicenter cooperative trial for evaluation of a vaccine to prevent coccidioidomycosis, the mycosis endemic to the southwest portion of the USA and parts of Mexico and South America, has been completed (PAPPAGIANIS 1986). Vaccinated subjects were not protected from developing coccidioidomycosis, and the severity of the disease did not differ between vaccinees and placebo recipients. The reasons for the lack of vaccine efficacy are not entirely clear. However, any subsequent studies of fungal vaccines need to account for the presence of components of the vaccine that may elicit immunosuppressive activity, as well as potentially protective immunologic responses. Thus, specific antigenic fungal-derived material will need to be identified and purified, so that a more predictable effect may occur.

In experimental systems, ribosomal vaccines have been used with some beneficial effects on the susceptibility of mice to invasive candidosis and histoplasmosis (LEVY et al. 1981, 1983; KHARDORI et al. 1986; SHARMA et al. 1986). However, the vaccine preparations are still relatively crude and would probably not be acceptable for use in humans. Moreover, the mechanism of action of these vaccine preparations is still not entirely clear. Thus, differences in the responses of rodents and humans to the same preparation may occur, and without direct experimentation or evidence as to the mechanisms of action in the animal model, the role of these preparations in the prevention of human disease is hard to determine. It will be a very long time before vaccines and their proposed mechanisms of action are sufficiently well defined to justify human studies.

F. The Future

The field of antifungal chemotherapy has reached a stage at which new agents in different classes of compounds and with differing modes of action are being synthesized and studied in preclinical and clinical trials. On the other hand, advances in diagnostic capabilities have not kept pace with those in new drug development. As a result, the clinician must frequently institute therapy empirically without knowing the definitive diagnosis; often the diagnosis of invasive fungal infection is never firmly established. Since some of the newer agents have a limited spectrum of activity (e.g., cilofungin), their use in these situations is problematic. Attempts at antibody or antigen detection have met with varying degrees of success; the sensitivity and specificity of currently available commercial or research assays are not good and certainly not satisfactory for routine use in patient care. Moreover, these assays are primarily directed at *Candida* and *Aspergillus*, rather than the less frequently isolated pathogens. Progress in DNA probe technology as one means of identifying fungal infection may hold some promise in this area (MASON et al. 1987; SCHERER and STEVENS 1987; OLIVO et al. 1987), although experience is still limited, so that the ultimate use of this methodology is not yet clear.

In future years we can expect antifungal therapy to be less toxic and, hopefully, more efficacious than that which is presently available. In particular, drugs useful in treating fungal diseases of the immunocompromised patient are particularly needed, since amphotericin B is not only extremely toxic but has questionable activity in many mycoses in the immunosuppressed patient. The newer agents will be selected for their increased activity against fungi currently relatively resistant to available options, e.g., *Aspergillus*, the Mucorales, and dematiaceous fungi, and for their ability to be taken orally not more than once daily.

Advances in antifungal drug development have catalyzed efforts in clinical investigation of the mycoses. Properly designed and controlled studies are a prerequisite for obtaining approval of a compound for general medical use. Because of a myriad of seemingly unresolvable aspects of many mycoses, rigorous studies of different therapeutic options have not been done for most of the medically important fungal diseases. The problems inherent in making a definitive diagnosis of candidosis, for example, have successfully impeded the initiation of studies designed to evaluate the effects of therapy on the natural history of disease. The result of incomplete evaluation of a potentially useful new drug is exemplified by miconazole, an intravenous imidazole studied and licensed in the 1970s, about 10 years before ketoconazole. Miconazole has an uncertain place in our pharmacopoeia vis-á-vis other agents, in large part because suitable comparative trials have never been performed. In contrast, ketoconazole and newer investigational agents (e.g., itraconazole, fluconazole, cilofungin, SCH 39304 liposomal amphotericin B) have been or soon will be studied in a comparative fashion in experimental animal mycoses and in humans with a variety of important fungal infections. The outcome of these trials will dictate how each is used in the more common mycoses. However, there are certain diseases, such as chromoblastomycosis and those caused by the agents listed in Table 1, that are uncommon enough so that comparative or even uncontrolled studies with sufficient numbers of patients will never be conducted. In that event, the guidance of experts in the field should be sought when treating patients with these diseases. Where studies are available, eligible patients should be enrolled so that results obtained in treating patients with rare mycoses can be pooled, and some idea about the relative efficacy of one drug versus another can be made.

In conclusion, physicians in most areas of medical and surgical practice have to diagnose and treat many different fungal infections. The therapeutic possibilities have already more than doubled over the past several years and that trend seems likely to continue for the foreseeable future. The challenge now confronting investigators is not only finding the correct use for each new agent; definitive, rapid, and accurate diagnosis must be the next area to be elucidated.

References

Anaissie E, Kantarjian H, Ro J, Hopfer R, Rolston K, Fainstein V, Bodey G (1988) The emerging role of *Fusarium* infections in patients with cancer. Medicine 67:77–83

Arena FP, Perlin M, Brahman H, Weiser B, Armstrong D (1981) Fever, rash, and myalgias of disseminated candidiasis during antifungal therapy. Arch Intern Med 141:1233

Arroyo J, Medoff G, Kobayashi GS (1977) Therapy of murine aspergillosis with amphotericin B in combination with rifampin or 5-fluorocytosine. Antimicrob Agents Chemother 11:21–25

Bailey JW, Sada E, Brass C, Bennett JE (1985) Diagnosis of systemic candidiasis by latex agglutination for serum antigen. J Clin Microbiol 21:749–752

Beaman L, Benjamani E, Pappagianis D (1983) Activation of macrophages by lymphokines: enhancement of phagosome-lysosome fusion and killing of *Coccidioides immitis*. Infect Immun 39:1201–1207

Bennett JE (1981) Treatment of cryptococcal, candidal, and coccidioidal meningitis. In: Remington JS, Swartz MN (eds) Current clinical topics in infectious diseases. McGraw-Hill, New York, pp 54–67

Bennett JE (1987) Rapid diagnosis of candidiasis and aspergillosis. Rev Infect Dis 9:398–402

Bennett JE, Dismukes WE, Duma RJ (1979) A comparison of amphotericin B alone and combined with flucytosine in the treatment of cryptococcal meningitis. N Engl J Med 301:126–131

Bronnimann DA, Adam RD, Galgiani JN, Habib MP, Petersen EA, Porter B, Bloom JW (1987) Coccidioidomycosis in the acquired immunodeficiency syndrome. Ann Intern Med 106:372–379

Brummer E, Stevens DA (1987) Activation of pulmonary macrophages for fungicidal activity by gamma-interferon or lymphokines. Clin Exp Immunol 70:520–528

Brummer E, Morrison CJ, Stevens DA (1985) Recombinant and natural gamma-interferon activation of macrophages in vitro: different dose requirements for induction of killing activity against phagocytizable and nonphagocytizable fungi. Infect Immun 49:724–730.

Brummer E, Hanson LH, Restrepo A, Stevens DA (1988) In vivo and in vitro activation of pulmonary macrophages by IFN-gamma for enhanced killing of *Paracoccidioides brasiliensis* or *Blastomyces dermatitidis*. J Immunol 140:2786–2789

Burnie J (1987) Latex tests in the early diagnosis of systemic candidosis. Serodiag Immunother 1:3–5

Cairns MR (1988) Fungal infections in the acquired immunodeficiency syndrome. J Electron Microscopy Techniques 8:115–131

Calhoun DL, Roberts GD, Galgiani JN, Bennett JE, Feingold DS, Jorgensen J, Kobayashi GS, Shadomy S (1986) Results of a survey of antifungal susceptibility tests in the United States and interlaboratory comparison of broth dilution testing of flucytosine and amphotericin B. J Clin Microbiol 23:298–301

Deepe GS Jr, Taylor CL, Harris JE, Bullock WE (1986) Modulation of cellular immune responses in mice with disseminated histoplasmosis by recombinant interleukin-2. Infect Immun 53:6–12.

Deng Z, Ribas JL, Gibson DW, Connor DH (1988) Infections caused by *Penicillium marneffei* in China and Southeast Asia: review of eighteen published cases and report of four more Chinese cases. Rev Infect Dis 10:640–652

De Repentigny L, Reiss E (1984) Current trends in immunodiagnosis of candidiasis and aspergillosis. Rev Infect Dis 6:301–312

De Repentigny L, Marr LD, Keller JW, Carter AW, Kuykendall RJ, Kaufman L, Reiss E (1985) Comparison of enzyme immunoassay and gas-liquid chromatography for the rapid diagnosis of invasive candidiasis in cancer patients. J Clin Microbiol 21:972–979

Deresinski SC, Stevens DA (1975) Coccidioidomycosis in compromised hosts. Experience at Stanford University Hospital. Medicine 54:377–395

Dick JD, Merz WG, Saral R (1980) Incidence of polyene-resistant yeasts recovered from clinical specimens. Antimicrob Agents Chemother 18:158–163

Dick JD, Rosengard BR, Merz WG, Stuart RK, Hutchins GM, Saral R (1985) Fatal disseminated candidiasis due to amphotericin-B-resistant *Candida guilliermondii*. Ann Intern Med 102:67–68

Dismukes WE, Cloud G, Gallis HA, Kerkering TM, Medoff G, Craven PC, Kaplowitz LG, Fisher JF, Gregg CR, Bowles CA, Shadomy S, Stamm AM, Diasio RB, Kaufman L, et al. (1987) Treatment of cryptococcal meningitis with combination amphotericin B and flucytosine for four as compared with six weeks. N Engl J Med 317:334–341

Drutz DJ (1986) Antigen detection in fungal infections. N Engl J Med 314:115–117

Dupont B, Huber M, Kim SJ, Bennett JE (1987) Galactomannan antigenemia and antigenuria in aspergillosis: studies in patients and experimentally infected rabbits. J Infect Dis 155:1–10

Edwards JE Jr (1985) *Candida* species. In: Mandell GL, Douglas RG, Bennett JE (eds) Principles and practice of infectious diseases. Wiley, New York, pp 1435–1447

Edwards JE Jr, Morrison J, Henderson DK, Montgomerie JZ (1980) Combined effect of amphotericin B and rifampin on *Candida* species. Antimicrob Agents Chemother 17:484–487

Fromtling RA (1987) (ed) Recent trends in the discovery, development and evaluation of antifungal agents. JR Prous, Barcelona

Galgiani JN, Reiser J, Brass C, Espinel-Ingroff A, Gordon MA, Kerkering TM (1987) Comparison of relative susceptibilities of *Candida* species to three antifungal agents as determined by unstandardized methods. Antimicrob Agents Chemother 31:1343–1347

Goering P, Berlinger NT, Weisdorf DJ (1988) Aggressive combined modality treatment of progressive sinonasal fungal infections in immunocompromised patients. Am J Med 85:619–622

Gold JWM (1984) Opportunistic fungal infections in patients with neoplastic disease. Am J Med 76:458–463

Greenfield RA, Troutt, DL, Rickard RC, Altmiller DH (1988) Comparison of antibody, antigen, and metabolite assays in rat models of systemic and gastrointestinal candidiasis. J Clin Microbiol 26:409–417

Henderson DK, Edwards JE Jr, Montgomerie JZ (1981) Hematogenous *Candida* endophthalmitis in patients receiving parenteral hyperalimentation fluids. J Infect Dis 143:655–661

Iwata K, Vanden Bossche H (1986) In vitro and in vivo evaluation of antifungal agents. Elsevier, NY

Johnson PC, Sarosi GA, Septimus EJ, Satterwhite TK (1986) Progressive disseminated histoplasmosis in patients with the acquired immune deficiency syndrome: a report of 12 cases and a literature review. Sem Respir Infect 1:1–8

Kahn FW, Jones JM (1986) Latex agglutination tests for detection of *Candida* antigens in sera of patients with invasive candidiasis. J Infect Dis 153:579–585

Karp JE, Burch PA, Merz WG (1988) An approach to intensive antileukemia therapy in patients with previous invasive aspergillosis. Am J Med 85:203–206

Khardori N, von Behren L, Chaudhary S, McConnachie P, Strano A, Tewari RP (1986) Cellular mediators of anti-histoplasma immunity: I. Protective immunity and cellular changes in spleens of mice immunized by sublethal infection with yeast cells of *Histoplasma capsulatum*. Mykosen 29:103–115

Levy R, Segal E, Eylan E (1981) Protective immunity against murine candidiasis elicited by *Candida albicans* ribosomal fractions. Infect Immun 31:874–878

Levy R, Segal E, Eylan E, Barr-Nea L (1983) Cell-mediated immunity following experimental vaccinations with *Candida albicans* ribosomes. Mycopathologia 83:161–168

Lew MA, Beckett KM, Levin MS (1977) Antifungal activity of four tetracycline analogs in vitro: potentiation by amphotericin B. J Infect Dis 136:263–270

Mason MM, Lasker BA, Riggsby WS (1987) Molecular probe for identification of medically important *Candida* species and *Torulopsis glabrata*. J Clin Microbiol 25:563–566

Matthews R, Burnie J (1988) Diagnosis of systemic candidiasis by an enzyme-linked dot immunobinding assay for a circulating immunodominant 47-kilodalton antigen. J Clin Microbiol 26:459–463

Matthews RC, Burnie JP, Tabaqchali S (1984) Immunoblot analysis of the serological response in systemic candidosis. Lancet ii:1415–1418
McManus EJ, Jones JM (1985) Detection of a *Trichosporon beigelii* antigen cross-reactive with *Cryptococcus neoformans* capsular polysaccharide in serum from a patient with disseminated *Trichosporon* infection. J Clin Microbiol 21:681–685
Medoff G, Kobayashi GS (1980) Strategies in the treatment of systemic fungal infections. N Engl J Med 302:145–155
Meunier F (1987) Prevention of mycoses in immunocompromised patients. Rev Infect Dis 9:408–416
Meunier-Carpentier F, Kiehn TE, Armstrong D (1981) Fungemia in the immunocompromised host. Changing patterns, antigenemia, high mortality. Am J Med 71:363–370
Olivo PD, McManus EJ, Riggsby WS, Jones JM (1987) Mitochondrial DNA polymorphism in *Candida albicans*. J Infect Dis 156:214–215
Pappagianis D (1986) Evaluation of the protective efficacy of the killed *Coccidioides immitis* vaccine in man. 26th Interscience Conference on Antimicrobial Agents and Chemotherapy, New Orleans (Abstr 784)
Polak A, Scholer HJ, Wall M (1982) Combination therapy of experimental candidiasis, cryptococcosis and aspergillosis in mice. Chemotherapy 28:461–479
Powderly WG, Kobayashi GS, Herzig GP, Medoff G (1988) Amphotericin B-resistant yeast infection in severely immunocompromised patients. Am J Med 84:826–832
Sabetta JR, Miniter P, Andriole VT (1985) The diagnosis of invasive aspergillosis by an enzyme-linked immunosorbent assay for circulating antigen. J Infect Dis 152: 946–953
Salzman SH, Smith RL, Aranda CP (1988) Histoplasmosis in patients at risk for the acquired immunodeficiency syndrome in a nonendemic setting. Chest 93:916–921
Scherer S, Stevens DA (1987) Application of DNA typing methods to epidemiology and taxonomy of *Candida* species. J Clin Microbiol 25:675–679
Sharma D, Khardori N, Chaudhary S, von Behren L, McConnachie P, Tewari RP (1986) Cellular mediators of anti-histoplasma immunity: II. Protective immunity and delayed hypersensitivity in mice immunized by sublethal infection with yeast cells of *Histoplasma capsulatum*. Mykosen 29:116–126
Sugar AM, Levitz SM (1988) Treatment of cryptococcal meningitis. N Engl J Med 318:381
Talbot GH, Weiner MH, Gerson SL, Provencher M, Hurwitz S (1987) Serodiagnosis of invasive aspergillosis in patients with hematologic malignancy: validation of the *Aspergillus fumigatus* antigen radioimmunoassay. J Infect Dis 155:12–27
Walling DM, McGraw DJ, Merz WG, Karp JE, Hutchins GM (1987) Disseminated infection with *Trichosporon beigelii*. Rev Infect Dis 9:1013–1019
Wu-Hsieh BA, Howard DH (1987) Inhibition of the intracellular growth of *Histoplasma capsulatum* by recombinant murine gamma interferon. Infect Immun 55: 1014–1016

CHAPTER 16

Management of Fungal Infections in Patients with Neoplastic Diseases

THOMAS J. WALSH and PHILIP A. PIZZO

A. Introduction

Systemic mycoses are life-threatening infections in granulocytopenic patients with neoplastic diseases (HORN et al. 1985; WALSH and PIZZO 1988). The problems of nosocomial outbreaks, clinical resistance, microbiological resistance, emergence of new pathogens, and difficulty in establishing an early diagnosis present formidable challenges to the successful management of these patients. Progress in treating these infections is being achieved through greater understanding of established available antifungal agents such as amphotericin B, flucytosine, miconazole, and ketoconazole. Promising investigational agents such as fluconazole and intraconazole will require careful clinical investigation in order to define their role in granulocytopenic patients. This chapter will review the management of fungal infections in granulocytopenic patients with neoplastic diseases.

Wc will review essential aspects of host defense against fungi relevant to granulocytopenic patients, define and classify their nosocomial fungal infections, discuss the management of their specific fungal infections, and review the current status of antifungal agents which demonstrate promise for use.

B. Principles of Host Defense in Patients with Neoplastic Diseases

Granulocytes maintain an essential role in host defense against opportunistic fungi, especially *Candida* spp., *Aspergillus* spp., the Mucoraceae, and *Trichosporon* spp. T-cell-mediated immunity is more critical in maintaining host defense against the primary pathogenic fungi, such as *Histoplasma capsulatum* and *Coccidioides immitis*. SCHAFFNER et al. (1986) demonstrated the critical role of granulocytes against germinated stages of opportunistic fungi including *Candida* and *Aspergillus* in comparison with the pathogenic fungi such as *Histoplasma* and *Coccidioides*, in which mononuclear cells were more active. This distinction between opportunistic fungi and the primary pathogenic dimorphic fungi is reflected in the epidemiologic pattern of invasive fungal infections in granulocytopenic patients. *Candida* spp., *Aspergillus* spp., and the Mucoraceae are the most common life-threatening systemic fungi causing disease in granulocytopenic patients. The frequency of systemic fungal infections, especially aspergillosis, increases with longer durations of granulocytopenia. By contrast, infections due to *C. neoformans*, *H. capsulatum*, and *C. immitis* are unusual in granulocytopenic patients but are the most common systemic fungal infections in patients with the acquired immune deficiency syndrome (AIDS), whose defect is that of profound impairment of T-cell-mediated immunity with usually intact granulocyte function and number.

Cancer patients may have a combination of immunological deficits. For example, granulocytopenic patients such as those with lymphocytic leukemia or lymphoma who are receiving corticosteroids as part of their chemotherapy protocol may develop systemic infections due to *C. neoformans*, *H. capsulatum*, or *C. immitis*. Broad-spectrum antibiotics, intravascular catheters, total parenteral nutrition, and disruption of mucosal barriers by cytotoxic chemotherapy further abrogate host defenses in the granulocytopenic patient.

The administration of broad-spectrum antibiotics, which are necessary to prevent or treat bacterial infections, may also increase the degree of colonization of the alimentary tract by *Candida* spp. and other opportunistic yeast-like fungi. Cytotoxic chemotherapy commonly causes disruption of the mucosal barriers of the alimentary tract, thereby permitting *Candida* and other yeast-like fungi to invade more readily across the disrupted mucosal surface (WINGARD et al. 1980). Intravascular catheters are required for venous access in the granulocytopenic patient but are also portals of entry for *Candida* spp. and other fungi. Total parenteral nutrition may further increase the risk for fungemia due to *Candida* spp. and *Malassezia furfur*.

C. Definitions and Classification of Nosocomial Fungal Infections

Most invasive mycoses in granulocytopenic patients are nosocomial fungal infections. In order to clarify unifying and distinguishing factors of hospital epidemiology, mechanisms of transmission, and possible means of prevention, we previously proposed a classification of them (WALSH and PIZZO 1988).

A nosocomial fungal infection was defined as any superficial, locally invasive, or disseminated mycosis acquired from the hospital environment or developing during the course of a patient's hospitalization. We further classified nosocomial fungal infections as one of two types: hospital-acquired fungal infection (type I) and hospital-associated fungal infection (type II). Type I included any mycosis acquired from the hospital environment. Type II included any mycosis which develops during the course of hospitalization from a fungus previously colonizing or latently infecting a patient. Type II was further classified into subtypes IIA and IIB. Subtype IIA was defined as a hospital-associated fungal infection which developed from endogenous colonizing fungi. Subtype IIB was defined as a hospital-associated fungal

Table 1. Classification of principal nosocomial fungal infections

Type I	Type II	
	Type IIA	Type IIB
Aspergillus spp.	*Candida* spp.[a,e]	*Histoplasma capsulatum*
Mucoraceae *Mucor*	*Trichosporon* spp.	*Coccidioides immitis*[e]
Rhizopus *Absidia* *Rhizomucor*	*Malassezia furfur*	*Cryptococcus neoformans*
Pseudallescheria boydii	*Trichophyton*[e] *rubrum*	
Fusarium spp.	*Saccharomyces*[f] *cerevisiae*	
Dematiaceous hyphomycetes		
Candida spp.[b]		
Coccidioides immitis[c]		
Histoplasma capsulatum[d]		
Cryptococcus neoformans[d]		
Blastomyces dermatitidis[d]		
Dermatophytes[d]		

[a] Principal mechanism of nosocomial infection.
[b] *Candida* spp. have been transmitted from the hospital environment to patients in several outbreaks.
[c] Laboratory acquisition or transmission from wound dressings by hospital personnel.
[d] Laboratory acquisition by hospital personnel.
[e] May be transmitted from other patients or hospital personnel.
[f] Colonization is usually transient.

infection which developed from reactivation of latently infecting fungi. The fungi associated with these different groups are given in Table 1.

I. Aspergillosis

1. Microbiology

The genus *Aspergillus* is characterized in culture by hyaline septate hyphae, conidiophores, and phialoconidia. The conidia measure 2.5–3.5 μm in diameter in most pathogenic strains. The diameter and hydrophobic properties of these conidia allow them to be carried on air currents into the alveolar air spaces where they may invade the pulmonary parenchyma in a compromised host. *A. fumigatus* and *A. flavus* are the two most common species to infect granulocytopenic patients. Airborne penetration of the respiratory tract is the main route of transmission of *Aspergillus* within the hospital environment.

2. Hospital Epidemiology

Two mechanisms of transmission of *Aspergillus* to granulocytopenic patients have been described: airborne transmission via the respiratory tract or into an operative site and contact transmission through direct inoculation from occlusive materials. The former is the most common mechanism of nosocomial transmission of most filamentous fungi to granulocytopenic patients. Most cases of aspergillosis in granulocytopenic patients can be classified as type I (or hospital-acquired) nosocomial fungal infection.

Aspergillus may be cultured from multiple sources within the hospital environment including: unfiltered air, contaminated ventilation systems, construction sites, dust, horizontal surfaces, food, and plants. Rosen and Sternberg (1976) observed a reduction in the frequency of aspergillosis and zygomycosis from 145 instances in a 3-year period to 30 over the next 3 years after patients from a large oncology center were moved from an older building with no central ventilation to a new facility with centrally filtered ventilation.

Ventilation systems including intake ducts, exhaust ducts, or filters also serve as potential sources of growth and transmission of *Aspergillus* spp. Air supply ducts to four operating rooms were demonstrated to be the source of *A. flavus* causing primary cutaneous aspergillosis in nine granulocytopenic patients with leukemia or aplastic anemia (Allo et al. 1987). These patients were undergoing insertion of Hickman intravenous catheters, and all developed *A. flavus* infections of the catheter sites. No additional cases of postoperative cutaneous aspergillosis developed after the four operating rooms were renovated and the air supply ducts vacuumed.

Inadequate air intake filters may have contributed to nosocomial aspergillosis observed in the allogeneic bone marrow transplant recipients at Roswell Park Memorial Institute during a period of nearby construction outside of the hospital (Rhame 1985; Rotstein et al. 1985). Another outbreak of aspergillosis occurred on a pediatric oncology floor 10 days after an exhaust fan from four rooms was shut down for maintenance (Mahoney et al. 1979). *Aspergillus* spp. contaminated the air conditioning system, and five children with leukemia in these four rooms acquired invasive aspergillosis. Contaminated equipment and rooms were cleaned, and no further cases of aspergillosis developed.

Hospital construction and renovation are other sources of *Aspergillus* conidia. An environmental investigation implicated *Aspergillus* cultured from cellulose-based fireproofing material coating steel girders and pipes as the source of eight new cases of aspergillosis in granulocytopenic patients in a newly constructed hospital (Aisner et al. 1976). Another outbreak of nosocomial aspergillosis occurred during hospital renovation of a large military medical center (Opal et al. 1986). The incidence of invasive aspergillosis increased from 4 patients during the 30 months preceding construction to 11 over the 24 months during renovation without control measures ($P < 0.05$). The incidence decreased to 1 over 18 months after establishing airtight plastic and dry wall barriers around the construction sites, negative-pressure ventilation in the work area, environmental decontamination with copper-8-quinolinolate, and high efficiency particulate air (HEPA) filters in the rooms of immunocompromised patients.

On the other hand, construction or renovation in or near cancer centers is not inevitably followed by outbreaks of nosocomial aspergillosis. For example, considerable renovation at the National Institutes of Health (NIH) Clinical Center has been conducted during the plast 7 years; however, there has been no measurable increase in the incidence of nosocomial aspergillosis in cancer patients at this center.

Aspergillus conidia may be present in the inanimate hospital environment, including dressings and materials applied to the skin. For example, PRYSTOWSKY et al. (1976) reported locally invasive cutaneous aspergillosis developing under adhesive tape or paper-covered extremity boards in three granulocytopenic children. Cutaneous aspergillosis in granulocytopenic cancer patients may cause destruction of the skin, subcutaneous tissue, and bone and may provide a portal of entry for fatal disseminated aspergillosis in cancer patients.

3. Clinical Manifestations

An analysis of risk factors in cancer patients with pulmonary aspergillosis demonstrated that protracted duration of granulocytopenia, especially beyond 21 days, was the single most important independent variable associated with the development of pulmonary aspergillosis (GERSON et al. 1984). The magnitude of the problem of pulmonary aspergillosis in granulocytopenic patients at some centers was presented in a study from the University of Minnesota (PETERSON et al. 1983), in which pulmonary or disseminated aspergillosis was the single most important infection causing death in allogeneic bone marrow transplant recipients.

Pulmonary aspergillosis in persistently granulocytopenic patients is characterized by an unremitting fever which continues despite the administration of broad-spectrum antibacterial antibiotics; nonproductive cough, tachypnea, pleuritic pain, and pleural rub may ensue (MEYER et al. 1973). Pulmonary infiltrates on chest radiography are usually apparent but may be absent early in the course of aspergillosis in granulocytopenic patients. Computerized tomography (CT) scans of the lungs may reveal multiple pulmonary nodules and may later show a cavity with a crescentic configuration. Due to the propensity of *Aspergillus* spp. to invade blood vessels, pulmonary infarction, cavitation, hemorrhage, and hemoptysis may ensue. Massive hemoptysis is a catastrophic complication of pulmonary aspergillosis. This frequently lethal complication is due to hemorrhagic infarction during granulocytopenia or to rupture of an inflammatory mycotic aneurysm when the granulocytopenia is resolving (PETERSON et al. 1983).

Pulmonary aspergillosis in cancer patients may be followed by dissemination to other sites, including brain, kidney, liver, and bone. Aspergillosis of the central nervous system often presents with the acute onset of a focal neurologic deficit or as focal seizure activity (PANOS et al. 1988). A CT scan (with radiocontrast) of the brain often reveals a ring-enhancing lesion or a pattern of infarction. Aspergillosis of the CNS is often initially misdiagnosed as an intracerebral hemorrhage due to thrombocytopenia or as a progression of the underlying neoplasm, e.g. lymphoma (Walsh et al. 1985).

Diagnosis of invasive pulmonary or disseminated aspergillosis in a granulocytopenic patient is based upon clinical manifestations and isolation of the *Aspergillus* spp. in tissue. Nevertheless, a positive nasal surveillance culture or sputum culture yielding *Aspergillus* in a persistently febrile granulocytopenic patient with pulmonary infiltrates strongly suggests pulmonary aspergillosis. A culture of sputum or bronchoalveolar lavage fluid that yields *A. fumigatus*, *A. flavus*, or *A. terreus* in a persistently febrile granulocytopenic patient should not be regarded as contamination (Yu et al. 1986). Instead, such culture findings in a febrile granulocytopenic patient are indicative of pulmonary aspergillosis. An open lung biopsy may be necessary to establish the diagnosis of invasive pulmonary aspergillosis in granulocytopenic patients if less invasive procedures are nondiagnostic. Immunodiagnostic assays for invasive aspergillosis are promising but remain investigational.

The paranasal sinuses also are frequent sites of invasive aspergillosis in granulocytopenic cancer patients. Viollier et al. (1986) observed that *Aspergillus* sinusitis occurred in patients who had profound ($<500/\mu l$) and protracted (mean of 42 days) granulocytopenia. Initial treatment with systemic amphotericin B was usually successful. However, *Aspergillus* sinusitis often recurred when the primary neoplastic disease relapsed or another cycle of chemotherapy was administered.

4. Treatment

Measures designed to eliminate *Aspergillus* conidia from the environment of high risk granulocytopenic patients may prevent nosocomial aspergillosis. Laminar air flow environments also may prevent transmission of *Aspergillus* conidia (Bodey 1984; Rogers 1986); however, the prohibitive cost and inconvenience of these facilities preclude their routine use (Armstrong 1984). Administration of an intranasal aerosol of amphotericin B is another strategy that may be effective in the prevention of nosocomial pulmonary aspergillosis in cancer patients (Meunier et al. 1987).

Once a diagnosis of invasive aspergillosis is established, we suggest that amphotericin B be administered i.v. at 1.0 mg/kg daily with flucytosine for the duration of the granulocytopenia and for a total dose of at least 30 mg/kg (Table 2). Also the usual dose of flucytosine of 150 mg/kg daily in four divided doses should be used initially in a patient with normal renal function. However, this dose can be decreased during the 1 week to maintain serum levels between 50 and 75 µg/ml in order to avoid myelosuppression and gastrointestinal toxicity. A recent report by Burch et al. (1987) found that administration of high-dose amphotericin B (1.0–1.5 mg/kg daily) with flucytosine to granulocytopenic patients with leukemia was associated with nearly 90% survival. These findings are promising but await further corroboration.

Table 2. Treatment of selected fungal infections in granulocytopenic patients with neoplastic diseases

Infection	Antifungal agent	Dosage	Comments
Aspergillosis			
Pulmonary	Amphotericin B	1.0–1.5 mg/kg daily	Addition of flucytosine is controversial
Maxillary sinus	Amphotericin B	1.0–1.5 mg/kg daily	Surgical drainage may be indicated
Candidosis			
Oropharyngeal	Clotrimazole	50 mg troche five times per day	
	Ketoconazole	5–10 mg/kg daily	
Esophageal	Amphotericin B	0.5 mg/kg daily	May be portal of entry for systemic candidosis
Gastrointestinal	Amphotericin B	0.5 mg/kg daily	
Candidemia	Amphotericin B	0.5–1.0 mg/kg daily	Candidemia due to *C. tropicalis* may require higher dosage
Catheter-associated candidemia	Amphotericin B	0.5–1.0 mg/kg daily	Remove catheter
Hepatosplenic	Amphotericin B	0.5–1.0 mg/kg daily	Protracted course of 3–9 months
	plus		
	flucytosine (5-FC)[a]	75–150 mg/kg daily	
Trichosporonosis	Amphotericin B	1.0–1.5 mg/kg daily	Consider miconazole or investigational triazole
	plus		
	flucytosine	75–150 mg/kg daily	
Fusariosis	Amphotericin B	1.0–1.5 mg/kg daily	
	plus		
	flucytosine	75–150 mg/kg daily	
Malassezia furfur			
Fungemia	Ketoconazole	5–10 mg/kg daily	Removal of catheter and discontinuation of lipid emulsions
Pseudallescheriosis	Amphotericin B	1.0–1.5 mg/kg daily	Antifungal susceptibility studies may be useful in guiding therapy
	plus		
	miconazole	10 mg/kg Q 8 h	
Histoplasmosis	Amphotericin B	0.5 mg/kg daily	
Cryptococcosis	Amphotericin B	0.3 mg/kg daily	
	plus		
	flucytosine[a]	75–150 mg/kg daily	

[a] Maintain levels of 5-FC between 40 and 60 μg/ml.

Survival following pulmonary aspergillosis in granulocytopenic hosts is highly dependent upon recovery from the granulocytopenia or reversal of other immunological deficits. Nevertheless, following recovery from granulocytopenia, aspergillosis often recurs in sites of previous pulmonary infection during a subsequent bout of granulocytopenia (e.g., a second cycle of chemotherapy). We propose therefore that such patients with a history of pulmonary aspergillosis who become febrile during a later episode of granulocytopenia receive amphotericin B i.v.

Cavitation of pulmonary *Aspergillus* lesions may be followed by massive and fatal hemoptysis (PANOS et al. 1988). The role of surgery in the management of cavitary pulmonary aspergillosis in cancer patients is controversial. However, antifungal chemotherapy alone may not be adequate to prevent either cavitation or hemoptysis. We recommend that a solitary cavitary lesion complicating pulmonary aspergillosis in a cancer patient be surgically resected if the patient is thought to be a surgical candidate (BURCH et al. 1987).

New pulmonary infiltrates that develop in febrile granulocytopenic patients during administration of broad-spectrum antibiotics have a high probability (approximately 50%) of having a fungal cause (COMMERS et al. 1984). Early initiation of amphotericin B in these patients may improve their therapeutic outcome.

II. Zygomycosis

1. Microbiology

The term zygomycosis is defined as fungal infection due to members of the class Zygomycetes. The family Mucoraceae, which consists of the genera *Mucor*, *Rizopus*, *Absidia*, and *Rhizomucor*, are the most common pathogens in granulocytopenic patients (MEYER et al. 1972). *Cunninghamella* spp. and other non-Mucoraceae have rarely been reported as causes of infection in cancer patients (KWON-CHUNG et al. 1975).

2. Hospital Epidemiology

Zygomycosis is classified as a type I nosocomial fungal infection. Mucoraceae are not usually part of the normal human flora. The mechanisms of airborne and contact transmission of the sporangiospores of the Mucoraceae are similar to those of conidia of *Aspergillus* spp. (ENGLAND et al. 1981; EVERETT et al. 1979; GARTENBERG et al. 1987; KRASINSKI et al. 1985; SHELDON and JOHNSON 1979).

3. Clinical Manifestations

Zygomycosis in granulocytopenic cancer patients most commonly involves the respiratory tract as sinusitis, rhinocerebral mucormycosis, and pulmonary mucormycosis (MEYER et al. 1972; LEHRER et al. 1980). The clinical course of pulmonary zygomycosis is similar to that of pulmonary aspergillosis. Features of fever, progressive pulmonary infiltrates, infarction, and cavitation in a granulocytopenic patient receiving antibacterial antibiotic therapy are common to pulmonary mucormycosis and aspergillosis. Zygomycosis of the CNS may present as focal neurologic deficits or seizures.

4. Treatment

The mainstays of treating zygomycosis in granulocytopenic cancer patients include early initiation of amphotericin B i.v., early and complete surgical debridement of rhinocerebral lesions, resection of cavitary pulmonary lesions, and reversal of underlying granulocytopenia as well as other immunological deficits. Should the patient also have diabetes mellitus, correction of any concomitant ketoacidosis is important. Hyperbaric oxygen has been suggested as an adjunct to antifungal chemotherapy of rhinocerebral mucormycosis. However, hyperbaric oxygen in pancytopenic cancer patients remains investigational.

III. Other Type I (Hospital-Acquired) Nosocomial Fungal Infections in Cancer Patients

1. Pseudallescherosis

Infections caused by *Pseudallescheria boydii* have been reported with increasing frequency in immunocompromised patients (Smith et al. 1985; Rippon 1988). Little is known about the epidemiology of transmission of *P. boydii* to patients. However, since it is a soil saprophyte, generates conidia, and invades the respiratory tract in immunocompromised patients, airborne and contract transmission similar to that of *Aspergillus* spp. and the Mucoraceae seems likely. The range of susceptible hosts, clinical manifestations, and histopathology of pulmonary and disseminated pseudallescherosis are similar to those of disseminated aspergillosis. *P. boydii* is often resistant to amphotericin B and tends to be more susceptible to the antifungal azole compounds, especially miconazole (Lutwick et al. 1979).

2. Fusariosis

Pulmonary and disseminated *Fusarium* infections have become increasingly recognized in granulocytopenic patients (Anaissie et al. 1985; Chaulk et al. 1986; June et al. 1986; Kiehn et al. 1985). *Fusarium* spp. are soil saprophytes and usually produce both micro- and macroconidia. Little is known about their epidemiology; however, nosocomial airborne and contact transmission seems to be the likely mechanisms of patient acquisition of this emerging pathogen. Disseminated *Fusarium* infection in granulocytopenic patients is associated with prominent, erythematous, maculopapular to nodular lesions from which the fungus may be cultured. Biopsy of these lesions may reveal branching septate hyphae invading the dermal blood vessels. Amphotericin B currently remains the preferred antifungal agent for treatment of invasive *Fusarium* infection in granulocytopenic patients. Doses of amphotericin B of 1.0 mg/kg to 1.5 mg/kg daily with flucytosine are indicated in refractory infection.

3. Phaeohyphomycosis

Phaeohyphomycosis is defined here as deep tissue or subcutaneous infection by dematiaceous (brown-pigmented) hyphomycetes. Causative organisms include members of the genera *Exserohilum*, *Bipolaris*, *Curvularia*, *Cladosporium*, *Alternaria*, and *Dactylaria* (ANAISSIE et al. 1985; ADAM et al. 1986; DIXON et al. 1988). Phaeohyphomycosis is being reported with increasing frequency in immunocompromised patients. There is considerable geographic variation in the frequency with which these fungi are isolated as pathogens at different medical centers. The exact extent to which they contribute to fungal infections in cancer patients remains to be further studied. We recommend for management of phaeohyphomycosis a combination, where possible, of surgical resection of discrete lesions and systemic antifungal chemotherapy. Initial antifungal chemotherapy for phaeohyphomycosis should initially consist of amphotericin B and flucytosine. As little is known about the optimal management of these infections, treatment is often individualized. Experimental antifungal studies by DIXON et al. (1988) demonstrated that dematiaceous fungal infections respond differently depending upon the etiological agent. Patients who do not respond to the combination of amphotericin B and flucytosine may be candidates for one of the new antifungal triazole compounds such as itraconazole.

IV. Candidosis

1. Microbiology

The genus *Candida* is characterized microscopically by the presence of blastoconidia, pseudohyphae, and hyphae. The production of germ tubes is indicative of *C. albicans*. Germ-tube-negative *Candida* are distinguished by carbohydrate assimilation and fermentation.

2. Hospital Epidemiology

In contrast to *Aspergillus*, the Mucoraceae, and the other hyphomycetes previously described, *C. albicans* is a normal constituent of the human gastrointestinal tract and cutaneous flora. Broad-spectrum antibiotics suppress the gastrointestinal bacterial flora, which may promote further colonization by *Candida* spp. *Candida* may become invasive and disseminate from the gastrointestinal tract in patients receiving cytotoxic chemotherapy. Factors such as granulocytopenia and disruption of normal mucosal epithelial integrity promote this invasion.

Most cases of nosocomial candidosis are classified as type II as the infecting organism is considered part of the normal flora and progresses from colonization to infection. This pattern contrasts with the airborne and contact transmission of conidia applicable to type I infections due to *Aspergillus* and the Mucoraceae. Nevertheless, there are well-documented outbreaks of nosocomial candidosis in which transmission from the hospital environment (i.e., type I) also has been clearly demonstrated (Solomon et al. 1984, 1986; Weems et al. 1987; Plouffe et al. 1977).

C. albicans is the most frequently isolated nosocomial species of *Candida. C. tropicalis* is a more virulent pathogen in granulocytopenic patients than in nongranulocytopenic hosts (Horn et al. 1985; Walsh and Merz 1986; Wingard et al. 1979). *C. krusei* also has been associated with granulocytopenic patients receiving intensive cytotoxic chemotherapy (Merz et al. 1986). *C. parapsilosis* is frequently associated with infections of vascular catheters, especially those used for total parenteral nutrition. *C. guillermondi* and *C. lusitaniae* may be highly resistant to amphotericin B; both species have caused fungemia refractory to amphotericin B in granulocytopenic patients (Dick et al. 1980, 1985; Pappagianis et al. 1979). A recent study showed that the minimum inhibitory concentrations (MICs) of amphotericin B in *Candida* spp. isolated from granulocytopenic bone marrow transplant recipients were significantly higher than those isolated from nongranulocytopenic patients (Powderly et al. 1988). Moreover, isolates of *C. albicans* and *C. tropicalis* from positive blood culture with MICs > 0.8 μg/ml were associated with a fatal outcome in 10 of 10 patients, whereas fungemic isolates with MICs ≤ 0.8 μg/ml were fatal in 8 of 17 ($P = 0.04$).

3. Clinical Manifestations

Candidemia and certain syndromes of esophageal, hepatosplenic, mucocutaneous, CNS, and osteoarticular candidosis are especially relevant in cancer patients (Edwards et al. 1978; Thaler et al. 1988; Jarowski et al. 1978).

a) Candidemia

Candidemia is a common manifestation of disseminated candidosis in granulocytopenic patients. In our opinion, any blood culture positive for *Candida* in a granulocytopenic patient should be treated as representing disseminated candidosis. Horn et al. (1985) studied 200 episodes of fungemia in cancer patients and showed that fungemia in this patient population was associated with a 76% mortality. Among those patients autopsied, 72% had disseminated infection. Maksymiuk et al. (1984) studied 188 patients with systemic candidosis during a 4-year period. Patients with acute leukemia had the highest frequency of candidosis (11 of 100 patients) in comparison with those with lymphoma (1 of 100 patients). Blood cultures were positive in only 52% of patients with systemic candidosis. Survival was inversely related to the number of positive blood cultures, suggesting that a delay in treatment may further increase mortality.

Venous catheters, including central venous catheters and chronic indwelling silastic catheters, further contribute to the problem of candidemia in cancer patients (Klein and Watanakunakorn 1979; Turner et al. 1985; Rose 1978). *Candida* spp. may infect catheters by several routes: access to the intravascular portion of the catheter via contaminated solutions (type I nosocomial fungal infection); colonization of the percutaneous catheter wound (type II); or blood-borne *Candida* from another infected site. Peripheral venous catheters may also be the site for *Candida* suppurative thrombophlebitis and candidemia (Walsh et al. 1986a).

Blood cultures are frequently negative in the early stages of disseminated candidosis in granulocytopenic patients. Candidemia in granulocytopenic patients may become evident only after the infection has become well-established in the deep viscera. Several studies have shown that candidemia may be detected earlier and in a greater number of infected patients by means of the lysis centrifugation technique when compared with conventional broth techniques (Henry et al. 1983; Kiehn et al. 1983). The development of immunodiagnostic systems for *Candida* cell-wall or cytoplasmic antigens and chromatographic assays for the detection of fungal metabolites may become important adjuncts for improving early diagnosis and treatment follow-up of disseminated candidosis (Bennett 1987; De Repentigny and Reiss 1984).

Treatment of fungemia involving central venous catheters in our opinion should consist of removal of the catheter and administration of amphotericin B i.v.; the total dose of amphotericin B depends upon the probability that other sites may have been become infected.

b) Hematogenous Candida Endophthalmitis

Hematogenous *Candida* endophthalmitis (HCE) is a common complication of candidemia associated with vascular catheters (Montgomerie and Edwards 1978). Nongranulocytopenic patients with HCE have cottonball-like lesions, which extend from the chorioretina into the vitreous. These lesions are seldom present in granulocytopenic patients. Laboratory findings indicate that *Candida* does involve the eye during granulocytopenia but without typical ophthalmoscopically evident chorioretinal opacities due to the absence of granulocytic inflammation (Henderson et al. 1980; Aoki et al. 1987). Occasionally, HCE may become clinically evident, with vitreal opacifications and blurred vision in patients at the time of recovery from granulocytopenia. HCE should be treated with the combination of amphotericin B plus flucytosine. This combination in our opinion is also indicated in any granulocytopenic patient with CNS candidosis, renal candidosis, hepatosplenic candidosis, and *Candida* thrombophlebitis of the great veins.

c) Hepatosplenic Candidosis

Hepatosplenic candidosis in cancer patients is a complication of disseminated candidosis which has only been reported significantly within the past 10 years.

Thaler et al. (1988) recently reviewed 8 patients from the NCI and 65 others described in the literature. All but 5 of the 73 patients had a history of granulocytopenia, and 59 had acute leukemia. The clinical manifestations of hepatosplenic candidosis were usually apparent only after recovery from granulocytopenia. The underlying neoplastic disease was often in remission. Indeed, 21 of 68 (31%) evaluable patients had leukocytosis. Of these patients 34 (50%) had received some form of previous antifungal therapy, for systemic candidosis (in 6 patients) or for local *Candida* infection or fever with granulocytopenia (in 28 patients). Of these 68 patients 58 (85%) presented with fever and 39 (57%) with abdominal pain. An elevated serum alkaline phosphatase concentration was the most consistent biochemical abnormality.

CT examination appeared to be more sensitive than ultrasonography in detecting hepatic lesions. The two techniques may be complementary in certain cases. Magnetic resonance imaging offers another modality for identification. The hepatosplenic lesions range in diameter from approximately 1–2 mm (below the threshold of diagnostic imaging modalities) to several centimeters. A definitive diagnosis should be established by laparotomy and wedge biopsy. Laparoscopy-directed biopsy performed by a skilled physician is an alternative to laparotomy. Percutaneous needle biopsy is usually inadequate, often yielding normal liver or inflammatory tissue without fungal elements. A full wedge biopsy may reveal only scattered pseudohyphal fragments and blastoconidia in large areas of necrosis and inflammation. Culture of biopsy tissue is often negative, especially in patients who have received previous antifungal therapy.

We have suggested the combination of amphotericin B and flucytosine for the treatment of hepatosplenic candidosis. The total dose of amphotericin B usually required is at least 2 g in an adult, although total doses of as much as 9 g have sometimes been necessary. Progression of splenic lesions during the course of antifungal therapy may warrant splenectomy (Helton et al. 1986; Johnson and Raff 1984).

A liposomal formulation of amphotericin B was recently reported to be successful in the treatment of hepatosplenic candidosis (Lopez-Berestein et al. 1987). Despite the high total doses administered, there was virtually no nephrotoxicity, myelotoxicity, or neurotoxicity. The liposomal formulations of amphotericin B may not necessarily be more fungicidal but may be less toxic than amphotericin B desoxycholate. Further investigation of liposomal formulations of amphotericin B are necessary to establish optimal stability, safety, antifungal activity, and feasibility of large scale commercial production (see Chap. 10).

d) Esophageal Candidosis

The pathogenesis, diagnosis, and treatment of esophageal candidosis have been reviewed elsewhere (Walsh et al. 1988). Esophageal candidosis is a common infection in cancer patients and is definitively diagnosed by the culture and histopathology of an endoscopically directed mucosal biopsy. Febrile, granulocytopenic patients with biopsy-proven esophageal candidosis should receive amphotericin B i.v. for the duration of their granulocytopenia. Our approach to patients who have symptoms of esophagitis but who are not endoscopy candidates is to administer an empirical combination of oral clotrimazole and acyclovir i.v. If there is no clinical response within 48 h, then amphotericin B i.v. is instituted.

e) Candida Epiglottitis

Candida epiglottitis has only recently been well characterized in granulocytopenic cancer patients (WALSH and GRAY 1987). It presents initially as refractory odynophagia in the hypopharyngeal and epiglottic regions. The patient may point directly to these areas as the most intense locations of pain. Laryngeal stridor may develop in more advanced cases. Diagnosis is corroborated by laryngoscopy-guided visualization and swabbing of the epiglottis. The swab material is cultured, smeared, stained, and examined microscopically. Treatment consists of amphotericin B.

f) Candida Cholecystitis

Candida cholecystitis may develop in cancer patients who have recently undergone abdominal surgery and have received broad-spectrum antibiotics (ADAMSON et al. 1990). The treatment of choice is surgical drainage and amphotericin B i.v. Biliary concentrations of amphotericin B exceed those in serum two to fourfold.

4. Treatment

a) Empirical Amphotericin B in Persistently Febrile Granulocytopenic Patients

As previously discussed, disseminated fungal infections in granulocytopenic patients carry a high mortality. Fungemia or other signs of established systemic fungal infection may not be detected in the granulocytopenic host until the infection is refractory to treatment. The problems of clinical detection and concomitant delay in the treatment of invasive fungal infections in granulocytopenic patients prompted a clinical trial of early empirical amphotericin B in persistently or recurrently febrile granulocytopenic patients in a randomized clinical trial at the NCI (PIZZO et al. 1982). Granulocytopenic patients who are persistently or newly febrile on or after day 7 of initial empirical antibiotic therapy were randomized to (1) discontinuation of antibiotics, (2) continuation of antibiotics, or (3) addition of amphotericin B. Those receiving amphotericin B had fewer invasive fungal infections than those who did not. Nonrandomized clinical studies by other investigators, as summarized by HOLLERAN et al. (1985), corroborated the benefit of amphotericin B in febrile granulocytopenic patients.

When the period of conventional pathogen-directed antifungal therapy (1975–1981) was compared with that of amphotericin B therapy (1982–1985) in comparable patient populations at the NCI, the mortality due to systemic candidosis declined from 63% (33/52) to 23% (7/30), respectively. Amphotericin B also has been successfully incorporated into a modifiable empirical antibiotic program (Pizzo et al. 1986). This approach to antifungal therapy provides early treatment for patients with a high risk of clinically occult invasive mycoses.

b) Combination Antifungal Therapy

The most useful combination of antifungal agents in cancer patients is that of amphotericin B plus flucytosine. This combination is frequently synergistic against *Candida* in vitro and in vivo, depending upon the strain. Flucytosine achieves a high concentration in the urine and CSF, thereby permitting further antifungal activity at these sites. We use the combination in our center for renal candidosis, *Candida* endophthalmitis, CNS candidosis, and refractory candidosis (as may occur with disseminated infection). As previously mentioned, the combination is useful in the management of hepatosplenic candidosis.

V. Trichosporonosis

Trichosporon beigelii may normally colonize the skin and alimentary tract, may cause white piedra in normal hosts, and causes a frequently lethal disseminated infection in granulocytopenic cancer patients (Anaissie et al. 1985; Walsh et al. 1986b). The lungs, kidneys, skin, and eyes are the main targets of this pathogen. A fungemia refractory to amphotericin B therapy may develop. Serum, plasma, and CSF from patients with disseminated trichosporonosis may react in the cryptococcal latex agglutination test due to antigens shared between *T. beigelii* and *C. neoformans*. Early initiation of treatment with high dose amphotericin B and recovery from granulocytopenia are important factors for survival from trichosporonosis in cancer patients.

VI. Malassezia furfur Fungemia

Malassezia furfur (*Pityrosporum obiculare*) is considered part of the normal skin flora and is the cause of tinea versicolor. *M. furfur* may infect central venous catheters, especially those used for TPN parenteral lipid emulsions, which is another example of a type IIA nosocomial fungal infection. *M. furfur* is lipophilic and grows best in vitro and in vivo in a lipid-rich microenvironment. Usually, *M. furfur*-associated catheter sepsis has developed in patients receiving parenteral lipid emulsions. A syndrome of progressive pulmonary infiltrates, hypoxia, and thrombocytopenia was originally described in neonates (Redline et al. 1985). *M. furfur* fungemia, however, may also develop in adults with neoplastic diseases. Infection of other tissue sites, such as the kidneys and eyes, generally does not occur. Treatment consists of discontinuing the parenteral lipid emulsion and removal of the central venous catheter. Systemic antifungal therapy is seldom effective unless these two measures are implemented. Nonimmunocompromised patients seldom require systemic antifungal therapy once the lipid emulsion is discontinued and the central catheter removed. If an antifungal agent is considered necessary in a granulocytopenic cancer patient, a systemic antifungal azole such as ketoconazole would be considered more active than amphotericin B.

VII. Reactivation of Latent Fungal Infections

The development of histoplasmosis and coccidioidomycosis in granulocytopenic cancer patients is unusual. Nevertheless, patients from endemic areas who receive corticosteroids as part of their antineoplastic therapy may reactivate these latent fungal infections (DERESINSKI and STEVENS 1977; DRUTZ 1983; WALSH et al. 1983). This form of nosocomial fungal infection is classified as type IIB. Disseminated histoplasmosis and coccidioidomycosis in cancer patients may be especially virulent. Early diagnosis and initiation of therapy are essential. Amphotericin B should be initiated promptly in granulocytopenic patients with suspected or proven histoplasmosis or coccidioidomycosis. We suggest that amphotericin B for coccidioidomycosis should be continued throughout the entire course of cycles of antineoplastic therapy.

VIII. Fungal Infections in Patients with Combined Neoplastic Diseases and AIDS

Patients with AIDS may develop large cell lymphomas requiring antineoplastic therapy. The most common systemic fungal infections complicating AIDS are cryptococcosis, histoplasmosis, and coccidioidomycosis (MINAMOTO and ARMSTRONG 1988; GRANT and ARMSTRONG 1988; GLATT et al. 1988). Amphotericin B generally does not cure these infections in patients with AIDS but only brings about clinical remission; maintenance antifungal therapy is therefore necessary to prevent relapse of infection. Amphotericin B is usually used for the initial treatment of these infections. Maintenance therapy consists of weekly or twice weekly amphotericin B or daily fluconazole for cryptococcosis. The role of azoles in maintenance therapy for coccidioidomycosis and histoplasmosis in AIDS is investigational.

D. Future Directions

In the foregoing discussion we have described the various mycoses which may cause problems in cancer patients and the current chemotherapeutic approach to treating these conditions. We are, however, living in an exciting era of change and new developments which may revolutionize the prophylaxis and treatment of our patients. Among the compounds in development may be mentioned itraconazole and fluconazole (see Chaps. 17 and 19), another azole, SCH 39,304, a cell-wall inhibitor, cilofungin (see Chap. 22), and liposomal formulations of amphotericin B which allow increased dosage with a marked reduction in toxicity (see Chaps. 10 and 18).

The trend of increasing nosocomial fungal infections in granulocytopenic patients will continue as aggressive interventions increase and the population of high risk patients expands. Comprehensive research efforts directed at improved prevention, diagnosis, and treatment of fungal infections complicating granulocytopenia will require effort in the following areas: (1) environmental and nosocomial infection control; (2) rapidly performed, highly predictive, immunodiagnostic and biochemical assays for early diagnosis and treatment follow-up of invasive fungal infections; (3) augmentation of host defenses with immunomodulatory agents; (4) more effective, pharmacologically versatile, antifungal agents with less toxicity; and (5) elucidation of the pathogenesis and biology of the well-recognized and newly emerging nosocomial fungal infections in granulocytopenic patients.

References

Adam RD, Paquin ML, Petersen EA, Sauballe MA, Rinaldi MG (1986) Phaeohyphomycosis caused by the fungal genera *Bipolaris* and *Exserohilum*. A report of 9 cases and review of the literature. Medicine 65:203–217

Adamson P, Rinaldi MG, Pizzo PA, Walsh TJ (1990) Amphotericin B in the treatment of *Candida* cholecystitis. Rev Infect Digest (in press)

Aisner J, Schimpff SC, Bennett JE, Young VM, Wiernik PH (1976) *Aspergillus* infections in cancer patients: association with fireproofing materials in a new hospital. JAMA 235:411–412

Allo MD, Miller J, Townsend T, Tan C (1987) Primary cutaneous aspergillosis associated with Hickman intravenous catheters. N Engl J Med 317:1105–1108

Anaissie EA, Hoy J, Jones P, Rolston K, Bodey GP (1985) New fungal pathogens in immunocompromised patients. 25th Intersci Conf Antimicrob Agents Chemother, Minneapolis, Abstr 870, p 253

Aoki S, Walsh TJ, Mechinaud F, Rubin M, Pizzo PA (1987) Effects of granulocytopenia and antifungal therapy in an experimental rabbit model of *Candida* endophthalmitis. 27th Intersci Conf Antimicrob Agents Chemother, New York, Abstr 775, p 232

Armstrong DA (1984) Protected environments are discomforting and expensive and do not offer meaningful protection. Am J Med 76:685–689

Bennett JE (1987) Rapid diagnosis of candidiasis and aspergillosis. Rev Infect Dis 9:398–402

Bodey GP (1984) Current status of prophylaxis of infection with protected environments. Am J Med 76:678–684

Burch PA, Karp JE, Merz WG, Kuhlman JE, Fishman EK (1987) Favorable outcome of invasive aspergillosis in patients with acute leukemia. J Clin Oncol 5:1985–1993

Chaulk CP, Smith PW, Feagler JR, Verdirame J, Commers JR (1986) Fungemia due to *Fusarium solani* in an immunocompromised child. Pediatr Infect Dis 5:363–366

Commers J, Robichaud KJ, Pizzo PA (1984) New pulmonary infiltrates in granulocytopenic patients being treated with antibiotics. Pediatr Infect Dis 3:423–428
De Repentigny L, Reiss E (1984) Current trends in immunodiagnosis of candidiasis and aspergillosis. Rev Infect Dis 6:301–312
Deresinski SC, Stevens DA (1977) Coccidioidomycosis in compromised hosts. Medicine 54:377–395
Dick JD, Merz WC, Saral R (1980) Incidence of polyene-resistant yeasts recovered from clinical specimens. Antimicrob Agents Chemother 18:158–163
Dick JD, Rosengard BR, Merz WG, Stuart RK, Hutchins GM, Saral R (1985) Fatal disseminated candidiasis due to amphotericin B resistant *Candida guilliermondii*. Ann Int Med 102:67–68
Dixon DM, Polak A, Walsh TJ (1988) Phaeaohyphomycosis. In: Torres-Rodríguez JM (ed) Proceedings of the X congress of the international society for human and animal mycology(-ISHAM). JR Prous, Barcelona, pp 84–92
Drutz DJ (1983) Amphotericin B in the treatment of coccidioidomycosis. Drugs 26:337–346
Edwards JE, Lehrer RI, Stiehm ER, Fischer TJ, Young LS (1978) Severe candidal infections. Clinical perspective, immune defense mechanisms, and current concepts of therapy. Ann Intern Med 89:91–106
England AC, Weinstein M, Ellner JJ, Ajello L (1981) Two cases of rhinocerebral zygomycosis (mucormycosis) with common epidemiologic and environmental features. Am Rev Respir Dis 124:497–498
Everett ED, Pearson S, Rogers W (1979) *Rhizopus* surgical wound infection associated with elasticized adhesive tape dressings. Arch Surg 114:738–739
Gartenberg G, Bottone EJ, Keusch GT, Weitzman (1987) Hospital-acquired mucormycosis (*Rhizopus rhizopodiformis*) of skin and subcutaneous tissue. N Engl J Med 299:1115–1118
Gerson SL, Talbot GH, Hurwitz S, Strom BL, Lusk EJ (1984) Prolonged granulocytopenia: the major risk factor for invasive pulmonary aspergillosis in patients with acute leukemia. Ann Int Med 100:345–351
Glatt AE, Chirgwin K, Landesman SH (1988) Current concepts: treatment of infections asociated with human immunodeficiency virus. N Engl J Med 318:1439–1448
Grant IH, Armstrong D (1988) Fungal infections in AIDS. Cryptococcosis. Infect Dis Clin NA 2:457–464
Helton WS, Carrico CJ, Zaveruha PA, Schaller R (1986) Diagnosis and treatment of splenic fungal abscesses in the immunosuppressed patient. Arch Surg 121:580–586
Henderson DK, Hockley LJ, Vukalcic LJ, Edwards JE (1980) Effect of immunosuppression on the development of experimental hematogenous *Candida* endophthalmitis. Infect Immun 27:628–631
Henry NK, McLimans CA, Wright AJ, Thompson RL, Wilson WR, Washington JA (1983) Microbiologic and clinical evaluation of the isolator lysis-centrifugation blood culture tube. J Clin Microbiol 17:864–869
Holleran WM, Wilbur JR, DeGregorio MW (1985) Empiric amphotericin B therapy in patients with acute leukemia. Rev Infect Dis 7:619–624
Horn R, Wong B, Kiehn TE, Armstrong D (1985) Fungemia in a cancer hospital: changing frequency, earlier onset, and results of therapy. Rev Infect Dis 7: 646–655
Jarowski CI, Fialk MA, Murray HW, Gottlieb GJ, Coleman M, Steinberg CR, Silver RT (1978) Fever, rash, and muscle tenderness. Arch Int Med 138:544–546
Johnson JD, Raff MJ (1984) Fungal splenic abscess. arch Int Med 144:1987–1993
June CH, Beatty PG, Schulman HM, Rinaldi MG (1986) Disseminated *Fusarium moniliforme* infection after allogeneic marrow transplantation. S Med J 79: 513–515
Kiehn TE, Wong B, Edwards EF, Armstrong D (1983) Comparative recovery of

bacteria and yeasts from lysis-centrifugation and a conventional blood culture system. J Clin Microbiol 18:300–304
Kiehn TE, Nelson PE, Bernard EM, Edwards FF, Koziner B, Armstrong D (1985) Catheter-associated fungemia caused by *Fusarium chlamydosporum* in a patient with lymphocytic lymphoma. J Clin Microbiol 21:501–504
Klein JJ, Watanakunakorn C (1979) Hospital-acquired fungemia: its natural course and clinical significance. Am J Med 67:51–58
Krasinski K, Holzman RS, Hanna B, Greco MA, Graff M, Bhogal M (1985) Nosocomial fungal infection during hospital renovation. Infect Control 6:278–282
Kwon-Chung KJ, Young RC, Orlando MV (1975) Pulmonary mucormycosis caused by *Cunninghamella elegans* in a patient with chronic myelogenous leukemia. Am J Clin Pathol 64:544–548
Lehrer RI, Howard DH, Sypherd PS, Edwards JE, Segal GP, Winston DJ (1980) Mucormycosis. Ann Int Med 93:93–108
Lopez-Berestein G, Bodey GP, Frankel LS, Menta K (1987) Treatment of hepatosplenic candidiasis with liposomal amphotericin B. J Clin Oncol 5:310–317
Lutwick LI, Rytel MW, Yanez JP, Galgiani JN, Stevens DA (1979) Deep infections from *Petriellidium boydii* treated with miconazole. JAMA 241:272–273
Mahoney DH, Steuber CP, Starling KA, Barrett FF, Goldberg J, Fernbach DJ (1979) An outbreak of aspergillosis in children with acute leukemia. J Pediatr 95:70–72
Maksymiuk AW, Thongprasert S, Hopfer R, Luna M, Fainstein V, Bodey GP (1984) Systemic candidiasis in cancer patients. Am J Med 77:20–27
Merz WG, Karp JE, Schron D, Saral R (1986) Increased incidence of fungemia caused by *Candida krusei*. J Clin Microbiol 24:581–584
Meunier F, Leleux A, Gerain J, Ninove D, Snoeck R, Klastersky J (1987) Prophylaxis of aspergillosis in neutropenic cancer patients with nasal spray of amphotericin B: a prospective randomized study. 27th Intersci Conf Antimicrob Agents Chemother, New York, Abstr 1346, p 331
Meyer RD, Rosen P, Armstrong D (1972) Phycomycosis complicating leukemia and lymphoma. Ann Intern Med 77:871–879
Meyer RD, Young LS, Armstrong D, Yu B (1973) Aspergillosis complicating neoplastic disease. Am J Med 54:6–15
Minamoto G, Armstrong D (1988) Fungal infections in AIDS. Histoplasmosis and coccidioidomycosis. Infect Dis Clin NA 2:447–456
Montgomerie JZ, Edwards JE (1978) Association of infection due to *Candida albicans* with intravenous hyperalimentation. J Infect Dis 137:197–201
Opal SM, Asp AA, Cannady PB, Morse PL, Burton LJ, Hammer PG (1986) Effect of infection control measures during a nosocomial outbreak of disseminated aspergillosis associated with hospital construction. J Infect Dis 153:634–637
Panos RJ, Barr LF, Walsh TJ, Silverman HJ (1988) Factors associated with fatal hemoptysis in cancer patients. Chest 94:1008–1013
Pappagianis D, Collins MS, Hector R, Remington J (1979) Development of resistance to amphotericin B in *Candida lusitaniae* infecting a human. Antimicrob Agents Chemother 16:123–126
Peterson PK, McGlave P, Ramsay NKC, Rhame F, Cohen E, Perry GS, Goldman AI, Kersey J (1983) A prospective study of infectious diseases following bone marrow transplantation: emergence of *Aspergillus* and cytomegalovirus as the major causes of mortality. Infect Control 4:81–89
Pizzo PA, Robichaud KJ, Gill FA, Witebsky F (1982) Empiric antibiotic and antifungal therapy for cancer patients with prolonged fever and granulocytopenia. Am J Med 72:101–110
Pizzo PA, Hathorn JW, Hiemenz J, Browne M, Commers J, Cotton D, Gress J, Longo D, Marshall D, McNight J, Ribin M, Skelton J, Thaler M, Wesley R (1986) A randomized trial comparing ceftazidime alone with combination antibiotic therapy in cancer patients with fever and neutropenia. N Engl J Med 315:552–558

Plouffe JF, Brown DG, Silva J Jr, Eck T, Stricof RL, Fekety R (1977) Nosocomial outbreak of *Candida parapsilosis* fungemia related to intravenous infusions. Arch Int Med 137:1686–1689

Powderly WG, Kobayashi GS, Herzig GP, Medoff G (1988) Amphotericin B-resistant yeast infection in severely immunocompromised patients. Am J Med 84:826–832

Prystowsky SD, Vogelstein B, Ettinger DS, Merz WG, Kaizer H, Sulica VI, Zinkham WH (1976) Invasive aspergillosis. N Engl J Med 295:655–658

Redline RW, Redline SS, Roxenbaum B, Dahms BB (1985) Systemic *Malassezia furfur* infection in patients receiving intralipid therapy. Hum Pathol 16:815–822

Rhame FS (1985) Lessons from the Roswell Park bone marrow transplant aspergillosis outbreak. Infect Control 6:345–346

Rippon JW (1988) Pseudallescheriasis. In: Rippon JW (ed) Medical mycology, 3rd edn. Saunders, Philadelphia, pp 651–680

Rogers TR (1986) Infections in hematologic malignancy. Infect Control 7:140–142

Rose HD (1978) Venous catheter-associated candidemia. Am J Med Sci 275:265–270

Rosen PP, Sternberg SS (1976) Decreased frequency of aspergillosis and mucormycosis. N Engl J Med 295:1319–1320

Rotstein C, Cummings KM, Tidings J, Killion K, Powell E, Gustafson TL, Higby D (1985) An outbreak of invasive aspergillosis among allogeneic bone marrow transplants: a case control study. Infect Control 6:347–355

Schaffner A, Davis CE, Schaffner T, Markert M, Douglas H, Braude AI (1986) In vitro susceptibility of fungi to killing by neutrophil granulocytes discriminates between primary pathogenicity and opportunism. J Clin Invest 78:511–524

Sheldon DL, Johnson WC (1979) Cutaneous mucormycosis. Two documented cases of suspected nosocomial cause. JAMA 241:1032–1034

Smith AG, Crain SM, Dejongh C, Thomas GM, Vigorito RD (1985) Systemic pseudallescheriasis in a patient with acute myelocytic leukemia. Mycopathologia 90:85–89

Solomon SL, Khabbaz RF, Parker RH, Anderson RL, Geraghty MA, Furman RM, Martone WJ (1984) An outbreak of *Candida parapsilosis* bloodstream infections in patients receiving parenteral nutrition. J Infect Dis 149:98–107

Solomon SL, Alexander H, Eley JW, Anderson RL, Goodpasture HC, Smart S, Furman RM, Martone WJ (1986) Nosocomial fungemia in neonates associated with intravascular pressure monitoring devices. Pediatr Infect Dis J 5:680–685

Thaler M, Pastakia B, Shawker TH, O'Leary TO, Pizzo PA (1988) Hepatic candidiasis in cancer patients: the evolving picture of the syndrome. Ann Int Med 108:88–100

Turner RB, Donowitz LG, Hendley JO (1985) Consequences of candidemia for pediatric patients. Am J Dis Child 139:178–180

Viollier A-F, Peterson DE, De Jongh CA, Newman KA, Gray WC, Sutherland JC, Moody MA, Schimpff SC (1986) *Aspergillus* sinusitis in cancer patients. Cancer 58:366–371

Walsh TJ, Gray W (1987) *Candida* epiglottitis in immunocompromised patients. Chest 91:482–485

Walsh TJ, Merz WG (1986) Pathologic features in the human alimentary tract associated with invasiveness of *Candida tropicalis.* Am J Clin Pathol 85:498–502

Walsh TJ, Pizzo PA (1988) Nosocomial fungal infections: a classification for hospital-acquired fungal infections mycoses arising from endogenous flora or reactivation. Ann Rev Microbiol 42:517–545

Walsh TJ, Catchatourian R, Cohen H (1983) Disseminated histoplasmosis complicating bone marrow transplantation. Am J Clin Pathol 79:509–511

Walsh TJ, Caplan LR, Hier DB (1985) *Aspergillus* infections of the central nervous system: a clinicopathologic analysis. Ann Neurol 18:574–582

Walsh TJ, Bustamente CI, Vlahov D, Standiford HC (1986a) Candidal suppurative peripheral thrombophlebitis, recognition, prevention, and management. Infect Control 7:16–22

Walsh TJ, Newman KR, Moody M, Wharton RC, Wade JC (1986b) Trichosporonosis in patients with neoplastic disease. Medicine 65:268–279

Walsh TJ, Hamilton SR, Belitsos N (1988) Esophageal candidiasis. Diagnosis and treatment of an increasingly recognized fungal infection. Postgrad Med 84:193–205

Weems JJ, Chamberland ME, Ward J, Willy M, Padhye AA, Solomon SL (1987) *Candida parapsilosis* fungemia associated with parenteral nutrition and contaminated blood pressure transducers. J Clin Microbiol 25:1029–1032

Wingard JR, Merz WG, Saral R (1979) *Candida tropicalis*: a major pathogen in immunocompromised patients. Ann Int Med 91:539–543

Wingard JR, Dick JD, Merz WG, Sanford GR, Saral R, Burns WH (1980) Pathogenecity of *C. tropicalis* and *C. albicans* after gastrointestinal inoculation in mice. Infect Immun 29:808–813

Yu VL, Muder RR, Poorsattar A (1986) Significance of isolation of *Aspergillus* from the respiratory tract in the diagnosis of invasive pulmonary aspergillosis. Results from a three-year prospective study. Am J Med 81:249–254

CHAPTER 17

Fungal Infections and AIDS

Bertrand Dupont

A. Introduction

Fungi feature prominently among the opportunistic organisms which can cause disease during the development of infection with HIV virus. The fungi encountered are the same as those found in other situations characterized by depressed cell-mediated immunity. Some mycoses are superficial – cutaneous or mucocutaneous – and generally benign, e.g. candidosis, dermatophytosis, pityrosporosis; others are deep-seated and potentially serious, e.g. cryptococcosis, histoplasmosis, coccidioidomycosis (Armstrong 1988; Holmberg and Meyer 1986; Schaffner 1984; Spencer and Jackson 1989). Aspergillosis and disseminated candidosis are rarely found in this situation, but a number of more obscure fungal infections are now being reported in the literature.

By their unexpected occurrence, relapsing nature or resistance to treatment, fungal superinfections are often the first indication of an underlying AIDS problem. Less severe (thrush) or more serious (cryptococcosis) infections have prognostic significance and may indicate the stage of development from HIV infection to full-blown AIDS (Holmberg and Meyer 1986; Klein et al. 1984). As with other infections, mycoses possibly play a co-factor role in the development of AIDS: activation of T_4 lymphocytes due to stimulation by fungal antigens may enhance cellular infection by the virus, and the fungal infection itself may occasionally cause immunosuppression.

B. Candidosis

Candidosis is the most frequently encountered fungal infection associated with AIDS (Barr and Torosian 1986; Holmberg and Meyer 1986; Torssander et al. 1987); *Candida albicans* is responsible for almost all the infections, and its origin appears to be endogenous. There have not, however, been any epidemiological studies concerning possible sources of infection, mode of transmission or pathogenicity of the particular strains isolated.

The most frequent clinical manifestation is oral thrush, which is often preceded for several weeks or months by asymptomatic carriage. The lesions are sometimes located at the rear of the buccal cavity and are frequently very widespread. In our experience with HIV-positive subjects, white plaques of more or less confluent thrush are not limited to the tongue but are found also covering the lining of the cheeks, palate and/or gums. This distribution helps in differential diagnosis from a simple dirty tongue or hairy leucoplakia. Functional effects are variable, from absence of symptoms to a scalded buccal cavity to a pharyngeal dysphagia which makes eating difficult. There may be associated angular cheilitis (perlèche). The presence of thrush indicates stage IVC_2 of the CDC classfication of AIDS. The occurrence of unforeseen and repeated thrush in a subject without known or admitted risk factors should alert the physician to the possibility of HIV infection. The unexpected appearance of thrush is an indication of the progression of an HIV infection (KLEIN et al. 1984). In our experience, all patients presenting with this type of condition have progressed over a period of months or years to full-blown AIDS. Numerous studies have shown a high frequency of opportunistic infections or Kaposi's sarcoma among patients first presenting with thrush (KLEIN et al. 1984).

Candidal oesophagitis manifests itself by a painful retrosternal dysphagia and is often associated with buccal thrush. Some cases are febrile and may have associated blood-stained vomit. Sometimes the oesophagitis is completely asymptomatic and is only discovered on endoscopy (CLOTET et al. 1986; JOY 1984; TAVITIAN et al. 1986). Fiberscopic exploration, taking material for culture and biopsy, aids in diagnosis (WHEELER et al. 1987). In our experience, diagnosis can usually be made on the basis of oropharyngeal thrush associated with retrosternal dysphagia. If symptoms persist beyond 5–7 days in spite of systemic anti-candidal treatment, we carry out further endoscopy to look for an alternative explanation such as herpes or cytomegalovirus. Candidal oesophagitis puts the infection in stage IVC_1 (full-blown AIDS) of the CDC classification of AIDS.

The CDC classification is arbitrary. Some patients show thrush and transient oesophagitis when first infected with HIV (stage I) (PEDERSEN et al. 1987). On the whole the majority of patients classified as IVC_2 on the basis of thrush would also be found to have an associated latent oesophagitis, resulting in a classification as IVC_1 if systematic endoscopy is performed (CLOTET et al. 1986; JOY 1984; TAVITIAN et al. 1986).

Candidosis can contribute to the nutritional status of the patient but does not explain any diarrhoea. It is interesting that septicaemia or deep-seated infections with *Candida* do not occur, illustrating the role of phagocytosis in visceral dissemination. MATTHEWS et al. (1988) have shown that the presence or production of antibodies to the 47Kd antigen of *C. albicans* plays a role in the prevention of dissemination. These antibodies are found in HIV-positive patients and in those suffering from chronic mucocutaneous candidosis but are frequently absent in fatal infections in leucopenic patients. Only the latter are susceptible to disseminated candidosis. In rare cases of deep-seated candidosis in HIV-positive patients, other associated factors such as catheterization or iatrogenic agranulocytosis are usually responsible. Recovery of yeasts by bronchoalveolar lavage is without diagnostic significance and does not allow diagnosis of pulmonary candidosis ahead of radiological investigation.

Table 1. Treatment schedule of oropharyngeal and esophageal candidosis in HIV-positive patients

Drugs	Dose per day	Duration	Remarks
Nystatin (topical)	10^6 units × 5	2–3 weeks	These drugs can be used for first episode thrush when patient's compliance is good, and as preventive therapy
Amphotericin B (topical)	200–400 mg × 5	2–3 weeks	
Clotrimazole (troche)	5–10 mg × 3–5	2–3 weeks	
Miconazole (buccal gel)	× 3–5	2–3 weeks	
Ketoconazole (oral)	200–400 mg	10–15 days	Used for relapsing or chronic thrush or oesophagitis and for preventive therapy
Fluconazole (oral)	50–100 mg	10–15 days	
Amphotericin B (i.v.)	15–20 mg	10–15 days	

Vaginal candidosis occurs much less frequently than oral thrush (Rhoads et al. 1987); onychomycosis and candidal intertrigo are likewise rare. Among the majority of patients delayed cutaneous hypersensitivity tests are negative; serological precipitation tests are of little interest.

Treatment of the first episode of oral thrush or pharyngitis may be with topical antifungals (Table 1). Whatever the drug used, it should be formulated so as to allow prolonged contact with the affected mucosa. Medication should be given 4–6 times a day, administered apart from meals, swallowed after several minutes contact with the lesions and should be continued for 2–3 weeks. Suitable drugs include the polyenes, amphotericin B and nystatin, or the topical azoles, clotrimazole and miconazole. Numerous commercial formulations are available in different countries as suspensions, powders, oral gels and tablets for chewing or sucking.

When thrush appears during antibiotic, antitubercular or antiparasitic treatment, antifungal medication should be given for a prolonged period of time covering the duration of the other medication. In practice, clinical control is sufficient. Mycological investigation shows an abundance of blastospores and mycelia when fresh smears are examined in 10% KOH, and confluent cultures are obtained. After several days of treatment the fungal population is reduced considerably. At the end of treatment a direct smear may be negative or may show no more than a few blastospores. Cultures may be negative or show rare colonies. In patients showing the persistence of 50–100 colonies on culture in spite of apparent clinical control of the thrush, rapid relapse of the condition may be anticipated.

In cases of relapse of oropharyngeal candidosis, the same topical treatment may be used. Overall patient compliance is likely to be poor due to the disagreeable taste of the medications and the necessity of frequent repeated application. An alternative is to give ketoconazole tablets 200–400 mg per day for 10-day periods or for a longer period of time during prolonged antibiotic or sulphonamide treatment. In cases of relapsing or chronic oropharyngeal candidosis, topical antifungal treatment is likely to be less effective and may in fact be refused by the patient. Recourse to ketoconazole is a suitable alternative, 200–400 mg daily over several months usually becoming necessary during the terminal stages of HIV infection (Table 1).

Certain problems, however, are associated with ketoconazole: the cost is high, and there may be interference with other drugs such as antacids, H_2 blockers or rifampicin (CLISSOLD 1987). In some patients failure of ketoconazole may be ascribed to decreased acid secretion in the stomach and a failure of the drug to dissolve (LAKE-BAKAAR et al. 1988). It is nevertheless essential to establish patient compliance, particularly in cases with cerebral malfunction. Administration of ketoconazole with dilute acid or with Coca Cola may solve the problem of malabsorption. Particular care is needed if hypoglycemic sulphonamides or anti-vitamin K drugs are being used, since ketoconazole may potentiate their action. Adrenal insufficiency is another possibility (CLISSOLD 1987). In our experience, hepatic toxicity is rare, and moderate elevations of transaminases or alkaline phosphatase may have other explanations. In cases of doubt it may be prudent to suspend treatment with ketoconazole and try to reintroduce it later. If ketoconazole is ineffective, poorly tolerated or toxic, few alternatives are available. Topical antifungals will probably have been declined, and recourse to intravenous amphotericin B is unrealistic for prolonged treatment. Fluconazole, recently introduced commercially in some European countries, may provide an interesting and useful alternative (Table 2). In our experience it has shown efficacy in cases of thrush clinically resistant to ketoconazole. The dose is 50–100 mg per day. It is also an excellent prophylactic treatment using a dose of 50 mg on alternate days. In a randomised, multicentre clinical trial with 150 patients comparing the efficacy of 50 mg/day fluconazole with 200 mg/day ketoconazole, results were slightly better with fluconazole. (DE WIT et al. 1989; DUPONT et al., to be published). Treatment with antiviral agents or immunomodulators such as zidovudine in our experience reduces the frequency of relapse of oropharyngeal candidosis. One problem not yet resolved is the prophylaxis of patients without clinical thrush, but who show heavy parasitisation by direct examination or culture of material obtained from the mouth and throat. Our attitude

Table 2. Clinical efficacy of fluconazole in HIV-positive patients with symptomatic oropharyngeal candidosis

Symptoms	Number of patients	Number cured	Days of treatment for 100% clinical cure
Thrush	34	34	5
Glossitis	5	5	7
Perlèche	3	3	7
Oesophagitis[a]	4	4	5–7
Perlèche[a]	5	5	7

[a] associated with thrush or glossitis.

is not to treat such patients systematically; however, it may be theoretically desirable to limit for as long as possible antigenic stimulation of CD_4 lymphocytes by fungal antigens.

Treatment of candidal oesophagitis by topical antifungals is rarely effective. Ketoconazole by mouth at 200–400 mg daily is the treatment of choice (Table 1). The classic treatment with moderate doses of amphotericin B i.v. (15–20 mg daily for 10–15 days) is an alternative possibility (HOLMBERG and MEYER 1986). Fluconazole at 50–100 mg daily for 10–15 days has given excellent results and provides an alternative to ketoconazole in cases of clinical failure or contraindication (DUPONT and DROUHET 1988). An intravenous formulation of fluconazole at the same dosage is used in patients who vomit. The perlèche which generally accompanies oral thrush responds well to local treatment with topical antifungals as a cream or ointment in association with topical or systemic treament of the thrush. Vaginitis can be controlled by topical treatment with polyenes or azoles; we prefer treatment for 5–10 days rather than the shorter courses of treatment now available. Difficult cases can be managed by oral treatment with ketoconazole (200–400 mg/day) or fluconazole (100 mg/day).

C. Cryptococcosis

Depression of cell-mediated immunity due to diseases such as Hodgkin's disease or sarcoidosis favours infection with *Cryptococcus neoformans*; AIDS is an extreme example and is today the leading predisposing factor for cryptococcosis. The incidence of cryptococcosis in HIV-positive North Americans is 6%–10%, with a rather higher rate in Haitians and black Africans. Cryptococcosis is the fourth most important infection causing death in AIDS patients, and it is the meningeal form which occurs most frequently (ENG et al. 1986; KOVACS et al. 1985; ZUGER et al. 1988). Cryptococcosis can be the first indication of HIV infection or may complicate the development of an already recognised infection or may complicate the development of an already recognised infection. Thus, CHUCK and SANDE (1989) observed cryptococcosis in 7% of 2087 AIDS patients seen over a 7-year period; in 45% of the cases of cryptococcosis, the fungal infection had been the first clinical manifestation of AIDS. The disease often runs an acute course, with marked symptoms of meningitis and/or encephalitis. However, as with non-HIV-positive patients, recognisable symptoms are sometimes limited to fever or headache. Likewise, neurological disease can exist with no recognisable clinical symptoms and is only confirmed by lumbar puncture provoked by the finding of a positive blood culture, broncho-alveolar lavage, cutaneous biopsy, or detection of antigen in the serum (BOURÉE et al. 1984; ROUX et al. 1985, 1986; VIVIANI and TORTORANO 1986).

Infection outside the nervous system is frequent, autopsy often showing marked dissemination to the lungs (GALL et al. 1986; MORIN et al. 1987; ROUX et al. 1987), lymph nodes, spleen, and liver (DISMUKES 1988; ENG et al. 1986; KOVACS et al. 1985; SPENCER and JACKSON 1989). Blood culture is positive in around 50% of cases, and the finding of cutaneous manifestations and yeasts in the urine suggests a systemic infection (BRANDICOURT et al. 1986; ROUX et al. 1985). One of the peculiarities of the cerebrospinal fluid (CSF) during the course of meningo-encephalitis is the frequent absence of any indication of an inflammatory response. The CSF may appear completely normal (KOVACS et al. 1985) on biochemical or cellular analysis, although in the majority of patients numerous yeasts can be found by direct microscopy or by culture. Cryptococcal antigen is present in frequently high titre and forms an invaluable aid to diagnosis. Intracerebral lesions (cryptococcomas), which can be detected by direct scanning, are rare.

Epidemiological studies show exclusively serotypes A or D, including geographical regions in which serotypes B and C are clinically predominant in non-HIV-positive patients (BOTTONE et al. 1987; SHIMIZU et al. 1986); there are few exceptions to this rule (KAPEND'A et al. 1987). Infection is characterized by a high mortality in spite of treatment, a relapse rate exceeding 60% in some studies and survival rarely exceeding 1 year (KOVACS et al. 1985). A fall in serum and CSF antigen during treatment suggests a good prognosis, although some subjects with an apparent cure of their meningitis continue to show a positive titre of around 1/100 (personal observations).

The treatment generally advised during the course of AIDS is amphotericin B i.v. at the rate of 0.5–1 mg/kg over 24 h (ARMSTRONG 1988). Because of its potential toxicity, the addition of 5-fluorocytosine (5-FC) is not usually recommended, but if given the daily dose should be no more than 100 mg/kg, and dosing should not be carried on beyond the first 10–15 days of amphotericin treatment. Toxic effects should be monitored by regular blood and liver function tests. Dosage should be adjusted so that peak 5-FC levels do not exceed 100 μg/ml and are preferably in the range 50–75 μg/ml (ARMSTRONG 1988). The duration of treatment with amphotericin B in AIDS is ill-defined. Given a favourable mycological response, a total dose of 1–2 g seems reasonable for therapy, but 0.5 mg/kg once or twice weekly or 100 mg once weekly should be continued prophylactically for life. Because of the toxicity associated with this classic treatment and poor patient compliance, great interest has been generated in the new antifungals with activity against *Cryptococcus*, particularly itraconazole and fluconazole (SAAG and DISMUKES 1988; GRANT and CLISSOLD 1989).

Itraconazole (Table 3) is a triazole which is very active in vitro against *Cr. neoformans*; 60.6% of strains are inhibited by 0.01 μg/ml and 100% by 0.1 μg/ml (VAN CUTSEM et al. 1987). However, in vitro results with azole derivatives are not necessarily indicative of activity in vivo (see Chap. 4). In animal models of infection using mice or guinea pigs VAN CUTSEM et al. (1987) have shown that treatment with itraconazole is able to prolong life, reduce the number of cfu (colony-forming units) recoverable on organ culture and produce negative brain cultures in an appreciable percentage of infected

Table 3. Biochemical and pharmacokinetic properties of three systemic azoles

	Molecular weight	Water soluble	Protein binding (%)	$t_{1/2}$ (h)	t_{max} (h)	urinary excretion	Percentage concentration (CSF/serum)
Ketoconazole	531	No	99	8	2–4	low	<10
Itraconazole	706	No	99	19	4	low	<10
Fluconazole	305	Yes	11	25	1	high	60–80

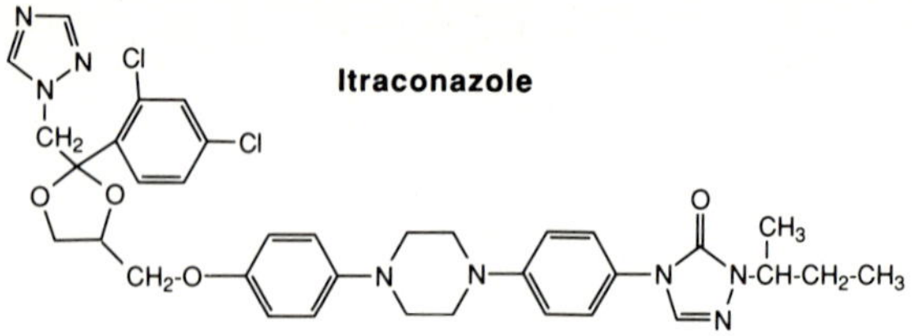

animals. In an experimental model of cryptococcal meningitis in cortisone-treated rabbits, PERFECT et al. (1986) found that itraconazole treatment results in an appreciable decline in the number of cfu recoverable from the CSF in spite of the apparently poor penetration of the drug into the CSF.

Publications concerning the treatment of cryptococcosis in AIDS patients with itraconazole are few in number. In three patients, one of whom had relapsed and another who failed to respond to amphotericin B plus 5-FC, treated with itraconazole at 200 mg daily for one month, clinical symptoms disappeared, and CSF cultures became negative (VIVIANI et al. 1987). Itraconazole has been used prophylactically to prevent relapse in five patients whose CSF had been sterilised by classic treatment with amphotericin B. Using a daily dosage of 200 mg for four patients and 400 mg daily for the fifth, no relapses were observed over a period of 3–12 months, and titres of cryptococcal antigen in the CSF fell during the period of observation (DE GANS et al. 1988). DENNING et al. (1989) reported favourably on the use of itraconazole at 400 mg daily in the suppression of cryptococcaemia in 10 patients, clinical and mycological cure in 10/15 patients meningitis, 2/2 cures of pulmonary infection and 3/5 cures of urinary tract infection.

Fluconazole is likewise a new triazole, but it is unique among these derivatives in its biochemical and pharmacokinetic profiles (Table 3). Of particular significance is its ability to penetrate the CSF, giving levels 70%–80% of those found in the serum (GRAYBILL 1987; SAAG and DISMUKES 1988). However, in vitro activity is poor; we have found MICs of 3–25 μg/ml for 30 isolates of *Cr. neoformans*. The activity of fluconazole in vitro is markedly inhibited by many of the constituents of the culture medium, and it provides the extreme example of the lack of in vitro-in vivo correlation discussed previously. Fluconazole prolongs the survival of mice inoculated intravenously

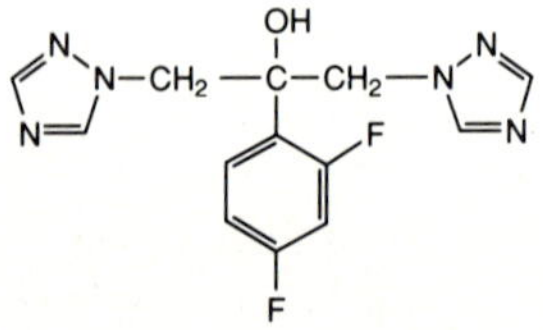

or intracerebrally with *Cr. neoformans* (GRAYBILL 1987). In the rabbit model of cryptococcal meningitis of PERFECT et al. (1986) previously mentioned, fluconazole showed comparable activity to itraconazole, causing a 1000-fold reduction of cfu in the CSF of some animals and bringing about complete sterilisation of the CSF in others.

Having experienced spectacular success in the treatment of one AIDS patient whose cryptococcal meningitis had relapsed following standard treatment with amphotericin B plus 5-FC (DUPONT and DROUHET 1987), we decided to treat a further series of patients. The results were so encouraging that we have extended the investigations to an open, multicentre French study. Thus, 35 AIDS patients with cryptococcal meningitis have been treated with oral or intravenous fluconazole; all had culture-positive CSF before treatment. After a loading dose of 400 mg, treatment was continued at 150–200 or in some cases 400 mg daily for 45–60 days. Three of the 29 patients died (at days 18, 50 and 51 days of treatment), two with progressive cryptococcosis. After 2 months of treatment 26/29 evaluable patients were still alive and asymptomatic or much improved; negative CSF cultures were obtained in 7/13 patients treated with 150–200 mg/day and in 11/13 treated with 400 mg/day. Prophylaxis using fluconazole at 100–200 mg/day has been practised in the 18 patients with culture-negative CSF. Two of them treated with 100 mg/day and one with 200 mg/day relapsed with culture-positive CSF; two have died. Seven of the 18 patients have died of causes other than cryptococcosis. Among the nine patients still living and on maintenance treatment, none have relapsed. Among those who have died, mean survival time from the start of fluconazole treatment was 5.6 months (range 2.4–13 months) and for those still living, 4.6 months (range 5–9 months).

As a result of these studies our recommendation is to treat with 400 mg fluconazole daily and following a response, to give a maintenance dose of 200 mg daily. Fluconazole is well tolerated. Other researchers have obtained similar good results in short series of patients (BYRNE and WAJSZCZUK 1988; VANT WOUT et al. 1988).

Recently, STERN et al. (1988) described a clinical and mycological response in 4/7 patients with doses of 50–400 mg daily; 3 of the 4 who responded had an active meningitis. They have also shown that 14/15 patients treated successfully with amphotericin B could be maintained without relapse on a daily dose of 50–200 mg fluconazole for 11–64 weeks. SUGAR and SAUNDERS (1988) have studied the efficacy of prophylactic fluconazole at 50–200 mg/day in 20 patients, 19 of whom had had meningitis. Only 2 relapses have been observed, and the period of treatment has exceeded 6 months in 13 patients.

In addition to oral or intravenous administration, the question of intrathecal or intraventricular injection remains. Only amphotericin B and miconazole have been used in this way. The majority of investigators conclude that there are more problems than advantages with intrathecal administration, particularly from irritation and local toxicity such as arachnoiditis and myelitis. With a basal meningitis progressing to give intracerebral foci, intrathecal treatment seems rather futile. In our opinion the procedure is inappropriate for primary treatment, and its value is likewise debatable for use in patients in whom alternative treatment has proved unsuccessful and CSF cultures have remained positive. Drugs can be administered via a subcutaneously implanted cranial reservoir (Armstrong 1988), but there is a major risk of bacterial contamination (pyogenic staphylococci), diffusion of the drug is uncertain, and in cases of ventriculitis the communication between the two ventricles is no longer patent.

In cases of unfavourable clinical response to treatment in spite of apparent control of the cryptococcosis, particularly where acute intracranial hypertension is evident, concominant cerebral toxoplasmosis should be considered. In our experience, this is a common occurrence, particularly presenting with abscesses or a diffuse encephalitis.

For HIV-positive subjects developing cryptococcal meningitis, therapeutic treatment can be summarized this:

(a) amphotericin B alone at 0.5 mg/kg every day or on alternate days
(b) amphotericin B in association with 5-FC (100 mg/kg) for the first 10–15 days
(c) fluconazole 400 mg daily
(d) itraconazole 400 mg daily

The duration of treatment is empirical but will be about 2 months. In order to prevent subsequent relapse, prophylactic treatment is desirable. Because of their ease of administration and good tolerance, both fluconazole and itraconazole at daily doses of 200 mg, presumably for life, are suitable (Table 4). Further study is necessary to define the current role of amphotericin B.

D. Histoplasmosis

The Center for Disease Control (Atlanta) classifies HIV-positive subjects who develop disseminated histoplasmosis as full-blown AIDS victims. The endemic zone for histoplasmosis (*Histoplasma capsulatum*) in the USA does not overlap with the main foci of AIDS (Los Angeles, New York, San Francisco). On the other hand in South America and Haiti (*H. capsulatum*) and in black Africa (*H. capsulatum* and *H. duboisii*), both conditions co-exist. No more than several dozen USA patients with histoplasmosis associated with AIDS have been published (Brivet et al. 1986; Deluol et al. 1987; Dupont et al. 1984; Dupouy-Camet et al. 1987; Graybill 1988; Huang et al. 1987; Taylor et al. 1984; Wheat et al. 1985), and only one involving *H. duboisii* has been reported (Peeters et al. 1987). Graybill (1988) mentioned more than 80 cases up to June 1988, but this condition will become more prevalent with the geographical spread of AIDS.

Table 4. Suggested treatments for cryptococcal meningitis in AIDS patients

Curative therapy:
1. Amphotericin B i.v. 0.5–1 mg per 24 or 48 h; total dose 2–3 g ± flucytosine 100 mg/kg daily for 10–15 days
2. IV or oral fluconazole, 400 mg/day for 2 months
3. Oral itraconazole 400 mg/day for 2 months

Prophylaxis to prevent relapse:
1. Amphotericin B i.v. 50 mg twice weekly, or 50–100 mg once weekly for life
2. Oral fluconazole 200 mg/day for life
3. Oral itraconazole 200 mg/day for life

The same schedules can be used in patients with non-meningeal cryptococcosis. Fluconazole and itraconazole are under investigation.

Symptoms are often acute and more severe than in other types of immunodeficiency (Wheat et al. 1982). The clinical picture usually includes fever, adenopathy, splenomegaly, cough, pulmonary infiltration and sometimes cutaneous involvement. Contrary to the classic description of histoplasmosis, it is surprising to observe disseminated intravascular coagulation, leukopenia or aplasia, respiratory distress, encephalitis or renal insufficiency. Nevertheless, the symptoms of histoplasmosis are similar to those of HIV or several other opportunistic infections. It is important to establish whether the patient has lived, even a long time ago, in an endemic zone of histoplasmosis. Diagnosis may be confirmed by blood culture, and sometimes yeasts can be found in granulocytes in a blood smear, or following sternal puncture, fibroscopic bronchoscopy, or biopsy of the skin, liver or lymph nodes. Serodiagnosis may be negative, and antigen detection in serum or urine is best left for specialised laboratories (Wheat et al. 1988).

Treatment is unsatisfactory, with high mortality or frequent relapses. One possible approach is to give amphotericin BIV at 35 mg daily up to a total dose of 2 g, followed by ketoconazole at 400 mg daily for a protracted period (Wheat et al. 1985). The numbers of patients treated are insufficient to establish this as a preferred scheme, and of course the problems associated with ketoconazole in AIDS patients (depressed absorption due to achlorhydria, adrenal insufficiency and gastric upset) limit its use. McKinsey et al. (1989) appear to have achieved very satisfactory results using long-term intermittent maintenance amphotericin B therapy following control of the acute disseminated disease with the same drug. Graybill (1988) has reported encouraging results in 63% of his patients following the use of itraconazole and fluconazole. The good tolerance allows daily dosing with 200–400 mg, which seems more effective than lower doses.

E. Coccidioidomycosis

Southern California is one of the most important foci for AIDS and overlaps the endemic zone of coccidioidomycosis; surprisingly, the number of published descriptions is small (KOVACS et al. 1984; ABRAMS et al. 1984; ROBERTS 1984; LEVY et al. 1985; SALBERG and VENKATACHALAM 1986). BRONNIMANN et al. (1987) reported on 7 cases among 27 HIV positive patients and suggested that 25% of AIDS victims in the endemic zone could be affected. CDC includes this condition among the opportunistic infections which allow an AIDS classification for HIV positive subjects. As with histoplasmosis the disease may result from the reactivation of a latent infection or may be due to increased susceptibility to primary infection. Haematogenous dissemination is the general rule in AIDS. The condition presents as a bilateral diffuse interstitial pneumonia or a unilateral infiltrate. Extrathoracic involvement is the rule: liver, bone marrow, blood, kidney, spleen, lymph nodes. Interestingly in a series of 7 patients only one cerebral location was mentioned and no cutaneous or osteoarticular metastases (BRONNIMANN et al. 1987). Symptoms are relatively mild considering the degree of dissemination: fever, cough, emaciation, general debility. Diagnosis is established by demonstration of spherules in the sputum or broncho-alveolar lavage fluid or by transbronchial or liver biopsy. Blood, urine, sputum or biopsy material are culture positive. Complement fixation tests are more often positive than precipitin reactions.

Mortality is high, with no patient having survived beyond 14 months. Among 5 who were autopsied, visceral dissemination to the lungs, liver, spleen, kidneys, lymph nodes and thyroid was observed (BRONNIMANN et al. 1987). One may hope for improvement or at least arrest of the disease by treating with amphotericin B i.v. at 0.5 mg/kg daily or on alternate days to a total dose of 2–3 g. This treatment will not produce cure, so it needs to be followed by further treatment to prevent clinical relapse; ketoconazole at 400 mg daily or amphotericin B 3 times weekly are the only available possibilities in spite of their limited efficacy and toxicity. The new triazoles, itraconazole and fluconazole, are potentially interesting because of their activity in vitro or in animal models. Encouraging results have been obtained in HIV-negative patients (TUCKER et al. 1990), and trials in AIDS patients are in progress.

F. Dermatophytes

The incidence of dermatophyte infections in the general population is around 2.8% (BADILLET and TRAORÉ 1987), but in HIV-positive subjects this rises to 18%–30% (BADILLET and TRAORÉ 1987; GOODMAN et al. 1987). As with the general population, *Trichophyton rubrum* predominates, while *T. interdigitale* and *Epidermophyton floccosum* are also frequent. Lesions are found in the classic sites: between the toes, in the groin and armpits, and on glabrous skin. Cases of wide dissemination are rare, and some clinical lesions are very circumscribed. Toenail infections are usually due to *T. rubrum* and can develop rapidly, often resembling leukonychia (Badillet and Traoré 1987). Diagnosis is easily confirmed by direct examination and culture of skin and nail scrapings. Treatment with topical agents such as azole derivatives, tolnaftate or ciclopiroxolamine is appropriate, although nail infections will require oral griseofulvin, ketoconazole or terbinafine.

G. Seborrhoeic Dermatitis

Seborrhoeic dermatitis with erythema, pruritis and greasy scales, and often associated with scalp pityriasis, is frequent among HIV-positive subjects; an incidence of 20%–46% has been reported, with lesions becoming more florid as the immunodeficiency becomes more pronounced (Farting et al. 1985; Goodman et al. 1987). It is disfiguring and sometimes associated with painful smarting. There is no consensus on the involvement of *Pityrosporum* (*Malassezia furfur*). Nevertheless, this yeast is often found in great abundance, clinical lesions can be reproduced by mouse inoculation, and oral ketoconazole is often remarkably effective (Drouhet et al. 1980). We have seen many cases of folliculitis due to *M. furfur* in AIDS patients respond to oral ketoconazole (400 mg daily), but relapses are frequent when treatment is stopped.

H. Other Mycoses

Anecdotal reports of other fungal infections in association with AIDS are continually appearing. Cutaneous alternariosis and alternariosis associated with necrotic ulceration of the nasal septum has been reported in two AIDS patients (Levy-Klotz et al. 1985; Wiest et al. 1987); surgical excision and amphotericin B i.v. resulted in cure in both. A fatal case of disseminated penicillinosis due to *Penicillium marneffei* has been described from an AIDS victim in the Far East (Ancelle et al. 1988). Another which showed temporary remission following amphotericin B treatment has been documented by Peto et al. (1988). Descriptions of patients with disseminated sporotrichosis (Bibler et al. 1986) and mucormycosis (Mostaza et al. 1989) have been published.

References

Abrams DI, Robia M, Blumenfeld W, Simonson J, Cohen MB, Hadeley WK (1984) Disseminated coccidioidomycosis in AIDS, N Engl J Med 310:986–987

Ancelle T, Dupouy-Camet J, Pujol F, Nassif X, Ferradini L, Lapierre J (1988) Un cas de pénicilliose disséminée à *Penicillium marneffei* chez un malade atteint de SIDA. Bull Soc Fr Mycol Méd 17:73–76

Armstrong D (1988) Life-threatening fungal infections in patients with the acquired immunodeficiency syndrome. Ann N Y Acad Sci 544:443–450

Badillet G, Traoré F (1987) Dermatophytes et sérologie HIV positive. Bull Soc Fr Mycol Med 16:95–98

Barr CE, Torosian JP (1986) Oral manifestations in inpatients with AIDS or AIDS-related complex. Lancet ii:288

Bibler MR, Luber HJ, Glueck HI, Ester SA (1986) Disseminated sporotrichosis in a patient with HIV infection after treatment for acquired factor VII inhibitor. JAMA 156:3125–3126

Bottone EJ, Salkin IF, Hurd NJ, Wormser GP (1987) Serogroup distribution of *Cryptococcus neoformans* in patients with AIDS. J Inf Dis 156:242

Bourée P, Thulliez P, Le Bras P, Ellrodt A, Palazzo L, Quillard J, Caquet R, Drouhet E (1984) Cryptococcose diffuse chez un Zairois atteint de SIDA. Bull Soc Fr Mycol Méd 13:195–200

Brandicourt O, Datry A, Rosenbaum W, Rosenheim M, Duflo B, Denis M, Brucker G, Gentilini M (1986) Cryptococcose et SIDA: à propos de 11 observations. Bull Soc Fr Mycol Méd 15:349–352

Brivet F, Roulot D, Naveau S, Delfraissy JF, Goujard C, Tertian G, Cartier I, Drouhet E, Dupont B (1986) The acquired immunodeficiency syndrome: B-cell lymphoma, histoplasmosis, and ethics and economics. Ann Int Med 104:447

Bronnimann DA, Adam RA, Galgiani JN, Habib MP, Petersen EA, Porter B, Bloom JW (1987) Coccidioidomycosis in the acquired immunodeficiency syndrome. Ann Int Med 106:372–379

Byrne WR, Wajszczuk CP (1988) Cryptococcal meningitis in AIDS: successful treatment with fluconazole after failure of amphotericin B. Ann Int Med 108: 384–385

Chuck SL, Sande MA (1989) Infections with *Cryptococcus neoformans* in the acquired immunodeficiency syndrome. N Engl J Med 321:794–799

Clissold SP (1987) Safety in clinical practice. In: Jones HE (ed) Ketoconazole today. A review of clinical experience. ADIS Press, Manchester, pp 79–91

Clotet B, Grifol M, Parra O, Boix J, Junca J, Tor J, Foz M (1986) Asymptomatic esophageal candidiasis in the acquired immunodeficiency-syndrome-related complex. Ann Int Med 105:145

De Gans J, Eeftinck Schattenkerk JKM, Van Ketel RJ (1988) Itraconazole as maintenance treatment for cryptococcal meningitis in the acquired immunodeficiency syndrome. Br Med J 296:339

Deluol AM, Marche C, Bizet C, Katlama C (1987) Histoplasmose disséminée au cours du SIDA. Bull Soc Fr Mycol Méd 16:363–366

Denning DW, Tucker RM, Hanson LH, Hamilton JR, Stevens DA (1989) Itraconazole therapy for cryptococcal meningitis and cryptococcosis. Arch Int Med 149:2301–2308

De Wit S, Weerts D, Goossens H, Clumeck N (1989) Comparison of fluconazole and ketoconazole for oropharyngeal candidiasis in AIDS. Lancet i:746–748

Dismukes WE (1988) Cryptococcal meningitis in patients with AIDS. J Inf Dis 157: 624–628

Drouhet E, Dompmartin D, Papachristou-Morati A, Ravisse P (1980) Dermatite expérimentale à *Pityrosporum ovale* et/ou *Pityrosporum orbiculare* chez le cobaye et la souris. Sabouraudia 18:149–156

Dupont B, Drouhet E (1987) Cryptococcal meningitis and fluconazole. Ann Int Med 106:778

Dupont B, Drouhet E (1988) Fluconazole in the management of oropharyngeal candidosis in a predominantly HIV antibody-positive group of patients. J Med Vet Mycol 26:67–71

Dupont B, Sansonetti P, Fleury J, Ravisse P, Drouhet E (1984) Histoplasmose septicémique au cours d'un SIDA, présence inhabituelle de *H. capsulatum* dans les polynucléaires. Med Mal Inf 14:261

Dupouy-Camet J, Vilette B, Thulliez M, Noizat F, Moyal M, Vedel G, Lapierre J (1987) Histoplasmose disséminée chez un malade grand voyageur atteint de SIDA. Bull Soc Fr Mycol Méd 16:81–83
Eng RHK, Bishburg E, Smith SM, Kapita R (1986) Cryptococcal infections in patients with acquired immune deficiency syndrome. Am J Med 81:19–23
Farting CF, Staughton RCD, Rowland Payne CME (1985) Skin disease in homosexual patients with acquired immune deficiency syndrome (AIDS) and lesser forms of human T cell leukemia virus (HTLV III) disease. Clin Exp Dermatol 10:3–12
Gall AA, Koss MN, Hawkins J, Evans S, Einstein H (1986) The pathology of pulmonary cryptococcal infections in the acquired immunodeficiency syndrome. Arch Pathol Lab Med 110:501–507
Goodman DS, Teplitz ED, Wishner A, Klein RS, Burk PG, Hershenbaum E (1987) Prevalence of cutaneous disease in patients with acquired immunodeficiency syndrome (AIDS) or AIDS-related complex. J Am Acad Derm 17:210–220
Grant SM, Clissold SP (1989) Itraconazole: a review of its pharmacodynamic and pharmacokinetic properties and therapeutic use in superficial and systemic mycoses. Drugs 37:310–344
Graybill JR (1987) Fluconazole efficacy in animal models of mycotic diseases. In: Fromtling RA (ed) Recent trends in the discovery, development and evaluation of antifungal agents. JR Prous, Barcelona, pp 113–124
Graybill JR (1988) Histoplasmosis and AIDS. J Inf Dis 158:623–626
Holmberg K, Meyer RD (1986) Fungal infections in patients with AIDS and AIDS related complex. Scand J Inf Dis 18:179–192
Huang CT, McGarry T, Cooper S, Saunders R, Andavoen R (1987) Disseminated histoplasmosis in the acquired immunodeficiency syndrome. Report of five cases from a non-endemic area. Arch Int Med 147:1181–1184
Joy M (1984) Oral candidiasis and AIDS. N Engl J Med 311:1378–1379
Kapend'a K, Komichelo K, Swinne D, Vandepitte J (1987) Meningitis due to *Cryptococcus neoformans* biovar *gattii* in a Zairean AIDS patient. Eur J Clin Microbiol 6:320–321
Klein RS, Harris CA, Small CB, Moll B, Lesser M, Friendland GH (1984) Oral candidiasis in high-risk patients as the initial manifestation of the acquired immunodeficiency syndrome. N Engl J Med 311:354–358
Kovacs A, Forthal DN, Kovacs JA, Overturf GD (1984) Disseminated coccidioidomycosis in a patient with acquired immune deficiency syndrome. West J Med 140:447–449
Kovacs JA, Kovacs AA, Polis M, Wright WC, Gill VJ, Tuazon CV, Gelmann EP, Lane HC, Longfield R, Overturf G, Macher AM, Fauci AS, Parrillo JE, Bennett JE, Masur H (1985) Cryptococcosis in the acquired immunodeficiency syndrome. Ann Int Med 103:533–538
Lake-Bakaar G, Tom W, Lake-Bakaar D, Gupta N, Beidas S, Elsakr M, Straus E, (1988) Gastropathy and ketoconazole malabsorption in the acquired immunodeficiency syndrome (AIDS). Ann Int Med 109:471–475
Levy RM, Bredesen DE, Rosenblum ML (1985) Neurological manifestations of the acquired immunodeficiency syndrome (AIDS): experience at UCSF and review of the literature. J Neurosurg 62:475–495
Levy-Klotz B, Badillet G, Cavelier-Balloy B, Chemaly P, Leverger G, Civatte J (1985) Alternariose cutanée au cours d'un SIDA. Ann Dermatol Venereol 112: 739–740
McKinsey DS, Gupta MR, Riddler SA, Driks MR, Smith DL, Kurtin PJ (1989) Long-term amphotericin B therapy for disseminated histoplasmosis in patients with the acquired immunodeficiency syndrome (AIDS). Ann Int Med 111:655–659
Matthews R, Burnie J, Smith D, Clark I, Midgley J, Conolly M, Gazzard B (1988) Candida and AIDS: evidence for protective antibody. Lancet ii:263–266
Morin O, Barrier J, Haloun A, Buzelin F, Baron D (1987) Détresse respiratoire aiguë due à une cryptococcose foudroyante mortelle chez un malade atteint du SIDA. Bull Soc Fr Mycol Méd 16:325–328

Mostaza JM, Barbado FJ, Fernandez-Martin J, Pena-Yanez J, Vasquez-Rodriguez JJ (1989) Cutaneoarticular mucormycosis due to *Cunninghamella bertholletiae* in a patient with AIDS. Rev Inf Dis 11:316–318

Pedersen C, Gerstoft J, Lindhardt BO, Sindrup J (1987) Candida esophagitis associated with acute human immunodeficiency virus infection. J Inf Dis 156:529–530

Peeters P, Depré G, Rickaert F, Coremans-Pelseneer J, Serruys E (1987) Disseminated African histoplasmosis in a white heterosexual male patient with the acquired immune deficiency syndrome. Mykosen 30:449–453

Perfect JR, Savani DV, Durack DT (1986) Comparison of itraconazole and fluconazole in treatment of cryptococcal meningitis and *Candida* pyelonephritis in rabbits. Antimicrob Agents Chemother 29:579–583

Peto TEA, Bull R, Millard PR, Mackenzie DWR, Campbell CK, Haines ME, Mitchell RG (1988) Systemic mycosis due to *Penicillium marneffei* in a patient with antibody to human immunodeficiency virus. J Infection 16:285–290

Rhoads JL, Wright DC, Redfield RR, Burke DS (1987) Chronic vaginal candidiasis in women with human immunodeficiency virus infection. JAMA 257:3105–3107

Roberts CJ (1984) Coccidioidomycosis in acquired immune deficiency syndrome: depressed humoral as well as cellular immunity. Am J Med 76:734–736

Roux P, Basset D, Delacourt T, Mayaud C, Touboul JL, Fouret P, Feuilhade M, Revuz J, Poirot JL, Marteau M, Lancastre F (1985) Problèmes posés par la cryptococcose au course du SIDA. Bull Soc Fr Mycol Méd 14:255–260

Roux P, Feuilhade M, Touboul JL, Basset D, Delacour T, Revuz T, Fouret P, Mayaud C, Lancastre F (1986) Interêt de la recherche systématique d'antigène sérique cryptococcique au cours du SIDA: à propos d'un cas de cryptococcose disséminée asymptomatique. Bull Soc Fr Mycol Méd 15:361–364

Roux P, Touboul JL, Basset D, Delacour T, Mayaud C, England D, Lancastre F (1987) Localisation pulmonaire de la cryptococcose au cours du SIDA: à propos de 6 cas. Bull Soc Fr Mycol Méd 16:113–116

Saag MS, Dismukes WE (1988) Azole antifungal agents: emphasis on new triazoles. Antimicrob Agents Chemother 32:1–8

Salberg DJ, Venkatachalam H (1986) Disseminated coccidioidomycosis presenting in AIDS. VA Practitioner 3:89–93

Schaffner A (1984) Acquired immune deficiency syndrome: is disseminated aspergillosis predictive of underlying cellular immune deficiency? J Inf Dis 149:828–829

Shimizu RY, Howard DH, Clancey MN (1986) The variety of *Cryptococcus neoformans* in patients with AIDS. J Inf Dis 154:1042

Spencer PM, Jackson G (1989) Fungal and mycobacterial infections in patients infected with the human immunodeficiency virus. J Antimicrob Chemother 23 (Suppl A):107–125

Stern JJ, Hartman BJ, Sharkey P, Rowland V, Squires KE, Murray HW, Graybill JR (1988) Oral fluconazole therapy for patients with acquired immunodeficiency syndrome and cryptococcosis: experience with 22 patients. Am J Med 85:477–480

Sugar AM, Saunders C (1988) Oral fluconazole: a suppressive therapy of disseminated cryptococcosis in patients with acquired immunodeficiency syndrome. Am J Med 85:481–489

Tavitian A, Raufman JP, Rosenthal LE (1986) Oral candidiasis as a marker for esophageal candidiasis in the acquired immunodeficiency syndrome. Ann Int Med 104:54–55

Taylor MN, Baddour L, Alexander JR (1984) Disseminated histoplasmosis associated with the acquired immune deficiency syndrome. Am J Med 77:579–580

Torssander J, Morfeld-Manson L, Biberfeld G, Karlson A, Putkonen PO, Wasserman J (1987) Oral *Candida* albicans in HIV infection. Scand J Inf Dis 19:291–295

Tucker RM, Denning DW, Dupont B, Stevens DA (1990) Itraconazole therapy of chronic coccidioidal meningitis. Ann Int Med 112:108–112

Van Cutsem J, Van Gerven F, Janssen PAJ (1987) The in vitro and in vivo antifungal activity of itraconazole. In: Fromtling RA (ed) Recent trends in the discovery, development and evaluation of antifungal agents. JR Prous, Barcelona, pp 177–192

Vant Wout JW, De Graeff-Meeder ER, Paul LC, Kuis W, Van Furth R (1988) Treatment of two cases of cryptococcal meningitis with fluconazole. Scand J Inf Dis 20:193–198

Viviani MA, Tortorano AM (1986) Surveillance de la cryptococcose chez les sujets à risque ou atteints de SIDA. Bull Soc Fr Mycol Méd 15:105–108

Viviani MA, Tortorano AM, Giani PC, Arici C, Goglio A, Crocchiolo P, Almaviva M (1987) Itraconazole for cryptococcal infection in the acquired immunodeficiency syndrome. Ann Int Med 106:166

Wheat LJ, Slama TG, Norton JA, Kohler RB, Eitzen HE, French MLV, Sathapatayavongs B (1982) Risk factors for disseminated or fatal histoplasmosis. Ann Int Med 96:159–163

Wheat LJ, Slama TG, Zeckel M (1985) Histoplasmosis in the acquired immune deficiency syndrome. Am J Med 78:203–210

Wheat LJ, Kohler RB, Tewar RP (1988) Diagnosis of disseminated histoplasmosis by detection of *Histoplasma capsulatum* antigen in serum and urine specimens. N Engl J Med 314:83–88

Wheeler RR, Peacock JE, Cruz JM, Richter JE (1987) Esophagitis in the immunocompromised host: role of esophagoscopy in diagnosis. Rev Inf Dis 9:88–96

Wiest PM, Wiese K, Jacobs MR, Morrissey AB, Abelson TI, Wilt W, Lederman MM (1987) *Alternaria* infection in a patient with acquired immunodeficiency syndrome: case report and review of invasive *Alternaria* infections. Rev Inf Dis 9:799–803

Zuger A, Lonie E, Molzman RS, Simberkoff MS, Rahal JJ (1988) Cryptococcal disease in patients with the acquired immunodeficiency syndrome. Ann Int Med 104:234–240

CHAPTER 18

Older Drugs

DONALD ARMSTRONG and HEINZ J. SCHMITT

A. Introduction

For one of us (D.A.), one of the pleasures of growing graciously older is being asked to write chapters on 'older drugs'. I assume the graciousness, otherwise I presume an editor wouldn't ask.

I first administered amphotericin B to a patient as an intern in 1958. It was a hot summer in New York. The patient was obese and diabetic and had one available vein with an intravenous needle in it. Because of fever, a sample for blood culture was drawn through that vein, and it yielded a *Candida* species. For presumed invasive candidosis (an even more tenuous diagnosis then than now), I administered amphotericin B. I don't remember the dose, but after 3 days of chills and fever the vein was no longer available. I removed the needle, and the patient did fine. What I didn't realize was that the trouble I had then in establishing a diagnosis of invasive candidosis would be with me more than 30 years later. Nor did I realize that the indications for stopping therapy would never again be so clear cut.

In 1990, we have a better idea when to use amphotericin B – or when not to – and we have improved guidelines as to when to stop a course of therapy (LOURIA 1967; ARMSTRONG 1989; SCHMITT and ARMSTRONG 1990). We have a far greater understanding of the pharmacokinetics of amphotericin B (BINDSCHADLER and BENNETT 1969; CHRISTIANSEN et al. 1985). It remains a toxic but manageable drug which has become the 'gold standard' in the treatment of most invasive fungal infections. It was the first antifungal agent to be used in combination chemotherapy of fungal diseases resulting in proven greater clinical efficacy (BENNETT et al. 1979; DISMUKES et al. 1987). The other drug is 5-fluorocytosine (flucytosine; 5-FC), which will also be discussed as an 'older drug' in this chapter.

B. Amphotericin B

I. History

By the early 1950s, few fungal infections were recognized as serious, and those that were common (dermatophytosis) could be managed with available modalities. Unlike the situation with antibacterial agents, where active screening programs had been started and were tremendously successful, until recently only few agents with useful antifungal activity had been discovered.

Fungicidin was the first polyene antifungal to be described (HAZEN and BROWN 1951), and it was later called nystatin (for New York State). Other polyenes such as fracidin, endomycin, and ricomydin were discovered in the same year, while ascocin, antimycoin, and trichomycin were described in 1952. Amphotericin B was first isolated from rotting vegetation on the banks of the Orinoco River in Venezuela by GOLD et al. (1956). Like the other polyenes, it was produced by a member of the genus *Streptomyces* (*S. nodosus*).

The preparation of almost pure amphotericin B containing less than 2% amphotericin A was accomplished by VANDEPUTTE et al. (1956). Within a few years after discovery, intravenous amphotericin B had become the treatment of choice for most invasive fungal infections (LOURIA 1967; PROCKNOW 1962). However, the remarkable toxicity of amphotericin B prompted a search for alternatives. Since no better class of antifungals was on the horizon, diminution of amphotericin toxicity and improved drug delivery became the main areas of research.

Esterification of amphotericin B resulted in a water-soluble micellar preparation (amphotericin B methyl ester). It seemed to be less nephrotoxic but also had reduced antifungal activity. Unfortunately, leukoencephalopathy occurred in the first human trials, and this prompted the end of the studies (ELLIS et al. 1982; HOEPRICH 1982). Recently, liposomal-encapsulated amphotericin B has shown promise in reducing amphotericin toxicity, and two preparations have reached the clinical trials stage. Apparently, higher doses of liposomal amphotericin B are tolerated than those that can be given with amphotericin B deoxycholate. It is not yet known whether this will result in an improved clinical outcome (LOPEZ-BERESTEIN et al. 1985; MEUNIER 1986; but see also Chap. 10).

Local treatment was another way to circumvent systemic toxicity and to achieve higher amphotericin B concentrations at the site of infection. Intrathecal administration has become the rule for coccidioidal meningitis, and in one retrospective study it was beneficial in immunocompromised patients with cryptococcal meningitis (POLSKY et al. 1986; but see Chap. 17). Recently, we have shown that aerosol amphotericin B improved survival in experimental pulmonary aspergillosis (SCHMITT et al. 1988). After approximately 30 years of laboratory investigation and clinical use, it seems that the full therapeutic possibilities inherent in amphotericin B have not yet been fully exploited. Amphotericin B has recently been shown to enhance antitumor effects and possesses immunomodulatory properties (BLANKE et al. 1975).

II. Mode of Action

Addition of polyenes to fungal cultures results in an increase of cellular constituents detectable in culture media and ultimately in cell death (KINSKY

1961a,b). These findings led to studies concentrating on the cell membrane, which is responsible for permeability. It was subsequently found that the inhibition of fungal growth was dependent on the binding and accumulation of polyenes by the cells. Furthermore, only cells that contain sterols (such as yeasts, molds, protozoa, algae, flatworms, and mammalian cells) are susceptible to polyenes, whereas resistant cells do not contain sterols. Conversely, adding sterols to the culture medium may protect polyene-sensitive organisms from growth inhibition (FEINGOLD 1965; WEBER and KINSKY 1965; BULDER 1971). Later, additional evidence for the interaction between sterols and polyenes was found using spectrophotometry (LAMPEN et al. 1959; SCHROEDER et al. 1971).

Electron microscopy studies have demonstrated defects in various experimental and natural membranes after exposure to polyenes, but no holes, pores, or channels were found (VERKLEIJ et al. 1973; TILLACK and KINSKY 1973). Today it appears that the binding of polyenes to sterols results in a more permeable membrane, and this is believed to be the main cause for the antifungal effect of polyenes.

The permeability effect of amphotericin B has been used to infiltrate other agents into fungal cells, resulting in synergism against the organism. Thus by combining amphotericin B with 5-FC, an increased uptake of ^{14}C-labelled 5-FC could be demonstrated. Combining amphotericin B with rifampin resulted in an inhibition of RNA synthesis, and combination with tetracycline, in decreased protein synthesis (MEDOFF et al. 1971, 1972; KWAN et al. 1972).

In addition, independent of this energy-dependent, reversible, permeability effect achievable with lower concentrations, a lethal effect has been described which is irreversible and not energy-dependent and which can be achieved with higher concentrations (KOTLER-BRAJTBURG et al. 1974, 1977).

It was shown recently that the lethal effect of amphotericin B is oxygen dependent and may involve peroxidative damage. Besides the permeability effect, synergy may be seen when amphotericin B is combined with compounds that increase oxidative metabolism (SOKOL-ANDERSON et al. 1986a,b; VERTUT-CROQUIN et al. 1986).

Another possible mechanism of action of amphotericin B is immunomodulation. It has been shown in mice that amphotericin B has potent immunoadjuvant and antitumor properties. The interactions with host cells that result in these immune effects are augmented by oxygen metabolites including hydrogen peroxide (BLANKE et al. 1977; LIN et al. 1977; MEDOFF et al. 1974). Thus, not only its effects on fungi but also those on host cells may contribute to the antifungal properties observed.

III. Resistance

Although amphotericin B has been the drug of choice for invasive fungal infections for almost 3 decades, emergence of acquired or primary resistance seems not to be a significant clinical problem; resistance has only rarely been seen (DROUHET 1970; WOODS et al. 1974). Such strains possess a decreased amount of ergosterol, grow more slowly in vitro, show cross-resistance to other polyenes but not to other antifungal agents, and seem to be less virulent. In vitro, however, several polyene-resistant *Candida* spp. have been selected (BONDRU 1969; HEJZLAR and VYMOLA 1970) or produced (HAMILTON-MILLER 1972; PATEL and JOHNSTON 1968).

While true (in vitro) resistance is rare, therapeutic failures to amphotericin B are common. Several explanations are possible. Amphotericin B binds to ergosterol in fungal membranes, but it also binds to cholesterol in the membranes of mammalian cells. In vivo, the drug is in an environment in which the intended targets, the infecting fungi, are few in number compared with competing sites. Association of amphotericin B with tissue or serum components, such as cholesterol or lipoproteins, may thus limit its availability and thereby its activity (BENNETT 1977).

This concept is further supported by an autopsy study. Amphotericin B at concentrations between 2.5 and 166 μg/g was found in organs from which *Aspergillus* and *Candida* spp. could be recovered by culture. The MICs of these organisms when tested in vitro were below 0.4 μg/ml. Thus, despite an adequate concentration of amphotericin B at the site of infection, susceptible organisms could be recovered (CHRISTIANSEN et al. 1985).

The explanation that a lack of bioavailability is an important mechanism of amphotericin B failure was further supported in this study by determining amphotericin concentrations in the liver and spleen. When aqueous homogenates, an ethanol extract and a bioassay, or HPLC to detect amphotericin B were used (Table 1), the aqueous homogenate revealed considerably lower amphotericin concentrations than the ethanol extract and bioassay.

Another mechanism for failure of amphotericin B therapy may be conditions at the site of infection which promote phenotypic changes in the fungi, thus conferring partial or even complete resistance. Oxygen is required for the production of sterols, and fungi growing in the absence of oxygen will be sterol-deficient. As said before, most amphotericin-resistant strains are deficient in ergosterol. Thus, lack of oxygen, which is to be anticipated in infected tissues, may result in a decreased production of ergosterol – which is necessary for the action of amphotericin B.

Other factors that are less well examined, but which may also contribute to amphotericin B failures, are too low concentrations at the site of infection; beginning therapy too late during infection to change the inflammatory damage done; and pretreatment or concomitant treatment with drugs that prevent the production of ergosterol, such as ketoconazole.

IV. Pharmacokinetics

Amphotericin B is poorly absorbed: After p.o. administration of 3 g/day, plasma concentrations between 0.1–0.5 μg/ml can be reached. Peak serum

Table 1. Comparison of concentrations of amphotericin B in the liver and spleen by bioassay and high-performance liquid chromatography (HPLC)[a]

Patient organ	Bioassay of aqueous homogenate	Bioassay of ethanol extract	HPLC of ethanol extract
1			
Liver	6.8 ± 5.5	95.0 ± 23.8	166.5 ± 18.5
Spleen	4.2 ± 2.4	57.1 ± 12.6	47.7 ± 3.9
2			
Liver	6.6 ± 4.6	105.3 ± 12.9	188.1 ± 11.0
Spleen	3.7 ± 2.8	61.6 ± 13.4	70.6 ± 6.8
3			
Liver	8.8 ± 3.2	36.6 ± 24.3	27.4 ± 3.3
Spleen	4.8 ± 2.8	18.8 ± 4.9	17.6 ± 9.9
4			
Liver	6.4 ± 4.2	102.8 ± 8.6	93.9 ± 5.9
Spleen	2.7 ± 1.1	89.5 ± 44.8	189.5 ± 8.8

Data are expressed as the mean ± SD of three separate experiments.
[a] Christiansen et al. (1985).

concentrations after i.v. administration range initially between 0.5 and 2.0 μg/ml but fall with additional treatments, and the average steady-state concentrations approach 0.5 μg/ml (Bindschadler and Bennett 1969). Renal or hepatic failure does not influence blood levels, nor does hemodialysis (except in a rare patient with lipemic plasma, who may lose the drug by its adherence to the dialysis membrane). Routine measurement of amphotericin B concentrations in serum is clinically not useful.

After iv infusion, amphotericin B separates from deoxycholate and binds to serum proteins, mainly to β-lipoproteins; according to Bennett (1977) it is presumed that the amphotericin binds mainly to cholesterol. Most of the amphotericin B administered rapidly leaves the vascular system and binds to cholesterol-containing membranes.

Among the various tissues, the highest amphotericin B concentrations can be found in liver, spleen, kidney and lungs. The liver is the major site of storage, containing as much as 41% of the total dose recovered (Table 1) (Christiansen et al. 1985). There is little accumulation in adipose tissue and muscle. Metabolites of the drug cannot be detected.

The fate of amphotericin B in the body is not exactly known. Only about 3% is excreted into urine (Atkinson and Bennett 1978). Bile may be a major route of elimination (Craven et al. 1979). Details of possible pathways or metabolism are not known. After the administration of amphotericin B is stopped, the drug can still be detected in urine for 7–8 weeks.

Concentrations of amphotericin B in fluids from inflamed aqueous humor, pleura, peritoneum, and synovium are about two-thirds of the serum

Table 2. Indications for therapy of selected fungal infections in the appropriate clinical setting

Candidosis	Sterile body site positive Blood culture positive Persistent fever with neutropenia despite antibacterial therapy Antigenemia Arabinitol/creatinine ratio increased
Aspergillosis	Sterile body site positive Blood culture positive Undiagnosed pulmonary infiltrate with neutropenia Positive sputum with neutropenia Antigenemia Antibody seroconversion
Cryptococcosis	Sterile body site positive Respiratory isolate in immunocompromised host Antigenemia CSF antigen
Mucormycosis	Sterile body site positive Mucous membrane smear with rhinocerebral presentation
Histoplasmosis	Sterile body site positive Respiratory isolates Rise in antibody titer Antigenemia Antigenuria
Coccidioidomycosis	Sterile body site positive Respiratory isolates Antibody present
Blastomycosis	Sterile body site positive Respiratory isolates
Others	Sterile body site positive[a]

[a] Susceptibility studies should be done – isolates such as *Fusarium*, *Petrolydium*, etc. may be resistant.

concentration; urine concentrations are similar to serum concentrations. Penetration into normal or inflamed meninges, vitreous humor and normal amniotic fluid is poor.

V. Indications

The indications for the administration of amphotericin B vary with the fungal infection suspected and will not be covered in detail here. A summary is included in Table 2, and the topic has recently been reviewed in detail (SCHMITT and ARMSTRONG 1990). The best indication is an isolate presumed to be susceptible, visualized and recovered from a sterile body site. With some infections (coccidioidomycosis) antibody determinations can be used as indications, with others (cryptococcosis, histoplasmosis) antigen detection, while with those such as candidosis and aspergillosis the indications are most often not clear, and presumptive or empirical therapy in the immunocompromised host is common (ARMSTRONG 1989). Once the decision to treat with amphotericin B is made, it is only reasonable to move rapidly (within 24 h) to adequate doses.

VI. Administration

Amphotericin B must be administered intravenously to treat systemic infections. The dose varies according to the type of infection (Table 2). There is disagreement among clinicians about the appropriate dose for a given infection. For invasive candidosis or aspergillosis we aim at 1 mg/kg daily, but others recommend 0.5 mg/kg daily. There are no studies available to settle this issue. Our schedule of administration is detailed in Table 3 along with a simpler alternative method. After 2 weeks of treatment, blood levels become stable, tissue levels begin to accumulate, and a schedule of every other day administration can be established. This is usually given at 1½ times the daily dose. For example, if we are giving a dose of 1 mg/kg per day, we will switch to 1.5 mg/kg every other day. The higher dose is usually tolerated by patients after daily administration for 2 weeks. Reactions become less severe, and patients are grateful for the 'day off.'

The administration of saline before amphotericin B treatment has been found beneficial in some studies. A 'washout' dose of 500–1000 ml normal saline before the administration of amphotericin B in 500–1000 ml of 5% dextrose and water is suitable. The washout appears to decrease renal toxicity and potassium wasting. The amphotericin B must be given in dextrose and water because it will precipitate out in saline. There is no need to protect the solution from light because there is insignificant loss of potency during the period used for administration, even over 24 h. Although there have been

Table 3. Amphotericin B administration schedules

	Test Dose 1 mg i.v. in 250 ml 5% D/W over 2 h
	If no reaction, then
Regimen I:	10 mg i.v. in 500 ml 5% D/W over 4–6 h to be followed immediately by 20 mg i.v. in 500 ml 5% D/W over 4–6 h to be followed immediately by 40 mg i.v. in 500 ml 5% D/W over 4–6 h
	or
Regimen II:	49 mg[a] i.v. in 1000 ml 5% D/W over 6 h
Regimen I or II should then be followed by: 1 mg/kg/day in 500 to 1000 ml 5% D/W over 4–6 h to 14 days then 1.5 mg/kg every other day in 500 to 1000 ml 5% D/W over 4–6 h[b]	

[a] The remainder of the vial after removing the 1 mg test dose.
[b] A 'priming' dose of 500 ml saline and a 'washout' dose of 500 ml saline has been recommended to decrease renal toxicity.

recommendations for relatively rapid infusion periods of up to 1 to 2 h, the tolerance varies considerably among patients and even in a given patient. Tolerance usually increases with prolonged experience with the drug. We find it is better to work out the regimen with the patient rather than to try rapid infusions on everybody.

VII. Toxicity

The adverse reactions and toxicity of amphotericin B are well known to both patients and physicians. Our patients refer to it as 'shake and bake' which aptly describes the most commonly observed adverse reactions, chills and fever. The chills may resemble the rigors of malaria, and the fever may reach 40°C. The reactions usually become less extreme with each daily dose, and slowing the administration may diminish the severity. Administration of acetaminophen (Tylenol) 650 mg every 4 h, or meperidine (Demerol) 50 mg, or diphenhydramine (Benadryl) 100 mg usually ameliorates the reactions. These can be given separately, but often two or three given together may be necessary. They are usually given ½ h before the amphotericin B administration, but patients often learn when the best time is for dosing these 'premedications'. In the face of extreme and persistent reactions we may be forced to give 50 mg of hydrocortisone, but would rather avoid this because of the potential immune suppression. Nausea and vomiting occur less often, and just as with chills and fever may be controlled by decreasing the rate of administration from 4 to 6 h.

Some patients will tolerate all of these reactions, and they can receive – if they choose to – the dose over 1 h or even less. Other patients may prefer longer periods of administration and elect to receive the drug during the night. The premedications often make patients sleepy, and if the reactions can be controlled, night-time administration can be very convenient.

Electrolyte imbalances occur, with hypokalemia and hypomagnesemia the most common and troublesome. Renal potassium and magnesium loss may well reach symptomatic proportions, particularly in patients on long-term therapy. Profound weakness including partial paralysis may be seen but responds well to replacement therapy. Cardiac arrhythmias due to hypokalemia are a concern, and potassium replacement should be given at the first low potassium level seen on careful monitoring. If serial determinations show a steady decline, replacement should start before reaching low levels; up to and more than 100 MEQ per day may be necessary. In especially difficult instances, usually seen with long-term therapy, measurement of urinary potassium losses can be helpful in anticipating daily requirements. A rising creatinine level is also seen regularly with amphotericin B administration. Since renal excretion is low – in the 5% range – this rise is not necessarily an indication to decrease the dose of amphotericin B. Continuing treatment will cause a further decrease in creatinine clearance but relatively little difference in the amount of amphotericin B excreted.

C. 5-Fluorocytosine

I. History

5-Fluorocytosine (flucytosine; 5-FC) is a fluorine analogue of cytosine, a normal body constituent. It is a 'designer drug', synthesized to be used as an antitumor agent in 1957 by DUSCHINKSY et al. It was, however, not effective against tumors (HEIDELBERGER et al. 1958). Further routine screening revealed that 5-FC possessed antifungal activity in vitro (BERGER and DUSCHINKSY 1962). In 1964 GRUNBERG et al. found that the compound was active in experimental candidosis and cryptococcosis in mice. It was used subsequently in humans and first reported to be successful in the treatment of human candidosis and cryptococcosis by GRUNBERG et al. (1967). It was finally marketed in the USA in 1972 as an oral preparation.

II. Mode of Action

The 'active principle' of 5-FC is not 5-FC itself, but 5-fluorouracil (5-FU). 5-FC is changed into 5-FU in susceptible cells, a process which requires several prerequisites:

1. 5-FC has to be taken into the cell by an enzyme, cytosine permease.
2. Intracellularly, 5-FC has to be deaminated by cytosine deaminase to 5-fluorouracil (5-FU).

These two enzymatic steps take place rapidly in a first 'uptake phase' of about 1–2 h after exposure of a susceptible organism to 5-FC. Large quantities of both 5-FC and 5-FU can be found in the internal pool of *Candida albicans* at that time (POLAK and SCHOLER 1973).

If either one of the above-mentioned enzymes is not present or is inactive, 5-FC will have no effect. 5-FU on its own cannot be used as an antifungal agent (1) because it exerts remarkable toxicity in mammalian cells and (2) because its uptake into fungal cells is poor (POLAK and GRENSON 1973).

After uptake into a susceptible cell and conversion into 5-FU, there are at least two mechanisms by which the latter may act against fungi. The first one involves a disturbance in the amino acid pool and/or inhibition of protein synthesis. This is achieved by the replacement of uracil by 5-FU in fungal RNA. The second mechanism involves inhibition of DNA synthesis. This is achieved by the inhibition of thymidylate synthetase by 5-fluorodeoxyuridine monophosphate, a metabolite of 5-FU.

Some 2–6 h after exposure to 5-FC ('incorporation phase') 5-FU appears in hydrolysates of ribosomal and transfer RNA and may replace up to 50% of the uracil. No fluorinated pyrimidine or 5-FC can be found in exposed fungi at this time (POLAK and SCHOLER 1973; GIÉGÉ and WEIL 1970; NORMARCK and SCHÖNEBECK 1972; BLOCK et al. 1973; WAGNER and SHADOMY 1976).

The presence of 5-FU in RNA does not necessarily mean that it interferes with protein synthesis. However, POLAK and SCHOLER (1975) demonstrated a relationship between the presence of 5-FU in fungal RNA and antifungal activity. It seems that incorporation of 5-FU into RNA is at least in part responsible for the antifungal activity of 5-FC. In addition, disturbances in the amino acid pool can be observed in fungi exposed to 5-FC (GIÉGÉ and WEIL 1970), and this may further contribute to the inhibitory effects of 5-FC on susceptible fungi.

In the experiments of POLAK and WAIN (1977) a decreased amount of DNA and RNA was detectable in *C. albicans* cells exposed to 5-FC. In other experiments, *C. albicans* converted 5-FC to FUdRMP, which was responsible for a pronounced inhibition of thymidylate synthetase (DIASIO et al. 1978a). Thus, inhibition of DNA synthesis is considered another mechanism of action of 5-FC.

III. Resistance

Two basic mechanisms of resistance are known. 5-FC-resistant fungi may have a deficiency in one of the enzymes necessary for the different metabolic changes of the molecule as described above. Alternatively, an increased de novo synthesis of physiological cell constituents competing with 5-FC or its metabolites may abolish its antifungal activity.

In mutant strains at least six types of resistance have been characterized biochemically; some of these have also been observed among clinical isolates (SCHOLER 1980). Primary and secondary resistance seem to be due to the same mechanisms.

The degree of resistance to 5-FC may either be complete or partial (NORMARCK and SCHÖNEBECK 1972). In the latter case, organisms are inhibited by relatively low concentrations of 5-FC but start growing after a prolonged period of incubation. Conversely, completely resistant strains are not inhibited by 5-FC concentrations up to 1 mg/ml.

The exact incidence of primary 5-FC resistance is controversial: About 8% of *Candida* spp. may be resistant (SCHOLER 1980), but other authors report rates as high as 44% (SHADOMY et al. 1973). Differences in the technique used, local factors, and differences among the various *Candida* spp. all may contribute to the variability of the results published.

Since fungi may be resistant to 5-FC due to many different biochemical mechanisms, it is assumed that in any fungal population there is a minority of mutants having one of them. 5-FC does not appear to induce resistance; it acts rather as a selection tool allowing only multiplication of resistant strains.

It has been shown that the overall incidence of resistance is (1) species specific, (2) correlated with the length of incubation, and (3) inversely correlated with the amount of 5-FC in the test medium (SCHOLER 1980). The clinical implications of these findings are important since they should help to identify risk factors for the occurrence of treatment failures.

A high number of infecting fungi, infection with a species or a strain with a high resistance frequency, treatment with 5-FC doses that achieve only low concentrations of the compound at the site of infection, and the clinical necessity to treat for a prolonged period of time (such as in immunocompromised patients) may all contribute to the emergence of resistance and to treatment failures if 5-FC monotherapy is used.

The high incidence of secondary resistance observed with 5-FC concentrations below 25 μg/ml is the support for the recommendation to aim at serum levels at or above 50 μg/ml – despite the fact that the MICs for most susceptible strains of yeasts are only about 1 μg/ml (NORMARCK and SCHÖNEBECK 1972). Except perhaps for chromomycosis, 5-FC should never be used as a single agent for the treatment of fungal infections. To our knowledge, cross-resistance with other antifungal agents has not yet been described.

IV. Pharmacokinetics

After oral administration, 5-FC is rapidly and completely absorbed. Almost no protein binding is seen in serum. The peak plasma concentration after a single dose of 37.5 mg/kg is 70–80 μg/ml after 1–2 h. The serum half-life is 3–6 h, but it increases extensively in renal failure (CUTLER et al. 1978). 5-FC is widely distributed with a volume of distribution that equals that of the total body water. In the CSF about three-quarters of the corresponding serum concentrations are achieved. More than 80% of 5-FC is excreted unchanged into the urine by glomerular filtration.

V. Indications

The indications for 5-FC are included in Table 2, along with those for amphotericin B. The most clearcut indication is in combination with amphotericin B in the treatment of cryptococcal meningitis in non-HIV-infected people (BENNETT et al. 1979). The exact dose and duration of either amphotericin B or 5-FC are uncertain (DISMUKES et al. 1987), but it is evident from these two studies that 5-FC added to amphotericin B is superior to amphotericin B alone and therefore indicated. Whether this is true for patients with HIV infection is not yet settled (CHUCK and SANDE 1989). At the Memorial Sloan-Kettering Cancer Center we use 5-FC with amphotericin B for patients with HIV infection and cryptococcosis as well as for those without. Trials are underway to compare amphotericin B with fluconazole for treatment of cryptococcosis in AIDS patients, and these should include studying the subset of patients treated with amphotericin B plus 5-FC.

Candidemia in the neutropenic as well as other immunocompromised hosts is not a clearcut indication. In a retrospective study of patients with fungemia due to *C. tropicalis*, we found that mortality was significantly decreased from 73% to 44% by adding 5-FC to amphotericin B (HORN et al. 1985). This was not a prospective, randomized study and that sort of scrutiny is required to convince many investigators.

VI. Administration

5-FC should not be given alone because fungi develop resistance regularly and rapidly. The recommended dose of 150 mg/kg daily is too high. Most people do not tolerate this because of gastrointestinal upset. Immunocompromised patients cannot tolerate this dose either because of marrow suppression. The MICs of clinical isolates of yeasts usually sensitive to 5-FC indicate that the 50–100 μg/ml levels attained at 150 mg/kg daily are not necessary to inhibit the yeast. Blood levels of 25–50 μg/ml are ample to inhibit isolates with MICs of 0.05–1.0 μg/ml (STAMM et al. 1987). We initiate therapy at 100 mg/kg daily in four divided doses and follow blood levels. If the marrow is obviously suppressed or even suspected of being suppressed, then 75 mg/kg daily should be used and levels ascertained after 24 h and every 72 h thereafter or according to the creatinine level or creatinine clearance, increasing the number of determinations as the creatinine level increases and decreasing the dose or withholding the drug if in doubt. 5-FC is removed from the body by hemodialysis and also by peritoneal dialysis; after each dialysis, a dose of 37.5 mg/kg should be administered.

VII. Toxicity

5-FC produces symptoms in three areas of toxicity (DIASIO et al. 1978b; HARRIS et al. 1986). The first and least serious is nausea and vomiting. The second and more serious is liver toxicity manifested by cell necrosis, but this is rarely fatal. The most serious is bone marrow toxicity. This is usually reversible but not always; marrow aplasia and death have resulted. The toxicity of 5-FC may at least in part be due to 5-FU. The latter may derive from conversion of 5-FC to 5-FU within the human body or from bacteria in the GI tract, from which it is absorbed.

References

Armstrong D (1989) Problems in the treatment of opportunistic fungal infections. In: Holmberg K, Meyer RD (eds) Diagnosis and therapy of systemic fungal infections. Raven Press, New York, pp 149–158

Atkinson AJ, Bennett JE (1978) Amphotericin B pharmacokinetics in humans. Antimicrob Agents Chemother 13:271–276

Bennett JE (1977) Amphotericin B binding to serum β-lipoprotein. In: Iwata K (ed) Recent advances in medical and veterinary mycology. Proc 6th ISHAM, University Park Press, Baltimore, USA, pp 107–109

Bennett JE, Dismukes WE, Duma RJ, Medoff G, Sande MA, Gallis H, Leonard J, Fields BT, Bradshaw M, Haywood H, McGee ZA, Cate TR, Cobbs CG, Warner

JF, Alling DW (1979) A comparison of amphotericin B alone and combined with flucytosine in the treatment of cryptococcal meningitis. N Engl J Med 301:126–131
Berger J, Duschinksy R (1962) Control of fungi with 5-fluorocytosine. US Pat Appl Ser No 181, p 822
Bindschadler DD, Bennett JE (1969) A pharmacologic guide to the clinical use of amphotericin B. J Infect Dis 120:427–436
Blanke PJ, Little JR, Shirley SF, Lynch RG (1977) Augmentation of murine immune responses by amphotericin B. J Cell Immunol 33:180–190
Blanke T, Lynch R, Little JR (1975) Mechanisms of antitumor effects of amphotericin B. Surg Forum 26:126–128
Block ER, Jennings AE, Bennett JE (1973) 5-Fluorocytosine resistance in *Cryptococcus neoformans*. Antimicrob Agents Chemother 3:649–656
Bondru I (1969) De la résistance des *Candida albicans* à la nystatine. J Pharm Belg 24:162–185
Bulder CJEA (1971) Anaerobic growth, ergosterol content and sensitivity to a polyene antibiotic of the yeast *Schizosaccharomyces japonicus*. Antonie van Leeuwenhoek 37:353–358
Christiansen KJ, Bernard EM, Gold JWM, Armstrong D (1985) Distribution and activity of amphotericin B in humans. J Infect Dis 152:1037–1043
Chuck SL, Sande MA (1989) Infections with *Cryptococcus neoformans* in the acquired immunodeficiency syndrome. N Engl J Med 321:794–799
Craven PC, Ludden TM, Drutz DJ, Rogers W, Haegele KA, Skrdlant HB (1979) Excretion pathways of amphotericin B. J Infect Dis 140:329–341
Cutler RE, Blair AD, Kelly MR (1978) Flucytosine kinetics in subjects with normal and impaired renal function. Clin Pharmacol Ther 24:333–342
Diasio RB, Bennett JE, Myers CE (1978a) Mode of action of 5-fluorocytosine. Biochem Pharmacol 27:703–707
Diasio RB, Lakings DE, Bennett JE (1978b) Evidence for conversion of 5-fluorocytosine to 5-fluorouracil in humans: possible factor in 5-fluorocytosine clinical toxicity. Antimicrob Agents Chemother 14:903–908
Dismukes WE, Cloud G, Gallis HA, Kerkering TM, Medoff G, Craven PC, Kaplowitz LG, Fisher JF, Gregg CR, Bowles CA, Shadomy S, Stamm AM, Diasio RB, Kaufman L, Soong S-J, Blackwelder WC and the National Institute of Allergy and Infectious Diseases Mycoses Study Group (1987) Treatment of cryptococcal meningitis with combination amphotericin B and flucytosine for four as compared with six weeks. N Engl J Med 317:334–341
Drouhet E (1970) Basic mechanisms of antifungal chemotherapy. Mod Treat 7: 539–564
Duschinsky R, Pleven E, Heidelberger C (1957) The synthesis of 5-fluoropyrimidines. J Am Chem Soc 79:4559–4560
Ellis WG, Sobel RA, Nielsen SL (1982) Leukoencephalopathy in patients treated with amphotericin B methyl ester. J Infect Dis 146:125–137
Feingold DS (1965) The action of amphotericin B on *Mycoplasma laidlawii*. Biochem Biophys Res Commun 19:261–267
Giégé R, Weil JH (1970) Etude des tRNA de levure ayant incorporé du 5-fluorouracile provenant de la désamination in vivo de la 5-fluorocytosine. Bull Soc Chim Biol 52:135–144
Gold W, Stout HA, Pagano JF, Donovick R (1956) Amphotericins A and B, antifungal antibiotics produced by a streptomycete. I. In vitro studies. In: Welch H, Marti-Ibañez F (eds) Antibiotics Annual 1955–1956. Medical Encyclopedia Inc, New York, pp 579–586
Grunberg E, Titsworth E, Bennett M (1964) Chemotherapeutic activity of 5-fluorocytosine. Antimicrobial Agents and Chemotherapy 1963. Am Soc Microbiol, pp 566–568
Grunberg E, Prince HN, Utz JP (1967) Observations on the activity of two newer antifungal agents, saramycetin (X-5079C) and 5-fluorocytosine. Proc 5th Int Cong Chemother, Vienna, 4:69–76

Hamilton-Miller JMT (1972) Physiological properties of mutagen-induced variants of *Candida albicans* resistant to polyene antibiotics. J Med Microbiol 5:425–440
Harris BE, Manning BW, Federle TW, Diasio RB (1986) Conversion of 5-fluorocytosine to 5-fluorouracil by human intestinal microflora. Antimicrob Agents Chemother 29:44–48
Hazen EL, Brown R (1951) Fungicidin, antibiotic produced by soil actinomycete. Proc Soc Exp Biol Med 76:93–97
Heidelberger C, Griesbach L, Montag BJ, Mooren D, Cruz O, Schnitzer RJ, Grunberg E (1958) Studies on fluorinated pyrimidines. II. Effects on transplanted tumors. Cancer Res 18:305–317
Hejzlar M, Vymola F (1970) Comparative study of pimaricin and fungicidin activity in vitro. J Hyg Epidemiol Microbiol Immun 14:211–213
Hoeprich PD (1982) Amphotericin B methyl ester and leukoencephalopathy: the other side of the coin. J Infect Dis 146:173–176
Horn R, Wong B, Kiehn TE, Armstrong D (1985) Fungemia in a cancer hospital: changing frequency, earlier onset, and results of therapy. Rev Infect Dis 7: 646–655
Kinsky SC (1961a) The effects of polyene antibiotics on permeability in *Neurospora crassa*. Biochem Biophys Res Commun 4:353–357
Kinsky SC (1961b) Alterations in the permeability of *Neurospora crassa* due to polyene antibiotics. J Bacteriol 82:889–897
Kotler-Brajtburg J, Price HD, Medoff G, Schlessinger D, Kobayashi GS (1974) Molecular basis for the selective toxicity of amphotericin B for yeast and filipin for animal cells. Antimicrob Agents Chemother 5:377–382
Kotler-Brajtburg J, Medoff G, Kobayashi GS, Schelssinger D, Atallah A (1977) Sensitivity to amphotericin B and the cholesterol: phospholipid molar ratios of 3T3. L, BHK and HeLa cells. Biochem Pharmacol 26:705–710
Kwan CN, Medoff G, Kobayashi GS, Schlessinger D, Raskas HJ (1972) Potentiation of the antifungal effects of antibiotics by amphotericin B. Antimicrob Agents Chemother 2:61–65
Lampen JO, Morgan ER, Slocum A, Arnow P (1959) Adsorption of nystatin by micro-organisms. J Bacteriol 78:282–289
Lin H-S, Medoff G, Kobayashi GS (1977) Effects of amphotericin B on macrophages and their precursor cells. Antimicrob Agents Chemother 11:154–160
Lopez-Berestein G, Fainstein V, Hopfer R, Mehta K, Sullivan MP, Keating M, Rosenblum MG, Mehta R, Luna M, Hersh EM, Reuben J, Juliano RL, Bodey GP (1985) Liposomal amphotericin B for the treatment of systemic fungal infections in patients with cancer: a preliminary study. J Infect Dis 151:704–710
Louria DB (1967) Deep-seated mycotic infections, allergy to fungi and mycotoxins. N Engl J Med 277:1065–1071, 1126–1134
Medoff G, Comfort M, Kobayashi GS (1971) Synergistic action of amphotericin B and 5-fluorocytosine against yeast-like organisms. Proc Soc Exp Biol Med 138:571–574
Medoff G, Kobayashi GS, Kwan CN, Schlessinger D, Venkov P (1972) Potentiation of rifampin and 5-fluorocytosine as antifungal antibiotics by amphotericin B. Proc Natl Acad Sci USA 69:196–199
Medoff G, Valeriote F, Lynch RG, Schelssinger D, Kobayashi GS (1974) Synergistic effect of amphotericin B and 1,3-bis(2-chloro-ethyl)-1-nitrosourea (BCNU) against a syngenic transplantable AKR leukemia. Cancer Res 34:974–978
Meunier F (1986) Serum fungistatic and fungicidal activity in volunteers receiving antifungal agents. Eur J Clin Microbiol 5:103–109
Normarck S, Schönebeck J (1972) In vitro studies of 5-fluorocytosine resistance in *Candida albicans* and *Torulopsis glabrata*. Antimicrob Agents Chemother 2:114–121
Patel PV, Johnston JR (1968) Dominant mutation for nystatin resistance in yeast. Appl Microbiol 16:164–165

Polak A, Grenson M (1973) Evidence for a common transport system for cytosine, adenine and hypoxanthine in *Saccharomyces cerevisiae* and *Candida albicans*. Eur J Biochem 32:276–282

Polak A, Scholer HJ (1973) Fungistatic activity, uptake and incorporation of 5-fluorocytosine in *Candida albicans*, as influenced by pyrimidines and purines. II. Studies on distribution and incorporation. Pathologia Microbiol 39:334–347

Polak A, Scholer HJ (1975) Mode of action of 5-fluorocytosine and mechanisms of resistance. Chemotherapy 21:113–130

Polak A, Wain WH (1977) The inhibition by 5-fluorocytosine of nucleic acid synthesis in *Candida albicans*, *Cryptococcus neoformans*, and *Aspergillus fumigatus*. Chemotherapy 23:243–259

Polsky B, Depman MR, Gold JWM, Galicich JH, Armstrong D (1986) Intraventricular therapy of cryptococcal meningitis via a subcutaneous reservoir. Am J Med 81:24–28

Procknow JJ (1962) Treatment of opportunistic fungus infections. Lab Invest 11: 1217–1230

Scholer HJ (1980) Flucytosine. In: Speller DCE (ed) Antifungal chemotherapy. Wiley & Sons, Chichester, pp 35–106

Schmitt HJ, Armstrong D (1990) Antifungal chemotherapy. In: Kass EH, Platt R (eds) Current therapy in infectious disease, 3rd ed. BC Decker Inc., Philadelphia, pp 12–17

Schmitt HJ, Bernard EM, Häuser M, Armstrong D (1988) Aerosol amphotericin B is effective for prophylaxis and therapy in a rat model of pulmonary aspergillosis. Antimicrob Agents Chemother 32:1676–1679

Schroeder F, Holland JF, Bieber LL (1971) Fluorometric evidence for the binding of cholesterol to the filipin complex. J Antibiot (Tokyo) 24:846–849

Shadomy S, Kirchoff CB, Ingroff AE (1973) In vitro activity of 5-fluorocytosine against *Candida* and *Troulopsis* species. Antimicrob Agents Chemother 3:9–14

Sokol-Anderson ML, Brajtburg J, Medoff G (1986a) Sensitivity of *Candida albicans* to amphotericin B administered as single or fractionated doses. Antimicrob Agents Chemother 29:701–702

Sokol-Anderson ML, Brajtburg J, Medoff G (1986b) Amphotericin B-induced oxidative damage and killing of *Candida albicans*. J Infect Dis 154:76–83

Stamm AM, Diasio RB, Dismukes WE, Shadomy S, Cloud GA, Bowles CA, Karam GH, Espinel-Ingroff A and members of the National Institute of Allergy and Infectious Diseases Mycoses Study Group (1987) Toxicity of amphotericin B plus flucytosine in 194 patients with cryptococcal meningitis. Am J Med 83:236–242

Tillack TW, Kinsky SC (1973) A freeze-etch study of the effects of filipin on liposomes and human erythrocyte membranes. Biochim Biophys Acta 323:43–54

Vandeputte J, Wachtel JL, Stiller ET (1956) Amphotericins A and B, antifungal antibiotics produced by a streptomycete: II. The isolation and properties of the crystalline amphotericins. Antibiotic Annual 1955–1956. Medical Encyclopedia Inc, New York, pp 587–591

Verkleij AJ, De Kruijff B, Gerritsen WF, Demel RA, Van Deenen LLM, Ververgaert PHJ (1973) Freeze-etch electron microscopy of erythrocytes, *Acholeplasma laidlawii* cells and liposomal membranes after the action of filipin and amphotericn B. Biochim Biophys Acta 291:577–581

Vertut-Croquin A, Brajtburg J, Medoff G (1986) Two mechanisms of synergism when amphotericin B is used in combination with actinomycin D or 1-(2-chloroethyl)-3-cyclohexyl-1-nitrosurea against the human promyelocytic leukemia cell line HL-60. Cancer Res 46:6054–6058

Wagner G, Shadomy S (1976) Mode of action of flucytosine in *Aspergillus* species. In: Williams JD, Geddes AM (eds) Chemotherapy. Proc 9th Int Cong Chemother, London 1975. Plenum Press, New York, 3:211–215

Weber MM, Kinsky SC (1965) Effect of cholesterol on the sensitivity of *Mycoplasma laidlawii* to the polyene antibiotic filipin. J Bacteriol 89:306–312

Woods RA, Bard M, Jackson IE, Drutz DJ (1974) Resistance to polyene antibiotics and correlated sterol changes in two isolates of *Candida tropicalis* from a patient with an amphotericin B-resistant funguria. J Infect Dis 129:53–59

CHAPTER 19

Systemic Azole Antifungal Drugs – Into the 1990s

JOHN R. GRAYBILL

A. The Evolution of Azole Antifungals in Clinical Use

I. Introduction: Why Not Stay with 'Good Old' Amphotericin B?

Amphotericin B marked the beginning of the real antifungal era. Beginning with the 1960s, there was a broad spectrum antifungal drug that could be administered parenterally and could arrest the course of devastating systemic fungal infections. Amphotericin B revolutionized the treatment of the major endemic mycoses (histoplasmosis, coccidioidomycosis, blastomycosis, and paracoccidioidomycosis) and also provided the first effective therapy for cryptococcal meningitis. Were efficacy the only relevant question today, it would still be difficult to find treatment significantly superior to amphotericin B. However, the toxicity of amphotericin B and the need for intravenous administration have made prolonged therapeutic regimens difficult to administer. In addition, the relative rarity of systemic fungal infections was an insufficient stimulus for pharmaceutical companies to undertake the increasingly costly investment required to identify and develop new classes of drugs for systemic mycoses.

One motivation that did prompt development of more benign antifungals was the desire for a systemically administered agent which could be effective (and nontoxic) in the much broader market for superficial dermatophytes and vaginal candidal infections. The search for such benign agents led in part to the initial exploration of azoles in coccidioidomycosis, histoplasmosis, paracoccidioidomycosis, and blastomycosis; these are often severe infections in which mild toxicity is less of an issue than efficacy. Azole antifungals all act to impair synthesis of the fungal cell membrane ergosterol (VANDEN BOSSCHE 1985). This process has many secondary 'ripple' effects on the fungus, but much less effect on mammalian cell membrane synthesis. Early data showed the relative lack of toxicity of azoles and their good efficacy in systemic mycoses. The expansion of these drugs into the superficial mycoses then began and continues today.

II. The Dawn of the Era of Azole Antifungals

Development of azoles might have occurred very slowly without the impetus of major changes in medical practice, changes only indirectly related to the mycoses. During the 1970s there were dramatic advances in the treatment of leukemia; immunosuppressive and cytotoxic therapies were introduced for the treatment of a variety of diseases; organ transplantation became commonplace; prolonged intravenous catheterization was widely used for hospitalized patients; antibacterial agents with an increasingly broad spectrum were used in more and more patients; finally, the AIDS pandemic was recognized in the early 1980s. All of these events provided fertile soil for an increase of the major opportunistic fungal diseases.

The opportunistic systemic mycoses may be conveniently divided into those which take advantage of defects in host polymorphonuclear leukocytes and those which exploit deficits of cell-mediated immunity. In the former group the major contenders are *Candida* and *Aspergillus* and, to a lesser degree, the zygomycetes. Mycoses caused by these agents often occur in the settings of neutropenia, uncontrolled diabetes mellitus, use of broad-spectrum antibacterials and of catheters of the intravascular or urinary tract types. Although there are distinguishing characteristics for diseases caused by the specific fungal pathogens, they share important features. Among these are a rapidly progressive course and refractoriness to therapy with amphotericin B if treatment is delayed. Mortality is in excess of 80% among neutropenic patients with 'documented' fungal infection and is not significantly lowered by the administration of amphotericin B (HORN et al. 1985). In the 1980s, fungal infections caused up to 25% of deaths in severely neutropenic patients, so this was a major clinical problem (BODEY 1984). Treatment has turned in recent years to initiating antifungal therapy empirically in the persistently febrile, neutropenic patient (PIZZO et al. 1982). High doses of amphotericin B have been used, and toxicity has been less of a concern than efficacy. One might ask whether antifungal azoles, with their slower onset of action and fungistatic activity, will have much role in these emergent situations. The answer is not yet clear but may be surprising.

The other major arena has been the fungal opportunists exploiting defects in cell-mediated immunity. These have commonly involved patients on corticosteroid therapy, those with lymphoproliferative diseases, and those with organ transplants. In the past 5 years these have been overshadowed by AIDS. Among the first appreciated fungal opportunists were dermatophytes and mucocutaneous *Candida* infections. These occur in more than half of patients with AIDS. They can be cosmetically devastating and cause severe thrush and esophagitis, with significant dysphagia as a consequence. There is clearly a role for azoles in suppressing these superficial infections.

In addition to the above, however, there are major life-threatening fungal infections. Cryptococcosis was the first appreciated of these (DISMUKES 1988). It most commonly takes the widely disseminated form and occurs in 5%–7% of AIDS patients. The initial reports of response to amphotericin B were extremely discouraging, with 60% failure of initial therapy, and 40% relapses occurring among those who did respond (KOVACS et al. 1985). Recently, there has been more optimism occasioned by initial treatment with daily amphotericin B, followed by weekly suppressive doses for an indefinite period

(ZUGER et al. 1988). The necessity of weekly dosing, the problems inherent in catheter management, and the toxicity of amphotericin B are all factors which prompt a re-examination of whether amphotericin B is appropriate primary or suppression treatment for cryptococcosis in the setting of AIDS. Because of the limited prognosis of AIDs patients, even if mycoses are suppressed, and because quality of life is a very important issue, prolonged treatment with fungistatic agents such as azoles may be an acceptable alternative to amphotericin B.

Another mycosis more recently associated with AIDS is aggressive, disseminated histoplasmosis. This can occur in the endemic areas and can also reactivate long after the patient has left the central USA. Initially, histoplasmosis was thought to occur in only about 0.5% of patients with AIDS, but physicians in Texas, Louisiana, Arkansas, and Oklahoma are now encountering histoplasmosis in as many as 5% of their AIDS patients (JOHNSON et al. 1988). Initial therapy was amphotericin B, which is curative in >80% of patients without AIDS but was effective in less than half of those with AIDS (JOHNSON et al. 1988). Relapses were also a major problem, prompting chronic suppressive therapy with amphotericin B in a similar fashion to cryptococcosis (MCKINSEY et al. 1989). There has been some preliminary exploration of antifungal azoles for histoplasmosis, although roles for either suppression or primary therapy are not yet established.

Thus, the development of antifungal azoles is presently undergoing a very rapid evolution. Indications for antifungal azoles are expanding, and new drugs are being developed at a surprising pace. The present text captures this dynamic story only at a moment in time. Nevertheless, it is worth considering the present status of the azole antifungals, as this will provide some basis for anticipating what the coming decade will bring in uses for this remarkable class of compounds.

1. The First Efforts 'Fail' – Clotrimazole

Clotrimazole was the initial venture into systemically administered antifungal azoles. The drug was given intravenously for a variety of infections, including coccidioidomycosis (JR GRAYBILL, unpublished observations). Initial unpublished observations were promising, but a number of later studies (including mine), also unpublished, were not so encouraging. The reason for this was stimulation of hepatic degrading enzymes. Clotrimazole levels in the bloodstream became undetectable within a week or two of commencing therapy. Instead of developing clotrimazole analogues to use systemically, Bayer adapted clotrimazole to topical use, where it rapidly became highly successful in the treatment of dermatophyte infections. Intravenous clotrimazole came and went with merely a hint of the success to follow.

2. The Potential Is Demonstrated – Miconazole

The next entry was miconazole (Monistat IV), developed by Janssen Pharmaceutica (STEVENS 1977). Miconazole suffered from water insolubility, which is a major problem common to the azoles. Miconazole is poorly absorbed after oral administration and can be solubilized only by using amphophilic carriers. The one chosen for clinical development was Cremophor, an agent used for solubilizing anesthetic agents. Miconazole is prepared as 200 mg in 20 ml of Cremophor. With a dose up to 3600 mg miconazole per day for coccidioidomycosis, the Cremophor dose became rather massive (STEVENS 1977, 1983). The relatively rapid clearance of miconazole necessitated 3 times daily intravenous administration, which meant hospitalization of the patient. Further more, prolonged therapy given for coccidioidomycosis was associated with significant toxicities, including thrombophlebitis, rash, dizziness, interaction with coumarin anticoagulants, hypertriglyceridemia, intense pruritus, and a syndrome of hypotension and bronchospasm (STEVENS 1983). A clinical report suggesting that these effects may be mediated by histamine release also suggested that slow infusion over 2 h was much safer than rapid infusion (FAINSTEIN and BODEY 1980). Although it is not entirely clear, much of the toxicity of miconazole may be caused by the carrier rather than the drug itself.

The greatest experiences with miconazole were accumulated in coccidioidomycosis and in disseminated candidosis. In several reports STEVENS and his colleagues (1977, 1983) found that miconazole treatment caused remissions in osteoarticular, pulmonary, and cutaneous lesions of patients with coccidioidomycosis. The drug was also found effective in patients with coccidioidal meningitis, although it is peculiar that the best results occurred in patients treated intravenously rather than intrathecally (DERESINSKI et al. 1977). These studies were confirmed by others (SUNG et al. 1978; HARRISON et al. 1983). However, STEVENS' group also noted that relapses arose very frequently after miconazole was discontinued, and others reported failures with miconazole (STEVENS 1983; MEYER et al. 1978; SUNG et al. 1977). Extension of treatment for more than 2 months may be associated with fewer relapses (DERESINSKI and STEVENS 1979). Even so, the responses of these patients, many of whom had failed or relapsed after amphotericin B, gave a clear indication that antifungal azoles could be beneficial in one of the most severe of the endemic mycoses.

Concurrent with studies in coccidioidomycosis were occasional reports of success in cryptococcal meningitis and candidal infections (JORDAN et al. 1979; WEINSTEIN and JACOBY 1980; MORGANS et al. 1979; GRAYBILL and LEVINE 1978; BENNETT and REMINGTON 1981). The patients treated for cryptococcosis improved dramatically but were too few in number for this to be more than suggestive of efficacy (MORGANS et al. 1979; GRAYBILL and LEVINE 1978; BENNETT and REMINGTON 1981; SUNG et al. 1977). Results in neutropenic patients treated for candidemia were conflicting (JORDAN et al. 1979; BENNETT and REMINGTON 1981; MAKSYMIUK et al. 1984).

Since these initial reports in the later 1970s and early 1980s, there have been only a few scattered case reports of intravenous miconazole use. The well-documented toxicity, high cost, need for hospitalization, failures, and relapses all combine to make miconazole at best a secondary agent. It is available today for parenteral use. Like clotrimazole, however, miconazole has become much more important as a topical agent for the treatment of superficial mycoses.

III. The Dam Breaks with Ketoconazole

Ketoconazole (Nizoral) was introduced in 1979–1980 as the first orally administered antifungal azole. The critical advantages of ketoconazole were its broad spectrum (VAN CUTSEM 1983), markedly increased water solubility in an acid milieu (which permits absorption from the gastrointestinal tract), lack of significant autoinduction of hepatic degrading enzymes, broad tissue distribution, and long serum half-life. The range of serum half-lives in different reports varies from 1 to 11 h. The half-life may be dose-dependent, suggesting some autoinhibition of degradation (DANESHMEND and WARNOCK 1988). Ketoconazole is also highly protein bound and penetrates poorly into the cerebrospinal fluid (CRAVEN et al. 1983).

The initial studies were conducted in coccidioidomycosis, histoplasmosis, blastomycosis, mucocutaneous candidosis, and paracoccidioidomycosis (NEGRONI et al. 1980; RESTREPO et al. 1983; STEVENS et al. 1983; GALGIANI et al. 1988; BRADSHER et al. 1985; DEFELICE et al. 1982; GRAYBILL et al. 1980). Reports of high efficacy and low toxicity were most encouraging for all of these, although coccidioidomycosis was still among the more refractory.

Larger prospective studies examined ketoconazole as a primary treatment for the endemic mycoses. While ketoconazole efficacy was confirmed in three of these, in coccidioidomycosis there were frequently modest improvements but relatively few remissions (National Institute of Allergy and Infectious Diseases Mycoses Study Group 1985; GALGIANI et al. 1988).

Penetration of ketoconazole into the cerebrospinal fluid was relatively low at 3%–7% of the serum concentration (CRAVEN et al. 1983). Nevertheless, doses of 1200 mg per day and above were associated with clinical remission of coccidioidal meningitis, the worst form of the disease.

The use of higher doses also brought out several of its problems. These included clearly dose-related gastrointestinal toxicity, with up to 50% of patients experiencing dose-limiting nausea and vomiting above 800 mg per day (SUGAR et al. 1987). It became apparent that high doses of ketoconazole impaired not only fungal sterol synthesis but also blocked synthesis of mammalian sterols (BRITTON et al. 1988). The most sensitive of these enzymes was C17–20 lyase, important in the synthesis of testosterone. The consequences of this included oligospermia, impotence, and gynecomastia (PONT et al. 1984). Effects on estrogen hormones are uncertain, but alopecia, loss of hair color, and irregular menses have all occurred in women. Higher doses of ketoconazole also suppress serum cortisol. This suppression is generally transitory and occurs several hours after high peak concentrations of the drug. The higher the dose of ketoconazole, the more prolonged the suppression. This does not persist for the full 24 h between doses, and perhaps for this reason, cortisol suppression has not been a major clinical problem with ketoconazole treatment, even with high doses (CRAVEN et al. 1983). Very few cases of adrenal hypocortisolism have been associated with ketoconazole (TUCKER et al. 1985; WHITE and KENDALL-TAYLOR 1985; PILLANS et al. 1985). One should be cautious, however, in using high doses of ketoconazole in patients with tuberculosis, histoplasmosis, paracoccidioidomycosis, or AIDS. The reason is that all of these problems are associated with hypoadrenalism, and ketoconazole may further aggravate this. Fortunately, even after prolonged courses of ketoconazole, its endocrine suppressive effects are gone within 2 days of discontinuing the drug.

On the other hand, endocrine suppressive effects have also been turned to a positive effect, both in testosterone suppression in patients with prostatic carcinoma and in the treatment of Cushing's syndrome (FARWELL et al. 1988; SONINO 1987). In a final 'twist,' it has been found that high doses of ketoconazole block cholesterol synthesis. When combined with cholestyramine, ketoconazole can sharply decrease low density cholesterol concentrations (MIETTINEN 1988). This suggests the use of such agents in the treatment of patients with hypercholesterolemia.

Another significant problem is hepatotoxicity (JANSSEN and SYMOENS 1983; LEWIS et al. 1984). This has been documented by liver function tests above the upper limits of normal in as many as 11% of patients. However, in one series 8% had elevated liver function tests before treatment (JANSSEN and SYMOENS 1983). For many patients with abnormal liver function tests, even if continued on ketoconazole, these tests return to normal. In one survey only 1:10000 developed symptomatic hepatitis (JANSSEN and SYMOENS 1983). A few deaths have been reported (DUARTE et al. 1984). It is generally accepted that the hepatitis is not dose related. However, relatively few patients have been treated at doses of 800 mg per day or higher, so the absence of dose dependence may in part reflect insufficient data for higher doses. Other adverse effects include rashes, dizziness, headache, and a variety of less common effects, which may be less clearly caused by ketoconazole.

In addition to the direct adverse effects of ketoconazole, there are a number of drug interactions which are relevant to the clinician. Ketoconazole is cleared largely by hepatic degradation, and all of the metabolic products are inactive. However, when combined with alcohol ingestion, ketoconazole may cause a disulfiram-like effect (FAZIO et al. 1983); I have also encountered a patient with this reaction (unpublished observation). A potentiation of the anticoagulant effects of warfarin has been reported by SMITH (1984). Other agents which stimulate hepatic enzymes may also accelerate the breakdown of ketoconazole. These include phenytoin (BRASS et al. 1982), rifampin (BRASS et al. 1982; MEUNIER-CARPENTIER et al. 1983; ENGLEHARD et al. 1984), barbiturates (STOCKLEY et al. 1983), and possibly isoniazid (ENGLEHARD et al. 1984). Furthermore, ketoconazole interferes with clearance of cyclosporin A; and when given together, cyclosporin A serum concentrations can rise into the toxic range (DIEPERINK and MØLLER 1982; SMITH et al. 1983; MORGEN-

STERN et al. 1982; FERGUSON et al. 1982). Ketoconazole also interferes with the clearance of chlordiazepoxide (BROWN et al. 1985).

Although ketoconazole is water soluble in the presence of acid, this imposes significant restraints on oral administration. Concurrent use of antacids or H2 blockers markedly reduces absorption, and clinical failures have been associated with low drug absorption (LELAWONGS et al. 1988). A practical point concerning ketoconazole treatment of immunosuppressed patients is that many of them on steroid treatment have concurrent antacid or H2 blocker treatment, and this must be stopped. An alternative is administering ketoconazole along with 3 acidulin tablets. This provides exogenous acid and helps to increase absorption. More recently we have learned that AIDS is associated with relative achlorhydria and a marked decrease in ketoconazole absorption (LAKE-BAKAAR et al. 1988). This undoubtedly contributes to some of the failures of ketoconazole treatment of thrush and *Candida* esophagitis in the AIDS patient. A significant additional problem arises from the malabsorption associated with mucositis induced by chemotherapy (STOCKLEY et al. 1983).

Despite the limitations noted above, ketoconazole has revolutionized antifungal therapy. For the first time we have an oral agent with broad spectrum antifungal activity and vastly less toxicity than amphotericin B. As more was learned about both the uses and the limitations of ketoconazole, however, it became apparent that there was still considerable room for improvement.

IV. The 'Second Generation' Azoles

1. Itraconazole – Broad Spectrum with Less Toxicity

Itraconazole offered an expanded in vitro spectrum, and animal studies also suggested efficacy in aspergillosis (VAN CUTSEM et al. 1987). Additionally, when compared with ketoconazole in animal studies, greater milligram for milligram potency was evident. Thus, itraconazole was introduced as a newer, more potent 'son of ketoconazole.' Several additional characteristics became apparent (VAN CAUTEREN et al. 1987). One of these was its markedly prolonged clearance time, with $t_{1/2}$ increasing from 20–30 h after the first dose to more than 40 h after a steady state had been achieved (about 2 weeks of therapy) (HARDIN et al. 1988). Absorption appears to be increased by acid and lipid meals, and I have unpublished results which strongly suggest that itraconazole absorption is significantly reduced by antacids given orally. Unpublished studies at Janssen imply that antacids may reduce absorption by 20%. There is no information on whether AIDS patients have decreased itraconazole absorption, as they do with ketoconazole. However, from unpublished experience, patients undergoing cancer chemotherapy had reduced itraconazole absorption.

Virtually all drug disposition occurs by hepatic degradation, and no drug is excreted in the urine. Also, cerebrospinal fluid penetration is virtually zero. The clinical importance of these characteristics in humans is uncertain.

Because of its expanded in vitro spectrum, itraconazole has been evaluated in the endemic mycoses, sporotrichosis, chromoblastomycosis, aspergillosis, and phaeohyphomycosis. Results have been mixed for aspergillosis, in part because of the difficulty in making a diagnosis and also because of the vagaries in determining what is and is not disseminated disease. For the other infections itraconazole has been quite promising.

One reason for encouragement is the relative paucity of adverse reactions. At 400 mg doses, the maximum presently permitted, itraconazole has been associated with a series of side reactions, most of which are quite minor. These include in one series of almost 50 patients nausea and vomiting, depressed libido (normal testosterone levels), headaches, dizziness, and leukopenia (GRAYBILL, for the Mycoses Study Group, unpublished observations). While a number of patients in this study had one or more 'reactions,' these were so minor that only 3 left the protocol for reasons of possible toxicity.

There are fewer data available, but Janssen in-house reviews suggest that itraconazole has only about half of the potential for hepatotoxicity as ketoconazole (LEGENDRE, Janssen Pharmaceutica, personal communication). One case of icteric hepatitis has been seen.

Itraconazole also has the potential for hepatic enzyme induction, and hepatic degradation may be accelerated by other agents which induce these enzymes. I have recently treated a patient with itraconazole over many months for pulmonary coccidioidomycosis. When he developed concurrent mycobacterial infection, rifampin was added to his regimen. Itraconazole serum concentrations, which had been quite stable, promptly became undetectable, returning to their prior range only after the rifampin had been discontinued.

Endocrine adverse effects are fewer than for ketoconazole and are of a different nature. Limited experience with patients treated at 600 mg per day for unusually severe disease showed that itraconazole was associated with hypertension, hypokalemia, and in one patient hypocortisolism (SHARKEY et al. 1988). These findings suggest that a block may occur at site another than those affected by ketoconazole.

In general, itraconazole has fewer adverse reactions than ketoconazole, and considerable promise in a wide variety of systemic mycoses. Itraconazole has already become the drug of choice for paracoccidioidomycosis and chromoblastomycosis and is likely to assume this role for a number of other serious fungal infections.

2. Fluconazole – Targeting a Disease Based on Preclinical Studies

Fluconazole was developed by Pfizer, with clinical studies introduced shortly after Janssen commenced theirs with itraconazole. Like itraconazole, fluconazole has been studied extensively in humans, and licensing in the USA is anticipated in the near future. Fluconazole is also a triazole, but with several characteristics which distinguish it from ketoconazole and itraconazole.

One of these, unfortunately, is the difficulty of demonstrating activity in vitro. Poor activity in the test tube is in sharp contrast to its good efficacy in a number of animal models. This also means that it may be difficult to predict the efficacy of some antifungal drugs based only on their in vitro profile (see Chap. 4). A second characteristic, and highly desirable, is its excellent water solubility. Unlike either ketoconazole or itraconazole, fluconazole can be given either orally or intravenously. Furthermore, oral absorption does not seem to depend on having a low intragastric pH. A third characteristic is good tissue penetration, including cerebrospinal fluid concentrations as high as 80% of concurrent serum concentrations (ARNDT et al. 1988). At a dose of 100 mg per day, peak serum concentrations ranged from 4.5 to 8 mg/ml, with 89% penetration into the cerebrospinal fluid (TUCKER et al. 1988b). Fourth, fluconazole is excreted primarily in the urine, making it a possible candidate for treatment of fungal urinary tract infections (HUMPHREY et al. 1985). Fifth, the clearance time is also prolonged, of the order of 30 h in humans. This means that there is progressive drug accumulation, with a steady state achieved after about 2 weeks.

The high penetration of the cerebrospinal fluid suggested that fluconazole would be a useful agent in the treatment of cryptococcal meningitis. This led to a series of studies is exploring the potential role for fluconazole in AIDS and non AIDS patients with cryptococcal meningitis. Other roles are less well defined.

Toxicities of fluconazole appear, like itraconazole, to be less than for ketoconazole. In studies of rat liver, HOUSTON et al. (1988) found fluconazole to interact less with hepatic P-450 enzymes than ketoconazole, and on this basis they believe that it may be more selective for fungal than mammalian enzymes. It is possible that fluconazole may produce less hepatotoxicity than ketoconazole in humans, but there are no clear data on this yet.

3. SCH39304 – Potent 'New Kid on the Block'

SCH39304 (SM 8668) is presently just completing animal studies and phase I trials in humans. This agent is much less soluble than fluconazole and has great potency in vitro and in animal models against a variety of fungal pathogens (HOBBS et al. 1988; RESTREPO et al. 1988c; KOBAYASHI et al. 1988; WALSH et al. 1988b; LOEBENBERG et al. 1988; SCHMITT et al. 1988; see chapter 22). However, like fluconazole SCH39304 is not highly protein bound and is excreted in the urine. There are no major metabolites known. In animal models, cerebrospinal fluid penetration is as much as 30% of serum. This suggests possible value in cryptococcal meningitis. The clearance is extremely slow, with a serum half-life of more than 60 h in humans (KRAMER et al. 1988). An intravenous preparation is under development. Efficacy in animal models of aspergillosis suggests that this agent may be useful in the treatment of neutropenic febrile patients (SCHMITT et al. 1988).

V. Further out on the Horizon

1. BAYER 3783

At present there are only the most preliminary in-house data available for this agent, developed by Bayer (HECTOR 1988; PLEMPEL and BÜCHEL 1988). In contrast with other azoles, some of the metabolites of this drug appear to have potent antifungal activity. There have as yet been no human studies with this drug (see also chap. 22).

2. Saperconazole – Son of Itraconazole

This drug is under development by Janssen. Like itraconazole, it shares a slow clearance time and is effective in animal models of aspergillosis and a variety of other fungal infections (VAN CUTSEM and JANSSEN 1988). A parenteral form is under development. The spectrum is apparently very broad. There are no data in humans as of this time (see also chap. 22).

VI. A Drug That was Retired Before Its Time – ICI 153,066

This agent has broad antifungal activity and appears quite effective in animal models of cryptococcosis and other mycoses (GRAYBILL et al. 1983b). However, its toxicity in animals led to a decision not to develop this drug further.

B. Interrelation of the Azoles

Among the uncertainties regarding the antifungal azoles is the correlation of in vitro animal models, and clinical efficacy. For most of the era of amphotericin B there had been no serious effort to address this relationship, in part because we had no other choices. Now that there is a variety of antifungal azoles, it is appropriate to address the relationship of in vitro sensitivities and clinical applications. To do so requires standardization of in vitro testing procedures among laboratories and selection of the procedures that best correlate with in vivo results (GALGIANI 1987). Such studies are being started for amphotericin B, and the effort is simply to standardize susceptibility studies among laboratories. The relationships among the azoles are considerably less clear. In vitro tests depend upon a host of conditions during the procedure and may not predict in vivo efficacy (see Chap. 4). What may be needed is a systematic examination of various azoles in multiple isolates of various fungal pathogens. In vitro susceptibilities appear to span broad ranges for *Candida* spp. *Cryptococcus neoformans*, and *Aspergillus* spp. It would seem reasonable to determine a 50% protective dose for each isolate, and then take the most responsive and least responsive isolates for comparison by a series of in vitro assays. With many azoles coming into clinical investigations, now would be an appropriate time to undertake such studies.

C. Patterns of Use of the Antifungal Azoles in the 1990s

I. Use in Neutropenic Patients

1. Treatment of Established Candidosis and Aspergillosis

Studies in the early 1980s showed that treatment with amphotericin B in neutropenic patients with documented systemic mycoses was ineffective (HORN et al. 1985). A later study was conducted by the group at MD Anderson Hospital, using miconazole (JORDAN et al. 1979); in all, 183 patients were treated with miconazole. Of these, 33 had documented *Candida* infections, of whom 12 survived, leading the researchers to comment that miconazole was as effective as amphotericin B. However, a short time later the group published their expanded observations (MAKSYMIUK et al. 1984). In contrast to the first report, they found neither amphotericin B nor miconazole effective in candidemia. Since these studies there have been only limited efforts to explore miconazole therapy of documented mycoses.

Until the advent of fluconazole there was no intravenous azole alternative to miconazole. Studies with fluconazole are presently in progress, and no results are available. The orally administered azoles have not been seriously pursued for treatment of documented fungal infection in these patients. The whole area is open for further study, with no therapeutic approach being clearly superior.

Hepatosplenic candidosis is one distinct clinical entity which is manifested paradoxically in the neutropenic patient after recovery of leukocyte counts (THALER et al. 1988); it is characterized by local abscesses which are remarkably resistant to amphotericin B. Although liposomal amphotericin B has shown some benefit, there may be a major role for azoles in this situation. We have treated one patient successfully with fluconazole (GRAYBILL, unpublished observation). WALSH et al. (1988a) found fluconazole to be effective in an animal model of this condition. Although there are virtually no clinical data, this would seem to be one attractive place to evaluate azole therapy.

2. Empiric Antifungal Therapy for Candidosis and Aspergillosis

This approach was popularized initially by the group at the National Cancer Institute, using placebo versus amphotericin B (PIZZO et al. 1982). Their initial study demonstrated that neutropenic patients persistently febrile after 1 week of antibacterial therapy had fewer documented fungal infections when treated empirically with amphotericin B than patients receiving placebo.

Although effective, amphotericin B had significant toxicity, and in a follow-up study, oral ketoconazole was compared with amphotericin B for empirical treatment. Both agents were equally effective (FAINSTEIN et al. 1987). However, some patients were ineligible for the study because they could not take oral medication. Another problem is that ketoconazole is not effective against aspergillosis, a potential ‘hole’ for this drug. Confirmational studies are needed, but the data available suggest that when oral antifungals can be given, ketoconazole is effective. The dose used is 600 mg per day, somewhat higher than the ‘usual’ 200–400 mg doses in use.

3. Prophylaxis of Candidosis and Aspergillosis

A logical extension of antifungal therapy reasons: If mortality can be reduced by giving empirical therapy, perhaps it can be eliminated by prophylaxis for every neutropenic patient. However, prophylaxis involves treating many more patients than in empirical therapy for documented disease. These patients may have complex regimens, some including antacids or H2 blockers. Some may have acute mucositis from chemotherapy. There may be less absorption of drug and more chance for adverse interactions. Statistical considerations are more complex, as 5%–20% of patients may develop fungal gastrointestinal tract colonization, and separating these from the much small number with disseminated disease is a problem.

Miconazole has recently been evaluated in a large, prospective, placebo-controlled trial aimed at prophylaxis in leukopenic patients (WINGARD et al. 1987). In this study 208 treatment courses in 180 patients were evaluated. Of the 97 patients treated with miconazole, only 1 developed fungal sepsis (not fatal), versus 8 of 111 receiving placebo (4 fatal). Reduction of fungal infection was significant at P = 0.03, while reduction of fungal fatalities was close to significant (P = 0.08). Surprisingly, there were no major side reactions. The investigators also commented favorably on the lack of increase in *Aspergillus* infections among treated patients. However, this may not be valid, as aspergillosis appears to be much more of a problem in specific centers where it is a major environmental hazard. I remain somewhat skeptical about the value of miconazole in the prophylaxis of mycoses in granulocytopenic patients, in part because of the cost, requirement for hospitalization, and toxicity seen with other mycoses.

Ketoconazole has been evaluated rather extensively for prophylaxis, sometimes in comparison with placebo and sometimes with oral amphotericin B or nystatin (HANN et al. 1982; MEUNIER-CARPENTIER 1984). In one study ketoconazole was clearly associated with fewer fungal infections than polyene (HANN et al. 1982). Ketoconazole clearly reduces candidal counts in the stool. However, *Torulopsis glabrata* (usually nonpathogenic) commonly replaces *Candida* in the cultures and may be difficult to identify (SHEPP et al. 1985). Ketoconazole prophylaxis has not consistently been associated with decreased days of empirically used amphotericin B or fewer fungal infections than with amphotericin B (MEUNIER-CARPENTIER 1984).

Itraconazole has also been explored as a possible prophylactic agent. At doses of 400 mg per day, an outbreak of aspergillosis at a Europen Cancer Center which began during the use of ketoconazole prophylaxis was suppressed after switching to itraconazole (TRICOT et al. 1987). In this historical study, ketoconazole prophylaxis was associated with a number of aspergillosis deaths. In another European study, also uncontrolled, 72 patients were treated with itraconazole during remission induction. 'The incidence of fungal infections was 18% (12.5% fatal) which compares favorably with our historical ketoconazole treated group (= 36.5% fungal fatalities)' (BOOGAERTS et al. 1988). Switching to itraconazole was associated with many fewer deaths. However, more recent trials conducted in the USA have found less evidence of protection (LEGENDRE, personal communication). We suspect this may be because the drug is not suspended in an acid environment and may well not have been absorbed initially.

There are fewer data on fluconazole for prophylaxis. Fluconazole has the advantage of oral absorption without the necessity of acid, and the potential disadvantage of little anti-*Aspergillus* activity. In one recently reported study, 14 patients randomized to amphotericin B oral prophylaxis at 1600 mg per day were compared with 13 fluconazole recipients at 50 mg per day (ROZENBERG-ARSKA et al. 1988). Despite the small number of patients, colonization was significantly reduced from 9 patients receiving fluconazole to 1 patient receiving amphotericin B. The researchers concluded that fluconazole was effective in preventing fungal infections and that colonization with fluconazole did not lead to infection. The inferred cause and effect relationship seems unwarranted, both because there was no placebo group and there was only one with a fungal infection in the entire group of 27 patients.

II. Use in Fungal Infections in Other Immunocompromised States

1. AIDS

a) Candidosis

More than half of AIDS patients develop oral thrush, and many of these develop candidal esophagitis as well. Dissemination is rare. Candidal skin lesions may also occur and may be associated with dermatophyte infection. Azole antifungals are extremely useful in these infections. A first line of treatment is topical clotrimazole, administered as lozenges. This is successful in half or more patients. For the remainder, ketoconazole has been used with success in both thrush and esophagitis (DESCHAMPS et al. 1988; FAZIO et al. 1983). However, there are three cautions with the use of ketoconazole in patients with AIDS. First, patients are relatively achlorhydric, and doses up to 600 per day are often required. Second, nausea and vomiting are common side effects of ketoconazole and may aggravate the anorexia already present in many patients. Third, ketoconazole can suppress the adrenal gland. The AIDS patient may already have a marginal adrenal reserve from either cytomegalovirus, histoplasmosis, or tuberculosis, and addition of ketoconazole could tip the balance to adrenal failure. Ketoconazole or clotrimazole are the presently recommended drugs for thrush, but as neither is ideal, both fluconazole and itraconazole have been investigated. More patients have been treated with fluconazole than with itraconazole. FARROW et al. (1987) recently reported an open study in which 95 patients with oropharyngeal candidosis were treated with 50 mg fluconazole daily for a median of 9 days. Most patients had either AIDS or malignancy. At follow-up (median 16 days after treatment termination) 90% had clinical cure and 67% and eradication of *Candida*. In another study from Belgium, ketoconazole and fluconazole were compared in a double-blind prospective trial (DE WIT et al. 1988). Both clinical cure (100%) and mycological eradication (54%) were significantly greater with fluconazole than cure for ketoconazole (75%) or mycological eradication (22%). However, only 33 patients were studied. Side effects of fluconazole were few, and fluconazole at 50 or 100 mg per day may become the drug of choice for candidal infection in AIDS patients.

b) Cryptococcosis

Amphotericin B, with or without flucytosine, remains the 'traditional' treatment, at initial doses of 0.5–0.8 mg/kg daily (DISMUKES 1988). Failures and relapses have ocurred in well over half the patients treated (KOVACS et al. 1985). Accordingly, initial treatment is now usually supplemented by indefinite weekly 1–1.5 mg/kg suppressive doses (DISMUKES 1988; ZUGER et al. 1988; ENG et al. 1986). However, the need for chronic intravenous catheters and the general toxicity and dependency on clinic visits are major impediments. There is now extensive uncontrolled experience with several reports; these largely concern suppressive therapy. In two such studies, 41 patients were treated with fluconazole (STERN et al. 1988; SUGAR and SAUNDERS 1988). Some 7 patients were treated initially with fluconazole, 4 with success; 34 were given fluconazole for chronic suppressive maintenance, and only 3 of these relapsed. These studies are promising, but there is no late follow-up on many of the patients. Also, the doses used, 50 and 100 mg per day, were relatively low by present standards. At present there is a multicenter study comparing fluconazole with amphotericin B for primary treatment. There is also a study for amphotericin B primary treatment and then randomization to suppression with either amphotericin B (intravenously administered) or fluconazole 200 mg per day. Patient enrollment is completed and preliminary data suggests that fluconazole and amphotericin B each cause remission in about 50% of patients, but with disproportionate early deaths in the fluconazole group.

Many AIDS patients with cryptococcosis in the USA have been entered in the multicenter fluconazole/amphotericin B studies. However, there is also some evidence for efficacy of itraconazole in cryptococcosis in AIDS patients. In a preliminary report by CAUWENBERGH et al. 1987), six patients were treated with itraconazole at 200 mg per day for 8 to 90 days. The cultures from two patients converted to negative and clinically there was a marked improvement, and data are not presented for the others. Other reported European experiences have also been positive, with about 75% of patients responding (DE GANS et al. 1988; VIVIANI et al. 1987). These studies are small and not comparative, as are those with fluconazole.

Thus, currently there are two azoles competing to replace amphotericin B as primary or maintenance treatment of cryptococcosis in the AIDS patient. It is uncertain which will ultimately prove superior, though there are more anecdotes and comparative data with fluconazole than with itraconazole.

c) Histoplasmosis

In the southern central USA histoplasmosis occurs in as many as 5% of the AIDS patients in Houston (JOHNSON et al. 1988). Response to amphotericin B, with or without continuing ketoconazole suppression, has been of the order of 50%. Because of relapses after amphotericin B, either long-term amphotericin B suppression or ketoconazole has been used to prevent histoplasmosis recurrences (MCKINSEY et al. 1989). In 14 patients treated with weekly amphotericin B with a mean follow-up of 9 months, there has been only 1 relapse. Data are needed to confirm whether or not this is effective. As another alternative, in a small series with 9 patients, itraconazole at 400 mg per day was effective as primary treatment in 8 patients, with a mean follow-up of 1 year (GRAYBILL 1988). In the same series, 3 of 5 patients treated with fluconazole ultimately relapsed. The fluconazole dose, 50 or 100 mg per day, is now known to be inadequate, and it is possible that higher doses may be successful. Larger multicenter studies are running to determine whether itraconazole will be effective either primary or supressive treatment.

d) Other

Coccidioidomycosis occurs infrequently in AIDS patients. In one small series, all patients were treated with amphotericin B, and treatment ultimately failed uniformly (BRONNIMANN et al. 1987). Very few patients have been treated with azoles, and it is not possible to come to any conclusion.

2. Cryptococcosis

Cryptococcal meningitis is now being evaluated in non-AIDS patients. A multicenter trial is comparing amphotericin B with fluconazole as primary therapy. No results are yet available.

III. Use in Nonimmunocompromised Patients

1. Major Endemic Mycoses

a) Histoplasmosis

Early reports of success in scattered cases of histoplasmosis were followed by the 400/800 mg per day comparative study of ketoconazole done by the Mycoses Study Group (National Institute of Allergy and Infectious Diseases

Mycoses Study Group 1985). In this study 31 patients were treated with 400 mg per day, with 24 responses, and 23 patients were treated with 800 mg per day, with 10 responses. The lower response rate at 800 mg per day was not readily explained. The overall responses were considered to be in the same range as amphotericin B (34 of 54). Based on this response rate, and with reduced toxicity when compared with amphotericin B, the Mycoses Study Group recommended ketoconazole at 400 mg per day for 6 months as the primary treatment for non-life-threatening histoplasmosis. Only 4 patients relapsed after successful treatment.

Initial reports have suggested that itraconazole is also highly effective in histoplasmosis. Of 16 patients treated by NEGRONI et al. (1987) with 100 mg per day for 6 months, 12 were cured and 4 were markedly improved; there was relapse in this series. Of two evaluable patients with histoplasmosis reported by PHILLIPS et al. (1987), one improved. The Mycoses Study Group recently reported treatment results in 28 patients with histoplasmosis (SAAG et al. 1988). While 16 remained on treatment at the time of the report, there was only 1 failure and 1 relapse in the entire study group.

Fluconazole on the other hand has been studied only at the 50 and 100 mg per day doses; preliminary results have not been encouraging, with fewer than half of the patients showing remission (Mycoses Study Group, unpublished observations).

Therefore, the present recommendation of ketoconazole as the drug of choice is likely to undergo revision as itraconazole becomes available.

b) Blastomycosis

In Bradsher's large series, 43 patients were treated for 1 to >6 months with ketoconazole at 400 mg per day (BRADSHER et al. 1985). Of the 6 patients who relapsed, 4 had been noncompliant with treatment. The Mycoses Study Group trial comparing 400 and 800 mg per day ketoconazole for 6 months confirmed these results (National Institute of Allergy and Infectious Diseases Mycoses Study Group 1985). Blastomycosis responds well to 400 mg per day (26 successes of 33 treated for 6 months or more) and to 800 mg per day (32 successes of 32 treated for 6 months or more). Because of lower gastrointestinal intolerance, the 400 mg per day dose was recommended as the drug of choice for primary treatment of non-life-threatening blastomycosis. It is also possible that itraconazole may supplant ketoconazole on grounds of similar efficacy and reduced toxicity. Preliminary findings by the Mycoses Study Group are very encouraging for 38 evaluable patients with blastomycosis (SAAG et al. 1988). Although 12 patients were still on treatment at the time of the initial report, only 1 failure was noted.

c) Coccidioidomycosis

Initial reports of ketoconazole success in coccidioidomycosis were quite optimistic (STEVENS et al. 1983; GALGIANI et al. 1988; DEFELICE et al. 1982;

GRAYBILL et al. 1980; CATANZARO et al. 1982; HORSBURGH et al. 1983; ROSS et al. 1982). Responses were reported above 60% in osteoarticular, chronic pulmonary, and soft tissue disease. These reports included modest as well as marked improvements and remissions, and reflected the different criteria used by various investigators. The summary provided in Levine's book, '*Ketoconazole in the Management of Fungal Disease*,' was closer to present estimates, reporting 13% remissions and marked improvement in 22% (HEEL 1982). A more recent study by the Mycoses Study Group comparing 400 mg per day with 800 mg per day found only 23% remissions at 400 mg per day and 32% remissions at 800 mg per day (GALGIANI et al. 1988). Even when treatment of failures at the initial doses was raised to as high as 1600 mg per day, fewer than half of the patients achieved remission. Finally, of the 36 patients who did achieve remission, 15 relapsed during a 1-year follow-up period. It is of interest that the patients who responded to 400 mg per day had a significantly less chance of relapsing than those who required higher doses to achieve a remission. Thus, ketoconazole is recommended as an alternative but not a superior treatment to amphotericin B.

Itraconazole is also being investigated in coccidioidomycosis. The Mycoses Study Group reported preliminary findings in 43 patients with non-meningeal coccidioidomycosis treated with 100 – 400 mg per day itraconazole (GRAYBILL et al. 1986). By 7 months of treatment the pretreatment evaluation scores had declined by 57%. Toxicities were minor, and most patients were continuing on treatment at the time of this report. In subsequent evaluation more than 50% of patients have achieved a state of remission (GRAYBILL, unpublished observation). TUCKER et al. (1988a) have also reported their experience with itraconazole (400 mg per day) given to 62 patients with coccidioidomycosis. At 6 months, 61% improvement was noted in 38 treatment courses. Failures of itraconazole were noted more frequently in patients who had failed to respond to prior therapy. Itraconazole is thus quite promising for coccidioidomycosis.

The azoles are also being increasingly used in coccidioidal meningitis (CRAVEN et al. 1983; BUCHSBAUM et al. 1985; SHEHAB et al. 1988; DERESINSKI et al. 1977; SUNG et al. 1978; HARRISON et al. 1983). Miconazole was initially employed, but toxicity and the relapse rate have limited its value (DERESINSKI et al. 1977). CRAVEN et al. (1983) first reported the use of high doses of ketoconazole, 800–2000 mg per day, in coccidioidal meningitis. Their encouraging responses led BUCHSBAUM and others to investigate high-dose ketoconazole as an alternative to amphotericin B (BUCHSBAUM et al. 1985; SHEHAB et al. 1988). Responses have been in general good, although ketoconazole cannot be recommended as the drug of choice for coccidioidal meningitis. Part of the reason is that treatment must be very prolonged, and there is no information on relapses after cessation of therapy. We have treated one patient for 7 years, only to have him relapse 6 months after treatment was terminated. More recently there has been an interest in fluconazole treatment for coccidioidal meningitis. Of 14 evaluable patients treated with 50 – 400 mg per day,

8 responses have occurred. Nine of these patients received fluconazole with no intrathecal amphotericin B, and six responded, which is very encouraging (TUCKER et al. 1990).

d) Paracoccidioidomycosis

Paracoccidioidomycosis was the first of the endemic mycoses treated with ketoconazole. Responses have been consistently excellent, above 90%, with both RESTREPO and NEGRONI reporting excellent outcomes in their patients (RESTREPO et al. 1983; NEGRONI et al. 1980). Treatment with ketoconazole is 200 mg per day for 1 year. Even so, itraconazole has made some inroads, with its 6-month course being as effective as 1 year of ketoconazole (though direct comparative studies are lacking). In two series, 41 patients were treated with 100 mg per day for 6 months (RESTREPO et al. 1987; NEGRONI et al. 1987). Some 39 were cured or markedly improved. Relapses were rare. On the basis of great efficacy, low toxicity, and the abbreviation of treatment to 6 months, itraconazole would appear to be the drug of choice for paracoccidioidomycosis.

2. Miscellaneous Mycoses

a) Sporotrichosis

Potassium iodide is presently the drug of choice for cutaneous sporotrichosis and amphotericin B, for disseminated disease. However, many patients either develop intolerance to potassium iodide, or amphotericin B therapy fails. The published experience is still very limited with azoles, but it appears that ketoconazole is of uncertain efficacy (CALHOUN et al. 1986; DISMUKES et al. 1983). In contrast, itraconazole is highly efficacious at 100 mg per day for 6 months. RESTREPO has published the largest series, all cutaneous or lymphocutaneous disease, and has found itraconazole to give excellent responses (RESTREPO et al. 1986). In 14 of 17 patients treated for an average of 115 days, there were no relapses. LAVALLE has also had good responses in 4 of 5 patients treated in Mexico, with doses of 50–200 mg per day (LAVALLE et al. 1987). Both of Borelli's 2 patients were cured (BORELLI 1987). Seven patients treated by the Mycoses Study Group also responded to itraconazole (SAAG et al. 1988). I have an unpublished series of 5 patients, including 1 with pulmonary and 1 with osteomyelitis, with excellent responses in all. Not enough patients with sporotrichosis are likely to accrue to conduct a controlled comparative trial, but it is my suspicion that itraconazole will become the drug of choice for lymphocutaneous disease (except in cost, as azoles are very expensive) as soon as it becomes available. It is not possible at this time to predict a role in disseminated disease, but a very few cases suggest there will be a role for this drug.

b) Phaeohyphomycosis

The 'black' fungi are becoming increasing frequent pathogens in the immunocompetent host and also the immunosuppressed host. They are generally sensitive to amphotericin B in vitro, but the drug usually fails in vivo. They are usually susceptible to itraconazole in vitro (VAN CUTSEM et al. 1987). GANER et al. (1987) reported on one patient with sinonasal alternariosis in whom treatment with amphotericin B, miconazole, and ketoconazole had failed yet she improved markedly with itraconazole. Recently I and others have had dramatic successes in individual patients with itraconazole therapy. It is unlikely that there will ever be enough patients for comparative studies, but itraconazole is acquiring a major role. Doses up to 400 mg per day for protracted courses of more than a year may be needed in some patients with cerebral infection.

c) Pseudallescheria boydii

This pathogen causes infections ranging from pneumonia to mycetoma. It is resistant to amphotericin B in the test tube and also resistant in patients. There have been minimal reports of patients treated with the azoles, but both miconazole and ketoconazole appear effective (GALGIANI et al. 1984). Ketoconazole 400 mg per day for a prolonged course is the preferred agent at this time, though it may ultimately be replaced by other azoles.

d) Chromoblastomycosis

South American chromoblastomycosis is usually caused by *Fonsecaea pedrosoi* or *Cladosporium* spp. In earlier years this could only be treated with amputation when possible. More recently there have been good responses to flucytosine, but this was only irregularly effective. Several recent reports have suggested that itraconazole may be effective in both *Fonsecaea* and *Cladosporium* infections (LAVALLE et al. 1987; BORELLI 1987). Ten of 11 evaluable patients with *Cladosporium carrioni* were cured by itraconazole 100 – 400 mg per day (BORELLI 1987). Treatment was for a remarkably brief period, less than 2 months in a number of these patients. Five have successfully completed 5 months or longer follow-up. Similarly, 10 of 13 evaluable patients with *Fonsecaea pedrosoi* improved and 2 may have been cured (BORELLI 1987). The post-treatment follow-up in these patients was only a few months, however. GANER et al. (1987) also had 2 patients with *Fonsecaea*, both of whom improved on itraconazole. In another series by RESTREPO et al. (1988a), patients with chromoblastomycosis (caused by *F. pedrosoi*) responded very well to itraconazole 200 mg per day. Here the treatment was longer, up to 2 years, but results were encouraging. RESTREPO et al. (1988a) also demonstrated shrinkage of involved skin lesions on their patients and suggested that those with very large body surface involvement might not fare quite so well. In unpublished studies I have found that *F. pedrosoi* infection in athymic mice responds well to both itraconazole and SCH39304. However, SCH39304 has not been used yet in humans. Therefore, given the dismal performance of prior efforts to treat this uncommon disease, the record with itraconazole strongly suggests that it is already the agent of choice in South American chromoblastomycosis. Unfortunately, different pathogens cause chromoblastomycosis in Africa, and these may not be so responsive to itraconazole (HAY, personal communication).

e) Aspergillosis

The majority of nonimmunocompromised patients with deep infections have *Aspergillus* fungus balls, although a few with invasive aspergillosis, usually chronic, have been seen. *Aspergillus* is generally resistant to ketoconazole in vitro. Nevertheless, SHALE et al. (1987) reported serological improvement in six patients with allergic bronchopulmonary aspergillosis or mycetoma versus no improvement in four controls. The forms of disease treated and the small numbers involved are inconclusive. Another case report claims success for treatment of a cerebral aspergilloma with 1200 mg per day for 6 months (KWONG et al. 1987). *Aspergillus* spp. are sensitive in vitro to itraconazole. DUPONT and DROUHET (1988) and RESTREPO et al. (1988b) reported a combined experience with itraconazole treatment of seven patients with fungus balls and have found improvement or resolution in four. RESTREPO et al. (1988b) additionally reported resolution of cavities in four of six patients and some improvement of cough, sputum production, and hemoptysis in their series of eight patients with aspergilloma or chronic pulmonary aspergillosis. The problem here is difficulty of evaluation of these patients, most of whom have extensive destructive processes, which are unlikely to undergo much resolution with any treatment.

f) Fungal Keratitis

Perhaps a better assessment of itraconazole in aspergillosis comes from the large series of patients with mycotic keratitis studied by THOMAS and RAJASEKERAN (1988). In their series 15 of 23 patients with severe keratitis had ‘excellent or moderate’ improvement, with the same result in 12 of 13 patients with ‘non-severe’ *Aspergillus* keratitis. Both *A. fumigatus* and *A. flavus* responded well. It is of interest that their in vitro susceptibility testing predicted good responses to *Aspergillus* spp., while another pathogen, *Fusarium*, was highly resistant in vitro and, unfortunately, also in vivo. Of 24 patients with *Fusarium* keratitis, fewer than half improved with itraconazole. Fluconazole has been administered by intravitreal injection in rabbits, and there were no intraocular effects (SCHULMAN et al. 1987). Unfortunately, it has little activity against either *Aspergillus* or *Fusarium*.

g) Candida Infections

Candidemia has occurred in the nonimmunosuppressed patient, often in drug addicts. In a large outbreak which occurred in France, DUPONT and DROUHET (1985) reported remarkable success with oral ketoconazole given to a large number of addicts who developed candidemia, manifested often as subcutaneous abscesses. The syndrome was so distinct that the good results achieved are irrelevant to the question as to whether oral ketoconazole can be used more generally in hematogenously spread *Candida* infection.

The other major *Candida* infection in the nonimmunosuppressed patient is urinary tract infection. This is a common but very controversial problem. There is little agreement on how many organisms are diagnostic for an infection (versus colonization) or how often infection responds to drug therapy versus spontaneous cure. With these major caveats, evaluating treatment regimens is at best done with great caution. Nevertheless, there are several studies which suggest that ketoconazole, despite its poor penetration into urine, may be associated with resolution in half of the patients with fungal urinary tract infection studied (GRAYBILL et al. 1983a; WISE et al. 1985). Two studies have also suggested that fluconazole may be of value in fungal urinary tract infection (GRAYBILL et al. 1988; BRU et al. 1988). The drug concentrates to as high as 600 μg/ml in urine. Fourteen patients with fungal urinary tract infections (7 with *C. albicans*, 3 with *C. tropicalis*, 4 with *Torulopsis glabrata*) were treated, with 11 responses. None of these studies were placebo controlled, an important limitation to interpreting results.

D. Summary

The antifungal azoles all share a common mechanism of action, but they also show remarkable diversity. This includes not only fungal spectrum but also route of administration, tissue distribution, urinary versus hepatic excretion, clearance rates, and toxicities for some.

The variety of these agents has for the first time brought to the clinician a broad choice among antifungals of a non-polyene class. For some of these infections ketoconazole has already replaced amphotericin B as the drug of choice (SAAG and DISMUKES 1988). Itraconazole and fluconazole are both well into clinical evaluation and appear to have major roles developing for their use. Drugs in earlier stages of investigation offer yet more variety. The 1990s should see the continuing expansion of azole antifungals, with multiple new drugs becoming available.

References

Arndt CAS, Walsh TJ, McCully CL, Balis FM, Pizzo PA, Poplack DG (1988) Fluconazole penetration into cerebrospinal fluid: implications for treating fungal infections of the central nervous system. J Inf Dis 157:178–180

Bennett JE, Remington JS (1981) Miconazole in cryptococcosis and systemic candidiasis: a word of caution. Ann Int Med 94:708–709

Bodey GP (1984) Candidiasis in cancer patients. Am J Med 77 (Suppl 4D):13–19

Boogaerts MA, Van De Pitte K, Verhoef G, Zachee P, De Beule K (1988) Itraconazole (ITRA) prophylaxis of invasive fungal infection in prolonged neutropenia. Abstract 576. Twenty-eighth Interscience Conference on Antimicrobial Agents and Chemotherapy, Los Angeles (Abstr 576)

Borelli D (1987) A clinical trial of itraconazole in the treatment of deep mycoses and leishmaniasis. Rev Inf Dis 9:S57–S63

Bradsher RW, Rice DC, Abernathy RS (1985) Ketoconazole therapy for endemic blastomycosis. Ann Int Med 103:872–879

Brass C, Galgiani JN, Blaschke TF, DeFelice R, O'Reilly RA, Stevens DA (1982) Disposition of ketoconazole, an oral antifungal, in humans. Antimicrob Agents Chemother 27:151–158

Britton H, Shebab Z, Lightner E, New M, Chow D (1988) Adrenal response in children receiving high doses of ketoconazole for systemic coccidioidomycosis. J Pediatrics 112:488–492

Bronnimann DA, Adam RD, Gagliani JN, Habib MP, Peterson EA, Porter B, Bloom JW (1987) Coccidioidomycosis in the acquired immunodeficiency syndrome. Ann Int Med 106:372–379

Brown MW, Maldonado AL, Meredith CG, Speeg KV (1985) Effect of ketoconazole on hepatic oxidative drug metabolism. Clin Pharmacol Ther 37:290–297

Bru JP, Lebeau B, Stahl JP, Micoud M (1988) Oral fluconazole treatment of urinary mycoses. Revista Ibérica de Micológia 5(Supplement 1):34 (abstract 0–94)

Buchsbaum HW, Fahs JJ, Friedman BA (1985) Coccidioidal meningitis treated with high-dose ketoconazole. In: Einstein HE, Catazano A (eds) Coccidioidomycosis. Proceedings of the 4th International Conference. National Foundation for Infectious Diseases, Washington DC, p 438

Calhoun DL, Galgiani JN, Stevens DA, Waskin H, Bonner JR, White MP, Mulholland JH, Rumans LW (1986) Ketoconazole treatment of *Sporothrix schenckii* arthritis and other infections. Abstract 780. Twenty-sixth Interscience Conference on Antimicrobial Agents and Chemotherapy, New Orleans

Catanzaro A, Einstein H, Levine B, Ross JB, Schillaci R, Fierer J, Friedman PJ (1982) Ketoconazole for treatment of disseminated coccidioidomycosis. Ann Int Med 96:436–440

Cauwenbergh G, De Doncker P, Stoops K, De Dier AM, Goyvaerts H, Schuermans V (1987) Itraconazole in the treatment of human mycoses: review of three years of clinical experience. Rev Inf Dis 9:S146–S152

Craven PC, Graybill JR, Jorgensen JH, Dismukes WE, Levine BE (1983) High-dose ketoconazole for treatment of fungal infections of the central nervous system. Ann Int Med 98:160–167

Daneshmend TK, Warnock DW (1988) Clinical pharmacokinetics of ketoconazole. Clin Pharmacokinetics 14:13–34

DeFelice R, Galgiani JN, Campbell SC, Palpant SD, Friedman BA, Dodge RA, Weinberg MG, Lincoln LJ, Tennican PO, Barbee RA (1982) Ketoconazole treatment of nonprimary coccidioidomycosis. Am J Med 72:681–687

De Gans J, Eeftinck Schattenkert JKM, Van Ketel RJ (1988) Itraconazole as maintenance treatment for cryptococcal meningitis in the acquired immunodeficiency syndrome. Br Med J 296:339

Deresinski SC, Stevens DA (1979) Bone and joint coccidioidomycosis treated with miconazole. Am Rev Resp Dis 120:1101–1107

Deresinski SC, Lilly RB, Levine HB, Galgiani JN, Stevens DA (1977) Treatment of fungal meningitis with miconazole. Arch Int Med 137:1180–1185

Deschamps MM, Pape JW, Verdier RI, De Hovits J, Thomas F, Johnson W, (1988) Treatment of *Candida* esophagitis in AIDS patients. Am J Gastroenterol 83:20–21

De Wit S, Weeris D, Hermans P, De Cock F, Clumeck N (1988) Double-blind randomized study of oral fluconazole (F) versus ketoconazole (K) in 40 episodes of oropharyngeal candidiasis (OC) in ARC/AIDS patients. Abstract 572. Twenty-eighth Interscience Conference on Antimicrobial Agents and Chemotherpay, Los Angeles

Dieperink H, Møller J (1982) Ketoconazole and cyclosporin. Lancet ii:1217

Dismukes WE (1988) Cryptococcal meningitis in patients with AIDS. J Inf Dis 157:624–628

Dismukes WE, Stamm AM, Graybill JR, Craven PC, Stevens DA, Stiller RL, Sarosi GA, Medoff G, Gregg CR, Gallis HA, Fields BT, Maner RL, Kerkering TA,

Kaplowitz LG, Cloud G, Bowles C, Shadomy S (1983) Treatment of systemic mycoses with ketoconazole: emphasis on toxicity and clinical response in 52 patients. Ann Int Med 98:13–20
Duarte PA, Chow CC, Simmons F, Ruskin J (1984) Fatal hepatitis associated with ketoconazole therapy. Arch Int Med 144:1069–1070
Dupont B, Drouhet E (1985) Cutaneous, ocular, and osteroarticular candidiasis in heroin addicts: new clinical and therapeutic aspects in 38 patients. J Inf Dis 152:577–591
Dupont B, Drouhet E (1988) The treatment of aspergillosis with azole derivatives. In: Vanden Bossche H, Mackenzie DWR, Cauwenbergh G (eds) Aspergillus and aspergillosis. Plenum, New York, pp 243–251
Eng RHK, Bishburg E, Smith SM, Kapila R (1986) Cryptococcal infections in patients with acquired immune deficiency syndrome. Am J Med 81:19–23
Engelhard D, Stutman HR, Marks MI (1984) Interactions of ketoconazole with rifampin and isoniazid. N Engl J Med 311:1681–1683
Fainstein V, Bodey GP (1980) Cardiorespiratory toxicity due to miconazole. Ann Int Med 93:432–433
Fainstein V, Bodey GP, Elting L, Maksymiuk A, Keating M, McCredie KB (1987) Amphotericin B or ketoconazole therapy of fungal infections in neutropenic cancer patients. Antimicrob Agents Chemother 31:11–15
Farrow PR, Brammer KW, Feczko JM (1987) Fluconazole: a new treatment for oropharyngeal candidiasis in AIDS and malignancy. Abstract 949. Twenty-seventh Interscience Conference on Antimicrobial Agents and Chemotherapy, New York
Farwell AP, Devlin JT, Stewart JA (1988) Total suppression of cortisol excretion by ketoconazole in the therapy of the ectopic adrenocorticotropic hormone syndrome. Am J Med 84:1063–1066
Fazio RA, Wickremeshinghe PC, Arsura EL (1983) Ketoconazole treatment of *Candida* esophagitis: a prospective study of 12 cases. Am J Gastroenterol 78:261–264
Ferguson RM, Sutherland DER, Simmons RL, Najarian JS (1982) Ketoconazole, cyclosporin metabolism, and renal transplantation. Lancet ii:882–883
Galgiani JN (1987) Antifungal susceptibility tests. Antimicrob Agents Chemother 31:1867–1870
Galgiani JN, Stevens DA, Graybill JR, Stevens DL, Tillinghast AJ, Levine HB (1984) *Pseudallescheria boydii* infections treated with ketoconazole. Clinical evaluations of seven patients and in vitro susceptibility results. Chest 86:219–224
Galgiani JN, Stevens DA, Graybill JR, Dismukes WE, Cloud GA (1988) Ketoconazole therapy of progressive coccidioidomycosis. Comparison of 400- and 800-mg doses and observations at higher doses. Am J Med 84:603–610
Ganer A, Arathoon E, Stevens DA (1987) Initial experience in therapy for progressive mycoses with itraconazole, the first clinically studied triazole. Rev Inf Dis 9:S77–S86
Graybill JR (1988) Histoplasmosis and AIDS. J Inf Dis 158:623–626
Graybill JR, Levine HB (1978) Successful treatment of cryptococcal meningitis with intraventricular miconazole. Arch Intern Med 138:814–816
Graybill JR, Lundberg D, Donovan W, Levine HB, Rodriguez MD, Drutz DJ (1980) Treatment of coccidioidomycosis with ketoconazole: clinical and laboratory studies of 18 patients. Rev Inf Dis 2:661–673
Graybill JR, Galgiani JN, Jorgensen JH, Strandberg DA (1983a) Ketoconazole therapy for fungal urinary tract infections. J Urol 129:68–70
Graybill JR, Kaster SR, Drutz DJ (1983b) Comparative activities of BAY n7133, ICI 153,066, and ketoconazole in murine cryptococcosis. Antimicrob Agents Chemother 24:829–834
Graybill JR, Stevens DA, Galgiani JN, Dismukes WE, Cloud G, Ganer A, Arathoon E, Fetchick R, Diaz M (1986) Itraconazole treatment of coccidioidomycosis. Abstract 788. Twenty-sixth Interscience Conference on Antimicrobial Agents and Chemotherapy, New Orleans

Graybill JR, Sharkey PK, Watson C (1988) Fluconazole treatment of funguria. Revista Ibérica de Micológia 5(Supplement 1):p 34 (abstract 0–93)

Hann IM, Corringham R, Keaney M, Noone P, Fox J, Szawatkowski M, Prentice HG, Blacklock HA, Shannon M, Gascoigne E, Boesen E, Hoffbrand AV (1982) Ketoconazole versus nystatin plus amphotericin B for fungal prophylaxis in severely immunocompromised patients. Lancet i:826–829

Hardin TC, Graybill JR, Fetchick R, Woestenborghs R, Rinaldi MG, Kuhn JG (1988) Pharmacokinetics of itraconazole following oral administration to normal volunteers. Antimicrob Agents Chemother 32:1310–1313

Harrison HR, Galgiani JN, Reynolds AF, Sprenger LW, Friedman AD (1983) Amphotericin B and imidazole therapy of coccidioidal meningitis in children. Pediatr Infect Dis 2:216–221

Hector RF (1988) Evaluation of the azole BAY R 3783 in rodent models of candidiasis and cryptococcosis. Revista Ibérica de Micológia 5 (Suppl 1):11 (abstract 0–4)

Heel RC (1982) Coccidioidomycosis. In: Levine HB (ed) Ketoconazole in the management of fungal disease. ADIS Press, New York, pp 132–135

Hobbs MM, Wright KA, Perfect JR, Tso CY, Durack DT (1988) Efficacy of SCH39304 and fluconazole in the treatment of experimental fungal infections. Abstract 166. Twenty-eighth Interscience Conference on Antimicrobial Agents and Chemotherapy, Los Angeles

Horn R, Wong B, Kiehn TE, Armstrong D (1985) Fungemia in a cancer hospital: changing frequency, earlier onset, and results of therapy. Rev Inf Dis 7:646–655

Horsburgh CR, Cannady PB, Kirkpatrick CH (1983) Treatment of fungal infections in the bones and joints with ketoconazole. J Inf Dis 147:1064–1069

Houston JB, Humphrey MJ, Matthew DE, Tarbit MH (1988) Comparison of two azole antifungal drugs, ketoconazole and fluconazole, as modifiers of rat hepatic monooxygenase activity. Biochem Pharmacol 37:401–408

Humphrey MJ, Jevons S, Tarbit MH (1985) Pharmacokinetic evaluation of UK-49,858, a metabolically stable triazole antifungal drug in animals and humans. Antimicrob Agents Chemother 28:648–653

Janssen PAJ, Symoens JE (1983) Hepatic reactions during ketoconazole treatment. Am J Med 74 (Suppl 1B):80–85

Johnson PC, Khardori N, Najjar AF, Butt F, Mansell PWA, Sarosis GA (1988) Progressive disseminated histoplasmosis in patients with acquired immunodeficiency syndrome. Am J Med 85:152–158

Jordan WM, Bodey GP, Rodriguez V, Ketchel SJ, Henney J (1979) Miconazole therapy for treatment of fungal infections in cancer patients. Antimicrob Agents Chemother 16:792–797

Kobayashi G, Travis SJ, Medoff G (1988) In vitro evaluation of Sch39304, fluconazole (FLU), and amphotericn B (AmB) against 12 clinical isolates of *Histoplasma capsulatum* (Hc) and comparison of therapeutic efficacies in treating histoplasmosis in immunocompetent and immunosuppressed mice. Abstract 172. Twenty-eighth Interscience Conference on Antimicrobial Agents and Chemotherapy, Los Angeles

Kovacs JA, Kovacs AA, Polis M, Wright WC, Gill VJ, Tuazon CU, Gelmann EP, Lane HC, Longfield R, Overturf G, Macher AM, Fauci AS, Parillo JE, Bennett JE, Masur M (1985) Cryptococcosis in the acquired immunodeficiency syndrome. Ann Int Med 103:533–538

Kramer W, Kim H, Symchowicz S, Perentesis G, Affrime M, Lin C (1988) Pharmacokinetics of SCH39304 in man. Abstract 165. Twenty-eighth Interscience Conference on Antimicrobial Agents and Chemotherapy, Los Angeles

Kwong YL, Yu YL, Chan FL, Lam KSL, Woo E, Huang CY (1987) High dose ketoconazole in the treatment of cerebral aspergilloma. Clin Neurol Neurosurg 89:193–196

Lake-Bakaar G, Tom W, Lake-Bakaar D, Gupta N, Beidas S, Elsakr M, Straus E (1988) Gastropathy and ketoconazole malabsorption in the acquired immunodeficiency syndrome (AIDS). Ann Int Med 109:471–473

Lavalle P, Suchil P, De Ovando F, Reynoso S (1987) Itraconazole for deep mycoses: preliminary experience in Mexico. Rev Inf Dis 9:S64–S70

Lelawongs P, Barone JA, Colaizzi JL, Hsuan AM, Mechlinski W, Legendre RL, Guarnieri J (1988) Effect of food and gastric acidity on absorption of orally administered ketoconaole. Clin Pharmacol 7:228–235

Lewis JH, Zimmerman HJ, Benson GD, Ishak KG (1984) Hepatic injury associated with ketoconazole therapy: analysis of 33 cases. Gastroenterology 86:503–513

Loebenberg D, Parmegiani R, Cacciapuoti A, Antonacci C, Norris C, Menzel F, Moss EL, Yarosh-Tomaine T, Lin CC, Hare RS, Miller GH (1988) Sch 39304, a new antifungal agent. I. Oral treatment of systemic infections in mice. Abstract 167. Twenty-eighth Interscience Conference on Antimicrobial Agents and Chemotherapy, Los Angeles

Maksymiuk AW, Thongprasert S, Hopfer S, Luna M, Fainstein V, Bodey G (1984) Systemic candidiasis in cancer patients. Am J Med 77(Suppl 4D):20–27

McKinsey DS, Gupta MR, Riddler SA, Driks MR, Smith DL, Kurtin PJ (1989) Long-term amphotericin B therapy for disseminated histoplasmosis in patients with the acquired immunodeficiency syndrome (AIDS): Ann Int Med 111:655–659

Meunier-Carpentier F (1984) Chemoprophylaxis of fungal infections. Am J Med 76:652–656

Meunier-Carpentier F, Heymans C, Snoeck R, Taterman J (1983) Interaction of rifampin (Rif) with ketoconazole (Ke) and Bay n7133 (Bay) in normal volunteers. Abstract 987. Twenty-third Interscience Conference on Antimicrobial Agents and Chemotherapy, Las Vegas

Meyer RD, Sattler FR, Linne SR, Ruskin J (1978) Miconazole for treatment of disseminated coccidioidomycosis: unfavorable experience. Chest 73:825–831

Miettinen TA (1988) Cholesterol metabolism during ketoconazole treatment in man. J Lipid Res 29:43–51

Morgans ME, Thomas MEM, Mackenzie DWR (1979) Successful treatment of systemic cryptococcosis with miconazole. Br Med J 2:100–101

Morgenstern GR, Powles R, Robinson B, McElwain TJ (1982) Cyclosporin interaction with ketoconazole and melphalan. Lancet ii:1342

National Institute of Allergy and Infectious Diseases Mycoses Study Group (1985) Treatment of blastomycosis and histoplasmosis with ketoconazole. Ann Int Med 103:861–872

Negroni R, Robles AM, Arechavala A, Tuculet MA, Galimberti R (1980) Ketoconazole in the treatment of paracoccidioidomycosis and histoplasmosis. Rev Inf Dis 2:643–649

Negroni R, Palmieri O, Koren F, Tiraboschi IN, Galimberti R (1987) Oral treatment of paracoccidioidomycosis and histoplasmosis with itraconazole in humans. Rev Inf Dis 9:S47–S50

Phillips P, Fetchick R, Weisman I, Foshee S, Graybill JR (1987) Tolerance to and efficacy of itraconazole in treatment of systemic mycoses: preliminary results. Rev Inf Dis 9:S87–S93

Pillans PI, Cowan P, Whitelaw D (1985) Hyponatremia and confusion in a patient taking ketoconazole. Lancet i:821–822

Pizzo PA, Robichaud KJ, Gill FA, Witebsky FG (1982) Empiric antibiotic and antifungal therapy for cancer patients with prolonged fever and granulocytopenia. Am J Med 72:101–111

Plempel M, Büchel KH (1988) Antimycotic effects of BAY R 3783 in vitro and on dermatophytoses and opportunistic mycoses of the organs in vivo. Abstract 0–7. Revista Ibérica de Micológia 5 (Suppl 1):11

Pont A, Graybill JR, Craven PC, Galgiani JN, Dismukes WE, Reitz RE, Stevens DA (1984) High-dose ketoconazole therapy and adrenal and testicular function in humans. Arch Intern Med 144:2150–2153

Restrepo A, Gomez I, Canio LE, Arango MD, Gutierrez F, Sanin A, Robledo MA (1983) Treatment of paracoccidioidomycosis with ketaconazole: a three year experience. Am J Med 74(1B):48–52

Restrepo A, Robledo J, Gomez I, Tabares AM, Gutierrez R (1986) Itraconazole therapy in lymphangitic and cutaneous sporotrichosis. Arch Dermatol 122:413–417
Restrepo A, Gomez I, Robledo J, Patiño MM, Cano LE (1987) Itraconazole in the treatment of paracoccidioidomycosis: a preliminary report. Rev Inf Dis 9:S51–S56
Restrepo A, Gonzalez A, Gomez I, Arango M, De Bedout C (1988a) Treatment of chromoblastomycosis with itraconazole. Ann N Y Acad Sci 544:504–516
Restrepo A, Munera MI, Atreaga ID, Gomez I, Tabares AM, Patiño MM, Arango M (1988b) Itraconazole in the treatment of pulmonary aspergilloma and chronic pulmonary aspergillosis. In: Vanden Bossche H, Mackenzie DWR, Cauwenbergh G (eds) Aspergillus and aspergillosis. Plenum, New York, pp 253–265
Restrepo BI, Ahrens J, Graybill JR (1988c) Efficacy of SCH393904 (SCH) in murine cryptococcosis. Abstract 170. Twenty-eighth Interscience Conference on Antimicrobial Agents and Chemotherapy, Los Angeles
Ross JB, Levine B, Catanzaro A, Einstein H, Schillaci R, Friedman PJ (1982) Ketoconazole for treatment of chronic pulmonary coccidioidomycosis. Ann Int Med 96:440–443
Rozenberg-Arska M, Dekker AW, Verhoff J (1988) Efficacy of fluconazole (FL) for prevention of fungal infections (FI) in comparison to amphotericin B (AmB) in granulocytopenic patients (pts). Abstract 577. Twenty-eighth Interscience Conference on Antimicrobial Agents and Chemotherapy, Los Angeles
Saag MS, Dismukes WE (1988) Treatment of histoplasmosis and blastomycosis. Chest 93:848–851
Saag M, Bradsher R, Chapman S, Kauffman C, Girard W, Stevens D, Bowles-Patton C, Dismukes WE (1988) Itraconazole (I) therapy (Rx) for blastomycosis (B), histoplasmosis (H), and sporotrichosis (S). Abstract 574. Twenty-eighth Interscience Conference on Antimicrobial Agents and Chemotherapy, Los Angeles
Schmitt HJ, Barnard EM, Hauser M, Armstrong D (1988) Comparison of antifungal agents in a rat model of pulmonary aspergillosis. Abstract 171. Twenty-eighth Interscience Conference on Antimicrobial Agents and Chemotherapy, Los Angeles
Schulman J, Peyman G, Fiscella R, Small G, Coast M, Wajszczuk C, Steahly L (1987) Toxicity of intravitreal injection of fluconazole in the rabbit. Can J Ophthalmol 22:304–306
Shale DJ, Faux JA, Lane DJ (1987) Trial of ketoconazole in noninvasive pulmonary aspergillosis. Thorax 42:26–31
Sharkey PK, Rinaldi MG, Lerner C, Fetchick R, Dunn JF, Graybill JR (1988) High dose itraconazole in the treatment of severe mycoses. Abstract 575. Twenty-eighth Interscience Conference on Antimicrobial Agents and Chemotherapy, Los Angeles
Shehab ZM, Britton H, Dunn JH (1988) Imidazole therapy of coccidioidal meningitis in children. Pediatric Infect Dis J 7:40–44
Shepp DH, Klosterman A, Siegel MS, Meyers JD (1985) Comparative trial of ketoconazole and nystatin for prevention of fungal infection in neutropenic patients treated in a protective environment. J Inf Dis 152:1257–1263
Smith AG (1984) Potentiation of oral anticoagulants by ketoconazole. Br Med J 288:188–189
Smith JM, Hows JM, Gordon-Smith EC, Baughan A, Goldman JM (1983) Interaction of CyA and ketoconazole. Clin Sci 64:67P–68P
Sonino N (1987) The use of ketoconazole as an inhibitor of steroid production. N Engl J Med 317:812–818
Stern JJ, Hartman BJ, Sharkey PK, Rowland V, Squires KE, Murray HW, Graybill JR (1988) Oral fluconazole therapy for patients with acquired immunodeficiency syndrome and cryptococcosis: experience with 22 patients. Am J Med 85:477–480
Stevens DA (1977) Miconazole in the treatment of systemic fungal infections. Am Rev Resp Dis 116:801–806

Stevens DA (1983) Miconazole in the treatment of coccidioidomycosis. Drugs 26: 347–354

Stevens DA, Stiller RL, Williams PL, Sugar AM (1983) Experience with ketoconazole in three major manifestations of progressive coccidioidomycosis. Am J Med 74 (Suppl 1B):58–63

Stockley RJ, Daneshmend TK, Bredow MT, Warnock DW, Richardson MD, Slade RR (1983) Ketoconazole pharmacokinetics during chronic dosing in adults with hematological malignancy. Eur J Clin Microbiol 5:513–517

Sugar AM, Saunders C (1988) Oral fluconazole as suppressive therapy of disseminated cryptoccosis in patients with acquired immunodeficiency syndrome. Am J Med 85:481–489

Sugar AM, Alsip S, Galgiani JN, Graybill JR, Dismukes WE, Cloud GA, Craven PC, Stevens DA (1987) Pharmacology and toxicity of high dose ketoconazole. Antimicrob Agents Chemother 31:1874–1878

Sung JP, Grendahl JG, Fresno MA, Levine HB (1977) Intravenous and intratheal miconazole therapy for systemic mycosis. West J Med 126:5–13

Sung JP, Campbell GD, Grendahl JG (1978) Miconazole therapy for fungal meningitis. Arch Neurol 35:443–447

Thaler M, Pastakia B, Shawker TH, O'Leary T, Pizzo PA (1988) Hepatic candidiasis in cancer patients: the evolving picture of the syndrome. Ann Int Med 108: 88–100

Thomas PA, Rajasekaran J (1988) Treatment of *Aspergillus* keratitis with imidazoles and related compounds. In: Vanden Bossche H, Mackenzie DWR, Cauwenbergh G (eds) Aspergillus and aspergillosis. Plenum, New York, pp 267–279

Tricot G, Joosten E, Boogaerts MA, Vande Pitte J, Cauwenbergh G (1987) Ketoconazole vs itraconazole for antifungal prophylaxis in patients with severe granulocytopenia: preliminary results of two nonrandomized studies. Rev Inf Dis 9:S94–S99

Tucker RM, Denning DW, Rinaldi MG, Hanson LH, Stevens DA (1988a) Itraconazole (IZ) therapy (Rx) of progressive coccidioidomycosis (C). Abstract 573. Twenty-eighth Interscience Conference on Antimicrobial Agents and Chemotherapy, Los Angeles

Tucker RM, Williams PL, Arathoon EG, Levine BE, Hartstein AI, Hanson LH, Stevens DA (1988b) Pharmacokinetics of fluconazole in cerebrospinal fluid and serum in human coccidioidal meningitis. Antimicrob Agents Chemother 32:369–373

Tucker RM, Galgiani JN, Graybill JR, Denning DW, Hanson LH, Eckman MR, Salemi C, Stevens DA (1990) Treatment of coccidioidal meningitis with fluconazole. Rev Inf Dis (in press)

Tucker WS, Snell BB, Island DP, Gregg CR (1985) Reversible adrenal insufficiency induced by ketoconazole. JAMA 253:2413–2414

Van Cauteren H, Heykants J, De Coster R, Cauwenbergh G (1987) Itraconazole: pharmacologic studies in animals and humans. Rev Inf Dis 9:S43–S46

Van Cutsem J (1983) The antifungal activity of ketoconazole. Am J Med 74 (Suppl 1B):9–15

Van Cutsem J, Janssen PAJ (1988) Oral and parenteral treatment of invasive aspergillosis in non-predisposed and in immunocompromised guinea pigs with saperconazole (R66905) and parenteral treatment with amphotericin B. Abstract 176. Twenty-eighth Interscience Conference on Antimicrobial Agents and Chemotherapy, Los Angeles

Van Cutsem J, Van Gerven F, Janssen PAJ (1987) Activity of orally, topically, and parenterally administered itraconazole in the treatment of superficial and deep mycoses: animal models. Rev Inf Dis 9:S15–S32

Vanden Bossche H (1985) Biochemical targets for antifungal azole derivatives: hypothesis on the mode of action. In: McGinnis M (ed) Current topics in medical mycology. Springer-Verlag, Berlin Heidelberg New York, pp 313–351

Viviáni MA, Tortorano AM, Woenstenborghs R, Cauwenbergh G (1987) Experience with itraconazole in deep mycoses in northern Italy. Mykosen 30:233–244

Walsh TJ, Aoki S, Mechinaud F, Foulds G, Rubin M, Pizzo PA (1988a) Treatment of disseminated candidiasis with fluconazole in persistently granulocytopenic rabbits. Abstract P-165. Revista Iberíca de Micológia 5(Suppl 1):92
Walsh TJ, Lee JW, Peter J, Schaufele R, Rubin M, Pizzo PA (1988b) SCH-39304 in the treatment of disseminated candidiasis in persistently granulocytopenic and non-granulocytopenic rabbits. Abstract 169. Twenty-eighth Interscience Conference on Antimicrobial Agents and Chemotherapy, Los Angeles
Weinstein L, Jacoby I (1980) Successful treatment of cerebral cryptococcoma and meningitis with miconazole. Ann Int Med 93:569–571
White MC, Kendall-Taylor P (1985) Adrenal hypofunction in patients taking ketoconazole. Lancet i:44–45
Wingard JR, Vaughan WP, Braine HG, Merz WG, Saral R (1987) Prevention of fungal sepsis in patients with prolonged neutropenia: a randomized, double-blind, placebo-controlled trial of intravenous miconazole. Am J Med 83:1103–1110
Wise GJ, Goldberg PE, Kozinn PJ (1985) Do the imidazoles have a role in the management of genitourinary fungal infections? J Urol 133:61–64
Zuger A, Schuster M, Simberkoff MS, Rahal JJ, Holzman RS (1988) Maintenance amphotericin B for cryptococcal meningitis in the acquired immunodeficiency syndrome (AIDS). Ann Int Med 109:592–593

CHAPTER 20

Terbinafine

THOMAS C. JONES and VIOLETTE V. VILLARS

A. Introduction

Terbinafine (SF 86-327; Lamisil) is the most recently developed member of a new class of antifungal drugs referred to as allylamine derivatives (PETRANYI et al. 1984). The drug interferes with the integrity of the cytoplasmic membrane of fungi by blocking membrane sterol synthesis (RYDER 1985). In addition, accumulation of squalene in the fungi induces a fungicidal action. Terbinafine is particularly effective in the treatment of dermatomycoses and can be used both topically and orally. Its usefulness in systemic mycoses has not been evaluated in sufficient detail to draw conclusions about its efficacy; however, it may have a role in selected deep mycoses and protozoal infections as well.

The need for new antifungal drugs has become clear recently as there is a rather small number of drugs available for treating serious infections, as the number of immunocompromised patients requiring such drugs increases, and as complications of drug resistance and side effects associated with the presently available therapy are recorded (DROUHET and DUPONT 1987). Terbinafine resolves some of these needs in that it is among a new class of drugs with a different mode of action, it has a broad spectrum of antifungal activity by in vitro assay, it is fungicidal against most organisms, and it is not toxic to mammalian cell membranes or metabolic systems. It does not solve some problems of tissue distribution, it is not available as an intravenous formulation, and it utilises the inhibition of cytoplasmic membrane synthesis of fungi as the primary mechanism of action as do existing drugs. Therefore, new modifications of this new class of drug as well as more new antifungals will continue to be required. Terbinafine provides one step in this process of antifungal drug development. In this review we summarize the chemistry and mode of action of terbinafine, its antifungal spectrum in vitro and in animals, its toxicological profile, and the results of its use in clinical trials in patients with dermatomycoses.

B. Chemistry and Mode of Action

I. Chemistry

The two most commonly used antifungal drugs, amphotericin B and griseofulvin, are produced by microbes. Potassium iodide, flucytosine and the

Table 1. Relationship between drug structure and antifungal activity

		MIC (μg/ml) *Trichophyton mentagrophytes*	Oral Rx guinea pig (% mycological cure) 10 (mg/kg/day)	75	150
Naftifine	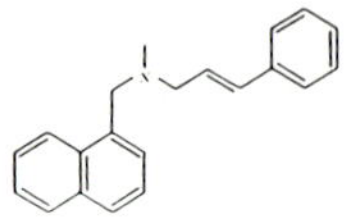	0.05	–	–	48
Two conjugated double bonds	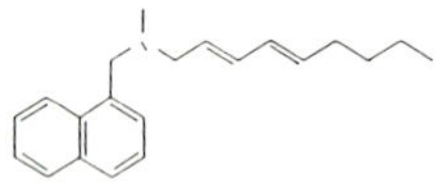	0.05	–	–	43
Substitution of the second double bond with a triple bond	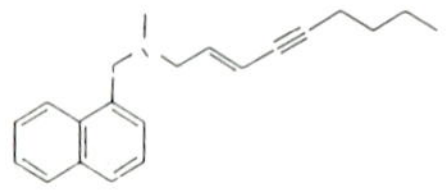	0.01	15	100	100
Terbinafine Addition of branched side chain to the triple bond	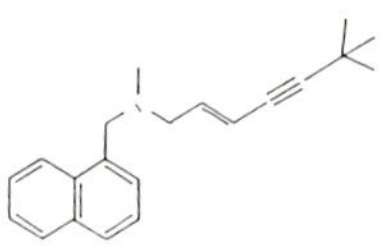	0.006	100	–	–

Rx = treatment,
MIC = mean inhibitory concentration.

azoles have been synthesised and selected for antifungal activity, and of these only the azoles have undergone detailed structure-activity analysis. Against this background, the impressive performance of a chemical substance discovered by accident in 1974 by BERNEY and developed at the Sandoz Forschungs Institut in Vienna provides a welcome addition. The process by which the activity of the first compound, naftifine, was identified, the reason the class of drugs was designated as 'allylamine derivatives' and the careful substitution analysis to identify basic structure-activity relationships which led to the synthesis of terbinafine have been recently recorded (STÜTZ 1987). A simplified summary is given in Table 1. The key structural modifications which led to an increase in antifungal activity both in vitro and in vivo are shown. It should be noted that over 1000 compounds were tested in the analysis of this structure-activity relationship; for details of the other compounds refer to STÜTZ and PETRANYI (1984), STÜTZ et al. (1984) and STÜTZ (1987, 1988). From the table it can be seen that antifungal activity in vitro required the allylamine group plus the structure imposed by the benzene ring (naftifine), an additional double bond or the unique triple bond (the acetylene group). Finally, the addition of the branched side chain, only in the *trans* form of the molecule, led to significantly increased antifungal activity in vitro and in vivo. Terbinafine was then selected for the extensive toxicological, mode of action, clinical efficacy and tolerability studies described below.

II. Mode of Action

Detailed studies have documented how terbinafine interferes with the growth of fungi and leads to their disintegration. These studies have shown that, like other important antifungal drugs such as amphotericin B and imidazoles, terbinafine interferes with cytoplasmic membrane synthesis, but it affects the synthetic process at an earlier step, and accumulation of metabolites lead to further toxicity to the fungal cell (RYDER 1986).

Terbinafine interacts with and inhibits the action of the enzyme squalene epoxidase, a key enzyme in the biosynthesis of ergosterol. Inhibition of this enzyme can fully account for the effects of terbinafine on ergosterol biosynthesis (RYDER 1986). Figure 1 shows a simplified representation of sterol synthesis in the fungal cytoplasmic membrane. The sites of inhibition by terbinafine and azoles are shown. Two additional features of this inhibition are of critical importance to the success of this drug in treating human fungal infections: it leads to marked accumulation of squalene within the fungi which in turn exerts a fungicidal effect, and it is highly specific for fungal squalene epoxidase, so that in mammalian cell systems 10000 times higher drug con-

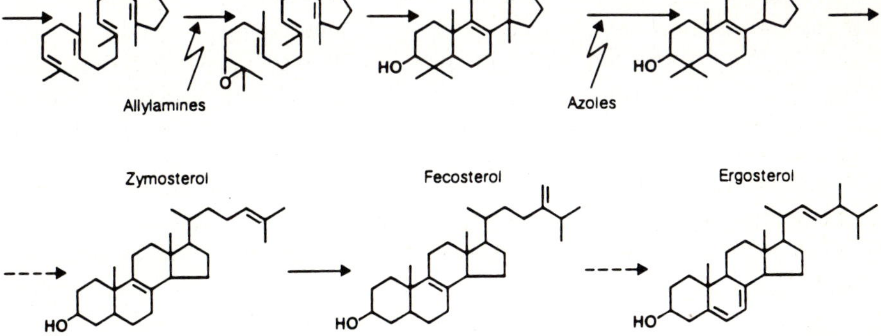

Fig. 1. Simplified presentation of sterol synthesis in the fungal cytoplasmic membrane showing the site of action of terbinafine (*allylamines*). From *Triangle*, Sandoz Zeitschrift für medizinische Wissenschaft, 25 (213), 1986, Sandoz AG, with permission

centrations are required to show significant inhibition (RYDER 1985; RYDER and DUPONT 1985). These two features, fungicidal action and fungal enzyme specificity, provide the most important and clinically relevant aspects of this new drug. For example, inhibition of sterol synthesis in the cytoplasmic membrane by azoles does not yield fungicidal products at doses relevant to systemic human use but does affect cytochromes P-450, a class of enzymes of high significance in human metabolic processes (BORGERS and VANDEN BOSSCHE 1982).

To evaluate further the relative contributions of inhibition of ergosterol biosynthesis and accumulation of squalene to the control of fungal infection, an analysis of the effects of terbinafine on the yeast and mycelial forms of *Candida albicans* has been presented (RYDER 1987). In this analysis it was seen that if the only pathway of control of fungi is inhibition of ergosterol biosynthesis, then complete inhibition of the process is required. This is not achieved with terbinafine on the yeast phase of *C. albicans*, hence the drug is fungistatic. However, ergosterol synthesis is inhibited to a high degree in the mycelial form of *C. albicans* with 0.025 μg/ml of terbinafine, a fact consistent with its high efficacy in treating cutaneous infections. *Candida* may have alternative mechanisms for dealing with squalene accumulation and its fungicidal action. In contrast, the accumulation of squalene may be the critical feature of the fungicidal action in organisms such as dermatophytes, *C. parapsilosis* and *Aspergillus* spp., since much lower concentrations of the drug are required, and complete inhibition of ergosterol biosynthesis does not appear to be necessary to achieve full fungicidal effects (RYDER 1987). Taken together the data suggest that two mechanisms are operative in the antifungal activity of terbinafine: a primarily fungicidal one associated with squalene accumulation, and a primarily fungistatic one dependent on inhibition of ergosterol biosynthesis.

Careful evaluation of the differences between terbinafine and azoles with regard to the binding of cytochrome P-450 has been conducted in view of the importance of this interaction in determining the side effect profile of azoles. In this evaluation it has been shown that terbinafine is metabolised by a small part of the cytochrome P-450 in liver microsomes (SCHUSTER 1987), the interaction with cytochrome P-450 is specific, with affinity for a small fraction of low affinity (type I) substrates, and there is no evidence of the non-specific, broad, high affinity (type II) binding which has been well recorded for azoles (SCHUSTER 1985). Thus, the absence of the drug interaction problems and of the effects on endocrine function recorded for azoles is well explained by the absence of high affinity, non-specific, cytochrome P-450 binding.

III. Measurement of Terbinafine in Plasma, Body Fluids and Tissue

Terbinafine and its metabolites can be measured in plasma, body fluids and tissues by a sensitive, quantitative method which involves extraction of the sample with hexane and chloroform and measurement on a high performance liquid chromatographic gradient system (HPLC) using either electrochemical detection or ultraviolet spectroscopy (SCHATZ et al. 1983; SCHATZ and HABERL 1989). With these methods nanogram amounts of the parent compound and numerous metabolites have been identified. The most important metabolites include a demethyl and a carboxy form, both of which are less lipophilic than the parent drug, and neither of which has significant antifungal activity. This method has been used to determine the pharmacokinetics of the drug in animals and humans and the concentrations in tissues referred to in subsequent sections of this review.

A bioassay for the presence of terbinafine in serum has also been described (KAN et al. 1986). By use of this technique a rather close correlation with HPLC methods has been demonstrated. This assay showed that the zone of inhibition around *Trichophyton mentagrophytes* was correlated in a logarithmic manner with the concentration of terbinafine. This method has been used to follow drug concentrations in animals and humans.

C. Antifungal Activity

I. Fungicidal and Fungistatic Actions

In in vitro studies terbinafine has proved to have a broad spectrum of antifungal activity. The allylamine derivatives, of which terbinafine is one, exert their selective action by inhibiting fungal ergosterol biosynthesis at the point of squalene epoxidation. Cell death follows the disruption of cell membranes and the interruption of cell wall synthesis as shown in the ultrastructural studies described below.

Antifungal activity in vitro was measured by determining the minimum inhibitory concentration (MIC) after serial dilution in Sabouraud dextrose broth. Incubation times were 48 h for yeasts and 7 days for dermatophytes, *Aspergillus* sp. and *Sporothrix schenckii*. The highest activity was recorded against dermatophytes such as *Trichophyton* spp., *Microsporum* spp. and strains of *Epidermophyton floccossum*, but against aspergilli, dimorphic and filamentous fungi, high levels of activity were also recorded. The activity of terbinafine against yeasts varied between different species and strains (PETRANYI et al. 1987a).

The high antifungal activity of terbinafine against dermatophytes, filamentous and dimorphic fungi, and some yeasts is associated with its primary fungicidal activity against these organisms (*T. mentagrophytes*, *M. canis*, *A. fumigatus*, *S. schenckii* and *C. parapsilosis*). Figure 2 shows the fungicidal effects of terbinafine in culture against these organisms. Fungicidal activity has also been shown against *Scopulariopsis brevicaulis*, *Histoplasma capsulatum* and *Blastomyces dermatitidis* (SHADOMY et al. 1985). Activity against yeasts is species dependent; in some it is primarily fungicidal (*C. parapsilosis*) while in others it is primarily fungistatic (*C. albicans*) (PETRANYI et al. 1987b).

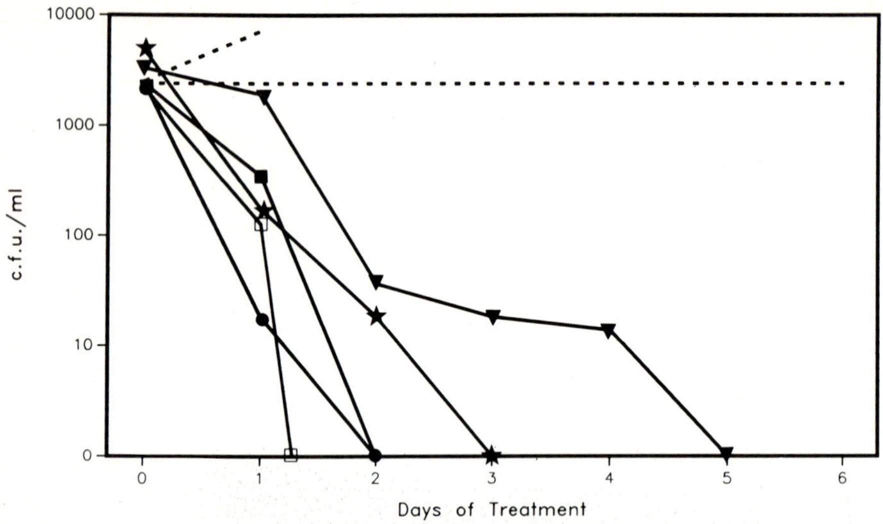

Fig. 2. Fungicidal action of terbinafine. Colony forming units (CFU) of fungi at fungicidal concentrations of terbinafine are shown on the ordinate and the days to killing of the microorganisms on the abscissa. Organisms treated with terbinafine (*solid lines*) are shown. Their identification and corresponding MICs are as follows: *circle*, *T. mentagrophtes (MIC = 0.006* µg/ml); *solid square*, *M. canis* (MIC = 0.006 µg/ml); *triangle*, *A. fumigatus* (MIC = 0.8 µg/ml); *star*, *S. schenckii* (MIC = 0.4 µg/ml); *open square*, *C. parapsilosis* (MIC = 0.4 µg/ml). Control, untreated cultures are shown (*dotted lines*). It is seen that sterile cultures occurred after 1–5 days of drug exposure

II. Morphological Effects of Terbinafine on Fungi

To determine the ultrastructural changes in the hyphae, germ tubes and microconidia, *T. mentagrophytes* was exposed to terbinafine. The effects of terbinafine on the ultrastructure was shown to be dose dependent. Exposure of the mycelia to terbinafine at a concentration of 0.005 µg/ml produced no changes after 24 h. However, after exposure to 0.01 µg/ml, only a few cells with normal architecture remained; the other cells were damaged to varying degrees. Their cell walls were thickened, and the cytoplasm contained numerous electron-dense bodies of different sizes. Many of these bodies were of a diameter similar to that of cross-sections of mitochondria (MEINGASSNER et al. 1983a). Smaller electron-dense particles were also found in the cell walls, and aggregates of particles were both embedded in and protruding from the cell wall (Fig. 3A,B). Treatment of the cultures with terbinafine at a concentration of 0.05 µg/ml showed even fewer normal cells. Changes in damaged cells were similar to those mentioned above. All cells were partially or completely autolysed in the cultures treated with 0.1 µg/ml or 0.5 µg/ml.

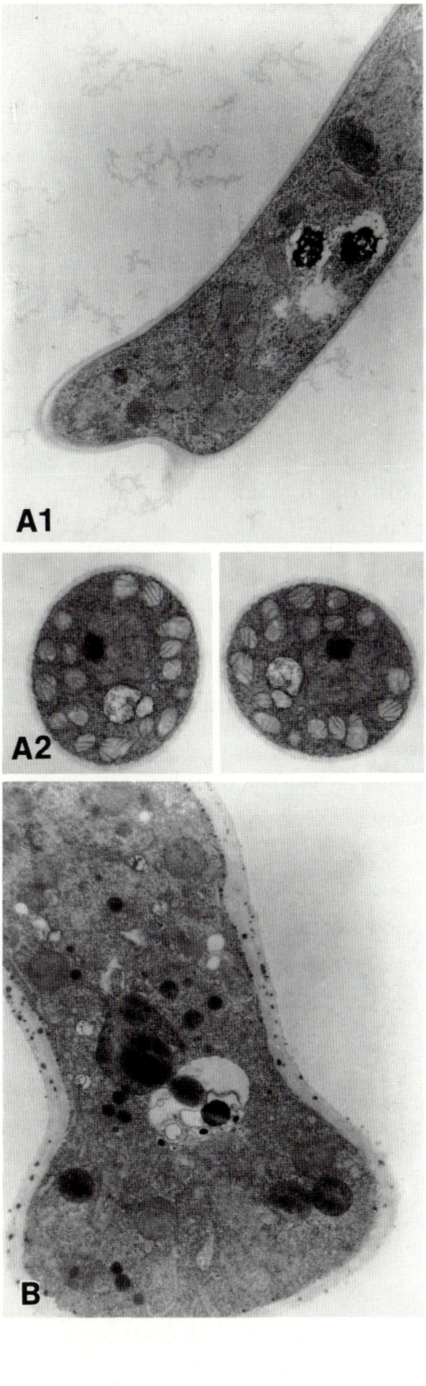

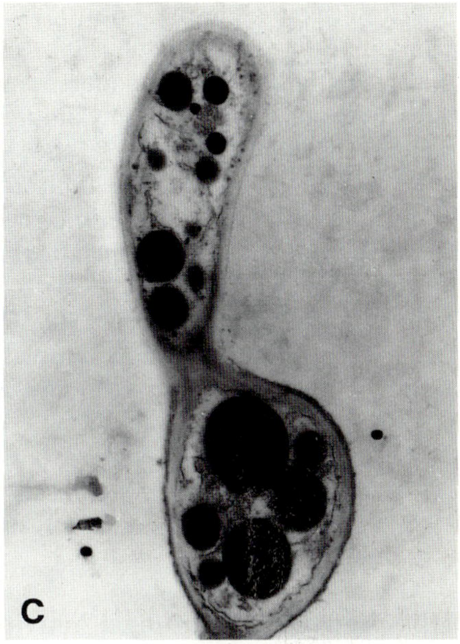

Fig. 3A–C. Electron micrographs of *T. mentagrophytes* in culture. **A1** and **A2** show untreated hyphae in longitudinal and cross sections (×9000). **B** shows hyphae after exposure to 0.01 μg/ml terbinafine for 24 h. The cell wall is thickened, and numerous electron-dense bodies of various sizes are present in thc cytoplasm, as well as in the cell wall (×16000). **C** shows a partially autolysed microconidium after exposure to 0.003 μg/ml of terbinafine for 39 h (×12700)

The effects of terbinafine (0.003 μg/ml for 15 h) on the microconidia included the persistence of short, plump germ tubes with enlarged tips. Changes in the cell walls and membranes were noted as described for mycelia. After an exposure of 39 h, only autolysed, germinated microconidia could be found in the culture. Figure 3C shows a microconidium treated for 39 h.

Exposure of *C. albicans* blastospores to terbinafine at 0.1 μg/ml produced no changes, but alterations were induced in the cell wall, the plasma membrane and the cytoplasm after exposure to 0.5 μg/ml. Oval vesicular inclusions of varying sizes were randomly distributed in the cell wall (MEINGASSNER et al. 1983b). Many cells also showed irregularly shaped nuclei. Small vesicles in the cytoplasm or within large vacuoles were observed. After exposure to 1.0 μg/ml the same changes were observed, but they were more prominent.

Ultrastructural changes in *Sc. brevicaulis* after exposure to terbinafine in low concentration (1 μg/ml) were also observed by MOULIN-TRAFFORT et al. (1987). These observations confirm the fungicidal action of terbinafine.

III. Spectrum of Antifungal Activity

As shown in Fig. 2 terbinafine is very active against various dermatophytes. The MICs recorded ranges from 0.003 to 0.01 μg/ml. In Table 2 it can be seen that dermatophytic, filamentous fungi and dimorphic fungi of various

Table 2. In vitro activities of terbinafine against pathogenic and opportunistic fungi

	MIC range (μg/ml)
I. Dermatophytic fungi	
Trichophyton mentagrophytes	0.001–0.01
T. rubrum	0.001–0.01
T. verrucosum	0.001–0.006
Epidermophyton floccosum	0.001–<0.06
Microsporum canis	0.005–0.01
M. gypseum	0.005–0.01
II. Filamentous fungi	
Aspergillus spp.	0.005–5.0
A. flavus	0.01–0.5
A. fumigatus	0.02–5.0
A. niger	0.005–0.5
Hendersonula toruloidea	1.0–4.0
Scopulariopsis brevicaulis	0.5–8.8
III. Dimorphic fungi	
Blastomyces dermatitidis	≤0.05–0.39
Histoplasma capsulatum	≤0.05–0.2
Sporothrix schenckii	≤0.05–2.0

MIC, minimum inhibitory concentration.

Table 3. In vitro activities of terbinafine against pathogenic yeasts

	MIC range (μg/ml)
Candida albicans (yeast form)	6.25–>128.0
C. albicans (mycelial form)	0.098–0.78
C. parapsilosis	0.1–3.13
C. tropicalis	10.0–128.0
C. pseudotropicalis	0.5–50.0
C. krusei	50.0–>100.0
C. guilliermondii	6.25–100.0
C. glabrata (*T. glabrata*)	>100.0–>128.0
Cryptococcus neoformans	0.25–2.0
Pityrosporum spp.	0.2–0.8

types are very sensitive to terbinafine. MIC ranges (0.1 → 100 μg/ml) for pathogenic yeasts varied much more between the different strains and species (Table 3). As noted in Table 3 blastospores of *C. parapsilosis* proved to be more sensitive than those of *C. albicans*. In contrast, the mycelia of *C. albicans*, which are important for the pathogenicity of this yeast, have proven to be very susceptible to the compound. Table 3 shows the results of an in vitro evaluation of terbinafine against mycelia and blastospores of yeast (SCHUSTER et al. 1988). Independent studies from SHADOMY et al. (1985) showed the same level of antifungal activity. In addition they showed that terbinafine was active against various isolates of *Cryptococcus neoformans*. These studies also confirmed the activity of terbinafine against *Aspergillus* sp. and *S. schenckii*.

D. Activity in Animals

I. Metabolism

To determine the compound's metabolism and pharmacokinetics in animals, ^{14}C-labelled terbinafine has been orally and topically administered to dogs and rats. Gastrointestinal absorption in rats ranged from 48% to 77% and in dogs from 21% to 94%. Peak levels of the parent drug were reached within the 1st hour after oral administration, but already 2 h after p.o. administration the parent drug represented less than 5% of total plasma ^{14}C. This decreased to <1% at 8 h, a finding consistent with the drug's rapid metabolism. In rats, the radioactivity decreased to 10% 2–3 days after administration and to 1% after 6 days. In both rats and dogs biliary excretion of the ^{14}C was predominant.

In rats that received ^{14}C-labelled terbinafine, a special study of absorption was done. One hour after the drug was administered into the proximal duodenum, HPLC analyses of blood, lymph and tissue extracts were performed. A twenty times higher concentration of radioactivity was found in the lymph than in the portal blood. The metabolic patterns derived from both fluids demonstrated a very important role of the lymph in the systemic delivery of the drug. In the lymph more than 90% consisted of parent compound, whereas in the portal blood this value was only 30%. After liver passage only 8% of the radioactivity could be assigned to the parent compound (GRIMUS and SCHUSTER 1983). After oral administration of terbinafine to male rats it was noted that maximal concentrations were found after 6 h in the liver, kidneys, fat tissue, skin and blood. Except for bones, no organ seemed to be free of radioactivity at that point.

The tissue distribution of the drug is an important feature of its potential antifungal activity in vivo. A slow elimination of radioactivity was observed from fat. Some 96 h after oral administration, two-thirds of the radioactivity still remained in the fat tissue. From most of the organs the radioactivity was eliminated 2–4 times slower than from blood. In vivo levels of active drug at sites of infection are controlled by the absorption and elimination from relevant tissues. In vitro it was shown that interaction with microsomal cytochrome P-450 led to extensive metabolic degradation of terbinafine (SCHUSTER 1987). As human liver only contains a low concentration of cytochrome P-450 isozymes capable of metabolising terbinafine, the drug is metabolised at a much slower rate than in the liver tissue of the rat and guinea pig. Therefore, a high metabolic stability leading to longer-lasting drug levels is expected for humans during therapeutic treatment with terbinafine.

II. Antifungal Activity

In assays in guinea pigs the excellent antimycotic efficacy of terbinafine (topically and orally) could be shown against trichophytosis caused by *T. mentagrophytes* and in microsporosis caused by *M. canis*. Treatment with orally administered terbinafine was started on the day of inoculation and continued for 9 days. Before inoculation the hair was shaved from guinea pigs and then 0.1 ml of the inoculum containing 10^6 colony forming units (cfu) was placed on the abraded skin. The results of therapy were assessed 24 h after the last treatment with the oral drug and are given in Table 4. The potential of the compound to protect the hair roots against persistent infection was used as a parameter of systemic activity (PETRANYI et al. 1987c).

Mycological parameters showed a daily dose of 6 mg/kg body weight to be the minimum protective one of terbinafine in guinea pig trichophytosis; 40 mg/kg body weight was found to be the minimum curative dose if treatment was started 48 h after inoculation. In microsporosis of the guinea pig the minimum protective dose was 40 mg/kg body weight (PETRANYI et al. 1987c). Similar studies in the same species using terbinafine topically applied showed that treatments with concentrations between 0.06% and 0.5% of terbinafine gave a high mycological cure rate. This indicates that the compound has an excellent ability to penetrate into the depths of the hair follicle and to kill the fungi during a short treatment period (PETRANYI et al. 1987c).

Table 4. Efficacy of orally administered terbinafine against dermatophytes in guinea pigs

	Treatment started (day)	Terbinafine dosage (mg/kg)	Proportion of animals with non-infected hair roots
Trichophyton mentagrophytes (MIC = 0.006 μg/ml)	0	2	4/10
	0	4	4/10
	0	6	10/10
	0	8	10/10
	0	Placebo	0/10
		Controls	0/10
	2	5	0/10
	2	8	0/10
	2	10	1/9[a]
	2	16	4/10
	2	20	5/9[a]
	2	40	10/10
Microsporum canis (MIC = 0.006 μg/ml)	0	2.5	0/10
	0	5	0/9[a]
	0	10	1/9[a]
	0	20	4/10
	0	40	10/10
	0	80	10/10

[a] One animal died during the course of treatment.

Efficacy of oral terbinafine has not been found in animal models of cryptococcosis, coccidioidomycosis, histoplasmosis and renal aspergillosis. The reasons for the absence of efficacy in these models are not clear, but they may involve factors such as tissue distribution, plasma protein or lipoprotein binding, and rapid drug metabolism by rodents. In a subcutaneous tissue model of sporotrichosis, activity was recorded after oral drug administration, suggesting that infections of the subcutaneous tissue may be effectively treated by terbinafine. This would include diseases such as blastomycosis, cutaneous leishmaniasis, sporotrichosis and chromoblastomycosis.

E. Toxicology

I. Acute and Chronic Toxicity

The acute intravenous toxicity (LD_{50}) of terbinafine in rats and mice was 213 mg/kg and 393 mg/kg, respectively, with an oral LD_{50} of over 4000 mg/kg for both species. Local tolerance to terbinafine when applied to skin or mucous membranes was also good. In a challenge test terbinafine did not provoke allergic skin reactions (Magnusson and Kligman 1969). Dermal administration of 1% and 2% cream formulations to rabbits for up to 26 weeks did not provoke adverse systemic effects. The only finding was mild to moderate skin irritation in all groups, including placebo controls. In rats treated for 26 weeks an increase in liver weight associated with enlargement of centrilobular hepatocytes was seen only at high doses. Studies of the exposure of rats to terbinafine during their life time (125 weeks) also showed effects in the liver at high doses which have been shown to be rat-specific. Effects have only been seen in animals treated with more than 10 times the dose recommended for human use. The results indicated that terbinafine would not have significant acute or long-term toxicity for humans.

II. Fertility, Reproduction, Teratogenicity and Mutagenicity

In a study of fertility and reproductive performance in rats, terbinafine was administered orally at daily doses of 10, 50 and 250 mg/kg. Animals receiving the 250 mg/kg dose showed impaired body weight gain, but fertility and general reproductive performance were normal. Treatment with 10 or 50 mg/kg daily showed no adverse effects. Terbinafine did not cause embryolethal or teratogenic effects in rats or rabbits at similar doses. In a peri- and post-natal study in rats using the same dose regimen, terbinafine did not produce any adverse effects on parturition and lactation or on the peri- and post-natal development and survival of the offspring.

In an in vitro teratogenicity study in rats, embryos were transferred on day 9.5 of gestation to a culture medium containing terbinafine at 1, 10, 100 or 300 μg/ml (BECHTER and SCHMID 1987). The embryos were grown extracorporally for a period of 48 h, after which time morphological features, degrees of differentiation and growth were examined. The development of embryos cultivated in the presence of terbinafine was comparable to that of control embryos at concentrations as high as 100 μg/ml, and no gross morphological changes were observed. From these results it was concluded that terbinafine does not adversely affect morphogenesis during the period of organ formation. In contrast, ketoconazole examined concurrently in this test system caused morphological lesions at concentrations as low as 1 μg/ml.

In mutagenicity studies using 5 *Salmonella typhimurium* strains terbinafine in concentrations ranging from 15–3000 μg/plate did not cause any mutagenic effects. In a micronucleus test in mice the oral administration of terbinafine (270, 900 and 2700 mg/kg) did not induce chromosomal damage. There was also no evidence of a mutagenic potential of terbinafine in a test for gene mutations in somatic mammalian cells (V79) using concentrations from 9 to 90 μg/ml, in a chromosome aberration test (concentrations from 1 to 20 μg/ml), in a sister chromatid exchange test (concentrations from 0.5 to 12 μg/ml) and in a test for DNA repair synthesis (concentrations from 0.0064 to 100 μg/ml).

In summary, toxicological investigations revealed a low toxic potential for terbinafine as recorded in acute and chronic toxicity, fertility, reproduction, teratogenicity and mutagenicity studies. From these data, no untoward effects are expected at the therapeutic doses and with the treatment duration recommended in humans.

F. Clinical Results; Efficacy and Tolerability

I. Pharmacokinetics in Humans

When applied topically as a 1% cream to skin, approximately 5% of the terbinafine is absorbed into the systemic circulation. This occurs slowly, with the peak amount of substance appearing as metabolites in the urine only 2–3 days after single-dose application. This slow absorption is believed to reflect the rate of entry of the drug into the subcutis and the persistence of the drug in the epidermis and dermis.

After oral administration of terbinafine at the doses recommended for clinical use (125 mg twice daily or 250 mg once daily) the drug is well absorbed, rapidly distributed to lipophilic tissue and slowly eliminated from tissue compartments (Stephen et al. 1987). The absorption of terbinafine is greater than 70%, and the absorption half-life after 250 mg orally is 0.8–1.2 h. A peak plasma concentration of 0.8–1.5 μg/ml is reached within 2 h of the drug being administered. The distribution half-life is 1.5 h, and the elimination half-life is 22 h. Pharmacokinetics are linear at doses between 50 mg and 750 mg. In multiple dose studies the steady state is reached after 10–14 days. These results indicate that terbinafine follows classic pharmacokinetics for a lipophilic drug and can be administered once daily. The drug's metabolism in elderly patients is similar to that in younger patients, so that no dosage adjustment is necessary. However, patients with severe renal (creatinine clearance less than 50 ml/min) or liver disease metabolise the drug more slowly, and dose reduction is necessary.

Unlike the situation with the azoles, there are with terbinafine no interactions that affect levels of other administered drugs. As has been well recorded, drugs such as cimetidine will inhibit terbinafine metabolism, and rifampicin will induce its metabolism; the use of these drugs would require adjustment of the terbinafine dose.

Terbinafine is strongly bound to plasma proteins in a non-specific way. The binding is to all plasma fractions including albumin, and high, low and very low density lipoproteins. This may alter its tissue and cellular distribution patterns.

Terbinafine appears to concentrate in the epidermis and subcutaneous fat tissue. This feature has led to its high level of clinical efficacy in treating fungal infections in these tissues, as described below.

II. Efficacy of Terbinafine

Clinical studies of terbinafine have been prompted by the high degree of efficacy demonstrated in vitro against a wide spectrum of dermatophytes and yeasts and its efficacy in curing dermatophyte and yeast skin infections in animal models. These organisms most commonly affect the skin of humans. They include the skin dermatophyte infections referred to as tinea corporis, tinea cruris and tinea pedis, the cutaneous yeast infections, candidosis and pityriasis versicolor, and infection of skin appendages, such as nails.

These diseases were therefore selected for study of the efficacy and tolerability of terbinafine. According to common dermatological practice, four of these diseases are usually treated by topical application: tinea cruris/ corporis (mild form), tinea pedis (interdigital type and mild plantar), localised cutaneous candidosis and pityriasis versicolor. The efficacy of topical terbinafine was therefore evaluated in them. Five diseases are often treated systemically by currently available drugs. These include: tinea corporis (moderate and severe forms), tinea pedis (plantar), cutaneous candidosis, more generalised pityriasis versicolor and onychomycosis. The efficacy of oral terbinafine was therefore evaluated in them. The duration of treatment selected was based on accepted practices and experience in the therapy of various dermatomycoses.

For topical studies the selection of a 1% cream was based on animal dose finding and tolerability studies, tolerability testing of 1%–3% cream in humans, and efficacy of the previously available allylamine, naftifine, at a 1% cream concentration. This concentration, which is frequently used for topical antifungal preparations, also met all requirements for pharmaceutical development. The dose of the drug for use systemically by oral administration was determined by the no-toxic-effect level of 30 mg/kg daily, defined in animal models after chronic drug administration, and by a study of experimental dermatophyte infection in humans, which showed that a dose of 250 mg b.i.d. was effective in curing three different dermatophyte skin infections but that 50 mg b.i.d. was inadequate for successful cure. Therefore, two doses (250 mg per day and 500 mg per day) were evaluated in the clinical trials.

There are two major issues in the resolution of a fungal infection, both of which can be carefully measured: (a) the mycological test for the presence of the organism must revert from positive at the beginning of therapy to negative at the end and remain negative at follow-up; (b) the signs and symptoms must rapidly diminish coincident with the disappearance of the microbe. To evaluate these two parameters all studies with terbinafine were analysed by measuring (1) the rate of conversion of documented positive microscopy and fungal culture to negative, (2) the resolution of signs and symptoms common to the disease by measuring a sum of scores of all signs and symptoms during the study and at follow-up, and (3) an overall efficacy rating which reflected in an objective manner combined mycological results and clinical signs and symptoms.

Prior to therapy, material for mycological diagnosis was obtained by gently scraping the lesion. A KOH wet mount was searched microscopically for fungal mycelium, the presence of which was a criterion for inclusion of a patient in the study. A KOH wet mount was also examined at each subsequent examination thereafter, a part of the specimen was inoculated on Sabouraud 2% glucose agar or an alternative recognised culture medium such as Mycosel, incubated at 30°C and examined over 2 weeks for fungal growth. Cultures and microscopy were rated as positive or negative at each visit, at the end of therapy and at follow-up. Clinical signs and symptoms of the disease were assessed at the initial clinical examination and at each subsequent examination.

Signs and symptoms including erythema, scaling, vesiculation, pustules, exudation, crusting and, pruritus were rated as absent, mild, moderate or severe. A total sum of scores for each visit was then recorded. The evaluation was done at follow-up, which was 2–6 weeks after the completion of topical or oral treatment. Only patients with negative mycology (microscopy and culture) who had in addition either none or only up to two mild symptoms were rated as being effectively treated. All other patients, including those with negative mycology but still persistent symptoms, were classified as ineffectively treated.

In a recent publication (Villars and Jones 1989) the efficacy of terbinafine has been presented. The paper reviewed 34 studies of either topical or oral use in the above-mentioned indications. The overall efficacy results obtained from these studies are shown in Table 5; 1258 patients have been treated in 24 studies with 1% terbinafine cream, and 580 patients in 17 studies have been treated orally.

In a double-blind trial comparing topical terbinafine with clotrimazole in interdigital tinea pedis it was observed that in patients treated with terbinafine fungal cultures became negative significantly faster than in those treated with clotrimazole. At the end of the study (2 weeks after the last application of the drug), significantly more patients were rated as effectively cured (Smith et al. 1987). All trials of topically applied 1% terbinafine showed high efficacy and a fast attainment of negative cultures consistent with the drug's fungicidal action (Greer et al. 1987; Ganzinger et al. 1986).

In an oral study comparing terbinafine with griseofulvin in patients with tinea pedis, plantar type, the quick attainment of negative cultures observed in the studies using topical terbinafine was repeated (Savin 1989). In this trial

Table 5. Cure rates in patients treated with terbinafine

Route	Disease	Percentage effectively treated
Topical	Tinea corporis	80–90
	Tinea pedis (Interdigital)	75–85
	Candidosis	75–85
	Pityriasis versicolor	70–80
Oral	Tinea corporis	80–90
	Tinea pedis (plantar)	75–85
	Candidosis	60–70
	Onychomycosis (fingernail)	90–100
	Pityriasis versicolor	0–5

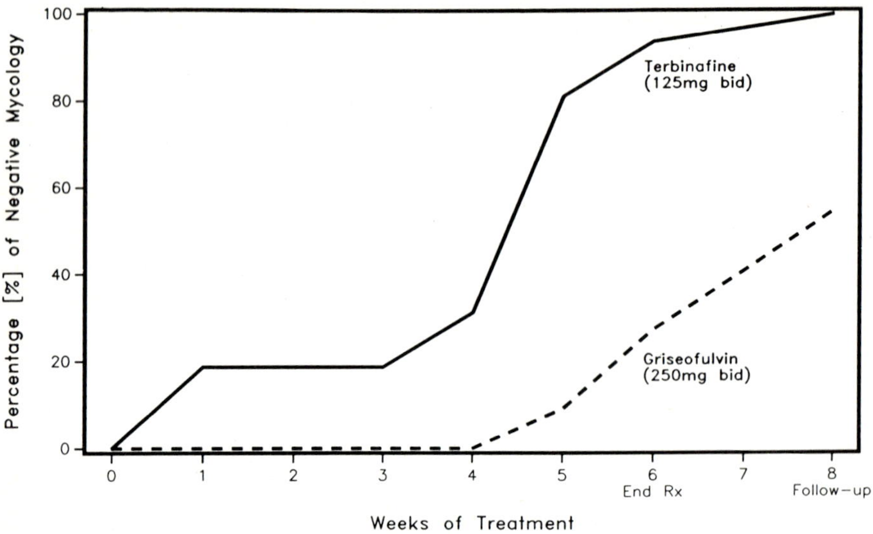

Fig. 4. Effect of treatment on mycological tests in patients with chronic tinea pedis, plantar type. The ordinate shows the percentage of patients with negative cultures for dermatophytes and microscopic identification of KOH preparations of skin scraping and the abscissa, the weeks of treatment (6 weeks) with terbinafine (*solid line*) or griseofulvin (*broken line*) plus evaluation at follow-up 2 weeks later

28 patients were evaluated: 16 were treated with 125 mg terbinafine b.i.d. and 12, with 250 mg griseofulvin also b.i.d. The mean duration of the disease of the patients prior to the start of the study was 9 years. The evaluation of the mycological results is shown in Fig. 4. There was a rapid attainment of negative culture and microscopy in the terbinafine group. The difference compared with the griseofulvin group is statistically significant and clinically impressive. At the follow-up evaluation all patients in the terbinafine group were mycologically cured compared with only 50% in the griseofulvin group.

The high efficacy of terbinafine is seen not only in its ability to induce mycological cure but also in its ability to promote clinical cure. This is illustrated by Fig. 5, which shows the disappearance of the most important symptom (desquamation) in this disease. At the end of the study all but one patient in the terbinafine group were cured according to this parameter compared with only 30% in the griseofulvin group. A follow-up after 6–15 months showed continued resolution of signs and symptoms in terbinafine-treated patients, but relapse of infection occurred in griseofulvin-treated patients; 94% of the terbinafine group stayed cured compared with only 30% in the griseofulvin group (SAVIN 1989).

Terbinafine also showed high efficacy in treating finger- and toenail onychomycosis. In a study done by ZAIAS and SERRANO (1989) all 11 patients

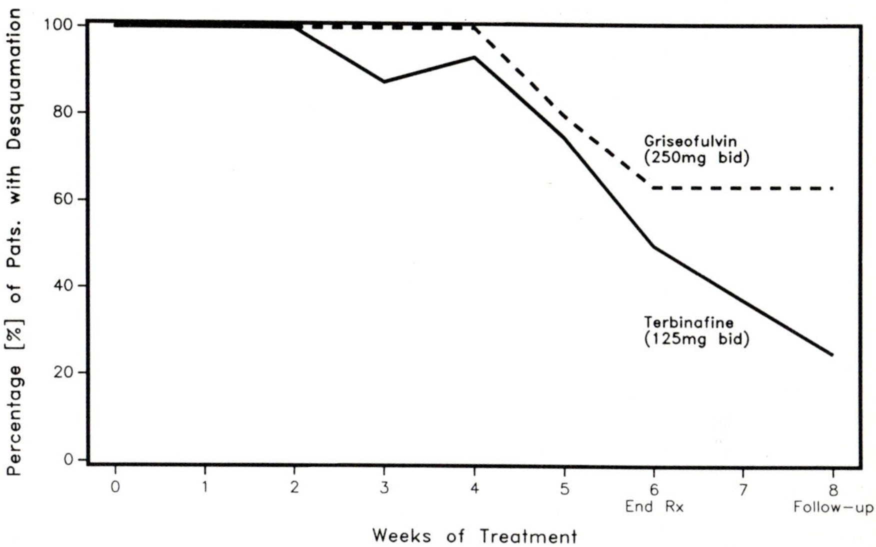

Fig. 5. Effect of treatment on one chronic sign of infection in patients with tinea pedis, plantar type. Percentage of patients showing desquamation is correlated with the weeks of treatment with terbinafine or griseofulvin

treated for fingernail onychomycosis with 125 mg terbinafine twice daily were cured after a treatment of 6 months (Fig. 6). Ten months after the last treatment, all but one patient remained cured. One patient had an infection of a nail which was not previously infected. Negative mycology in this study was obtained between months 2 and 4. In another study, the mean time to mycological cure in the treatment of toenail infections was 6 months and in treatment of fingernails, only 3 months. Again the fungicidal action of terbinafine appears to provide an important advantage in allowing a short duration of treatment of this chronic condition.

III. Tolerability of Oral and Topical Terbinafine

Table 6 lists all side effects associated with orally used terbinafine. The comparative drugs used were ketoconazole, griseofulvin or placebo. A total of 694 patients treated with terbinafine were enrolled in these studies and available for assessment of drug tolerability. Several points are of particular interest. The most common side effects during oral therapy with terbinafine occurred in the gastrointestinal tract (3.5%) when the now recommended effective dose of 250 mg/day was used. These were mild and often transient. They included nausea, dyspepsia and stomach pains. These events were less

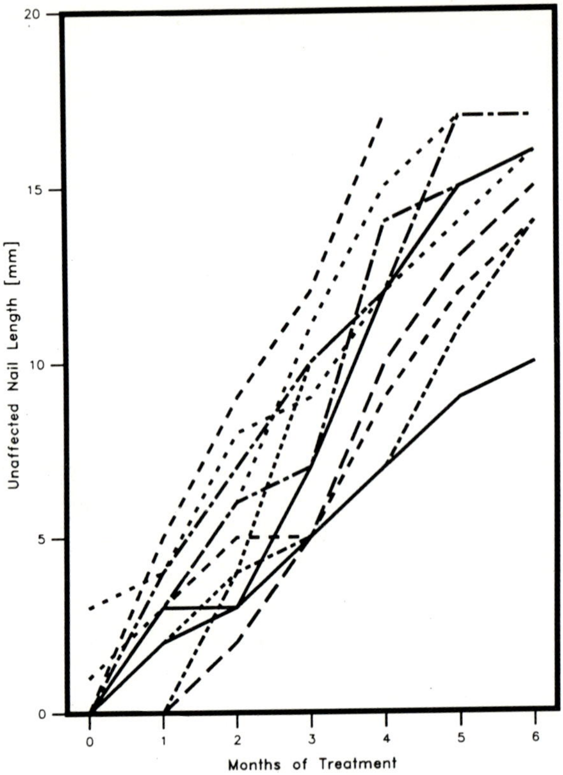

Fig. 6. Growth of normal, uninfected fingernails during treatment of onychomycosis. Ordinate shows the millimeters of normal nail measured from the cuticle to the beginning of diseased nail. Abscissa shows the months of treatment with terbinafine. It is seen that each of the 11 patients treated showed continuous outgrowth of normal nail from the first month of treatment until complete cure after 5–6 months of treatment

Table 6. Side effects in 1215 patients treated orally with terbinafine, comparative drugs or placebo

	Terbinafine		Comparative drugs[a] (n = 372)	Placebo (n = 149)
	250 mg/day (n = 452)	500 mg/day (n = 242)		
Gastrointestinal	16 (3.5%)	18 (7.4%)	25 (6.7%)	6 (4.0%)
Skin	5 (1.1%)	4 (1.7%)	7 (1.9%)	0 (0.0%)
Other	5 (1.1%)	14 (5.8%)	27 (7.3%)	2 (1.3%)
Total	26 (5.8%)	36 (14.9%)	59 (15.9%)	8 (5.4%)

[a] 500 mg/day of griseofulvin (15% total side effects) or 200 mg/day of ketoconazole (17% total side effects).

common than when the higher dose of terbinafine (500 mg) was used (7.4%), and when the comparative drugs were given in their standard recommended dose (6.7%). Skin reactions during oral treatment occurred in approximately 1% of patients in each group. At the dose of 250 mg/day recommended for terbinafine in all indications, its side-effects profile was similar to that of placebo. Oral terbinafine is therefore very well tolerated. No significant, clinically relevant, drug-related changes in haematological or biochemical tests were recorded during treatment with terbinafine. Side effects occurred in 2.2% of patients using topical 1% terbinafine cream. They consisted of local burning, itching or redness at the application site. Similar reaction rates were observed with each of the comparative drugs.

G. Summary

Terbinafine is a member of a new class of antifungal drugs called allylamine derivatives that act at a unique site in the inhibition of fungal membrane sterol synthesis. The drug binds to squalene epoxidase, which leads to the accumulation of squalene in the fungi and contributes to the fungicidal action of the drug.

The drug is effective in vitro and in vivo in animal models against a broad range of fungi. It is metabolised in animals and in humans in a classic way, with good oral absorption, rapid distribution and slow elimination from tissues. It does not bind to cytochrome P-450 in a non-specific manner; therefore, none of the side events associated with these drugs which inhibit this class of enzyme are expected, nor do they occur. The toxicology profile in animals and the absence of adverse events in humans show that the drug is very safe and well tolerated.

Clinical results to date in over 1000 patients indicate that it is a safe drug with a high cure rate when used either topically as a 1% cream or orally in a dose of 250 mg daily. When used topically it cures most patients (70%–90%) who have dermatomycoses. Orally it is ineffective against pityriasis versicolor, but it has high levels of efficacy against the classic dermatophytoses such as chronic tinea pedis, plantar type, and onychomycosis.

It is expected that terbinafine will provide an important addition to the treatment of dermatomycoses since it contributes a high degree of efficacy in chronic, recalcitrant dermatophyte infections and it is well tolerated without evidence of hepatic, renal or haematopoeitic toxicity in humans.

References

Bechter R, Schmid BP (1987) Teratogenicity in vitro – a comparative study of four antimycotic drugs using the whole-embryo culture system. Toxic In Vitro 1:11–15

Borgers M, Vanden Bossche H (1982) The mode of action of antifungal drugs. In: Levine HB (ed) Ketoconazole in the management of fungal disease. Adis Press, Sydney, pp 25–47

Drouhet E, Dupont B (1987) Evolution of antifungal agents: past, present, and future. Rev Inf Dis 9:S4–S14
Ganzinger U, Stütz A, Petranyi G, Stephen A (1986) Allylamines: topical and oral treatment of dermatomycoses with a new class of antifungal agents. Acta Derm Venereol (Stockh) (Supp 121):155–160
Greer D, Millikan L, Jolly H (1987) Effect of topical SF 86-327 1% cream in treatment of tinea cruris/tinea corporis. Abstracts, part II, 17th World Congress of Dermatology, Berlin, May 1987, p 130
Grimus R, Schuster I (1983) SF 86-327: uptake, distribution and metabolism in the rat. A comparison of in vitro and in vivo data. Proc 13th Int Cong Chemother, Vienna, part 116, PS 4.8/4–12
Kan VL, Henderson DK, Bennett JE (1986) Bioassay for SF 86-327, a new antifungal agent. Antimicrob Agents Chemother 30:628–629
Magnusson B, Kligman AM (1969) The identification of contact allergens by animal assay. The guinea-pig maximisation test. J Invest Dermatol 52:268–267
Meingassner JG, Sleytr UB, Petranyi G (1983a) SF 86-327: effects on the ultrastructure of *Trichophyton mentagrophytes* in vitro. Proc 13th Int Cong Chemother, Vienna, part 116, PS 4.8/4–7
Meingassner JG, Müller M, Sleytr UB (1983b) SF 86-327: Effects on the ultrastructure of *Candida albicans* in vitro. Proc 13th Int Cong Chemother, Vienna, part 116, PS 4.8/4–8
Moulin-Traffort J, Steinmetz MD, Régli P (1987) Étude ultrastructurale de l'action de la terbinafine sur *Scopulariopsis brevicaulis*. Bull Soc Fr Mycol Méd 16:269–272
Petranyi G, Ryder NS, Stütz A (1984) Allylamine derivatives: new class of synthetic antifungal agents inhibiting fungal squalene epoxidase. Science 224:1239–1241
Petranyi G, Stütz A, Ryder NS, Meingassner JG, Mieth H (1987a) Experimental antimycotic activity of naftifine and terbinafine. In: Fromtling RA (ed) Recent trends in the discovery, development and evaluation of antifungal agents. JR Prous, Barcelona, pp 441–450
Petranyi G, Meingassner JG, Mieth H (1987b) Antifungal activity of the allylamine derivative terbinafine in vitro. Antimicrob Agents Chemother 31:1365–1368
Petranyi G, Meingassner JG, Mieth H (1987c) Activity of terbinafine in experimental fungal infections of laboratory animals. Antimicrob Agents Chemother 31:1558–1561
Ryder NS (1985) Specific inhibition of fungal sterol biosynthesis by SF 86-327, a new allylamine antimycotic agent. Antimicrob Agents Chemother 27:252–256
Ryder NS (1986) Biochemical mode of action of the allylamine antimycotic agents naftifine and SF 86-327. In: Iwata K, Vanden Bossche H (eds) In vitro and in vivo evaluation of antifungal agents. Elsevier, Amsterdam, pp 89–99
Ryder NS (1987) Mechanism of action of the allylamine antimycotics. In: Fromtling RA (ed) Recent trends in the discovery, development and evaluation of antifungal agents. JR Prous, Barcelona, pp 451–459
Ryder NS, Dupont M-C (1985) Inhibition of squalene epoxidase by allylamine antimycotic compounds. A comparative study of the fungal and mammalian enzymes. Biochem J 230:765–770
Savin R (1989) Successful treatment of chronic tinea pedis (moccasin type) with terbinafine (Lamisil). Clin Expt Dermatol 14:116–119
Schatz F, Haberl H (1989) Analytical methods for the determination of terbinafine and its metabolites in human plasma, milk and urine. Arzneimittelforsch 39: 527–532
Schatz F, Haberl H, Czok R (1983) SF 86–327: methods for determination of the parent compound and metabolites in human plasma and urine. Proc 13th Int Cong Chemother, Vienna, part 116, PS 4.8/4–9
Schuster I (1985) The interaction of representative members from two classes of antimycotics – the azoles and the allylamines – with cytochromes P-450 in steroidogenic tissues and liver. Xenobiotica 15:529–546

Schuster I (1987) Metabolic degradation of terbinafine in liver microsomes from man, guinea pig and rat. In: Fromtling RA (ed) Recent trends in the discovery, development and evaluation of antifungal agents. JR Prous, Barcelona, pp 461–470

Schuster I, Schaude M, Schatz F, Mieth H (1988) Preclinical characteristics of allylamines. In: Berg D, Plempel M (eds) Sterol biosynthesis inhibitors. Ellis Horwood, Chichester, pp 449–470

Shadomy S, Espinel-Ingroff A, Gebhart RJ (1985) In-vitro studies with SF 86-327, a new orally active allylamine derivative. Sabouraudia: J Med Vet Mycol 23: 125–132

Smith EB, Zaias N, Savin R (1987) Successful treatment of tinea pedis (athlete's foot type) with 1% topical SF 86-327 cream. 15th Congress of Chemotherapy, Ecomed Verlagsgesellschaft, p 1017

Stephen A, Czok R, Male O (1987) Terbinafine: initial clinical results. In: Fromtling RA (ed) Recent trends in the discovery, development and evaluation of antifungal agents. JR Prous, Barcelona, pp 511–520

Stütz A (1987) Allylamine derivatives – a new class of active substances in antifungal chemotherapy. Angew Chem Int Ed Engl 26:320–328

Stütz A (1988) Synthesis and structure-activity correlations within allylamine antimycotics. Ann NY Acad Sci 544:46–62

Stütz A, Petranyi G (1984) Synthesis and antifungal activity of (E)-*N*-(6,6-dimethyl-2-hepten-4-ynyl)-*N*-methyl-1-naphthalenemethanamine (SF 86-327) and related allylamine derivatives with enhanced oral activity. J Med Chem 1984 27:1539–1543

Stütz A, Georgopoulos A, Granitzer W, Petranyi G, Berney D (1986) Synthesis and structure-activity relationships of naftifine-related allylamine antimycotics. J Med Chem 29:112–125

Villars V, Jones TC (1989) Clinical efficacy and tolerability of terbinafine (Lamisil), a new topical and systemic fungicidal drug for treatment of dermatomycoses. Clin Exp Dermatol 14:124–127

Zaias N, Serrano L (1989) The successful treatment of finger *Trichophyton rubrum* onychomycosis with oral terbinafine. Clin Exp Dermatol 14:120–123

CHAPTER 21

Amorolfine

ANNEMARIE POLAK and MICHEL ZAUG

A. Introduction

Amorolfine (3-[*p*-(1,1-dimethylpropyl)-phenyl]2-methyl-propyl-2,6-*cis* dimethylmorpholine hydrochloride; Ro 14-4767/002) shows activity against fungi pathogenic to plants, animals and humans (POLAK and DIXON 1987). Given here is a resume of preclinical findings with this drug as well as a summary of published clinical data. In vitro the spectrum against representative species pathogenic for humans was defined measuring fungistatic as well as fungicidal effects. In vivo studies were conducted using models of dermatophytosis, vaginal candidosis and various organ mycoses.

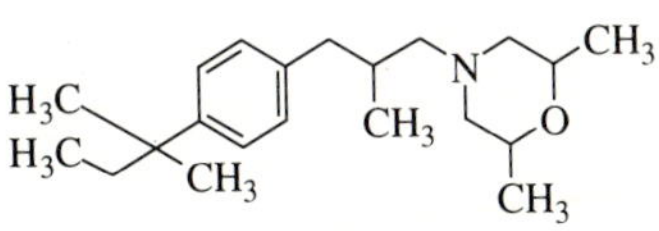

Amorolfine

B. Preclinical Results

I. Antifungal Activity of Amorolfine In Vitro

1. Fungistatic Activity

Amorolfine possesses remarkable antifungal activity against a broad spectrum of medically important fungi (Table 1). The dermatophytes, dematiaceous fungi, dimorphic fungi and yeasts were generally inhibited by less than 1 μg/ml, the dermatophytes being the most sensitive. The drug achieved variable results against moulds, the aspergilli were more or less resistant, while *Hendersonula*, *Alternaria* and *Scopulariopsis* showed sensitivity.

Amorolfine demonstrated the same considerable intraspecies variation against *Candida* spp. as is known for other sterol biosynthesis inhibitors like allylamine and especially azole derivatives (ODDS et al. 1984; HALLER 1979; ODDS and ABBOTT 1984; POLAK 1983; POLAK and DIXON 1987). The results of in vitro testing in these species are strongly dependent on the choice of medium and test conditions (HALLER 1979; ODDS and ABBOTT 1984; POLAK 1982a,b). Under standardised test methods performed in a single laboratory,

Table 1. Antifungal activity of amorolfine in vitro

Organism	No. of strains tested	MIC (μg/ml) Geometric mean	Range
Dermatophytes			
Microsporum canis	21	0.062	0.001–0.13
M. gypseum	7	0.026	0.01–0.1
Trichophyton mentagrophytes	39	0.029	0.001–0.13
T. rubrum	40	0.004	<0.001–0.13
Epidermophyton floccosum	13	0.088	0.03–6.2
Pityrosporum sp.	15	0.1	0.005–0.2
Yeasts			
Candida albicans	155	0.55	0.001–>100
C. tropicalis	36	0.22	0.001–>100
Torulopsis glabrata	23	25	0.06–>100
C. krusei	10	0.112	0.1–1
C. parapsilosis	35	1.09	0.03–30
C. pseudotropicalis	6	0.156	0.06–1
C. guillermondii	14	0.302	0.1–1
Cryptococcus neoformans	53	0.033	<0.001–8
Dematiaceous fungi			
Cladosporium bantianum	15	0.074	0.006–0.25
C. carrionii	10	0.29	0.1–1.56
Fonsecaea pedrosoi	28	0.100	0.01–0.39
Madurella mycetomatis	5	0.02	0.001–0.1
Phialophora verrucosa	3	0.47	0.1–>128
Wangiella dermatitidis	6	0.0125	0.01–0.025
Dactylaria constricta	2	0.034	0.03–0.05
Dimorphic fungi			
Histoplasma capsulatum	15	0.06	0.06
Coccidioides immitis	5	0.07	0.06–0.13
Blastomyces dermatitidis	22	0.21	0.001–0.5
Sporothrix schenckii	22	0.12	0.06–10
Moulds			
Aspergillus fumigatus	30	>100	30–>100
A. flavus	18	>100	30–>100
A. nidulans	5	21	3–>100
A. niger	9	44	3–>100
Absidia corymbifera	2	10	
Mucor circinelloides	10	45	30–>100
Rhizomucor pussillus	2	30	
Rhizopus oryzae	35	15.3	10–30
R. rhizopodiformis	4	3	1–10
Pseudallescheria boydii	4	0.06	0.06
Fusarium sp.	8	30	0.3–100
Hendersonula sp.	6	0.3	0.1–1
Alternaria sp.	5	0.35	0.05–1
Scopulariopsis brevicaulis	10	2.0	0.5–5

MIC, minimal inhibitory concentration.

Table 2. Fungistatic concentrations (geometric mean of MICs in μg/ml) of amorolfine in comparison with other antimycotics in casitone medium

Organism	Antifungal drug				
	Amorolfine	Ketoconazole	Oxiconazole	Miconazole	Terbinafine
Candida albicans	0.404	1.195	15.2	3.9	12.0
C. tropicalis	0.025	1.36	100	1	–
C. parapsilosis	0.937	0.096	1	5	0.27
Torulopsis glabrata	2.52	1.96	3	5	>100
Cryptococcus neoformans	0.003	–	0.025	–	–
Trichophyton spp.	0.009	1.0	0.41	1.0	0.0013
Aspergillus spp.	>100	10	1.46	1.0	3.0
Histoplasma capsulatum					
Mycelial phase	0.1	1.0	0.1	1.0	1.0
Yeast phase[a]	0.15	0.02	–	–	–

MIC, minimal inhibitory concentration.
[a] Determined on brain heart infusion agar supplemented with cysteine and blood.

the activity of amorolfine compares favourably with other antimycotics available today in all instances, except against *Aspergillus* spp. (Table 2).

2. Fungicidal Activity

Amorolfine possesses true fungicidal activity against *C. albicans*, *Cryptococcus neoformans*, dermatophytes, dimorphic fungi and dematiaceae (Table 3). The fungicidal activity is both concentration and time dependent (Fig. 1).

Table 3. Fungicidal activity of amorolfine: concentration (μg/ml) which kills more than 90% of the cells within 24 or 48 h incubation on casitone medium

	24 h	48 h
Candida albicans	3	1
Cryptococcus neoformans	100	30
Histoplasma capsulatum	10	1.7
Wangiella dermatitidis	5.0	0.25
Trichophyton mentagrophytes	3	0.001

II. Therapeutic Efficacy in Animal Models

1. Deep Mycoses

Amorolfine showed no more than slight activity in various models of systemic mycoses (including opportunistic as well as primary pathogenic fungi; Table 4). The lack of good systemic activity is most probably due to rapid metabolism of the drug in mice and/or very strong protein binding.

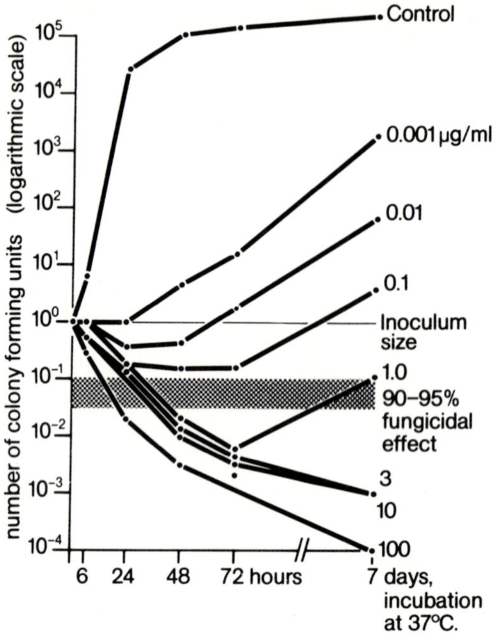

Fig. 1. Fungicidal activity of amorolfine against *Candida albicans*. Viability time determinations were made in casitone broth and are presented as the mean of seven strains

Table 4. Chemotherapeutic activity of amorolfine in various systemic fungal infections of mice

	Minimal dose significantly prolonging survival (mg/kg per day)
Candidosis	100 p.o.
Cryptococcosis	30 s.c.
Aspergillosis	>2000 p.o.
Histoplasmosis	100 s.c.
Phaeohyphomycosis	>200
Sporotrichosis	>200

2. Topical Mycoses

Amorolfine showed high efficacy in experimental trichophytosis when treatment was started either before or after the fungal foci were visible. In Table 5 the activity of amorolfine in prophylactic experiments is compared with other antimycotic treatments; animals were considered as cured when they were free of fungal lesions and cultures were negative. The only drug in the study that showed a greater effect was terbinafine. Results were similar in thera-

Table 5. Chemotherapeutic activity of amorolfine cream and other antimycotics in trichophytosis of the guinea pig (topical treatment for 11 days)

Compound	% active ingredient in cream	Percentage of animals totally cured
Amorolfine	0.01	100
	0.003	80
	0.001	60
	0.0003	20
	0.0001	10
Oxiconazole	0.3	100
Ketoconazole	0.5	100
	0.2	20
Bifonazole	1	100
	0.3	40
	0.1	10
Terbinafine	0.001	100

peutic experiments in which drug treatment was started on day 3 after inoculation (Fig. 2).

In experiments designed to investigate the persistence of amorolfine, lesions were scored in guinea pigs following a single application of 0.1% amorolfine cream on days 4, 3, 2 or 1 before inoculation. The severity of the lesions was directly proportional to the length of time between prophylactic

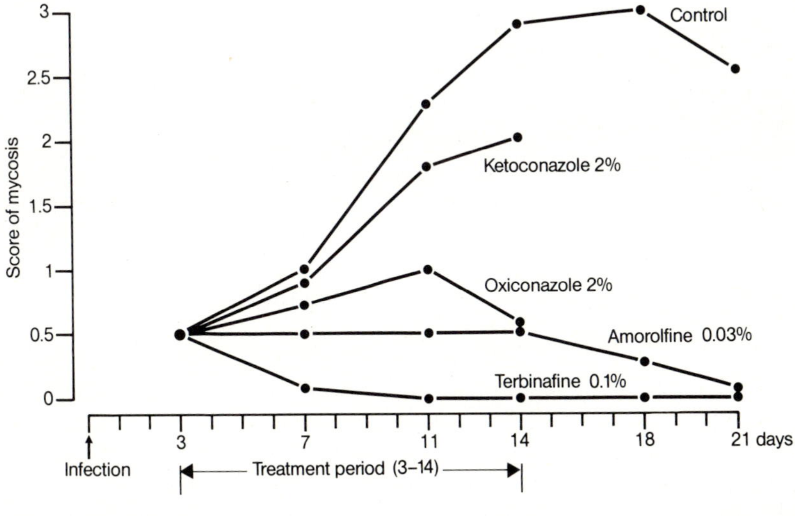

Fig. 2. Comparative antifungal activities of amorolfine and various other drugs against *Trichophyton mentagrophytes* strain 109 in the guinea pig. Treatment started on day 3 after inoculation

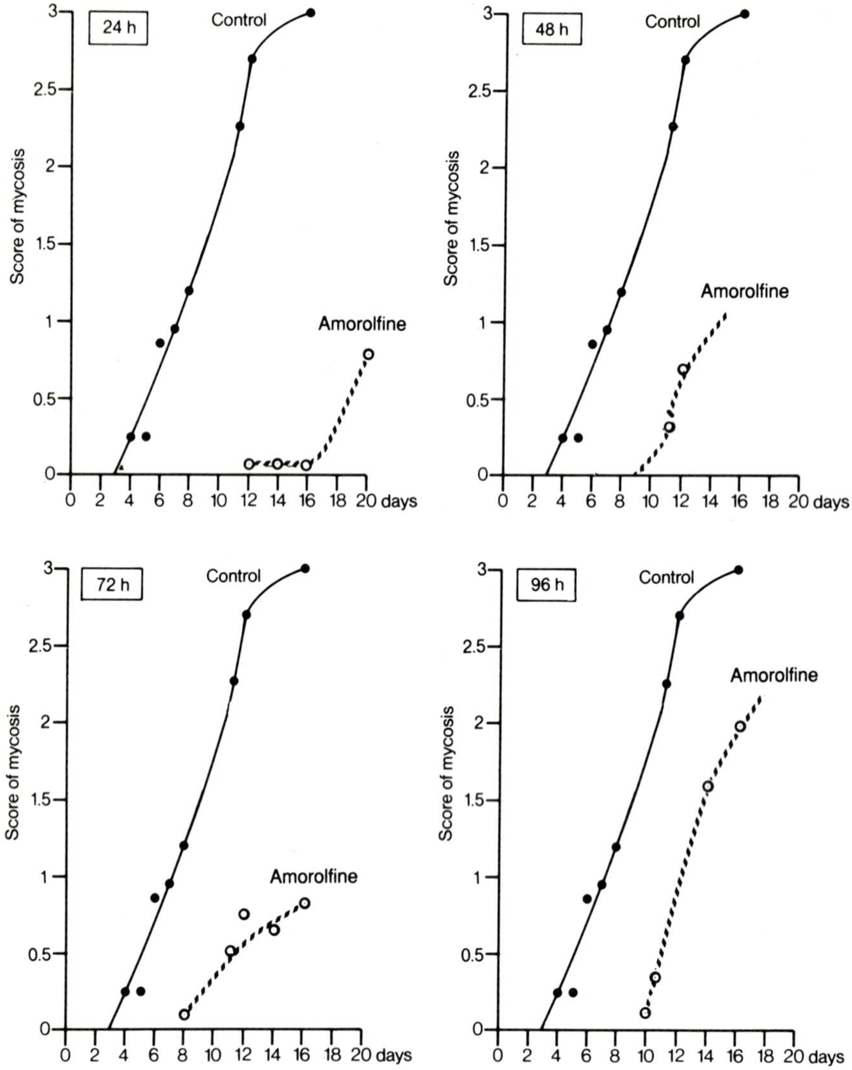

Fig. 3. Activity of amorolfine against trichophytosis in the guinea pig as measured in the cutaneous retention time test (time before inoculation)

treatment and experimental inoculation (Fig. 3; POLAK 1984). These results indicate that the activity of amorolfine persists for a considerable time in the skin, and therefore the frequency of therapeutic application can be significantly reduced.

In the treatment of vaginal candidosis of the rat, amorolfine was equally impressive. As little as 0.01% to topically applied drug resulted in a nearly two log reduction in viable *C. albicans* recoverable from the vaginas of

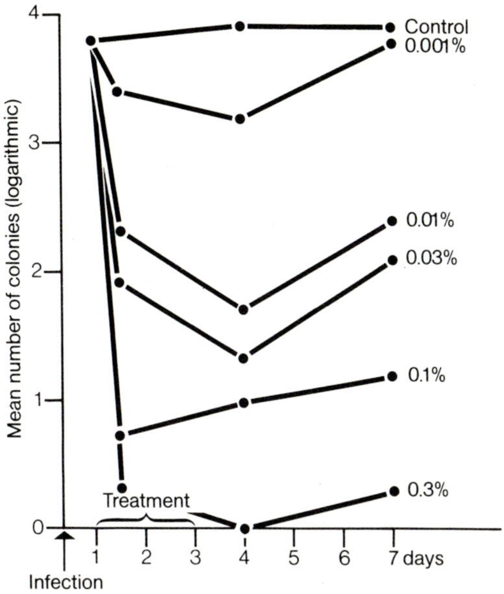

Fig. 4. Activity of amorolfine in reducing viable numbers of *Candida albicans* from the vaginas of experimentally infected rats

experimentally infected rats; 0.3% was more or less curative (Fig. 4). In this model amorolfine compared favourably with other antimycotics (Table 6).

C. Clinical Studies

I. Human Pharmacokinetics

1. Dermal Penetration

Eight healthy male volunteers were treated with 0.5 mg ^{14}C-labelled amorolfine (10 μCi) incorporated in a 0.5% amorolfine cream applied to an area of about 10 cm^2 of intact (two volunteers) or stripped (six volunteers) skin which remained uncovered for 8 h. After this period the remaining cream was removed from the skin, and the treated area was stripped ten times with Scotch tape. Recovered drug and skin strippings were assayed for total radioactivity. Blood samples were collected at intervals up to 72 h after treatment and total urine and faeces were collected separately in portions up to 120 h after treatment. No detectable levels of radioactivity were found in any of the plasma, urine or faecal samples collected. Between 0.8% and 2.6% of the administered dose was recovered from the stripped skin of the treated area. The overall recovery of radioactivity was 99% of the dose administered (ROHDE et al. 1987).

Table 6. Chemotherapeutic activity of amorolfine in comparison with other antifungals in vaginal candidosis in rats

Drug	Chemotherapeutic activity[a]
Amorolfine trial 1	0.029
trial 2	0.02
trial 3	0.019
trial 4	0.015
Amphotericin B	5
Candicidin	0.5
Ketoconazole	0.055
Tioconazole	0.24
Miconazole	1
Oxiconazole	0.09
Naftifine	>1
Terbinafine	>1

[a] % active ingredient in topical preparation required to produce 50% reduction of $\log_{10}$ of *Candida albicans* in the vagina.

2. Vaginal Absorption

A single dose of 50 mg ^{14}C-labelled amorolfine in the form of a tablet was administered intravaginally to six healthy volunteers. The tablet was held in the vagina for 24 h using a tampon, after which the remains of the tablet were washed out. Blood samples were collected after various times up to 96 h after administration; urine and faeces were collected separately in portions up to 168 h after administration. Peak plasma concentrations of radioactivity corresponding to 27–83 ng-equiv/ml amorolfine were found 36–72 h after administration. In one of the subjects the intact drug was also assayed; this reached a peak value of 8.8 ng/ml 48 h after administration. Unchanged drug accounted for only 16% of the total radioactivity (55 ng-equiv/ml) measured at the same time. Recovery of radioactivity from urine (8%–28%) and faeces (1.4%–3.8%) in these subjects could not be taken as a measure of vaginal absorption, since the radioactivity recovered in the urine was obviously due to unchanged drug which had remained in the vagina even after washing out the leftovers of the tablet (ROHDE et al. 1987).

II. Human Pharmacology

1. Persistence in the Skin

Twelve healthy volunteers were treated with a single application of 0.5% amorolfine cream or alcoholic solution on the skin; the treated area was then covered with a bandage. Tape strippings were taken at various intervals from the treated skin and applied to the surface of microculture slides which had previously been inoculated with *Trichophyton mentagrophytes* var. *granulosum* or *T. rubrum*. The persistent effects of the drug in the epidermis

Table 7. Residual antimycotic effects against *Trichophyton rubrum* following a single topical application of 0.5% amorolfine cream

Time in days between treatment of the skin and sampling	No. of samples with		
	Normal growth	Suppressed growth	No growth
1	0	0	3
2	0	1	2
3	1	2	0
4	3	0	0
7	3	0	0

were assessed by the degree of inhibition of growth of dermatophytes under the tape. Amorolfine cream 0.5% had a persistent antimycotic effect for at least 48 h, and a reduced effect was observed in some cases up to 3 days after application (Table 7). The corresponding figures for amorolfine 0.5% alcoholic solution were 3 and 4 days. These results suggest that topical treatment with amorolfine once every 2nd day may be adequate; this might result in better patient compliance than a treatment regimen once or twice per day (GIP 1989).

2. Dermal Tolerance

The local tolerance of 0.125%, 0.25% and 0.5% cream preparations of amorolfine was compared with that of the vehicle alone. Two models, the Duhring chamber and a scarification test, were used. Both trials were double-blind, randomized with simultaneous comparisons in 20 healthy subjects. In the first test, occlusion was produced by means of a Duhring chamber on healthy skin for 21 days. In the second test, the skin was scarified and the cream applied for 3 days under an occlusive dressing. Local tolerance, as established in 20 volunteers and assessed on a five point scale from 0 to 4, can be considered as good, since the reactions in both tests were of low-grade severity (Table 8). In neither test was dose dependence established (ROHDE et al. 1987).

3. Persistence Under the Nail

Ten patients who had onychomycosis (nine toenails, one fingernail) were treated with amorolfine. *T. rubrum* was isolated in all cases (Kimmig agar). Patients applied a 5% nail lacquer twice weekly for 1 month (eight applications). Nail lacquer was removed at the end of treatment, and material from under the nail was taken from each patient immediately, 24 h, 48 h, 76 h and 7 days after the end of treatment. This material was used not only for microscopical diagnosis and mycological culture but also to measure inhibition zones after being placed on plates freshly inoculated with *T. rubrum*.

In nine of ten patients cultures were negative immediately after and up to

Table 8. Duhring chamber and scarification tests with different concentrations of amorolfine cream

Score	Duhring chamber[a]				Scarification test[b]			
	Placebo	0.125%	0.25%	0.5%	Placebo	0.125%	0.25%	0.5%
0	11	10	8	7	7	9	9	10
1	8	8	10	9	12	11	11	10
2	1	2	1	4	1	0	0	0
3	0	0	1	0	0	0	0	0
4	0	0	0	0	0	0	0	0

[a] In the Duhring chamber test the score had the following meaning: 0 = no reaction; 1 = slight erythema; 2 = moderate erythema; 3 = severe erythema; 4 = very severe erythema (plus oedema, plus necrosis).
[b] The scarification test was evaluated according to the following criteria: 0 = negative, scratches invisible; 1 = slight erythema confined to scratches; 2 = broader bands of increased erythema with or without rows of vesicles, pustules or erosions; 3 = severe erythema with partial confluence, with or without other lesions; 4 = confluent severe erythema, sometimes associated with oedema, necrosis or blistering.

Table 9. Determination of inhibition zone (mm) induced by the material from under the nail after twice weekly applications of amorolfine lacquer for 1 month

Patient no.	At end of treatment	+24 h	+48 h	+76 h	+7 days
1	44[a]	44[a]	44[a]	44[a]	44[a]
2	35	40	40	38	35
3	44[a]	44[a]	44[a]	44[a]	44[a]
4	44[a]	44[a]	44[a]	44[a]	44[a]
5	44[a]	44[a]	44[a]	44[a]	44[a]
6	66	80	58	66	64
7	75	75	–	72	70
8	45	45	41	39	41
9	85	85	80	75	60
10	80	76	54	50	50

[a] Diameter size of inhibition zone was at least 44 mm.

7 days following the end of treatment. One patient showed a positive culture on the 7th day, although the first four cultures (up to 76 h) were negative. In the first series of five patients a 90 mm diameter dish was used for testing three samples; under these conditions the inhibition zones overlapped when their diameter exceeded 44 mm, making the interpretation of the results difficult. For this reason, only one sample per 90 mm dish was tested in the second series of five patients. The diameter of the inhibition zones in this second series ranged from 45 to 85 mm at the end of the 1-month treatment, and from 41 to 70 mm 7 days after the end of treatment (Table 9).

These data suggest that antifungal activity persists under the nails for at least 7 days after treatment and that a twice weekly application of 5% amorolfine nail lacquer is satisfactory for the therapy of onychomycosis (Mensing and Splanemann 1988).

4. Vaginal Tolerance

In a double-blind, placebo-controlled study, three groups of eight healthy female volunteers received a vaginal tablet containing either 50 mg amorolfine or placebo. Vaginal tablets were inserted either once or on 3 or 6 consecutive days. Local and systemic tolerance were evaluated 24 h and 7 days after the completion of treatment. Amorolfine was well tolerated in all cases. Neither objective nor subjective symptoms of intolerance nor clinically relevant changes in laboratory examinations were observed (Rohde et al. 1987).

III. Therapeutic Trials

1. Dermatomycosis

a) Mixed Mycoses

In four centres in the FRG, 232 patients with dermatomycoses such as foot mycosis, cutaneous candidosis, tinea inguinalis or tinea corporis were treated with 0.125%, 0.25% or 0.5% amorolfine cream or 1% bifonazole cream for 2–6 weeks. Mycological examinations were performed before, at the end of and 1 week after treatment. Clinical examinations were done before, each week during, and 1 week after the end of therapy.

Some 208 patients were evaluated for efficacy. A total of 217 pathogens were isolated: *T. rubrum* (77), *T. mentagrophytes* (65), *E. floccosum* (10), *M. canis* (4), *T. terrestre* (1), *Candida*, spp. (51), aspergilli (8) and *Rhodoturola*, spp. (1). One week after the end of treatment, 87.3% (n = 55), 91.7% (n = 48), 90.7% (n = 54) and 92.2% (n = 51) of the patients had negative cultures in the 0.125%, 0.25%, 0.5% amorolfine and 1% bifonazole treatment groups, respectively. The overall assessment made 1 week after the end of treatment is shown in Fig. 5. Local adverse effects were observed in 1, 2, 0 and 3 patients, respectively. There were no differences in mycological and clinical efficacy or tolerance between the groups (Nolting 1988).

b) Foot Mycoses

In a randomised, parallel study with three groups of 40 patients each, two alcoholic solutions (0.5% and 2%, double-blind) and a 0.5% cream (open) were compared. Diagnosis was established on the basis of the clinical picture and positive mycological findings in a fresh preparation and in a concurrently started culture. Patients with foot mycoses caused by dermatophytes and/or yeasts were included. Both the solutions and the cream were applied once daily for a period of 3 weeks. Clinical symptoms and local findings were

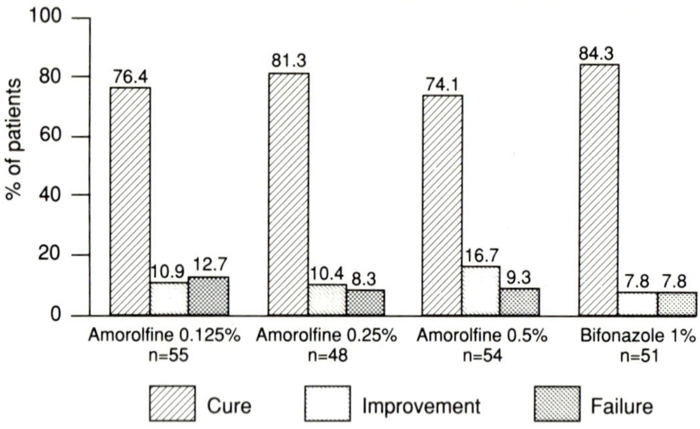

Fig. 5. Overall clinical results after once daily application of three different concentrations of amorolfine cream or 1% bifonazole cream in patients with dermatomycosis

evaluated at enrollment, once a week during the treatment, at the end of treatment and 2 weeks after therapy was completed. Microscopic investigations on fresh preparations and species identification by appropriate culture were performed at enrollment and 2 weeks after the end of treatment.

The following pathogens were isolated: *T. rubrum* (65), *T. mentagrophytes* (25), *E. floccosum* (19), *M. canis* (2) and *Candida* sp. (4), and there were four mixed infections. Five patients treated with the 2% solution and one patient with the 0.5% solution were prematurely withdrawn from the study due to lack of co-operation.

Two weeks after the end of treatment, 30/35 (86%), 34/39 (87%) and 39/40 (98%) of the patients treated with the 2% solution, the 0.5% solution and the 0.5% cream, respectively, had sterile mycological cultures. Table 10 shows the overall assessment for each group. The differences in results between the various formulations employed were not statistically significant ($P > 0.05$). Three patients treated with the 2% and three with the 0.5% alcoholic solution complained of burning sensations; in the latter group another patient reported increased pruritus, fissures and crusts. Two patients treated with the 0.5% cream complained of burning sensations (GALIMBERTI et al. 1988).

2. Onychomycoses

A total of 155 patients who had onychomycosis were treated with either 2% or 5% amorolfine nail lacquer for up to 6 months in a double-blind, randomised study. Clinical examinations were carried out before, each month during, and 1 and 3 months after therapy. Mycological examinations were performed before treatment, and 1 and 3 months after the end of treatment.

Table 10. Overall assessment 2 weeks after the end of amorolfine treatment in patients with tinea pedis

Result	0.5% Solution		2% Solution		0.5% Cream	
	n	%	*n*	%	*n*	%
Cure	27	69.2	24	68.6	37	92.5
Improvement	7	17.9	6	17.1	2	5.0
Failure	5	12.9	5	14.3	1	2.5

Samples for culture were taken from the most affected nail of the hand and/or the foot. Mycological cure was defined as both cultures negative, relapse/reinfection as negative at the first follow-up and positive at the second, and failure as positive culture(s) on at least one follow-up.

A total of 119 patients with a mean of three affected nails were evaluated. Since three patients were affected on both hands and feet, a total of 122 sites were assessed – 104 on toe- and 18 on fingernails. Of these sites, 58 were treated with 2% and 64 with 5% lacquer. Pathogens isolated were: *T. rubrum* (78), *T. mentagrophytes* (23), other dermatophytes (5), yeasts (10), other (4) and mixed infections (2). Three months after the end of therapy with the 5% lacquer there were 41 mycological cures, 9 relapses/reinfections, 11 failures and 3 not assessable for mycology. Corresponding figures were 27, 6, 14 and 11 with the 2% lacquer. The 5% concentration was thus significantly more effective than the 2% one. Three of the 149 patients assessed for tolerance experienced local adverse effects (vesicles, pruritus and burning sensation), but none of them showed adverse systemic symptoms (REINEL 1988).

3. Vulvovaginal Mycosis

Efficacy in vulvovaginal candidosis was assessed in three series of comparative trials using a single dose of amorolfine. Patients underwent one pretreatment examination and two follow-up examinations 7 days (first follow-up) and 4–5 weeks (second follow-up) after treatment. Cure was defined as complete clinical cure (apart from obviously residual symptoms) with negative mycological findings at the first and second follow-ups, or positive mycology at the first but negative findings at the second follow-up. Improvement was defined as improvement of signs and symptoms and mycology as described above. Failures were all cases with positive mycological findings at the first and/or at the second follow-up examinations.

a) Dose-Finding Trial

In a randomised, prospective, double-blind trial in five centres, 196 patients with vaginal mycosis were treated with a single vaginal tablet containing either 10 mg, 25 mg or 50 mg of amorolfine; external treatment of vulvitis with cream was not allowed. Partners were treated with 0.5% amorolfine

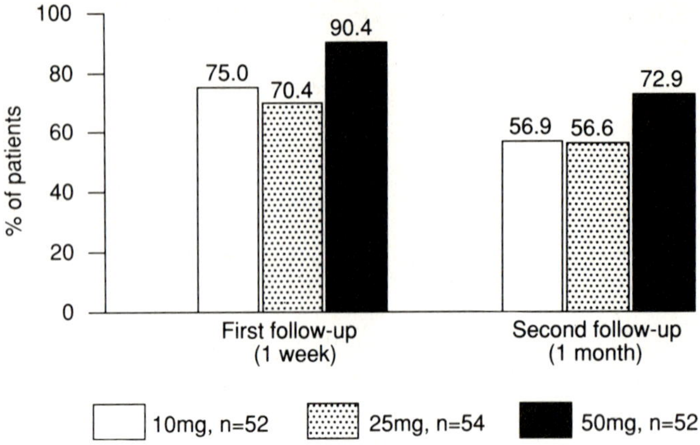

Fig. 6. Percentage of negative cultures after single-dose treatment of vaginal candidosis with amorolfine

cream for 2–7 days. Patients were equally distributed between the three groups.

A total of 158 patients were evaluated for efficacy: *C. albicans* was isolated in 154 patients, *S. cerevisiae* in 3 and *T. glabrata* in 1. At the first follow-up examination 75%, 70% and 90% (χ^2 test, P = 0.0327) and at the second 57%, 57% and 73% (P = 0.0374) of the cultures were negative in the 10, 25 and 50 mg groups, respectively (Fig. 6). Overall 56%, 56% and 73% of the patients had negative cultures at both examinations; 23%, 17% and 23% relapsed (negative at first and positive at second follow-up); and 21%, 28% and 4% were failures (positive at least at first follow-up). Statistics were in favour of 50 mg over the lower doses (P = 0.010). In an overall clinical and mycological assessment, 61% of the patients were cured, 9% improved and 29% were failures in the 10 mg group. The figures were 59%, 6% and 35% in the 25 mg group and 76%, 14% and 10% in the 50 mg group, respectively. Amorolfine was well tolerated by the patients. Local burning, possibly or probably related to the administration of the vaginal tablet, was reported by 4 patients in all, 2 each in the 25 and 50 mg groups (SCHARLAU et al. 1987).

b) Comparative Trial

A study to compare single-dose treatment with 50 mg or 100 mg vaginal tablets of amorolfine (double-blind) or 500 mg vaginal tablets of clotrimazole (open-labelled) was performed in 259 patients from ten trial centres. Additional use of cream externally was permitted for the treatment of vulvitis and of the partner. The results obtained are shown in Fig. 7. No obvious difference between the three treatment groups was seen regarding efficacy. Local adverse effects, probably due to the vaginal tablets, were reported in

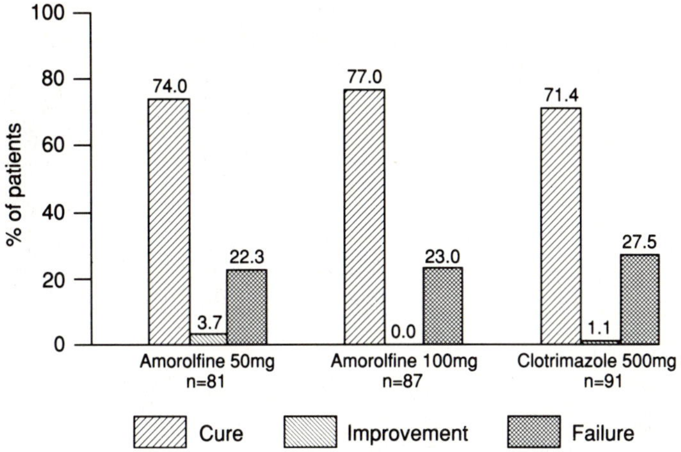

Fig. 7. Overall results in vaginal candidosis after a single vaginal tablet containing 50 mg or 100 mg amorolfine or 500 mg clotrimazole

2.2% ($n = 81$), 4.5% ($n = 87$) and 2.2% ($n = 91$) of the patients in the 50 mg and 100 mg amorolfine and 500 mg clotrimazole groups, respectively (ROHDE et al. 1987).

c) Vaginal Ovules

Single vaginal ovules containing 10, 25, 50 or 100 mg of amorolfine were administered to 80 patients who had vaginal candidosis in a double-blind study. Mycological and clinical examinations were carried out immediately before treatment, 1 week later and finally 2–5 weeks after treatment. Of these 77 patients were evaluable for efficacy in the overall therapeutic assessment. The cure-improvement rate (corresponding to the percentage of patients with negative cultures) ranged from 75% to 90% (Table 11). With the number of patients evaluated, no differences could be observed between the groups. In all four groups, regardless of the amount of active substance,

Table 11. Results obtained with vaginal ovules containing different amounts of amorolfine

	Single dose of amorolfine			
	10 mg	25 mg	50 mg	100 mg
Cure	9	12	13	11
Improvement	6	5	2	7
Failure	3	2	5	2

the signs and symptoms of vaginal candidosis were reduced within 6 days of the administration of the ovule. In no patient did the drug cause any adverse effects, and it was well accepted (PARISSIS et al. 1987).

IV. Conclusion

Amorolfine was administered as a nail lacquer (once or twice weekly) in patients suffering from onychomycosis, as a cream (once daily) in patients suffering from dermatomycosis, as a pump-spray for foot mycosis, or as single dose vaginal tablets or ovules in vaginal candidosis. In all these indications it was effective against both dermatophytes and yeasts, as would be expected from the pre-clinical data. In nail mycosis, applied once to twice weekly in the form of a nail lacquer, amorolfine proved to be a valuable adjunct to therapy in a field in which treatment efficacy has to be balanced with safety. Amorolfine was well tolerated. The local adverse effects observed were mainly burning and itching, with an incidence of 1%–6% according to the formulation used.

References

Galimberti R, Garcia A, Milicich R, Cuomo G, Bonino MV, Flores V, Traballi CA (1988) Amorolfine (Ro 14-4767) a new trend for the treatment of tinea pedis. In: Torres-Rodríguez JM (ed) Proceedings of X congress of international society for human and animal mycology, Barcelona. JR Prous, Barcelona, pp 223–226

Gip L (1989) In vitro studies of the antifungal activity of amorolfine, a phenylpropyl morpholine. Adv Ther 6:26–38

Haller I (1979) Zum Wirkungstyp von Imidazol-Antimykotika: Konsequenz für die Empfindlichkeitsbestimmung. Mykosen 22:423–430

Mensing H, Splanemann V (1988) Evaluation of the antimycotic activity of the pathological substance under the nail after treatment with Ro 14-4767 nail lacquer. Revista Ibérica de Micológia 5 (Suppl 1):20

Nolting S (1988) Double-blind, randomized study comparing 3 concentrations (0.125, 0.25, 0.5%) of Ro 14-4767 and bifonazole 1% creams in patients with dermatomycosis. Revista Ibérica de Micológia 5 (Suppl 1):19

Odds FC, Abbott AB (1984) Relative inhibition factors – a novel approach to the assessment of antifungal antibiotics in vitro. J Antimicrob Chemother 13:31–43

Odds FC, Webster CE, Abbott AB (1984) Antifungal relative inhibition factors: BAY l-9139, bifonazole, butoconazole, isoconazole, itraconazole (R 51211), oxiconazole, Ro 14-4767/002, sulconazole, terconazole, and vibunazole (Bay n-7133) compared in vitro with nine established antifungal agents. J Antimicrob Chemother 14:105–114

Parissis N, Noutsis C, Rigopoulos D (1987) A single dose treatment of vaginal mycosis with the morpholine derivative Ro 14-4767. In: Berkarda B, Kuemmerle H-P (eds) Progress in antimicrobial and anticancer chemotherapy, vol. II. Ecomed, Munich, pp 1576–1578

Polak A (1982a) Oxiconazole, a new imidazole derivative. Evaluation of antifungal activity in vitro and in vivo. Arzneimittelforsch 32:17–24

Polak A (1982b) Experimental activity of a new antimycotic. Curr Chem Immunother. Proceedings of the 12th international congress of chemotherapy, Florence, 19–24 July 1981, pp 1023–1025

Polak A (1983) Antifungal activity in vitro of Ro 14-4767/002, a phenylpropylmorpholine. Sabouraudia 21:205–213

Polak A (1984) Antifungal activity of four antifungal drugs in the cutaneous retention time test. Sabouraudia 22:501–503

Polak A, Dixon DM (1987) Antifungal activity of amorolfine (Ro 14-4767/002) in vitro and in vivo. In: Fromtling RA (ed) Recent trends in the discovery, development and evaluation of antifungal agents. JR Prous, Barcelona, pp 554–573

Reinel D (1988) Double-blind, randomized, multicentre trial of 2% vs. 5% Ro 14-4767 nail lacquer in patients suffering from onychomycosis. Revista Ibérica de Micológia 5 (Suppl 1):93

Rohde E, Zaug M, Hartmann D (1987) Preliminary clinical experience with Ro 14-4767 (Amorolfine) in superficial mycoses. In: Fromtling RA (ed) Recent trends in the discovery, development and evaluation of antifungal agents. JR Prous, Barcelona, pp 575–582

Scharlau L, Goldberg M, Lutziger H, Probst H, Schaal HJ (1987) Double-blind, randomized multicentre, dose-finding trial comparing three single doses (10, 25 and 50 mg) of amorolfine in patients suffering from vaginal mycosis. In: Berkarda B, Kuemmerle H-P (eds) Progress in antimicrobial and anticancer chemotherapy, vol. II. Ecomed, Munich, pp 1573–1575

Section IV. Where Next?

Introduction

JOHN F. RYLEY

'Where there is no vision, the people perish' (Proverbs 29:18). When inviting friends and colleagues to write for this volume, I also asked each one to provide some thoughts concerning the future of medical mycology and antifungal treatment. In spite of gentle reminders, the response has been poor; this fact could have several interpretations! From the limited feedback I have had and from enforced careful study of each chapter during editing, some things have, however, become clear. Fungal infections are not going away, and in spite of remarkable advances in treatment, entirely satisfactory drugs are not yet available.

Topical antifungal treatments abound, and there is little to choose between them from the point of view of efficacy. None are effective in every circumstance, but overall cure rates are generally high. Based on experience it is difficult to see how a new agent could do better than those already available, and with the abundance of basically good products on hand, commercial justification for developing yet another product would be hard to establish.

Oral treatment of superficial infections is attractive on both scientific and aesthetic counts, but it is discounted by many physicians on the grounds that it is foolish to risk toxicity for the treatment of what they regard as very minor conditions. Untoward experiences with ketoconazole – albeit in a very small proportion indeed of patients treated – has reinforced this view. Nevertheless, treatment of dermatophytoses with griseofulvin, and more recently with terbinafine, and the one-shot treatment of vaginal candidosis with fluconazole seem to me to be preferable alternatives to the inconvenience and messiness associated with topical medication. Even safer orally active drugs would support this approach.

In connection with the more serious systemic mycoses, three peripheral, but nevertheless important, issues require special attention. It is an unfortunate fact that fungal disease in very many patients who have become infected as a result of other serious medical problems is only diagnosed postmortem or at best when it is far too late to start treatment with any hope of a successful outcome. A great deal of research is already underway to try and remedy this situation, but so far rapid and reliable diagnostic tests are not available. Of less practical importance in the long run, but nevertheless frustrating to those who would like to have the facility, is the need for reliable and predictive in vitro antifungal susceptibility tests. Were it possible to devise and standardise such tests, it would make life at both the clinical and the research level so much easier. Although clinical trials with common fungal infections are relatively easy to set up, realistic assessment of a new drug in the more obscure fungal diseases is difficult. With few patients available it is impossible to set up large scale comparative trials, and with a wide variety of symptoms and responses in a small number of subjects it is difficult to evaluate and quantify the efficacy of a new treatment.

Azoles have predominated among the new drugs developed during the past decade, although it has been encouraging to see activity in other types of compounds such as terbinafine and cilofungin. The ideal drug should be quick-acting, fungicidal rather than fungistatic, wide-spectrum in its activity, formulatable for oral, intravenous, intramuscular or topical administration, widely distributed in the body (skin, vagina, internal organs, CSF and urine), palatable and free from toxicity. A tall order! Although fluconazole has shown some features unique for an azole (e.g. water solubility and distribution to the CSF and urine), it seems unlikely that the ideal drug will be found in this chemical class. I live in hope that the rational approach will lead to new and more effective chemical classes but realize that a more concerted effort with the empirical approach to chemical collections and natural product sources may in the long term be more successful. Recent experiences with liposomal amphotericin B alone and conjugated to monoclonal antibodies suggest that specific drug targeting may increase the utility of drugs already available. Not all drugs are wide spectrum in their activity, and it will be most interesting to see what impact cilofungin – whose activity is restricted to two species of *Candida* only – will have on the clinical scene. More effective utilisation of narrow-spectrum agents will depend on the development of rapid and accurate diagnostic tests.

But for the immediate future, interesting developments are in hand. A recent in-house survey of patent and commercial intelligence sources listed 64 products with antifungal activity supposedly in some stage of development or clinical evaluation. It is unrealistic to imagine that many of these are serious candidates for the clinical scene. However, in Chapter 22, with help from Bob GORDEE of Lilly and David LOEBENBERG of Schering-Plough, I have tried to summarise the data available at the time of writing (September 1989) on the status and properties of just a few of these newer compounds.

CHAPTER 22

Other Compounds in Development

JOHN F. RYLEY with ROBERT S. GORDEE and DAVID LOEBENBERG

A. Cilofungin

Echinocandin B is a lipopeptide produced by some species of *Aspergillus* which has activity against *Candida albicans*; it is, however, somewhat toxic, causing particularly haemolysis. Enzymatic removal of the linoleoyl side chain and chemical replacement with a 4-*n*-octyloxybenzoyl group have resulted in a compound, cilofungin (LY121019), which retains anti-*Candida* activity but is considerably less toxic (DEBONO et al. 1988, 1989; see also Chap. 3).

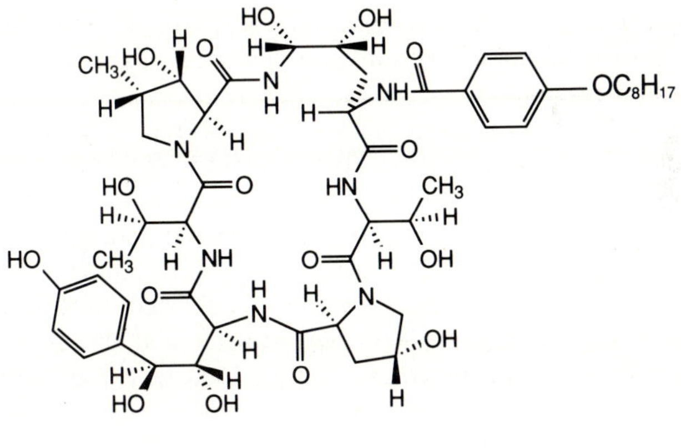

Cilofungin (LY121019)

I. Antifungal Activity In Vitro

In vitro testing shows that cilofungin is a narrow spectrum antifungal agent, with activity restricted to species of *Candida*. Its activity against *C. albicans* and *C. tropicalis* is similar to that of amphotericin B, but all other species of *Candida* are considerably less susceptible (BULO et al. 1988; GORDEE et al. 1988; HALL et al. 1988; PICARD et al. 1988; SPITZER et al. 1988). Minimum inhibitory concentrations, MIC_{90} and MIC_{50}, against 1047 isolates of *C. albicans* were 0.63 and 0.27 μg/ml, respectively. The MIC against one strain of *C. albicans* increased no more than 8-fold after 17 serial transfers in medium containing cilofungin (GORDEE et al. 1984). ODDS (1988) found RIFs (relative inhibition factors) in the range 41%–66% for strains of *C. albicans* and *C. tropicalis*, suggesting activity comparable to that of systemically active azole compounds but rather less than that of amphotericin B; RIFs for other *Candida* spp. were greater than 85%. Activity was reduced in media containing serum. According to ODDS (1988) cilofungin was generally less fungicidal than amphotericin B and only rarely fungicidal in media containing serum, although GORDEE et al. (1988) reckoned that fungicidal activity was similar to that of amphotericin B and that minimum fungicidal concentrations (MFCs) were no more than 4 times the MIC.

MCINTYRE and GALGIANI (1989a) found that susceptibility results did not change with inocula between 10^2 and 10^5 yeast cells per ml or temperature between 30° and 37°C, but that pH did have a significant influence on activity. As the pH decreased from 7.4 to 3.0, IC_{50}s increased up to 64-fold; broth microdilution results for 42 isolates of *C. albicans* in SAAMF (synthetic amino acid medium, fungal) showed IC_{50}s of 0.08–2.5 μg/ml at pH 7.4 and 5–10 μg/ml at pH 3.0. Fungicidal concentrations were closer to MIC results at the lower pH, i.e. an average of 16-fold above the MIC at pH 3.0 compared with an average 256-fold difference at pH 7.4. MICs in yeast nitrogen base broth and minimal essential medium were generally higher than in SAAMF or RPMI 1640 medium.

HALL et al. (1988) found that activity was clearcut in antibiotic medium no. 3, although it decreased with inocula greater than 10^5 yeasts per ml. Isolates of *C. albicans* and *C. tropicalis*, however, demonstrated a 'paradoxical' effect in Sabouraud dextrose broth or yeast nitrogen base broth in that growth was only partially inhibited at concentrations equivalent to those of the MIC in antibiotic medium no. 3, while at higher concentrations reduced growth took place. SPITZER et al. (1988) showed that the granular growth taking place at higher concentrations resulted in large clumps of cells, many of which were viable. RENNIE and HELLMAN (1989) investigated this 'paradoxical' effect further and noted that at high concentrations of cilofungin (20–40 μg/ml), the restricted growth resulted in cells sufficiently damaged to make them highly susceptible to killing by fresh cilofungin. The damaged cells also had increased susceptibility to other antifungal agents to which they were normally resistant. Thus, MICs for ketoconazole and econazole were at least 2–5 μg/ml for 7 strains of *C. albicans* but were uniformly reduced to ≤0.04 μg/ml when mixed with cilofungin at 20 μg/ml; effects with 5-fluorocytosine (5-FC) were more variable and less pronounced. BULO et al. (1989) investigated the possibility of synergism between cilofungin and 5-FC and amphotericin B using 50 strains of various *Candida* species. Synergistic inhibition of growth occurred only once with amphotericin B and cilofungin and only twice with 5-FC and cilofungin, although synergistic killing occurred in 5 strains with the amphotericin B-cilofungin combination and in 7 strains with the 5-FC-cilofungin combination. Antagonism occurred frequently with both combinations. Time-kill studies with *C. albicans* and *C. tropicalis* (PFALLER et al. 1989) showed that exposure to cilofungin 0.6 μg/ml resulted in a 2-log decrease in cfu by 12–24 h but that significant regrowth occurred by 48–72 h; non-metabolising *C. albicans* incubated in saline was killed at a similar rate. Combinations of cilofungin with amphotericin B, 5-FC or ketoconazole were less active than cilofungin alone, but marked synergism was observed between cilofungin and anticapsin, an inhibitor of chitin and mannoprotein synthesis.

II. Antifungal Activity In Vivo

Documentation of activity in vivo is as yet somewhat limited. Cream formulations containing 5% or 3% cilofungin have been shown to have topical activity against superficial infections with *C. albicans* of the skin of guinea pigs or the vagina of rats, respectively (GORDEE et al. 1984); as only systemic treatment of humans is envisaged, these studies have not been extended. In immunocompromised mice (*X*-irradiation) inoculated intravenously with *C. albicans*, the ED_{50} for cilofungin administered 0, 4 and 24 h after inoculation was 7–8 mg/kg; ED_{50}s for amphotericin B, 5-FC and ketoconazole were 2–4, 7–8 and 11 mg/kg, respectively (GORDEE et al. 1988). Doses of 50 mg/kg cilofungin or amphotericin B administered once daily for 5 days beginning 24 h after inoculation reduced the recovery of *C. albicans* from kidney homogenates by more than 3 orders of magnitude; lower doses were effective when treatment was started before inoculation. Although cilofungin has limited oral absorption, 50 or 100 mg/kg oral doses were effective in eradicating *Candida* from the gastrointestinal tract of colonised mice; this activity is superior to that of nystatin but not as good as that of modern azoles. POPE et al. (1988) established intestinal infections in infant mice with *C. albicans* and then induced dissemination to internal organs by treatment with cytoxan plus cortisone acetate. Animals receiving a total dose of 25 mg/kg cilofungin showed significantly fewer positive livers and kidneys than control animals. It should be noted that the extent of dissemination which can be achieved in this model is feeble (see Chap. 5).

MCINTYRE and GALGIANI (1989a,b) showed that two strains of *C. albicans* which gave very different IC_{50}s at pH 7.4 but identical IC_{50}s at pH 3.0 responded equally well to cilofungin therapy using a systemic infection in rats. By contrast GRAYBILL et al. (1988) found that the response of systemic infections with *C. albicans* in mice to cilofungin therapy as measured by kidney counts depended on the in vitro sensitivities of the strains; mice infected with *C. tropicalis* also responded to cilofungin treatment. Based on observations of mortality and kidney lesions and fungal counts MORRISON and STEVENS (1988) found that *C. albicans* infections in mice could be suppressed but not cured by treatment with cilofungin or amphotericin B; amphotericin B was more potent than cilofungin but was also considerably more toxic. SMITH et al. (1989) also found amphotericin B at daily doses of 1–4 mg/kg to be more effective than cilofungin at 25–100 mg/kg in systemic candidosis in normal mice, but KHARDORI et al. (1989) came to the opposite conclusion using neutropenic mice! An interesting compromise was suggested by HANSON et al. (1989) who investigated combinations of cilofungin and amphotericin B in normal mice: synergistic activity was noted with daily doses of cilofungin at 62.5 mg/kg and amphotericin B at 0.625 mg/kg, and pharmacokinetic studies revealed higher blood levels for cilofungin when dosed with amphotericin B than when administered alone.

Using a model of disseminated candidosis in rabbits, PERFECT et al. (1989b) found that intravenous treatment with amphotericin B at 1 mg/kg daily or cilofungin at 50 mg/kg twice daily starting 24 h after inoculation and continuing for 7 days was equally effective in controlling pyelonephritis and endophthalmitis, but that amphotericin B was considerably more effective than cilofungin in reducing yeast counts in cardiac vegetations. PADULA and CHAMBERS (1989) found that intravenous administration of cilofungin did not affect survival nor reduce fungal counts in aortic valve vegetations of rabbits, whereas all rabbits treated with amphotericin B survived, showing some reduction in candidal counts. Using visking chambers implanted under the skin of rabbits, CHAPMAN et al. (1989) studied the pharmacokinetic and antifungal activity of intravenously administered cilofungin. Although chamber levels of cilofungin were well above the MIC, growth of *C. albicans* was not prevented; the explanation may be due to protein binding rather than to the development of drug resistance.

III. Mode of Action

Like echinocandin B from which it is derived, cilofungin is a selective inhibitor of cell wall synthesis in *C. albicans* (GORDEE et al. 1988). Incorporation studies with radiolabelled precursors demonstrated that cilofungin inhibits the biosynthesis of the β-1,3-glucan cell wall component but has little effect on the synthesis of chitin, mannan, DNA, RNA or protein. PFALLER et al. (1989) observed an 80% decrease in glucan content and a 96% decrease in the incorporation of [^{14}C]-glucose into the glucan fraction of cells exposed to cilofungin at 0.6 μg/ml but additionally found a 15% decrease in the ergosterol and a 61% increase in the lanosterol content relative to control cells. In isolated enzyme studies cilofungin was shown to be a noncompetitive inhibitor of the β-1,3-glucan synthase of *C. albicans*; it had no effect on chitin synthase (TAFT et al. 1988).

IV. Toxicology

The LD_{50} of cilofungin administered intravenously is 292 mg/kg in mice and 125–180 mg/kg in rats. A single intravenous dose of 110 mg/kg in monkeys caused no clinical signs of toxicity over a 2-week period. Intravenous administration of 2.5, 10 or 50 mg/kg to rats had no effect on survival, clinical chemistry or histopathology; the 50 mg/kg dose caused sedation, cyanosis, scratching and excessive water consumption. Daily intravenous infusions of 5, 10 or 50 mg/kg in dogs were well tolerated. Treatment-related toxicity included minor clinical signs noted after the first and/or third dose, increased plasma histamine levels, and in high-dosed dogs minimal increases in liver weight, which were reversible after a 1-month recovery period. A 13-week fertility study in rats dosed with 2.5, 10 or 50 mg/kg i.v. revealed no differences in mating or fertility indices; the number of implanations, resorptions and the percentage pre-implantation or post-implantation losses were similar among all treatment groups. Cilofungin was negative in the Ames test. It did not induce sister chromatid exchange in bone-marrow cells of Chinese hamsters or DNA repair synthesis in rat hepatocytes and was not mutagenic in L5187Y mouse lymphoma cells. It was well tolerated in animals and did not show evidence of nephrotoxicity; toxicological studies indicate that cilofungin is at least 20-fold less toxic than amphotericin B (GORDEE et al. 1984).

V. Pharmacokinetics

Following the intravenous administration of 2.5, 10 or 50 mg/kg to rats, peak serum levels of cilofungin occurred immediately after the infusion dose and were 22.3, 75.4 and 162 μg/ml, respectively. The area under the curve increased with dose as did the serum half-life, which was less than 1 h in the rat. Cilofungin was administered to dogs to 10, 30 or 100 mg/kg i.v. 5 days a week for 3 months; serum samples were obtained at the end of infusion and 0.5, 1, 2, 4 and 6 h later after the first dose and again after 1, 2 and 3 months of treatment. The concentration of cilofungin was found to be directly related to the dose administered. Concentrations at the end of infusion ranged from 112–156, 344–622 and 558–1064 μg/ml for dogs receiving daily doses of 10, 30 and 100 mg/kg, respectively (GORDEE et al. 1984). Cilofungin was present in the serum of dogs receiving 30 or 100 mg/kg for 6 h after dosing. There was no evidence of accumulation or altered peak serum concentrations. Animal studies showed that the primary route of excretion of cilofungin is biliary. In pharmacokinetic studies in humans reported by BLACK et al. (1989), intravenous doses up to 4 mg/kg every 6 h for 14 days were well tolerated. Although plasma levels fell below the limits of detection following a single dose, plasma accumulation was noted with multiple dosing. Cilofungin pharmacokinetics were time- and dose-dependent, and less than 2% of the dose was recovered in the urine, again suggesting biliary excretion.

VI. Current Status

Cilofungin has completed phase I clinical trials successfully and is currently in phase II; no details of the latter are available. The clinical use of such a narrow-spectrum antifungal agent will largely be dependent on rapid and accurate diagnosis. It will be most interesting to see whether an agent with potential utility only for infections with *C. albicans* and *C. tropicalis* will find clinical acceptance and be economically viable.

B. SCH 39304 (SM 8668)

SCH 39304 (SM 8668) is an antifungal triazole being developed by Schering-Plough under licence from Sumitomo; it is active orally, parenterally and topically, and the information available is mainly in abstract form. SCH 39304 was selected from a series of 1-azolyl-alkylsulphonyl-alkanol derivatives; antifungal activity resides mainly in the (2*R*, 3*R*)-(-) isomer (SAJI et al. 1988). Preliminary evaluation in a number of animal models of fungal infection showed superior activity to fluconazole, good oral absorption and a half-life in mice and rats twice that of fluconazole (OKUDA et al. 1988).

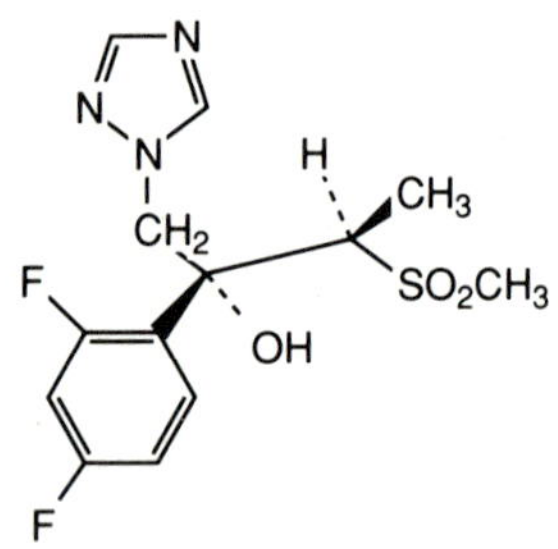

SCH 39304 (SM 8668)

I. Antifungal Activity In Vitro

The in vitro activity of SCH 39304 was compared with fluconazole, ketoconazole, itraconazole, miconazole and amorolfine against various yeasts, dermatophytes and opportunistic fungi; in general, activity was similar to fluconazole (LOEBENBERG et al. 1988a). In separate experiments MICs for SCH 39304 and fluconazole were similar (0.78–≥1000 μg/ml!) for 12 clinical isolates of *Histoplasma capsulatum* (KOBAYASHI et al. 1988). The lack of correlation between in vitro and in vivo activity for antifungals is well known (see Chap. 4) and also occurs here. Difficulties in interpretation may be due, in part, to the dependence of MICs and IC_{50}s on test conditions. With SCH 39304 and with fluconazole, MICs were shown to increase 16- to 512-fold when the inoculum size was increased from 10^2 to 10^5 yeasts/ml; IC_{50} values, however, remained stable as the inoculum size was varied. In vivo efficacy of SCH 39304 seems to correlate with MIC results when broth macrodilution testing is performed with a *small* inoculum and with IC_{50} results which are independent of inoculum size. A 4- to 32-fold increase in IC_{50}s for SCH 39304 was observed with increasing acidity when tested over the pH range 7.4 to 3.0. Two- to 16-fold differences were observed in IC_{50}s between four types of test media (McIntyre and Galgiani 1989b). In another study, MICs for SCH 39304 against five *C. albicans* isolates decreased from a range of 0.3–>80 μg/ml to 0.08–0.3 μg/ml with the addition of 25% human serum to the test media (Meunier et al. 1990).

II. Antifungal Activity In Vivo

Using the mouse kidney infection model, the activity of SCH 39304 in experimentally induced systemic *C. albicans* infection was compared with fluconazole and ketoconazole (Loebenberg et al. 1988a). In normal mice after oral administration, SCH 39304 was three times more potent than fluconazole and about 200 times more active than ketoconazole. In immunocompromised mice (γ-irradiation), oral SCH 39304 was 35 times more active than fluconazole. In experiments in which the size of the inoculum was varied, SCH 39304 was 3–12 times more active than fluconazole and far more active than ketoconazole. Excellent prophylactic activity was seen with oral SCH 39304 when dosing was carried out 1.5–24 h prior to inoculation; protection with fluconazole was only obtained when the drug was given within 6 h of inoculation. An intravenous formulation containing SCH 39304 was equally active when administered orally or intravenously to mice infected with *C. albicans*.

Treatment of experimental candidosis in rats with SCH 39304 and fluconazole resulted in ED_{50}s of 0.33 and 0.49 mg/kg daily, respectively. The ED_{50} for the azole-resistant KB isolate of *C. albicans* and SCH 39304 was 2.25 mg/kg daily; fluconazole was not tested. In a preliminary study using a disseminated *C. albicans* infection in granulocytopenic rabbits, oral SCH 39304 at 2 mg/kg daily, oral fluconazole at 2 mg/kg daily and intravenous amphotericin B 0.6 mg/kg daily plus intravenous 5-FC at 50 mg/kg daily were equally effective; complete clearance of *C. albicans* from vitreous, choroid and cerebrum was achieved, and a $\geqslant 10^4$ reduction in cfu/g was obtained in liver, spleen, lung and kidney tissues (Walsh et al. 1988). In a model of disseminated candidosis in rabbits, Perfect et al. (1989a) noted sterilisation of the choroid, retina and vitreous, and a marked reduction in fungal count in the renal cortex and cardiac vegetations following treatment with either SCH 39304 10–2.5 mg/kg or fluconazole 20–2.5 mg/kg for 1 week; in most instances SCH 39304 showed greater potency than fluconazole.

In the treatment of intracerebral cryptococcal infections in mice, oral SCH 39304 consistently prolonged survival longer than fluconazole at similar doses, while after intranasal challenge with *Cryptococcus neoformans* SCH 39304 was more active than fluconazole based on pulmonary colony counts (Restrepo et al. 1989). In the treatment of meningeal cryptococcal infections in rabbits, oral SCH 39304 was as effective as fluconazole and significantly reduced yeast counts in the CSF (Perfect et al. 1989a). In systemic infections with *Aspergillus* in mice, SCH 39304 was much more active than fluconazole as measured by prolongation of survival time (LOEBENBERG et al. 1988a), while in the treatment of pulmonary aspergillosis in rats, SCH 39304 was more active than any other azole tested but was not as active as amphotericin B (SCHMITT et al. 1988). SCH 39304 was shown to be far more effective than itraconazole or fluconazole in prolonging survival and reducing lung fungal counts of cortisone-treated mice inoculated intranasally with *A. fumigatus* (DEFAVERI and GRAYBILL 1989b). LOEBENBERG et al. (1989) described a most interesting model in which mice compromised with cortisone and tetracycline were forced to breathe air passed over a sporulating culture of *A. flavus*; untreated mice died within 6–9 days. SCH 39304 was considerably more active than itraconazole, fluconazole or ketoconazole in this model as measured by survival. Doses of SCH 39304 of 5 mg/kg daily or greater were able to sterilise the lungs; 50% of mice treated with itraconazole at 100 mg/kg still had culture-positive lungs.

Based on prolongation of survival, SCH 39304 was far more active than fluconazole in the treatment of *H. capsulatum* infections in mice, although amphotericin B was the most active agent tested; similar results were obtained in immunocompromised animals (KOBAYASHI et al. 1988). In a further study (TRAVIS et al. 1989), they showed that a strain of *H. capsulatum* resistant to azoles in vitro responded more or less normally to SCH 39304 in vivo (another inconsistency between in vitro and in vivo results).

SCH 39304 was more effective than fluconazole in murine pulmonary blastomycosis (SUGAR et al. 1989) and in intravenously induced coccidioidomycosis in mice (CLEMONS et al. 1989); in mice inoculated intracerebrally with *C. immitis* it was superior to fluconazole and itraconazole in terms of survival, and at doses of 10 mg/kg daily or above was able to sterilise the infection in the brain, which the other two drugs were unable to do. SCH 39304 and itraconazole at 20 mg/kg daily both significantly reduced the lesion size in athymic mice inoculated subcutaneously with *Fonsecaea pedrosoi* (chromoblastomycosis; DEFAVERI and GRAYBILL 1989a).

The activity of SCH 39304 administered orally or topically against *C. albicans* vaginal infections in hamsters was compared with fluconazole; in each experiment treatment began 4 days after inoculation. In treatment regimens employing oral administration for 4 days, SCH 39304 was about four fold more potent than fluconazole; 100% of the animals treated with SCH 39304 at 1.6 mg/kg were cured, while fluconazole required doses of 6.3 mg/kg to achieve 100% cures. In experiments using a single oral dose, SCH 39304 was again four fold more potent than fluconazole. At a dose of 2.5 mg/kg, 83% of animals treated with SCH 39304 were cured while only 67% of animals treated with a 10 mg/kg dose of fluconazole were cured. A cure rate of 100% was obtained with a single 10 mg/kg dose of SCH 39304. SCH 39304 was also more active than fluconazole against vaginal *C. albicans* infections in hamsters when applied intravaginally for 8 days; SCH 39304 produced a 100% cure rate at concentrations as low as 0.025% (LOEBENBERG et al. 1988b).

In guinea pigs with cutaneous *Trichophyton mentagrophytes* infections, SCH 39304 administered for 10 days at oral doses of 3.12–25 mg/kg starting 3 days after inoculation reduced lesion scores to 50%–59% of controls; lesions scores of animals treated with fluconazole at the same doses were 72%–81% of controls. When 0.5% SCH 39304 was applied topically for 10 days, 71% of total samples cultured were negative as compared with only 46% following treatment with the same concentration of fluconazole; with 0.25% concentrations of drug the figures were 69% and 14%, respectively (LOEBENBERG et al. 1988b).

III. Pharmacokinetic Studies in Animals

Bioavailability studies in various animals showed that SCH 39304 was well absorbed orally. Following a single oral dose of 10 mg/kg (rabbits only) or 20 mg/kg, the plasma $t_{1/2}$ of SCH 39304 in mice (6 h), rabbits (20 h), squirrel monkeys (40 h) and cynomolgous monkeys (61 h) was about 40%–180% longer than that of fluconazole. In all species plasma concentrations of SCH 39304 were higher than those of fluconazole for a longer period of time. The C_{max} ranged from 8.5 to 20.2 μg/ml for SCH 39304 and from 8.7 to 28.3 μg/ml for fluconazole (LIN et al. 1988). In rabbits, the pharmacokinetic parameters obtained for SCH 39304 were shown to be unaffected by the immune status of the animal. SCH 39304 penetrated into multiple tissues after oral administration, including the liver and central nervous system, in both normal and granulocytopenic rabbits (LEE et al. 1989). It crossed the blood-brain barrier of rabbits in the presence or absence of meningeal inflammation, reaching approximately 60% of the simultaneous concentrations in serum (PERFECT et al. 1989a).

In mice, the plasma $t_{1/2}$ of SCH 39304 was similar (6 h) following either intravenous or oral dosing at 2 mg/kg. The AUC observed in this experiment after oral dosing was higher than that obtained with intravenous dosing, indicating good oral absorption of the drug. SCH 39304 was also well absorbed in dogs following a single oral dose of 20 mg/kg. The plasma $t_{1/2}$ was 27 h and the cumulative excretion of unchanged drug in urine accounted for 57% of the dose. Serum levels of SCH 39304 obtained from beagle dogs, rats and monkeys receiving multiple daily doses during 2-week to 3-month toxicity studies showed that SCH 39304 was absorbed and eliminated slowly, in a dose proportional manner. Protein binding of SCH 39304 in both human serum and 4% human serum albumin was low and ranged from 10%–12% (LIN et al. 1988). Further pharmacokinetic studies in rhesus monkeys indicated that following a single oral dose of 2 mg/kg SCH 39304 effectively penetrated the CSF, achieving concentrations active against many opportunistic fungi and sustaining these concentrations for at least 24 h. A CSF $t_{1/2}$ of 39 h was calculated compared with a plasma $t_{1/2}$ of 72 h; maximal concentrations in the CSF and plasma were 1.34 and 1.96 μg/ml at 10 and 24 h, respectively (WALSH et al. 1989).

IV. Current Status

SCH 39304 has completed phase I clinical trials and phase II/III studies are in progress. The compound has been given 'high priority' status by the AIDS Clinical Drug Development Committee of the US National Institutes of Health. Tolerance studies in normal volunteers showed that single oral doses of 5, 15, 50, 100 or 200 mg SCH 39304 produced no significant clinical or laboratory abnormalities. The plasma C_{max} was 1.05, 2.00 and 4.04 μg/ml at doses of 50, 100 and 200 mg, respectively; serum half-lives ranged from 56.6–64.4 h. Renal excretion of unchanged drug was the primary route of elimination, accounting for approximately 80% of the dose (KRAMER et al. 1988). Following daily oral doses of 25, 50 or 100 mg SCH 39304 for 17 days in a further group of volunteers, steady-state half-lives of 54–93 h were observed (LIN et al. 1989). The long serum half-life suggests the possibility of a less frequent dosage regimen than other systemic antifungals, perhaps as infrequently as 2 or 3 times a week, or once a week as maintenance therapy.

C. ICI 195,739

ICI 195,739 is a wide-spectrum, orally active antifungal which has the distinction of being the most potent of all agents tests tested in animal models of fungal infection. It is a bistriazole discovered as a result of a synthetic campaign serviced by a screening cascade designed to identify compounds with high in vivo activity, acceptable pharmacokinetics and freedom from teratogenicity in vitro and in rats and rabbits (BOYLE et al. 1988). ICI 195,739 is currently the subject of licensing negotiations.

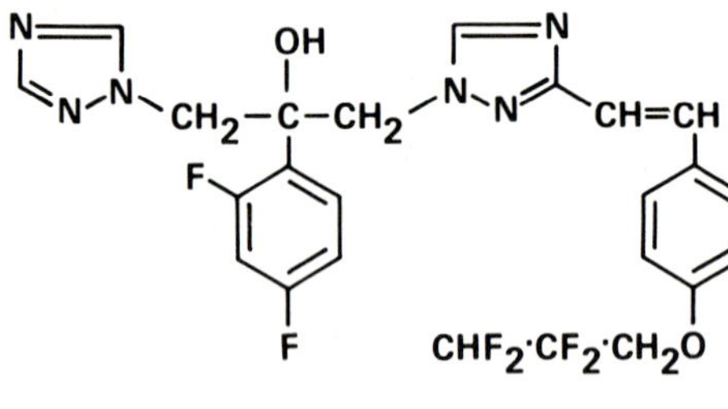

ICI 195,739

I. Antifungal Activity In Vitro

MIC assays were performed in Kimmig's agar using a Denley multipoint inoculator which delivers around 100 organisms per inoculation site; incubation was at 30°C for 24 h. Four isolates of *C. albicans*, eight species of dermatophyte, one isolate of *C. neoformans* and nine isolates of four species

Table 1. In vitro activities of ICI 195,739 and other azoles (minimum inhibitory concentrations in μg/ml)

(A) Agar dilution	*Candida*	Dermatophytes	*Cryptococcus*	*Aspergillus*
ICI 195,739	6.2	⩽1.6	⩽1.6	⩽8.7
Ketoconazole	50	0.8–3.1	0.4	4.2
Itraconazole	⩾100	⩽0.1	0.14	0.08
Fluconazole	⩾100	100	11	>100

(B) Broth dilution	*C. albicans* B 2630	*C. parapsilosis*		*Torulopsis glabrata*	*Cryptococcus neoformans*	*Aspergillus*		*Pityrosporum ovale*
		(9-1)	(9-2)			*flavus*	*fumigatus*	
ICI 195,739	8	0.008	0.125	8	0.08	1	16	⩽0.8
Ketoconazole	64	0.062	0.25	8	0.16	1.6	12.5	⩽0.1
Itraconazole	>256	0.25	4	256	1	0.8	1.6	⩽0.1
Fluconazole	>256	4	32	256	5	>100	>100	6.2

of *Aspergillus* were used. Part A of Table 1 gives the MICs obtained; the figures for *Aspergillus* are G-MICs for the nine isolates. MICs were also determined in yeast nitrogen base broth with glucose; microtitre plates were used for the assays. Inocula were 10^5/ml for *Pityrosporum ovale* and 1.2 × 10^3/ml for the other organisms. Incubation was at 37°C for *P. ovale* and *C. neoformans* and 30°C for the other organisms, for 6 days for *P. ovale* or 48 h for the rest. The resulting MICs are given in part B of Table 1. The in vitro activity of azoles can be very misleading when attempts are made to translate them to the in vivo situation (see Chap. 4); one would have reservations about taking ketoconazole, itraconazole or fluconazole to the clinic solely on the basis of the data in this table. As the figures stand, ICI 195,739 is markedly superior, but again not too much should be read into this situation at this stage. As would be expected, all four compounds are active against the mycelial form of *C. albicans*, with MICs of 0.1 μg/ml or less.

In company with most azole antifungals, ICI 195,739 does not have any fungicidal activity against *C. albicans*; incubation for 24 h with 100 μg/ml had no effect in reducing the size of the starting population. A similar lack of effect was seen with ketoconazole, itraconazole and fluconazole. However, ICI 195,739 does have some fungicidal activity against *C. parapsilosis*; Table 2 shows the concentration required to give >90% kill (MCC) relative to that which prevents visible growth over a 24-h period (MIC) using a starting inoculum of 2 × 10^3/ml. Initial experiments with dermatophytes, using *Trichophyton rubrum* as a representative organism, have shown that ICI 195,739 is more fungicidal than ketoconazole, itraconazole or fluconazole. Incubation with ICI 195,739 at 32 μg/ml resulted in >99% kill within 24 h. Some effect could be achieved with prolonged incubation in the presence of ketoconazole at 128 μg/ml, but no fungicidal activity was observed with itraconazole or fluconazole.

II. Antifungal Activity In Vivo

The extensive in vivo evaluation of ICI 195,739 in animal models of fungal infection has been detailed by RYLEY et al. (1988); some of these data are

Table 2. Fungicidal activity of ICI 195,739 against *Candida parapsilosis*

	C. parapsilosis (9-1)		*C. parapsilosis* (9-2)	
	MIC (μg/ml)	MCC (μg/ml)	MIC (μg/ml)	MCC (μg/ml)
ICI 195,739	0.125	1	0.5	8
Ketoconazole	0.06	128	0.06	32
Itraconazole	0.25	2	0.5	16
Fluconazole	32	>128	32	>128

MCC, concentration giving >90% kill; MIC, minimum inhibitory concentration.

Table 3. Activity of azoles in experimental in vivo models of fungal infection

Model	Host	ICI 195,739	Ketoconazole	Itraconazole	Fluconazole
Vaginal *C. albicans*	Mouse	0.5–2.5 × 6	25–10 × 6	25 × 6	5–2.5 × 6
Vaginal *C. albicans*	Rat	0.5 × 5	10–5 × 5	1 × 5	1–0.5 × 5
Intestinal *C. albicans*	Infant mouse	0.5 × 7	250 × 7	5 × 7	2.5 × 7
Dermatophyte	Mouse	0.5 × 6	25–10 × 6	5–2.5 × 6	5–2.5 × 6
Dermatophyte	Guinea pig	5 × 12	100 × 12	–	25 × 12
Systemic *C. albicans*	Mouse	0.5 × 90	50 × 90	–	2.5 × 90
Systemic *Cryptococcus neoformans*	Mouse	10 × 21	⩾100 × 21	⩾100 × 21	100 × 21
Systemic *Aspergillus fumigatus*	Mouse	10 × 21	100 × 21	100 × 21	25 × 21
Systemic *Trypanosoma cruzi*	Mouse	1 × 5	10 × 5	25 × 5	50 × 5

Figures are minimum effective doses expressed as mg/kg × number of daily doses.

summarised in Table 3, which gives minimum doses effective in the various models and indicates doses of other azoles required to produce equivalent responses. Independent confirmation of in vivo activity has been provided by POLAK (personal communication) and is summarised in Table 4.

Vaginal candidosis in the mouse or rat is eliminated by doses of 0.25–0.5 mg/kg ICI 195,739; intestinal candidosis, important in humans as a reservoir of infection and focus from which systemic dissemination or spread to the vagina can take place, is similarly eliminated by 0.5 mg/kg daily for a week. The figures in Table 3 indicate a potency for ICI 195,739 which is 10–500 times that of ketoconazole, 2–50 times that of itraconazole, and 2–10 times that of fluconazole. Superficial infections with dermatophytes in mice and guinea pigs likewise respond well to oral treatment with ICI 195,739. Although our primary interest has not been to discover yet another topical treatment for superficial fungal infections, ICI 195,739 displays remarkable topical activity; formulations containing 0.01% of the drug were as good as or better than proprietary formulations containing 1%–2% active ingredient in our models of vaginal candidosis, while a formulation containing 0.3% ICI 195,739 was very effective in guinea pig trichophytosis.

Treatment with oral ICI 195,739 has been effective in systemic infections in mice produced by intravenous inoculation of *C. albicans*, *C. neoformans* or *A. fumigatus* or intranasal inoculation with *C. neoformans*. Protection from death has been achieved with low daily doses of the compound, and fungal counts in appropriate internal organs much reduced; sterilisation of the infecton, as with other azoles, is rarely achieved. POLAK (personal communication; Table 4) has shown marked activity against *Histoplasma capsulatum* in mice, and TUCKER et al. (1989) have demonstrated activity against *Blastomyces dermatitidis* in mice. Interestingly enough, ICI 195,739 is the only azole they have ever tested which has produced complete sterilisation of the infection in this model. Because of similarities to fungi in sterol composition and biosynthesis, the protozoan *Trypanosoma cruzi* – the causative agent of Chagas' diseasee in South and Central America – is sensitive to azoles. ICI 195,739 has demonstrated very good activity against *T. cruzi* in mice (Table 3) and is in fact able to produce sterilisation of chronic infections. On the basis of its performance in animal models of infection, the projected human dose is 10–50 mg/day (0.2–1 mg/kg daily).

III. Mode of Action Studies

Biochemical mode of action studies have been described by BARRETT-BEE et al. (1988). Like other antifungal azoles, ICI 195,739 is a potent inhibitor of fungal C14 sterol demethylation; *C. albicans* incubated with the drug accumulates lanosterol and other methylated sterols. This inhibition is non-competitive with respect to the substrate. Kinetic studies suggest that the drug does not compete for the lanosterol binding site but binds to the P-450 enzyme at some other site, almost certainly to the heme. The relative

Table 4. Comparative activity of ICI 195,739 in experimental models of fungal infection

Model	Host	ICI 195,739	Ketoconazole	Itraconazole	Fluconazole	Terbinafine
Vaginal *C. albicans*	Mouse	0.8–1.8	20–25	10–22	3.5	–
Vaginal *C. albicans*	Rat	0.15	5	0.85	1–3	–
Trichophyton quinckeanum	Mouse	3.5	20	12	38	15
Systemic *C. albicans*	Mouse	2.5	–	50	50	–
Systemic *Cryptococcus neoformans*	Mouse	2.6	–	>80	20	–
Systemic *Aspergillus fumigatus*	Mouse	25	–	50	60	–
Systemic *Histoplasma capsulatum*	Mouse	0.55	–	3.5	5.5	–

Figures are ED_{50}s in mg/kg daily by mouth.
Personal communication from A Polak.

potencies against the enzyme in whole cells and broken cells are similar, indicating that the drug is freely permeable. This suggests that it may be more effective against ketoconazole-resistant isolates which have reduced azole uptake. Cholesterol biosynthesis is much less sensitive to ICI 195,739, demonstrating fungal specificity. This result is in agreement with others in mammalian systems where it was shown that the compound is not potent against steroid-metabolising enzymes: the cholesterol side chain cleavage enzyme, 11-hydroxylase, 17-hydroxylase and placental aromatase. In animal experiments no effect on testosterone biosynthesis was seen with conditions under which ketoconazole and fluconazole significantly reduced serum testosterone levels.

IV. Pharmacokinetics and Toxicology

Little published information is available on the toxicology and pharmacokinetics of ICI 195,739. The compound was identified by our screening cascade as being non-teratogenic in vitro and in rats and rabbits. Blood level determinations following six daily doses of 1 mg/kg in rats indicated an elimination half-life of 24 h (BOYLE et al. 1988). Pharmacokinetic studies indicate that the half-life depends on the size of dose and species of animal. Thus, TUCKER et al. (1989) observed a peak serum level of 17.6 μg/ml 12 h after a single oral dose of 50 mg/kg in mice, and a half-life in excess of 12 h. Mice dosed with 50 mg/kg daily for 21 days showed trough serum levels of 19.5 μg/ml and peak levels of 21.0 μg/ml; the half-life was markedly prolonged – in excess of 48 h.

D. Other Azoles

I. Saperconazole

Saperconazole (R 66905) is a close relative of itraconazole undergoing development by Janssen, currently in phase II. Scant published information is available. Chemically the compound is itraconazole with the two chlorine atoms replaced by fluorine; the compound is still lipophilic but is less insoluble and intractable than itraconazole, and there is a possibility of an intravenous formulation using dimethyl β-cyclodextrin. According to VAN

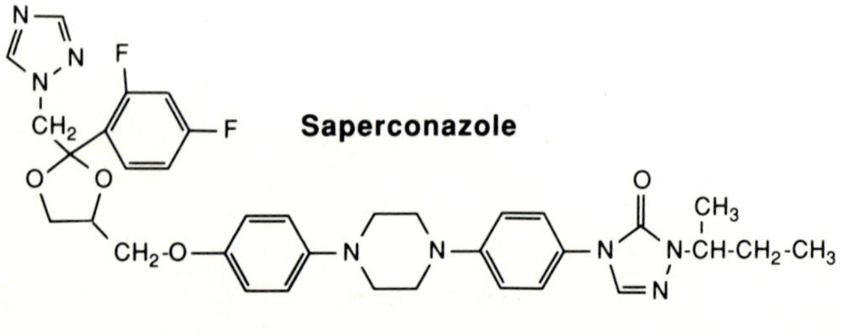

Saperconazole

CUTSEM et al. (1988) the compound has potent broad-spectrum antifungal activity; more than 1000 fungal strains belonging to 173 species of *Candida*, *Cryptococcus*, *Pityrosporum*, *Aspergillus*, dermatophytes, dimorphic fungi and phaeohyphomycetes have been tested in vitro. Activity was demonstrated in various animal models of infection including superficial dermatophytosis and candidosis in guinea pigs, disseminated trichophytosis in guinea pigs, systemic candidosis, cryptococcosis and aspergillosis in normal and immunodepressed guinea pigs, and vaginal candidosis in rats. Daily oral doses of 0.63–1.25 mg/kg were required to control the superficial infections, while 5–10 mg/kg was necessary to show activity in aspergillosis. Activity was on the whole superior to that of fluconazole; topical activity at low concentrations was also demonstrated in the skin and vaginal infections. Serum half-life in mice was reported to be 18 h. The drug is fungistatic. Activity in aspergillosis seems to be of particular interest, and this aspect has been studied in vitro by DENNING et al. (1989). In further work described by VAN CUTSEM et al. (1989a) guinea pigs inoculated i.v. with *A. fumigatus* died between days 4–7 if left untreated; some animals were compromised by prior injection with mechlorethamine HCl or cyclophosphamide. Early treatment with saperconazole at 1.25 mg/kg for 14 days was highly efficaceous, while delayed treatment with 5 mg/kg cured moribund animals. Immunocompromised guinea pigs responded equally well to intact ones. Parenteral treatment with amphotericin B was moderately efficaceous, but at therapeutic doses, toxic; drug-related side effects were not seen with saperconazole. Evaluation in vitro with a variety of organisms (MCGOUGH et al. 1989) and in a mouse model of pulmonary aspergillosis (RINALDI et al. 1989) suggests that saperconazole has activities very similar to those of itraconazole. Like itraconazole, saperconazole was inactive in experimental zygomycosis in guinea pigs (VAN CUTSEM et al. 1989b). The half-life of saperconazole in humans after a single 200 mg dose is 20 h (VAN CUTSEM et al. 1989a).

II. SDZ 89-485

SDZ 89-485 is a triazole antifungal synthesized by GRASSBERGER et al. (1988) at Sandoz; it is currently the subject of licensing negotiations. In vitro against

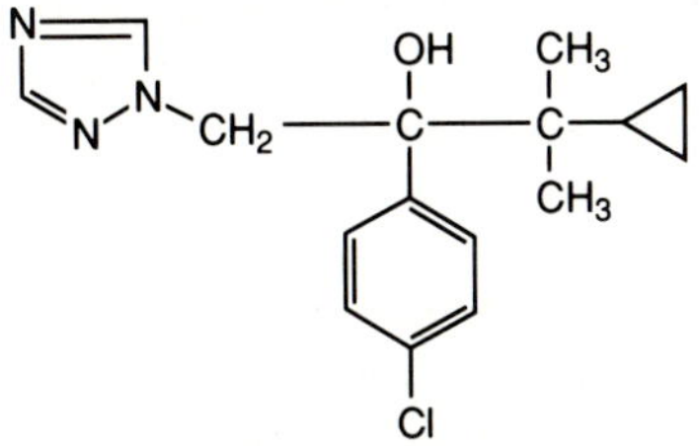

SDZ 89-485

a range of fungi the compound behaved similarly to ketoconazole and other azoles (SCHAUDE and MIETH 1988), while in vivo it showed outstanding oral activity in a number of animal models of superficial and systemic infection (SCHAUDE et al. 1988). The compound has limited activity against disseminated *Sporothrix schenckii* in mice (KAN and BENNETT 1988), and has recently been shown to be substantially more effective than fluconazole against experimental coccidioidomycosis in mice (FIERER et al. 1990). Doses of 5 mg/kg twice daily starting 48 h after ip inoculation with arthroconidia sterilized infections as did fluconazole at 50 mg/kg twice daily. When the start of treatment with 10 or 100 mg/kg/day was delayed until 8 days after inoculation, counts in the lungs, spleen and omentum were reduced or eliminated, indicating inhibition of spherule growth. Absorption following oral dosing is slower than with fluconazole, and the drug persists longer in the blood. Interestingly the compound did not demonstrate any teratogenic potential in vitro or in rats or rabbits (BECHTER et al. 1988). Biochemical studies (RYDER 1988; SCHUSTER and MEINGASSNER 1988) indicate that its mode of action is the same as for other azoles; activity against relevant enzymes from the host suggests that there is sufficient selectivity to preclude toxicity at therapeutic doses. Thus testicular and adrenal steroid synthesis in dogs was not affected by iv administration of the drug at 10 times the therapeutic dose. The (-) enantiomer is responsible for the bulk of the antifungal activity.

III. BAY R 3783 (Electrazole)

BAY R 3783 was reported by PLEMPEL and BÜCHEL (1988) to have broad spectrum, in vitro activity typical of azoles; evaluation in animal models of dermatophytosis, candidosis, cryptococcosis and aspergillosis showed activity similar to that of fluconazole and superior to that of ketoconazole, and in some cases itraconazole. Further details of its in vitro activity have been given by PLEMPEL et al. (1988) and by FOTHERGILL et al. (1989). HECTOR (1988) reported activity equivalent to that of fluconazole in rat vaginal candidosis and in systemic infections in mice with *C. albicans*, *C. tropicalis* and *C. neoformans*; although both drugs were equivalent in their ability to delay mortality in the model of meningo-cerebral cryptococcosis, neither was able to sterilise the brain infection. HECTOR and YEE (1990) extended these studies to compare Bay R 3783 with fluconazole, itraconazole, ketoconazole and amphotericin B in rodent models of superficial and systemic candidosis, meningocerebral cryptococcosis, and pulmonary aspergillosis. Overall, Bay R 3783 was comparable or slightly superior to fluconazole and markedly superior to itraconazole and ketoconazole in both survival and short-term organ load experiments in models of candidosis or cryptococcosis, but was less effective than amphotericin B. Of the antifungals tested, only Bay R 3783 and itraconazole showed any efficacy in the model of pulmonary aspergillosis. PAPPAGIANIS et al. (1988a, 1989) obtained somewhat better results than with fluconazole though not as good as with amphotericin B in murine models of aspergillosis, blastomycosis, candidosis, coccidioidomycosis, cryptococcosis and histoplasmosis.

BAY R 3783 is metabolised in vivo, and it is significant that two of the three primary metabolites which have been identified (BAY U 3624 and BAY U 3625) are also active in vitro and in vivo (RITTER, personal communication). LEE et al. (1989) have studied pharmacokinetics in rabbits; BAY R 3783 gave a half-life of 2.1 h following a dose of 40 mg/kg, but the metabolite BAY U 3625 showed a half-life of 48.3 h and gave blood levels in excess of 0.1 μg/ml at 144 h. According to WRIGHT et al. (1989), BAY R 3783 is effective in the treatment of experimental cryptococcal meningitis in rabbits, giving a reduction in CSF yeast counts slightly smaller than those obtained with equivalent doses (40 mg/kg) of itraconazole and fluconazole. Interestingly enough, in their pharmacokinetic studies they observed significant levels of BAY R 3783, BAY U 3624 and fluconazole in the CSF of rabbits but were unable to detect

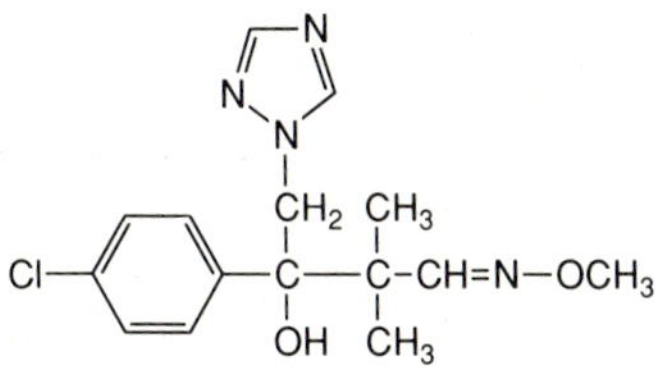

BAY R 3783
(Electrazole)

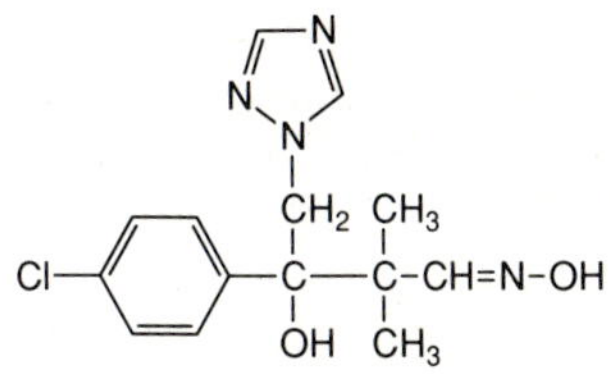

BAY U 3624

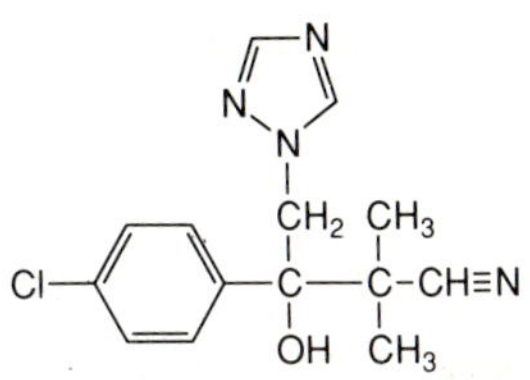

BAY U 3625

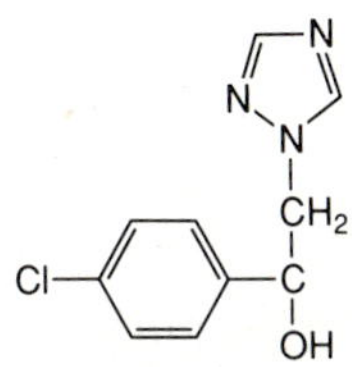

BAY V1637

any BAY U 3625 or itraconazole following single oral doses of 40 mg/kg of the five compounds. LEE et al. (1989) suggested that BAY U 3625 may be a major contributor to the antifungal effect of BAY U 3783 and also an inhibitor of its metabolism; it would be interesting to know whether BAY U 3625 given to rabbits would have any therapeutic effect on cryptococcal meningitis – as does itraconazole – in spite of its apparent inability to penetrate into the CSF. Pharmacokinetic studies in humans indicate that BAY R 3783 is nearly completely metabolised at first pass with a $t_{1/2}$ of less than 1 h. The initial metabolite, BAY U 3624, has a similarly brief half-life, but the product, BAY U 3625, is very persistent. Although no toxicity was observed, it was felt that the very long half-life of 7 ± 3 days and non-linear kinetics of BAY U 3625 posed an unpredictable and unacceptable risk, and phase I studies in humans were abandoned (RITTER, personal communication).

E. Non-Azoles

I. SDZ 87-469

Although terbinafine displays the potential for activity against a wide spectrum of fungi in in vitro tests, its clinical utility is effectively restricted to dermatophytes. The announcement by Stütz et al. (1988) that replacement of the naphthalene nucleus of terbinafine by a substituted benzo (b) thiophene resulted in significantly enhanced activity against *C. albicans* was therefore of considerable interest. Biological studies reported by Petranyi et al. (1988) indicated remarkable fungicidal activity against a variety of dermatophytes, aspergilli and *Sporothrix schenckii* in vitro and good fungistatic activity against *C. albicans*. Oral treatment of mouse sporotrichosis and guinea pig trichophytosis and microsporosis was effective, and guinea pig dermatophytosis and skin candidosis responded well to topical treatment. It is unfortunate, therefore, that development of the compound seems to have been abandoned during phase I studies in humans.

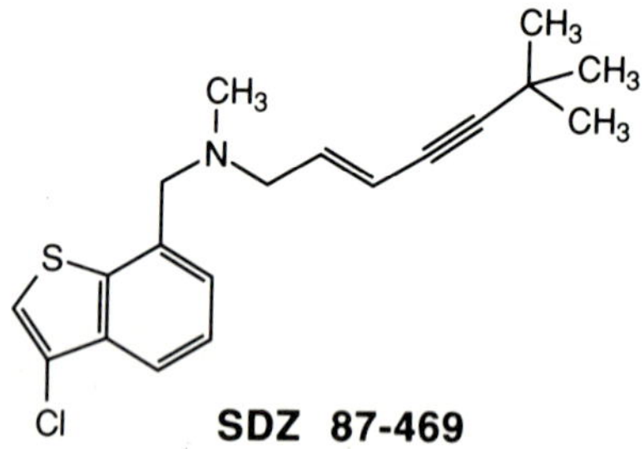

SDZ 87-469

II. BMY 28567 (Pradimycin)

BMY 28567 is a potent antifungal antibiotic produced by a new strain of *Actinomadura hibisca* (Tsunakawa et al. 1988). It exhibits fungicidal activity against a wide variety of fungi and yeasts, including many strains resistant to other antifungal agents (Oki et al. 1988); therapy of yeast infections seems to be of particular interest (Desiderio et al. 1988). PD_{50}s of 2.7–11.5 mg/kg were observed with systemic infections with several strains of *C. albicans*, *C. tropicalis*, *C. pseudotropicalis* and *C. paratropicalis* in mice. Although not as good as amphotericin B, it was effective against a number of strains resistant in vivo to fluconazole and/or 5-FC. Likewise, though not as effective as amphotericin B, it gave PD_{50}s of 7.6–25 mg/kg against two strains of *C. neoformans* in a murine model of cryptococcal meningitis in which fluconazole, itraconazole, ketoconazole and 5-FC were ineffective (Tsai et al. 1988). Although at an early stage of development, the compound is of double interest in the context of AIDS, since activity against the HIV virus has also been demonstrated.

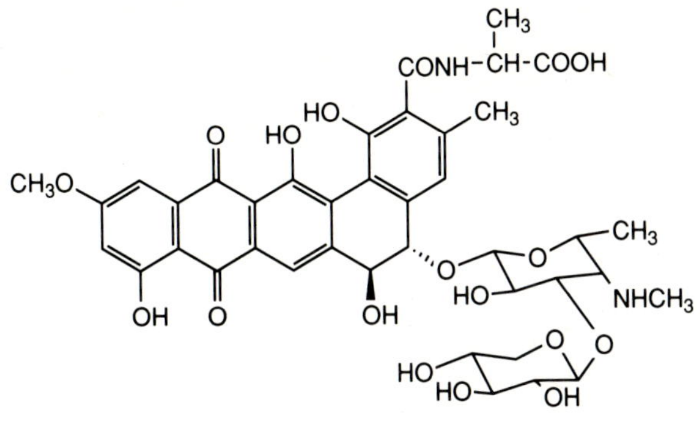

BMY 28567 (Pradimycin)

III. Nikkomycin Z

The advent of cilofungin, an inhibitor of β-1,3-glucan synthesis, emphasises the potential of the cell wall as the target for an antifungal drug. Nikkomycin Z is an inhibitor of chitin synthase which appears to have more potential than

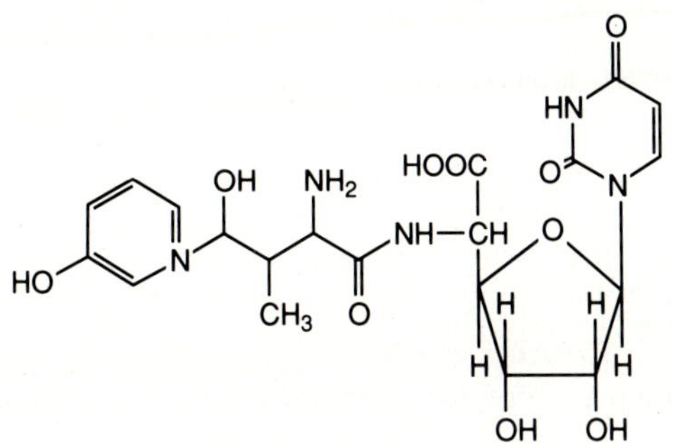

Nikkomycin Z

polyoxins for in vivo anti-*Candida* activity (see Chap. 3). Although hardly at this stage a development compound, recent reports from HECTOR et al. (1988) and PAPPAGIANIS et al. (1988b) suggest continuing interest and potential in this compound. Nikkomycin Z at doses of 20–75 mg/kg b.i.d. had activity in murine models of coccidioidomycosis and blastomycosis but not histoplasmosis. Mortality was reduced or prevented and striking reductions in lung colonisation observed; in some instances complete biocure was achieved.

References

Barrett-Bee K, Lees J, Pinder P, Campbell J, Newboult L (1988) Biochemical studies with a novel antifungal agent, ICI 195,739. Ann NY Acad Sci 544:231–244

Bechter R, Hamada M, Nakashima T (1988) SDZ 89-485; a systemic antimycotic azole derivative is non-teratogenic in vitro and in vivo. Revista Ibérica de Micológia 5(Suppl 1):Abst P-149

Black HR, Brier GL, Wolny JD, Dorrbecker SH (1989) Pharmacology and pharmacokinetics of cilofungin. 29th Intersci Conf Antimicrob Agents Chemother, Houston TX, (Abst 1357)

Boyle FT, Gilman DJ, Gravestock MB, Wardleworth JM (1988) Synthesis and structure-activity relationships of a novel antifungal agent, ICI 195,739. Ann NY Acad Sci 544:86–100

Bulo AN, Bradley SF, Kauffman CA (1988) Susceptibility of yeast-like fungi to a new antifungal agent, LY 121019. Mycoses 31:330–333

Bulo AN, Bradley SF, Kauffman CA (1989) The effect of cilofungin (LY 121019) in combination with amphotericin B or flucytosine against *Candida* species. Mycoses 32:46–52

Chapman R, Moody J, Fasching C, Sinn L, Gerding D, Peterson L (1989) In vitro and in vivo activity of cilofungin against clinical isolates of *Candida albicans* and *Candida parapsilosis*. 29th Intersci Conf Antimicrob Agents Chemother, Houston (Abst 819)

Clemons KV, Hanson LH, Perlman AM, Stevens DA (1989) Efficacy of SCH39304 in a systemic model of murine coccidioidomycosis. 29th Intersci Conf Antimicrob Agents Chemother, Houston TX, (Abst 823)

Debono M, Abbott BJ, Turner JR, Howard LC, Gordee RS, Hunt AS, Barnhart M, Molloy RM, Willard KE, Fukuda D, Butler TF, Zeckner DJ (1988) Synthesis and evaluation of LY 121019, a member of a series of semisynthetic analogues of the antifungal lipopeptide echinocandin B. Ann NY Acad Sci 544:152–167

Debono M, Abbott BJ, Fukuda DS, Barnhart M, Willard KE, Molloy RM, Michel KH, Turner JR, Butler TF, Hunt AH (1989) Synthesis of new analogs of echinocandin B by enzymatic deacylation and chemical reacylation of the echinocandin B peptide: synthesis of the antifungal agent cilofungin (LY 121019). J Antibiot 42:389–397

Defaveri J, Graybill JR (1989a) Treatment of chromoblastomycosis with antifungal azoles. 29th Intersci Conf Antimicrob Agents Chemother, Houston TX, (Abst 820)

Defaveri J, Graybill JR (1989b) SCH39304 in treatment of murine pulmonary aspergillosis. 29th Intersci Conf Antimicrob Agents Chemother, Houston TX, Abst 822

Defaveri J, Sun SH, Graybill JR (1989) Treatment of murine coccidioidal meningitis with SCH39304. 29th Intersci Conf Antimicrob Agents Chemother, Houston TX, Abst 824

Denning DW, Hanson LH, Stevens DA (1989) In vitro activity of saperconazole against *Aspergillus* sp. 29th Intersci Conf Antimicrob Agents Chemother, Houston TX, Abst 722

Desiderio J, Leonard G, Lamb L, Brutkiewicz R, Hibbard J, Beaudoin B, Kessler RE (1988) Activity of BMY 28567, a novel antifungal agent, against a variety of *Candida* species in vivo. 28th Intersci Conf Antimicrob Agents Chemother, Los Angeles CA, Abst 1002

Fierer J, Kirkland T, Finley F (1990) Comparison of fluconazole and SDZ89-485 for therapy of experimental murine coccidioidomycosis. Antimicrob Agents Chemother 34:13–16

Fothergill AW, McGough DA, Rinaldi MG (1989) In vitro activity of BAY R 3783, an investigational antifungal triazole. 29th Intersci Conf Antimicrob Agents Chemother, Houston TX, Abst 725

Gordee RS, Zeckner DJ, Ellis LF, Thakkar AL, Howard LC (1984) In vitro and in vivo anti-*Candida* activity and toxicology of LY 121019. J Antibiot 37:1054–1065

Gordee RS, Zeckner DJ, Howard LC, Alborn WE, Debono M (1988) Anti-*Candida* activity and toxicology of LY 121019, a novel semisynthetic polypeptide antifungal antibiotic. Ann NY Acad Sci 544:294–309

Grassberger MA, Meingassner JG, Schaub F (1988) Synthesis and structure-activity relationships of SDZ 89-485 and analogues. Revista Ibérica de Micológia 5(Suppl 1):Abst P-153

Graybill JR, Ahrens J, Rinaldi M (1988) LY 121019 in murine candidiasis: in vivo and in vitro correlations. 28th Intersci Conf Antimicrob Agents Chemother, Los Angeles CA, (Abst 1527)

Hall GS, Myles C, Pratt KJ, Washington JA (1988) Cilofungin (LY 121019), an antifungal agent with specific activity against *Candida albicans* and *Candida tropicalis*. Antimicrob Agents Chemother 32:1331–1335

Hanson LH, Perlman AM, Clemons KV, Stevens DA (1989) Synergy between cilofungin and amphotericin B in a murine model of candidosis. 29th Intersci Conf Antimicrob Agents Chemother, Houston TX, (Abst 818)

Hector RF (1988) Evaluation of the azole BAY R 3783 in rodent models of candidiasis and cryptococcosis. Revista Ibérica de Micológia 5(Suppl 1):Abst 0–4

Hector RF, Yee E (1990) Evaluation of Bay R 3783 in rodent models of superficial and systemic candidiasis, meningeal cryptococcosis, and pulmonary aspergillosis. Antimicrob Agents Chemother 34:448–454

Hector RF, Zimmer BL, Pappagianis D (1988) Use of the chitin synthase inhibitor nikkomycin Z in murine models of coccidioidomycosis, blastomycosis, and histoplasmosis. Revista Ibérica de Micológia, vol 5, suppl 1, Abst 0–5

Kan VL, Bennett JER (1988) Efficacies of four antifungal agents in experimental murine sporotrichosis. Antimicrob Agents Chemother 32:1619–1623

Khardori N, Kalvakuntla L, Wong E, Rosenbaum B, Bodey GP (1989) Comparative activities of cilofungin (Ly121019) and amphotericin B against disseminated *Candida albicans* infection in neutropenic mice. 29th Intersci Conf Antimicrob Agents Chemother, Houston TX, Abst 817

Kobayashi GS, Travis SJ, Medoff G (1988) In vitro evaluation of SCH 39304, fluconazole and amphotericin B against 12 clinical isolates of *Histoplasma capsulatum* and comparison of therapeutic efficacies in treating histoplasmosis in immunocompetent and immunosuppressed mice. 28th Intersci Conf Antimicrob Agents Chemother, Los Angeles CA, Abst 172

Kramer W, Kim H, Symchowicz S, Perentesis G, Affrime M, Lin C (1988) Pharmacokinetics of SCH 39304 in man. 28th Intersci Conf Antimicrob Agents Chemother, Los Angeles CA, Abst 165

Lee JW, Lin C, Loebenberg D, Rubin M, Pizzo PA, Walsh TJ (1989) Pharmacokinetics and tissue penetration of SCH 39304 in granulocytopenic and nongranulocytopenic rabbits. Antimicrob Agents Chemother 33:1932–1935

Lee J, Ritter W, Lecciones J, Kelly P, Pizzo P, Walsh TJ (1989) Plasma pharmacokinetics of Bay R 3783 and its metabolite, Bay U 3625, in rabbits. 29th Intersci Conf Antimicrob Agents Chemother, Houston TX, Abst 727

Lin C, Kim H, Lapiguera A, Loebenberg D, Miller GH, Symchowicz S (1988) Comparative pharmacokinetics of SCH 39304 and fluconazole in mice, rabbits, S. monkeys and C. monkeys. 28th Intersci Conf Antimicrob Agents Chemother, Los Angeles CA, (Abst 163)

Lin C, Kim H, Radwanski E, Affrime M, Symchowicz S (1989) Steady-state pharmacokinetics of SCH 39304 in man. 29th Intersci Conf Antimicrobial Agents Chemother, Houston TX, (Abst 1359)

Loebenberg D, Parmegiani R, Cacciapuoti A, Antonacci B, Norris C, Menzel F, Moss EL, Yarosh-Tomaine T, Lin CC, Hare RS, Miller GH (1988a) SCH 39304, a new antifungal agent. I. Oral treatment of systemic infections in mice. 28th Intersci Conf Antimicrob Agents Chemother, Los Angeles CA, (Abst 167)

Loebenberg D, Parmegiani R, Cacciapuoti A, Antonacci B, Norris C, Menzel F, Moss EL, Yarosh-Tomaine T, Hare RS, Miller GH (1988b) SCH 39304, a new antifungal agent. II. Oral and topical treatment of vaginal and skin infections. 28th Intersci Conf Antimicrob Agents Chemother, Los Angeles CA, (Abst 168)

Loebenberg D, Parmegiani R, Moss EL, Frank D, McHugh M, Yarosh-Tomaine T, Antonacci B, Menzel F, Hare RS, Miller GH (1989) SCH39304, a new antifungal agent. Oral activity in a murine model of pulmonary aspergillosis. 29th Intersci Conf Antimicrob Agents Chemother, Houston TX, (Abst 821)

McGough DA, Ayo S, Fothergill AW, Rinaldi MG (1989) Saperconazole, a new investigational antifungal triazole: in vitro activity and measurement by a modified bioassay. 29th Intersci Conf Antimicrob Agents Chemother, Houston TX, (Abst 723)

McIntyre KA, Galgiani JN (1989a) pH and other effects on the antifungal activity of cilofungin (LY 121019). Antimicrob Agents Chemother 33:731–735

McIntyre KA, Galgiani JN (1989b) In vitro susceptibilities of yeasts to a new antifungal triazole, SCH 39304: effects of test conditions and relation to in vivo efficacy. Antimicrob Agents Chemother 33:1095–1100

Meunier F, Lambert C, Van Der Auwera P (1990) In-vitro activity of SCH39304 in comparison with amphotericin B and fluconazole. J Antimicrob Chemother 25:227–236

Morrison CJ, Stevens DA (1988) Effect of LY 121019 on experimental murine candidosis. 28th Intersci Conf Antimicrob Agents Chemother, Los Angeles CA, (Abst 1530)

Odds FC (1988) Activity of cilofungin (LY 121019) against *Candida* species in vitro. J Antimicrob Chemother 22:891–897

Oki T, Saitoh K, Tomatsu K, Tomita K, Konishi M, Kawaguchi H (1988) Novel antifungal antibiotic BMY-28567. Ann NY Acad Sci 544:184–187

Okuda T, Tanio T, Ichise K, Nakajima T (1988) In vivo evaluation of SM-8668, a new orally active triazole antifungal agent. 28th Intersci Conf Antimicrob Agents Chemother, Los Angeles CA, (Abst 174)

Padula A, Chambers HF (1989) Evaluation of cilofungin (LY121019) for treatment of experimental *Candida albicans* endocarditis in rabbits. Antimicrob Agents Chemother 33:1822–1823

Pappagianis D, Zimmer B, Theodoropoulos G, Hector R (1988a) Evaluation of the azole BAY R 3783 in murine models of coccidioidomycosis, blastomycosis, and histoplasmosis. Revista Ibérica de Micológia 5(Suppl 1):Abst 0–64

Pappagianis D, Zimmer B, Hector RV (1988b) Nikkomycin therapy in experimental coccidioidomycosis, blastomycosis and histoplasmosis. 28th Intersci Conf Antimicrob Agents Chemother, Los Angeles CA, (Abst 1004)

Pappagianis D, Zimmer BL, Hector RF (1989) Comparative efficacy of the triazole Bay R 3783 in murine models of deep mycoses. 29th Intersci Conf Antimicrob Agents Chemother, Houston TX, (Abst 726)

Perfect JR, Wright KA, Hobbs MM, Durak DT (1989a) Treatment of experimental cryptococcal meningitis and disseminated candidiasis with SCH39304. Antimicrob Agents Chemother 33:1735–1740

Perfect JR, Hobbs MM, Wright KA, Durak DT (1989b) Treatment of experimental disseminated candidiasis with cilofungin. Antimicrob Agents Chemother 33: 1811–1812

Petranyi G, Meingassner JG, Schaude M (1988) Experimental chemotherapeutic activity of SDZ 87-469, a new allylamine antimycotic. Revista Ibérica de Micológia 5(Suppl 1): Abst P-150

Pfaller M, Riley J, Koerner T (1989) Effects of cilofungin (LY121019) on carbohydrate and sterol composition of *Candida albicans*. Eur J Clin Microbiol Infect Dis 8:1067–1070

Pfaller M, Gordee R, Gerarden T, Yu M, Wenzel R (1989) Fungicidal activity of cilofungin (LY 121019) alone and in combination with anticapsin or other antifungal agents. Eur J Clin Microbiol Infect Dis 8:564–567

Picard M, Meshulam T, Sugar AM (1988) In vitro activity of LY 121019 against *Candida* species and *Torulopsis glabrata*. Eur J Clin Microbiol Infect Dis 7:432–433

Plempel M, Büchel KH (1988) Antimycotic effects of BAY R 3783 in vitro and on dermatophytoses and opportunistic mycoses of the organs in vivo. Revista Ibérica de Micológia 5(Suppl 1):Abst 0–7

Plempel M, Berg D, Büchel K-H, Ritter W (1988) Experimental antimycotic activity of azole derivatives – experience, knowledge and questions. In: Berg D, Plempel M (eds) Sterol biosynthesis inhibitors. Pharmaceutical and agrochemical aspects. Ellis Horwood, Chichester, pp 349–396

Pope LM, Tanaka K, Cole GT (1988) Efficacy of LY 121019 in clearance of *Candida albicans* from body organs of persistently colonized, immunocompromised mice. 28th Intersci Conf Antimicrob Agents Chemother, Los Angeles CA, (Abst 1528)

Rennie RP, Hellman L (1989) Comparative activity in vitro of cilofungin (LY 121019) with other agents used for treatment of deep-seated *Candida* infections. Mycoses 32:145–150

Restrepo BI, Ahrens J, Graybill JR (1989) Efficacy of SCH39304 in murine cryptococcosis. Antimicrob Agents Chemother 33:1242–1246

Rinaldi MG, Allendoerfer R, Defaveri J, Graybill JR (1989) Therapy of experimental murine aspergillosis with a new antifungal triazole, saperconazole: initial investigations. 29th Intersci Conf Antimicrobial Agents Chemother, Houston TX, (Abst 724)

Ryder NS (1988) Biochemical mode of action and enantiomeric selectivity of SDZ 89-485. Revista Ibérica de Micológia 5(Suppl 1):Abst P-154

Ryley JF, McGregor S, Wilson RG (1988) Activity of ICI 195,739 – a novel, orally active bistriazole – in rodent models of fungal and protozoal infections. Ann NY Acad Sci 544:310–328

Saji I, Ohashi N, Tamoto K, Tanio T, Okuda T, Atsumi T (1988) Structure-activity relationships of SM-8668, a new orally active triazole antifungal, and related compounds. 28th Intersci Conf Antimicrob Agents Chemother, Los Angeles CA, (Abst 173)

Schaude M, Mieth H (1988) In vitro activity of SDZ 89-485, a new orally active triazole antifungal. Revista Ibérica de Micológia 5(Suppl 1):Abst P-152

Schaude M, Petranyi G, Meingassner JG, Ackerbauer H, Mieth H (1988) Biological activity of SDZ 89-485 in animal models. Revista Ibérica de Micológia 5(Suppl 1):Abst P-151

Schmitt HJ, Bernard EM, Hauser M, Armstrong D (1988) Comparison of antifungal agents in a rat model of pulmonary aspergillosis. 28th Intersci Conf Antimicrob Agents Chemother, Los Angeles CA, (Abst 171)

Schuster I, Meingassner JG (1988) SDZ 89-485: a study of interactions with mammalian cytochromes P-450 in vitro and in vivo. Revista Ibérica de Micológia 5(Suppl 1):Abst P-155

Smith K, Lank K, Cobbs G, Dismukes W (1989) Cilofungin vs amphotericin B therapy of murine candidiasis. 29th Intersci Conf Antimicrob Agents Chemother, Houston TX, (Abst 816)

Spitzer ED, Travis SJ, Kobayashi GS (1988) Comparative in vitro activity of LY 121019 and amphotericin B against clinical isolates of *Candida* species. Eur J Clin Microbiol Infect Dis 7:80–81

Stütz A, Nussbaumer P, Petranyi G (1988) SDZ 87-469: synthesis and structure-activity relationships of a novel allylamine antimycotic. Revista Ibérica de Micológia 5(Suppl 1):Abst P-156

Sugar AM, Picard M, Noble L (1989) Comparison of SCH 39304, fluconazole, and amphotericin B in the treatment of murine pulmonary blastomycosis. 29th Intersci Conf Antimicrob Agents Chemother, Houston TX, (Abst 825)

Taft CS, Stark , Selitrennikoff CP (1988) Cilofungin (LY 121019) inhibits *Candida albicans* (1–3)-β-D-glucan synthase activity. Antimicrob Agents Chemother 32:1901–1903

Travis SJ, Medoff G, Kobayashi GS (1989) In vitro susceptibility of a clinical isolate of *Histoplasma capsulatum* to two triazoles does not correlate with treatment outcome in murine histoplasmosis. 29th Intersci conf Antimicrob Agents Chemother, Houston TX, (Abst 1157)

Tsai YH, Kelly WA, Ferraro C, Kessler RE (1988) BMY 28567: therapeutic study in murine cryptococcal meningitis. 28th Intersci Conf Antimicrob Agents Chemother, Los Angeles CA, (Abst 1003)

Tsunakawa M, Nishio M, Ohkuma H, Tsuno T, Konishi M, Naito T, Oki T, Kawaguchi H (1988) A new antifungal antibiotic, BMY-28567. Structure elucidation. 28th Intersci Conf Antimicrob Agents Chemother, Los Angeles CA, (Abst 1001)

Tucker RM, Hanson LH, Brummer E, Stevens DA (1989) Activity of ICI 195,739, a new oral triazole, compared with that of ketoconazole in the therapy of experimental murine blastomycosis. Antimicrob Agents Chemother 33:573–575

Van Cutsem J, Van Gerven F, Janssen PAJ (1988) R66905, a new potent broad-spectrum antifungal with topical, oral and parenteral activity. Revista Ibérica de Micológia, vol 5, suppl 1, Abst 0–2

Van Cutsem J, Van Gerven F, Janssen PAJ (1989a) Oral and parenteral therapy with saperconazole (R 66905) of invasive aspergillosis in normal and immunocompromised animals. Antimicrob Agents Chemother 33:2063–2068

Van Cutsem J, Van Gerven F, Fransen J, Janssen PAJ (1989b) Treatment of experimental zygomycosis in guinea pigs with azoles and with amphotericin B. Chemotherapy 35:267–272

Walsh TJ, Lee JW, Peter J, Schaufele R, Rubin M, Pizzo PA (1988) SCH 39304 in the treatment of disseminated candidiasis in persistently granulocytopenic and non-granulocytopenic rabbits. 28th Intersci Conf Antimicrob Agents Chemother, Los Angeles CA, Abst 169

Walsh TJ, McCully C, Rinaldi MG, Balis F, Lee J, Pizzo PA, Poplack D (1989) Pharmacokinetics and penetration of SCH 39304 into cerebrospinal fluid of rhesus monkeys. 29th Intersci Conf Antimicrob Agents Chemother, Houston TX, Abst 1361

Wright KA, Perfect JR, Ritter W (1989) The pharmacokinetics and efficacy of BAY R3983 in experimental cryptococcal meningitis. 29th Intersci Conf Antimicrob Agents Chemother, Houston TX, Abst 728

Subject Index